Cognitive Communication Disorders

Fourth Edition

Cognitive Communication Disorders

Fourth Edition

Michael L. Kimbarow, PhD, CCC-SLP, FASHA
Sarah E. Wallace, PhD, CCC-SLP, FASHA

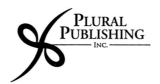

PLURAL
PUBLISHING
INC.

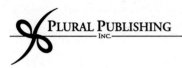

9177 Aero Drive, Suite B
San Diego, CA 92123

email: information@pluralpublishing.com
website: https://www.pluralpublishing.com

Typeset in 10.5/13 Palatino by Flanagan's Publishing Services, Inc.
Printed in the United States of America by Integrated Books International

For permission to use material from this text, contact us by
Telephone: (866) 758-7251
Fax: (888) 758-7255
email: permissions@pluralpublishing.com

*Every attempt has been made to contact the copyright holders for material originally
printed in another source. If any have been inadvertently overlooked, the publisher will
gladly make the necessary arrangements at the first opportunity.*

Library of Congress Cataloging-in-Publication Data:
Names: Kimbarow, Michael L., 1953- editor. | Wallace, Sarah E., editor.
Title: Cognitive communication disorders / [edited by] Michael L. Kimbarow,
   Sarah E. Wallace.
Description: Fourth edition. | San Diego, CA : Plural, [2025] | Includes
   bibliographical references and index.
Identifiers: LCCN 2023024964 (print) | LCCN 2023024965 (ebook) | ISBN
   9781635505115 (paperback) | ISBN 9781635504408 (ebook)
Subjects: MESH: Cognition Disorders--complications | Communication
   Disorders--etiology
Classification: LCC RD594 (print) | LCC RD594 (ebook) | NLM WM 204 |
DDC
   617.4/81044--dc23/eng/20230824
LC record available at https://lccn.loc.gov/2023024964
LC ebook record available at https://lccn.loc.gov/2023024965

Contents

Preface

Webster defines an inflection point as a moment when significant change occurs. This is an apt descriptor of the fourth edition of *Cognitive Communication Disorders* (*CCD*). After the release of the third edition of *CCD*, I enjoyed a personal inflection point when I retired from my academic position and became an Emeritus Professor in the Department of Communication Disorders and Sciences at San Jose State University. Consequently, I recognized it was time to hand the text over to my colleagues and friends who remain active in teaching, research, and clinical service. Thus, inflection point number two. With this new edition, I welcome Sarah E. Wallace on board as coeditor of the text. Sarah brings an astounding background of knowledge, teaching, research, and editorial experience to the enterprise and will be the sole editor of the book for future editions.

The field of cognitive communication disorders continues to advance with increasing focus on evidence-based assessment and intervention approaches. Readers will note that many of the authors from previous editions of *CCD* have remained with the text, and their commitment to updating and revising their contributions is evident in this fourth edition. Updated content addresses the broader societal impact of cognitive communication disorders and the importance of being inclusive in our research and treatment with individuals with cognitive communication disorders.

As noted in the preface to the third edition, the goal in creating any new edition of a textbook is to ensure that the work remains true to its core value and to remain relevant to the reader. I am confident that once again, thanks to our outstanding roster of international (Australia, Canada, Cyprus, and the United States) contributors, that we have indeed upheld and exceeded our goal.

We are grateful to the authors who remain with the text from the third edition, Margaret Blake, Jessica Brown, Fofi Constantinidou, Heather Dial, Kathryn Hardin, Maya Henry, Nidhi Mahendra, and Sarah Villard. I'm also delighted to welcome a remarkable roster of new contributors who share coauthor credit on many chapters (Marianna Devledian, Petrea Cornwell, Eduardo Europa, Ronelle Hewetson, Kelly Knollman-Porter, Katy O'Brien, Catherine Wiseman-Hakes, Maya Albin). These new additions to the contributors list represent a third inflection point; they are the best and brightest of the next wave of teacher-scholars, and we look forward to their future contributions to the book.

The book remains organized in the familiar fashion as the previous three editions. The first three chapters cover attention (Villard), memory (Constantinidou and Devledian), and executive functions (Purdy and O'Brien), and they provide the all-important and necessary foundational understanding of the cognitive systems that support communication. Learning how these cognitive systems work individually and synergistically is critical to understanding how these same systems are impacted by neurological damage. The book then explores the juncture between cognition and communication as manifested in right hemisphere damage (Cornwell, Hewetson, and Blake), primary progressive aphasia (Dial and Henry), the dementias (Mahendra and Europa), and mild traumatic brain injury/concussion (Hardin and

Wiseman-Hakes) and traumatic brain injury (Knollman-Porter, Brown, and Wallace). The book concludes with a new chapter that addresses the challenges and considerations associated with providing care to marginalized and underserved individuals with cognitive communication disorders (Wiseman-Hakes, Hardin, and Albin).

We thank all the readers of the text for your continued support of the book. The information explosion since the first edition was released in 2011 is an imperative for ensuring that this valuable text continues to serve as an up-to-date resource for students, instructors, researchers, and clinicians. The people with cognitive communication disorders and their families deserve nothing less.

Acknowledgments

To my wife, Joyce, for the love and joy of every day together. It's been a remarkable life journey with you, and I look forward to the adventures ahead.

With gratitude and appreciation to my coeditor, Sarah Wallace, for your friendship, your partnership, your contribution, and your keen editorial eye. I am comforted knowing that you'll be shepherding the text going forward.

My thanks to all the returning and new contributing authors for sharing your outstanding work and expertise for this edition. It's my privilege to know you and to work with you, and it's been great having you along for the fourth edition ride.

Finally, my thanks to the Plural Publishing team for your continued support of the book and your invitation to produce a fourth edition to ensure it remains current and relevant to the students, clinicians, and researcher-scholars who work with persons with cognitive communication disorders.

Michael L. Kimbarow

To my family and found family, to my village in Pittsburgh, my people in Michigan, and friends from around the world—thank you for your support. It means everything to me. Editing a text can be lonely work, and I'm grateful for my feline editorial assistant Oliver and his steadfast companionship. To my colleagues and the many people who have done much of the important work we are writing about in this text, thank you for your contributions to the area of cognitive communication disorders. I truly feel in this field I am standing on the shoulders of giants, and I only hope I can provide the same kind of support for those who come after me.

To my coeditor, Michael Kimbarow, thank you for the invitation to go on this journey with you and for trusting me with this important project moving forward. Most of all, thank you for your friendship, mentorship, patient guidance, and support. I will miss our regular chats.

To the many new and returning contributing authors, we could not do this important work without you. I am grateful that you have shared your expertise with us and am humbled by all that I have learned from you. The time you have invested to put together the high-quality chapters in this text is a testament to your dedication to improving the services provided to people with cognitive communication disorders and their families.

To the Plural Publishing team—I am honored to work with each of you and grateful for your support of this important work.

Sarah E. Wallace

Contributors

Maya Albin, MSc, Reg. CASLPO
Speech-Language Pathologist
McMaster University
School of Rehabilitation Science
Hamilton, Ontario, Canada
Chapter 9

Margaret Lehman Blake, PhD, CCC-SLP, FASHA
Professor
University of Houston
Department of Communication
    Sciences and Disorders
Houston, Texas
Chapter 4

Jessica A. Brown, PhD, CCC-SLP
Speech-Language Pathologist
Olentangy Local School District
Columbus, Ohio
Chapter 8

Fofi Constantinidou, PhD, CCC-SLP, CBIS
ASHA and ACRM Fellow
Professor of Language Disorders and
    Clinical Neuropsychology
Department of Psychology &
    Director of the Center for Applied
    Neuroscience
University of Cyprus
Nicosia, Cyprus
Chapter 2

Petrea L. Cornwell, PhD, BSpPath (Hons), CPSP
Associate Professor and Academic
    Lead Speech Pathology
School of Health Sciences and Social
    Work
Griffith University
Gold Coast, Australia
Chapter 4

Marianna Christodoulou Devledian, PhD, CCC-SLP
Lecturer, Speech and Language
    Therapy Program
School of Sciences, Department of
    Health Sciences
European University Cyprus
Nicosia, Cyprus
Chapter 2

Heather Dial, PhD
Assistant Professor
Department of Communication
    Sciences and Disorders
University of Houston
Houston, Texas
Chapter 5

Eduardo Europa, PhD, CCC-SLP
Assistant Professor
Department of Communicative
    Disorders and Sciences
San Jose State University
San Jose, California
Chapter 6

Kathryn Y. Hardin, PhD, CCC-SLP
Associate Professor
Department of Speech, Language,
Hearing Sciences
Metropolitan State University of
Denver
Denver, Colorado
Chapters 7 and 9

Maya Henry, PhD, CCC-SLP, FASHA
Associate Professor
Departments of Speech, Language,
and Hearing Sciences and
Neurology
The University of Texas at Austin
Austin, Texas
Chapter 5

Ronelle Hewetson, PhD, CPSP
Lecturer of Speech Pathology
School of Health Sciences and Social
Work
Griffith University
Gold Coast, Australia
Chapter 4

**Kelly Knollman-Porter, PhD,
CCC-SLP**
Associate Professor
Miami University
Department of Speech Pathology and
Audiology
Oxford, Ohio
Chapter 8

**Nidhi Mahendra, PhD, CCC-SLP,
FASHA**
Professor and Director of the Spartan
Aphasia Research Clinic (SPARC)
Department of Communicative
Disorders and Sciences
San Jose State University
San Jose, California
Chapter 6

Katy H. O'Brien, PhD, CCC-SLP
Senior Scientific Advisor
Courage Kenny Rehabilitation
Institute
Minneapolis, Minnesota
Chapter 3

**Mary H. Purdy, PhD, CCC-SLP,
BC-ANCDS**
Professor Emeritus
Department of Communication
Disorders
Southern Connecticut University
New Haven, Connecticut
Chapter 3

Sarah N. Villard, PhD, CCC-SLP
Research Assistant Professor
Department of Speech, Language and
Hearing Sciences
Boston University
Boston, Massachusetts
Chapter 1

**Sarah E. Wallace, PhD, CCC-SLP,
FASHA**
Professor
Director, Master's Degree Program in
Speech-Language Pathology
Department of Communication
Science and Disorders
School of Health and Rehabilitation
Sciences
University of Pittsburgh
Pittsburgh, Pennsylvania
Chapter 8

**Catherine Wiseman-Hakes, PhD,
Reg. CASLPO**
Assistant Clinical Professor
Speech Language Pathology Program
School of Rehabilitation Science
McMaster University
Hamilton, Ontario, Canada
Chapters 7 and 9

1

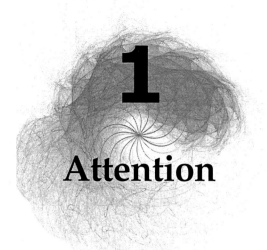

Attention

Sarah N. Villard

Chapter Learning Objectives

After reading this chapter you will be able to:

1. Explain why attention is relevant to assessment of language deficits in individuals with aphasia.
2. Compare the extent of attention deficits in different neurologically impaired populations, including dementia, aphasia, right hemisphere disorder, and traumatic brain injury.
3. Give examples of ways that attention can be incorporated into language treatment for patients with acquired neurological impairments.
4. Describe several tests of attention that may be used by speech-language pathologists and provide advantages and disadvantages of each.

Introduction

Interest in the cognitive skill of attention within the field of speech-language pathology has increased considerably over the past several decades, as researchers and clinicians have continued to uncover more and more about the complexity of language abilities and the ways in which they are intertwined with cognitive abilities. Attention, while not a language skill per se, is an example of an essential cognitive process that interacts with language and communication in a number of different ways. Impairments in attention have been observed in individuals with a number of different neurologically acquired and degenerative conditions, including stroke, traumatic brain injury, and various types of dementia. Even in aphasia, traditionally conceptualized as a language-specific impairment, attention deficits have frequently been noted and are becoming increasingly of interest.

Researchers in communication sciences and disorders are continuing to refine the ways in which attention can be applied to better understand neurogenic impairments, and clinicians who assess and treat cognitive communication disorders now routinely consider attention alongside other cognitive-linguistic abilities.

The aim of this chapter is to discuss the construct of attention as it relates to clinical practice in speech-language pathology for individuals with acquired and neurodegenerative impairments. In order to properly contextualize this discussion within the historical literature on attention, we will start with an overview of some basic principles of attention, as well as several major historical models and theories of attention from the neuropsychological literature on healthy populations. The discussion will then shift to the ways in which attention manifests in specific acquired and degenerative cognitive communication disorders, as well as the ways in which existing models of attention may be able to enhance our understanding of these disorders. Next, principles of assessment and treatment of attention within the field of speech-language pathology will be outlined, and some specific assessment tools will be described. Finally, a case study will be presented as an example of how these principles and tools might be applied to better understand the role of attention in the assessment and treatment of an individual patient.

Central Principles of Attention

A major challenge in studying the cognitive skill of attention is defining precisely what attention is. Most of us

have a general sense of what it entails —after all, "attention" is a familiar term that occurs frequently and flexibly in everyday conversation. We may casually comment that an individual has a short or long "attention span"; we may remind someone that important information is forthcoming ("Pay attention!"); we may talk about "attention to detail" or about "drawing someone's attention" to something. We may associate the idea of attention with concepts such as distraction or multitasking or meditation, or with the feeling of suddenly realizing we have just read the same paragraph over several times without absorbing any of its content. And particularly in recent years, with the ever-increasing ubiquity of scrolling, texting, video snippets, and social media, many of us report an increasing sense of concern about whether our habit of scanning and flitting from image to image and from page to page could be negatively impacting our ability to focus on a single topic for longer periods of time.

These everyday references to attention, however, are sprawling and imprecise, and it is difficult to extract from them a definitive definition of this construct. Is attention one thing or many things? Is it about how *long* we can pay attention? Is it about how *well* we can pay attention? Or is it more about how many things we (think we) can pay attention to at the same time? How can we measure an individual's attention, and what does that mean? And—most importantly for our discussion here—how does attention fit into the assessment and treatment of cognitive communication disorders?

The first step in considering how attention may manifest in clinical populations will be to consider the ways in which the neuropsychological literature has defined attention in healthy people. This is no small undertaking, as a wide variety of models and theories of attention have been proposed, and each one characterizes attention somewhat differently. We will consider a number of major historical models of attention in this chapter. However, before delving into specifics, it may be useful to first outline several broad, fairly universal principles of attention that are inherent in multiple models.

The first central principle of attention is that it is always defined in relation to a stimulus: You always pay attention *to* something. A stimulus can be either external (originating from the environment) or internal (originating from within the individual). Examples of external stimuli could include a funny story your sister tells you about her dog, the rapidly falling shapes in a game of Tetris, the lyrics of "Bohemian Rhapsody," or this chapter you're currently reading. Some examples of internal stimuli are a mental grocery list, a major decision you're trying to think through, or a childhood memory. In some cases, you might also be attending (or attempting to attend) to multiple stimuli at once. For example, you might be writing an email while also watching a talk show and dividing or switching your attention between the two. The important takeaway here, however, is that in order for attention to take place, at least one stimulus must be involved.

A second, related principle of attention that relates primarily to external stimuli is that the modality of the stimulus should be identified and noted. We can attend, for example, to an auditory stimulus such as a radio news program or an intercom announcement; likewise, we can also attend to a visual stimulus such as a silent film or a chess game. Many of the objects we attend to on a daily basis consist of a combination of auditory and visual stimuli; an action film, a live dance performance, a thunderstorm, and a family member speaking to us from across the dinner table all fall into this category. Additionally, although it is common to think of attention in terms of the visual, auditory, or combined visual-auditory modalities, it is certainly also possible to attend through other modalities—reading Braille, for example, requires attention through the tactile modality. We may also attend to simple everyday stimuli such as the wind on our face (another tactile stimulus), to the smell of something baking in the next room (an olfactory stimulus), or to the taste of an apple (a gustatory stimulus).

Another notable feature of attention is that it is thought to be closely connected to other processes such as memory and executive function, as well as to the effective use of language to communicate. From a certain perspective, you might even say that attention functions as a prerequisite that must be fulfilled before certain other cognitive-linguistic operations can be successfully carried out. For example, how could you possibly recall a set of verbal directions if you were not able to pay attention to the directions when they were originally given? How could you harness executive function to create and execute a plan without directing some attention toward that plan? How could effective communication occur without attention to the topic or attention to a communication partner's message? Attention is necessary for all of these cognitive-linguistic activities. This interconnectedness of attention with other cognitive-linguistic skills can present a challenge in studying attention in an experimental or evaluation context, as it can be difficult to cleanly separate from other processes. This issue will be further explored later when discussing the assessment of attention.

This brings us to perhaps the two most important features of attention as it is understood in the neuropsychological literature: **capacity limitation** and **selection**, concepts that are closely related to one another and should be considered in tandem. The first, capacity limitation, refers to the fact that the human attention system can only process a limited number or amount of stimuli at once. The second, selection, represents the ability of this system to focus on stimuli that are most relevant to its behavior, goals, or interests, while ignoring or filtering out stimuli that are less relevant (while continuing to monitor these less-relevant stimuli to some extent in case they should become relevant again). We can consider capacity limitation to be a weak point of the human attention system and selection to be a complementary strong point: We may not be able to attend to everything at once, but at least we can be somewhat selective about which stimuli we *do* want to attend to.

The psychologist William James, who wrote about attention in the late 19th century, summed up the ideas of capacity limitation and selection nicely in the following passage:

[Attention] is taking possession by the mind, in clear and vivid form, of one out of what seem several simultaneously possible objects or trains of thought. Focalization, concentration, of consciousness are of its essence. It implies withdrawal from some things in order to deal effectively with others and is a condition which has a real opposite in the confused, dazed, scatterbrained state which in French is called distraction. (James, 1890/1950, pp. 403–404)

While James's characterization is somewhat more philosophical than evidence based, it nicely expresses the idea that in many everyday situations, a multiplicity of different stimuli compete for our attention, and if we are to "deal effectively" with any of them, we must (consciously or subconsciously) select specific stimuli on which to focus our attention and find a way to ignore the others. As an illustration, think of all the many stimuli that might bombard you as you enter a busy restaurant: the sights of tables, chairs, lights, menus, the décor, the hostess, servers, and other patrons, as well as the sounds of clinking glasses and silverware, the music, and the numerous conversations unfolding simultaneously around you. Due to capacity limitations, it would be difficult if not impossible to attend fully to all of these stimuli at once. Even in a calmer, less complicated situation, for example, if you were sitting alone on the couch reading a book, capacity limitations would likely still be at play. In this case, the multiple stimuli competing for your attention might consist of the words on the page, the feel of the book in your hand, the light in the room, the ticking clock, your occasionally vibrating phone, and the distant hum of a lawn mower or of cars going by outside, as well as perhaps internal stimuli such as thoughts about dinner or about a conversation you had earlier in the day.

Typically, selection is based on which stimulus or stimuli are most relevant to the task or behavior we are currently engaged in. In the above example in which your chosen task is reading, presumably with the goal to finish the book, the book is the relevant stimulus and most other stimuli in your environment are irrelevant by comparison. In the restaurant example, the most relevant stimulus might be the hostess as she asks how many are in your party. Ideally, you would want to select and attend to these relevant stimuli, while ignoring or filtering out stimuli that are less relevant.

Theories and Models of Attention

Having outlined some fundamental principles of attention, we will now discuss several of the most influential theories and models of attention that have emerged in the neuropsychological literature since this cognitive skill began to be studied systematically and in depth, in the mid-20th century. In general, models of attention tend to fall into one of three categories: models that attempt to explain selection, models that focus on capacity limitations, and models that delineate different subtypes of attention. Major examples of each of these three types of models will be discussed in turn. Where relevant, important experimental findings will also be described.

Theories and Models of Selection

Much of the literature on attentional selection has been influenced by early investigations of the "cocktail party problem" in the 1940s and 1950s. The cocktail party problem, a term originally coined by Colin Cherry (1953), refers to the study of the factors and mechanisms that allow humans to selectively attend to an auditory stimulus—typically a target speech stream—in situations when other, less relevant, auditory information is also present. As the term suggests, this phenomenon is exemplified by the experience of engaging in conversation with a friend at a noisy cocktail party, surrounded by a bevy of other conversations, and trying to selectively attend to what that friend is saying while filtering out all the other audible talkers (for a review of the cocktail party problem, see Bronkhorst, 2015). Early work on the cocktail party problem sought to identify factors that make this type of selective listening more—or less—successful. An early experiment by Cherry (1953) included a dichotic listening task, in which two different speech streams were presented to a listener simultaneously, one in each ear via headphones. The listener was asked to attend to the ongoing message in one ear, repeating it aloud as it was heard (a task known as "shadowing"). It was found that when listeners were asked to shadow the message in one ear but were later asked about the voice and message played into the other, unattended ear, they were typically unable to report anything about that unattended message other than global acoustic information about the speaker (e.g., whether they had perceived a male or female voice). This is a clear example of selection, in which the listener selected one message to process, at the expense of the other.

A subsequent experiment by Broadbent (1952) added to this work, expanding the understanding of the role of attention in selective listening. In this experiment, subjects listened to two messages spoken by two different voices, but instead of the two messages being played simultaneously and funneled to different ears (as in the dichotic listening experiment above), the messages were serially interleaved, word by word. The subject heard the first word of the first message, followed by the first word of the second message, followed by the second word of the first message, followed by the second word of the second message, and so on. The subject was instructed at the start to listen and respond to only *one* of these two messages. Results suggested that presenting sentences in this way caused confusion for the subject or, as Broadbent termed it, "failures of attention in selective listening."

The finding that interleaved, non-overlapping speech could negatively impact processing of a target message was critical because previous work on selective listening had mostly asked listeners to attend to target speech in the presence of sustained, overlapping background noise (e.g., Egan & Wiener, 1946). In these experiments, difficulty understanding the target was usually attributed to time-frequency overlap between the target and the masker (i.e., the irrelevant or distractor stimulus). Because the auditory system processes sounds in time-frequency units, any time-frequency unit containing strong energy originating from the masker could result in a reduced ability of the listener to detect energy in that same unit originating from the target. This would not be considered a failure of the listener's attention abilities but rather a physiologically based inability of the listener's peripheral auditory system to effectively segregate target and masker. Broadbent's (1952) experiment, however, demonstrated that even in a paradigm with zero time-frequency overlap between target and masker, confusion could still occur. The existence of masking effects that cannot be explained by time-frequency overlap between target and masker has been confirmed by a number of more recent studies using more technologically advanced methods (e.g., Arbogast et al., 2002; Brungart et al., 2006). This additional level of masking, now known as "informational masking," is thought to be due to higher-order, central processing factors such as attention (for a review, see Kidd & Colburn, 2017). Researchers have also identified a number of factors that influence the extent to which listeners are able to selectively attend to target speech, including degree of spatial separation between target and masker (e.g., Freyman et al., 2001), degree of linguistic similarity of the target and masker (Brouwer et al., 2012), and familiarity of the target and masker languages (e.g., Van Engen & Bradlow, 2007). Such findings are highly relevant to attentional selection in everyday situations, particularly in relation to auditory stimuli.

Early work on auditory selective attention also produced three notable theories about the process whereby the human attention system may select relevant stimuli and filter out irrelevant stimuli. These theories are known as the early filter theory, the filter attenuation model, and the late filter model. These models were all designed to explain the steps involved in attentional selection; however, they differ from one another in the specifics of those steps. The early filter theory (Broadbent, 1958) suggests that all stimuli receive preliminary analysis of general features such as location or intensity but that irrelevant or unattended stimuli are filtered out at a relatively early stage of processing, while the attended stimulus is selected and goes on to receive additional processing. The filter attenuation model (Treisman, 1960) was developed later, based in part on results that called the early filter theory into question. Specifically, it was found that even though subjects in dichotic listening tasks were usually unable to report any content from the unattended ear, they were sometimes able to report part of this content if it was highly salient (Moray, 1959; Treisman, 1960). Like the early filter model, the filter attenuation model posits that relevant stimuli are selected early on for further processing; however, in the filter attenuation model, unselected stimuli are not completely filtered out but rather are attenuated, making them potentially available for further analysis later on. Finally, the late filter (or late selection) model (Deutsch & Deutsch, 1963) theorized that all stimuli are analyzed in the early stages of processing and that selection of the target stimulus occurs later and is based on "importance weighting." Although all three models have influenced the study of attention, a number of more recent studies have lent support to Treisman's filter attenuation model (e.g., Cowan, 1997; Driver, 2001).

In addition to the theories described above, which are all based on work in auditory attention, several influential theories of selection have developed from work on visual attention. One of these is the spotlight theory of attention (Posner et al., 1980), which suggests that visual cues can trigger the formation of a "spotlight" in a specific location of the visual field, and as a result, an object in that location receives enhanced processing. It has been argued that the idea of attention as a spotlight may have limitations in dynamic visual scenes (i.e., those involving object movement) (Driver & Baylis, 1989); however, the basic analogy of attention as a mechanism that highlights a specific visual object in a potentially complex scene is still highly intuitive and useful. Although the idea of a "spotlight" lends itself most easily to visual attention, it can also be applied to auditory attention (Fritz et al., 2007).

A related theoretical principle of visual attention is that of object formation. Object formation is the concept that humans, when presented with a complex mixture of sensory information (sometimes known as a visual or auditory "scene"), tend to perceptually group the sensory information in this scene into specific "objects" (Desimone & Duncan, 1995). This grouping is typically based on perceived spatial location, as well as on other qualities (e.g., color and contour in the visual modality). To give a simple visual example, if you see a blue circle on your left, a green square on your right, and a yellow circle straight ahead, you will almost certainly, and without thinking much about it, perceive these areas of color as three separate objects (rather than as 2 objects or 11 objects or as simply a cluttered mess) and will attend to them as such. Shinn-Cunningham

(2008) extended the theory of object formation to apply to auditory attention as well, defining an auditory object as "a perceptual entity that, correctly or not, is perceived as coming from one physical source" (p. 2). If you hear a bark that you perceive to be coming from your left, a meow that sounds like it's coming from your right, and a chirp straight ahead, therefore, your brain will use this information to form three auditory objects originating from three different animals. Object formation, whether visual or auditory, is relevant to attentional selection: The attention system may be considered to be selecting between competing perceptual objects.

Theories and Models of Capacity Limitation

Another group of theories of attention has focused not on selection per se but rather on the limits of attentional capacity. Attentional capacity has frequently been considered and studied in the context of dual-task experiments, in which a subject is asked to pay attention to two sets of stimuli at the same time and to split their attention between the two. Dual-task experiments are often thought to recruit divided attention processes and can be thought of as a form of multitasking. Because successful multitasking can (depending on the tasks) place high demands on the attention system, dual-task paradigms can be an effective way of determining at what point an individual's capacity limit has been reached. Researchers often manipulate the difficulty or salience of one or both tasks in order to determine how these changes will impact subjects' performance. Dual-task experiments in

the neuropsychological literature have also frequently been used to examine age-related differences in attentional capacity (e.g., Künstler et al., 2018; McDowd & Craik, 1988; Naveh-Benjamin et al., 2005).

One of the most well-known theories of attention, the **resource allocation theory** (Kahneman, 1973), offers an account of capacity limitations in the attention system, as well as an explanation of how attention functions during dual-task experiments. According to the resource allocation theory, humans are able to flexibly allocate resources from a single cognitive pool to various cognitive tasks. This cognitive pool of resources is considered to be limited in capacity, such that when more resources are taken up by one task, fewer resources remain to be allocated to other tasks. This may result in decreased task performance when multiple tasks are engaged in simultaneously, as in dual-task paradigms. Kahneman also noted that when two tasks required detection of stimuli through the same modality (e.g., visual), performance declined more than it did when the two tasks involved stimuli from different modalities. Kahneman termed this phenomenon "structural interference" and theorized that it occurs when both tasks use the same input channels. Other researchers, however, have proposed alternative explanations for structural interference, specifically that there may exist a number of different resource pools, each specialized for a cognitive processing domain (e.g., Gopher et al., 1982; Navon & Gopher, 1979; Wickens, 1980). For example, different resource pools might exist for verbal versus spatial processing or for visual versus auditory processing (Wickens, 1980).

A competing theory of attentional capacity limitations is the central bottleneck model (Pashler, 1994). This model argues that cognitive resources, particularly those related to response selection, must be sequentially allocated to specific tasks, rather than being simultaneously allocated to multiple tasks. The implication of the central bottleneck model is that attention capacity limitations are ultimately due to the "bottleneck" created when attention must be switched back and forth between one task and another.

Models Delineating Attentional Subtypes

A third group of models of attention has focused on dividing the vast and multifaceted construct of attention into different subtypes. Note that some of these models overlap to some extent in terms of the subtypes they identify.

An early theory put forth by Schneider and Shiffrin (1977) and Shiffrin and Schneider (1977) proposed a dichotomy between automatic versus controlled processing. Automatic processing is described as processing that is the result of learned sequences, is not impacted by capacity limitations, and requires no control from the individual. Controlled processing, conversely, is described as being controlled by the individual and subject to capacity limitations. Later studies have suggested that a simple dichotomy between automatic and controlled processes may be too oversimplified (Kahneman & Treisman, 1984); however, this binary distinction continues to persist. While Shiffrin and Schneider's model is not technically an attention model—in fact,

automatic processing is considered to be able to occur without attention—it has been influential in thinking about the ways attention may or may not be under voluntary control. It is also related to concepts of top-down versus bottom-up attention, which will be further discussed below.

One of the most influential attention models still in current use was proposed by Posner and Petersen (1990). This model, groundbreaking in part because it was based on findings from neuroimaging and lesion studies, included three components: **orienting**, **target detection**, and **alerting**. The first of these, orienting, involves the direction of attention toward a specific location. If a person is instructed or cued to direct their attention or gaze toward a particular location, subsequent stimuli that occur in that location will be processed and responded to sooner than stimuli in other locations. Cueing toward a target location can be either overt (in which the gaze is directed toward the location) or covert (in which attention but not gaze is directed toward the location). Subsequent work has described orienting as a process that can be either top-down (goal directed) or bottom-up (stimulus directed) (Corbetta & Shulman, 2002; Shulman & Corbetta, 2012). Later work has also built upon this model, describing ways in which the top-down and bottom-up attention systems may flexibly interact with one another (e.g., Itti & Koch, 2001; Vossel et al., 2014).

Posner and Petersen (1990) also discuss three specific mechanisms believed to be involved in the orienting subsystem: disengaging (detaching attention from a currently focused location), moving (shifting attention to a new location), and engaging (fixing attention on a new target). Evidence for orienting and for these three mechanisms has been provided by studies of covert visual attention (e.g., Posner et al., 1984, 1987). See the Assessment of Attention section in this chapter for a description of one such task, the Covert Orienting of Visual Attention (COVAT) (Posner & Cohen, 1980). The second component of Posner and Petersen's model, target detection, which was later renamed the **executive control system** in an update to the model (Petersen & Posner, 2012), is involved in the effortful control of attention, which includes processes such as conflict resolution and error detection. The third and final component of the model, alertness, is the ability to prepare for, and sustain alertness to, relevant stimuli. Alertness is thought to primarily impact response rate: States of higher alertness can facilitate faster response times but also higher error rates in response selection. Posner and Petersen's (1990) model was updated in 2012 to reflect more recent findings from neuroimaging, developmental, pharmacological, and genetic studies (Petersen & Posner, 2012); however, the basic principles of the model remain the same.

Another notable framework of attentional types was proposed by Mirsky and colleagues (Mirsky et al.,1991). This model comprised four subtypes: **focus, sustain, shift**, and **attention for outcomes**. In this model, focus refers to the ability to select target stimuli from an array; sustain refers to the ability to maintain focus on selected stimuli, as well as alertness; shift refers to the ability to flexibly adapt attentive focus; and attention for outcomes is the process by which we connect stimuli (input) with a response to that stimuli (output). This

model shares some basic concepts with Posner and Petersen's model discussed above. Rather than being rooted in neuroimaging studies, however, it was based on results of neuropsychological testing of a large sample of healthy adult control subjects, neuropsychiatric patients, and elementary school-age children.

One final model that has been particularly influential in the evolution of assessment and treatment of attention in individuals with cognitive communication disorders is the clinically based model developed by Sohlberg and Mateer (1987, 2001b). McKay Sohlberg, a speech-language pathologist, and Catherine A. Mateer, a clinical neuropsychologist, developed and proposed an attentional framework specifically for understanding and evaluating attention deficits in clinical populations. This model comprised a hierarchical taxonomy of types of attention based on the authors' clinical observations and experience and was intended to be useful for clinicians in classifying and treating patients' attentional impairments.

Sohlberg and Mateer's (1987, 2001b) original framework included five specific types of attention, which they arrange in a hierarchy based on task demands. The first and most basic type of attention in the model, **focused attention**, was defined as a fundamental, low-level ability to orient and respond to specific stimuli in any modality. The next, **sustained attention**, referred to the ability to maintain attention to an ongoing, repetitive task for a period of time. Sohlberg and Mateer noted that sustained attention might involve the recruitment of working memory to hold the task instructions in mind and might require a response set. The next type of attention in the model was **selec-**

tive attention, defined as the ability to sustain attention to a target stimulus in the presence of irrelevant or distractor stimuli; here, too, working memory and a response set might be involved. Next in the hierarchy came **alternating attention**, or the ability to flexibly switch back and forth between different tasks and task instructions. Finally, Sohlberg and Mateer included **divided attention**, or the ability to engage in multiple tasks simultaneously, as the most demanding type of attention in their model. Interestingly, recent work by Abdelrahman and colleagues (2019) has provided evidence from physiological measures (thermal imaging and eye tracking) supporting the distinctions between sustained, alternating, selective, and divided attention.

The original five-element version of Sohlberg and Mateer's model continues to be widely used in clinical settings; however, the authors updated their framework in 2010 to "reflect the functional importance of executive control and working memory, and the lack of clarity around the concept of divided attention" (Sohlberg & Mateer, 2010, p. 7). This updated framework is simpler, comprising two major components: sustained attention and **executive control of attention**, where executive control of attention is a category that includes working memory, selective attention, suppression, and alternating attention (Table 1–1). The revised framework no longer includes divided attention; instead, the skill of attending to two tasks simultaneously is thought

Table 1–1. Sohlberg and Mateer's (2010) Clinical Taxonomy of Attention

Attention Component	Description	Representative Task
Sustained	Ability to maintain attention during continuous and repetitive activities	Monitoring a spoken list for target words
Executive control		
Selective	Selectively process information while inhibiting responses to nontarget information	Listening to a spoken passage in the presence of background noise and/or distracting visual stimuli
Alternating	Ability to shift focus between tasks, stimuli, or response sets; mental flexibility	Switching back and forth between listening to a spoken passage and reading text
Suppression	Ability to control impulsive responding	Inhibiting automatic responses during a task; "thinking before acting"
Working memory	Ability to hold and manipulate information in mind	Doing math in one's head

Source: Hula and Biel (2014).

to be represented by alternating attention (a subcomponent of executive control of attention). Note that Sohlberg and Mateer's updated model reflects a change in the way that attention and working memory are conceptualized relative to one another. In the earlier model, working memory was considered to be a feature of sustained attention, whereas in the updated model, working memory is a subcomponent of executive control of attention. Other models have also begun to explore the constructs of attention and working memory as somewhat overlapping with one another.

Characterizing Attention: Other Considerations

Before moving on to examine the literature on attention in cognitive communication disorders, we will briefly discuss three additional concepts related to the characterization of attention that do not fit neatly into any of the above models but will be useful to keep in mind when considering the assessment and treatment of attention. They are the differences (and similarities) between visual attention and auditory attention, the consideration of variability, and the role of effort in attention.

Auditory Versus Visual Attention

Since many of studies on attention have been focused specifically on either visual attention or auditory attention, it is worth thinking about the ways in which visual and auditory attention can differ. Auditory attention is almost always time dependent, driven by the source of the stimulus. As an example, the experience of reading a book with your eyes is somewhat different from the experience of listening to an audiobook. With visual reading, you can read at any pace you like, but there may be only one speed at which you can listen to an audiobook (or possibly several, depending on the device you're using). Similarly, during visual reading, your eyes can jump around the page, whereas when listening to an audiobook, it may be harder to skip around or locate a particular sentence. Similar principles hold true for the ways in which visual and auditory attention can be studied in experimental settings or assessed by standardized tests. Some tasks in one modality may have no close equivalent in the other modality. A notable example is a visual search task, in which an individual might be given a sheet of paper with many letters of the alphabet scattered on it and asked to circle all of the Ks. The individual could use a variety of different strategies to find all the Ks: searching quickly or slowly, from left to right or from top to bottom, and so on. It would be difficult to create an auditory version of this task; the closest equivalent might be a task in which an individual is asked to listen to a series of letters spoken aloud and raise their hand whenever they hear a K. In this task, the individual must listen to the letters in the order they are spoken—they cannot formulate a strategy that involves listening to the letters at a certain speed or in a certain order. Likewise, some types of auditory attention tasks, such as the experiments described earlier in which an individual is asked to attend to target speech in the presence of an auditory masker, may have no clear visual equivalent.

Time-Based Variability in Attention

Another concept to keep in mind when considering how to measure attention is the extent to which attention in a given situation is expected to be sustained over time. In some situations, successful attention might involve orienting and responding to a single stimulus, but in many situations, successful attention requires sustained focus to an ongoing stimulus over a longer period of time: a minute, 2 minutes, 5 minutes. Attention could also vary from day to day: if an individual is given the same task to complete on several different days, performance may fluctuate to some degree from day to day. This concept of **intraindividual variability** has been shown to be related to age, with older individuals showing higher degrees of variability than younger individuals (Dykiert et al., 2012; MacDonald et al., 2009). It has also been shown to be elevated in individuals with neurocognitive disorders, including traumatic brain injury (e.g., Bleiberg et al., 1997; Stuss et al., 1994), dementia (Hultsch et al., 2000; Murtha et al., 2002), and aphasia (Villard & Kiran, 2015, 2018). On a related note, attention can also decrease over time, particularly during a longer task; this declining performance is known as a decrement in performance over time (Sarter et al., 2001). The literature on time-based fluctuations is continuing to evolve; recent work has revealed that these fluctuations in attentional state

may be predicted by functional connectivity (Rosenberg et al., 2020).

Attention and Effort

One final issue that may be useful to consider when assessing attention is the relationship between attention and effort. Effort—like attention—can be very difficult to define, making the relationship between the two challenging to measure. Kahneman's (1973) influential theory posits a very close relationship between attention and effort, even suggesting that the two terms are synonymous. As a result, attention and effort have often been equated in the psychological and neuropsychological literature, though this conceptualization has also been questioned (Bruya & Tang, 2018). While effort may be difficult to define in relation to attention, it is relevant to how taxing or fatiguing an individual perceives a task to be and may therefore be useful to consider in clinical contexts. Researchers have utilized a variety of different tools to study effort during tasks requiring attention. One example is pupillometry (e.g., Strauch et al., 2022; Wagner et al., 2019), which involves measuring involuntary changes in pupil diameter during a task and is considered to reflect the amount of cognitive effort put forth by an individual (Kahneman & Beatty, 1966). Pupillometry is thought to be particularly sensitive to changes in the allocation of attention (see Laeng et al., 2012, for a review). Functional magnetic resonance imaging (fMRI) has also been used to examine brain regions recruited during tasks requiring effortful attention (e.g., Hervais-Adelman et al.,

2012), as has functional near-infrared spectroscopy (fNIRS) (Wijayasiri et al., 2017). Effort during a variety of types of tasks can also been assessed through self-report (e.g., by asking the individual to subjectively rate their effort during a specific task or item; e.g., Schepker et al., 2016).

Attention in Neurogenic Cognitive Communication Disorders

This section summarizes the research on attention deficits that may occur in several acquired/degenerative neurological disorders. While attention may not necessarily be the most salient deficit in many patient profiles, it can interact closely with other cognitive-linguistic abilities and therefore can be important to consider when choosing assessment approaches and designing treatment programs. The diagnoses discussed in this section are traumatic brain injury, aphasia, and dementia. From this point forward, when possible, we will refer to subtypes of attention using Sohlberg and Mateer's (1987, 2001b) original taxonomy, as well as Posner and Petersen's (1990) model.

Traumatic Brain Injury

Traumatic brain injury (TBI) is a general term that refers to any damage to the brain caused by sudden trauma (see Chapter 8 of this book for more on TBI). As such, it encompasses a number of different types of injuries, as well as a wide range of resulting patterns of impairment and recovery. Depending on the specific case, TBI could involve a closed or open head injury, diffuse axonal injury (widespread shearing of white matter in the brain), contusion (bruising of the brain), increased intracranial pressure, hypoxia, and/or several other types of initial injuries or sequelae. In the most recent update to the *Diagnostic and Statistical Manual of Mental Disorders* (5th ed.; *DSM-5*; American Psychiatric Association, 2013), TBI has been reclassified as *neurocognitive disorder due to traumatic brain injury*, under the heading major or minor neurocognitive disorders, and may be marked by decreased cognitive skills in areas including complex attention, executive function, learning, and memory, among others.

While cognitive impairments in TBI can vary substantially from patient to patient, attention has very frequently been observed to be impacted. However, the manifestation and extent of cognitive impairments in TBI can vary based on a multitude of factors, including severity and type of initial injury, extent and type of complications, age of the patient, and premorbid functioning, making it difficult to draw general conclusions. For this reason and others, the available literature has yielded mixed results on the presence and extent of different types of attentional impairment in TBI patients.

Despite the variability within the TBI population, however, a number of studies have provided evidence that patients with TBI do exhibit impairments in sustained attention (Bonnelle et al., 2011; Chan, 2002; Manly et al., 2003; Whyte et al., 1995). Sleep disorders and disturbances are also widely studied in TBI, and some of the research on sustained attention in TBI has overlapped with research on arousal, fatigue, or sleepiness in this population. A number of studies examining sleep disturbances in TBI have suggested that these disturbances are associated with deficits in sustained attention (Bloomfield et al., 2010; Castriotta et al., 2007).

There is also some evidence that selective attention, or the ability to resist distraction, is impaired in TBI. One study found that individuals with TBI exhibited slower reaction times than controls when visual distractions were presented immediately following a target stimulus, suggesting distractibility during response preparation (Whyte et al., 1998). A subsequent study by the same group observed TBI patients and healthy controls completing tasks both with and without distractions and concluded that TBI patients were significantly less attentive than controls in both conditions (Whyte et al., 2000); however, evidence that distractions posed additional difficulties for patients (beyond the difficulties present when no distractions were involved) was weak. Other studies on selective attention in TBI have found evidence of visual selective attention deficits in patients relative to controls (Bate et al., 2001a), associations between selective attention and fatigue (Ziino & Ponsford, 2006), and evidence of deterioration of performance over time on a selective attention task (Schnabel & Kydd, 2012). Divided attention has often been found to be impaired in TBI as well, although findings regarding the specifics of this impairment have varied from study to study. It has been suggested that this is due to marked differences in the tasks used in different studies to examine divided attention and that tasks with fewer memory or controlled processing

components may not be sensitive to differences between TBI patients and controls (Park et al., 1999). Impairments in executive attention or executive control of attention have also been noted in TBI (e.g., Niogi et al., 2008; Ríos et al., 2004).

A key complication in assessing and understanding attention deficits in TBI stems from difficulty separating impaired (which sometimes means **slowed**) attention from slowed cognitive processing in general. Research suggests that patients with TBI do typically exhibit overall slowed cognitive processing relative to healthy controls (Ben-David et al., 2011; Ríos et al., 2004). Some studies have argued that slowed processing and attention are two separate impairments in TBI patients (Dymowski et al., 2015; Mathias & Wheaton, 2007). Other studies, however, have concluded that slowed processing speed may significantly contribute to the observed attention impairments in TBI (Ponsford & Kinsella, 1992) or may even fully explain them (Willmott et al., 2009). In short, results on this point are mixed, and the relationship between attention and slowed processing is still under discussion in the TBI literature.

Much of the research on attention in TBI has been motivated by understanding the ways in which individuals engage in everyday tasks such as activities of daily living (ADLs) and their level of competence or safety while doing so. Some studies have specifically examined the link between attention deficits and cognitive failures during everyday tasks in TBI patients, with somewhat mixed results. A widely cited study by Robertson and colleagues (1997) found significant associations between performance on a sustained attention task, severity of brain damage (assessed by a coma scale and posttraumatic amnesia duration), and everyday slips in attention (as reported by caregivers of the study participants). The particular sustained attention task used in this study was the Sustained Attention to Response Test (SART), which is described at greater length in the Assessment portion of this chapter. However, a later study was unable to replicate Robertson and colleagues' key findings (Whyte et al., 2006). Finally, a study by Dockree and colleagues (2006) found evidence that errors during a divided attention task were correlated with everyday cognitive failures.

There has also been a substantial amount of work on TBI and driving, a task considered to require higher-level forms of attention (e.g., a driver might recruit divided attention when checking to see if it is safe to change lanes while also maintaining safety in their current lane). There is some evidence that impaired divided attention following TBI may be associated with reduced safety in driving (Brouwer et al., 1989, 2002; Cyr et al., 2009). However, a systematic review on studies examining prediction of driving capacity after TBI concluded that due to methodological limitations in many studies, there is still no reliable way to predict driving abilities in TBI (Ortoleva et al., 2012).

Finally, a note on neglect. Brain injury—as well as other etiologies, notably right hemisphere stroke—can result in unilateral neglect, also known as hemispatial neglect. Patients with neglect have decreased abilities to detect, orient to, or respond to stimuli on the side of space contralateral to the lesion (in the majority of neglect cases, right hemisphere damage results in left neglect). Although neglect can be considered a form of impaired attention, it will not be discussed at length here. For a thorough discussion of right hemisphere disorder and neglect, the reader is referred to Chapter 4 of this book.

Aphasia

Aphasia in most cases results from a stroke or injury to the language-dominant hemisphere of the brain (the left hemisphere in most but not all individuals) and is characterized by a decrease in receptive and/or expressive language abilities. As a result, the bulk of the research on aphasia has centered on language impairments and on damage to language centers in the brain. However, while language deficits are typically considered the most salient feature of aphasia, many individuals with aphasia have been found to have attention deficits as well (for reviews, see Kurland, 2011; Murray, 1999). A growing body of research is examining the extent and role of decreased attention in this population, and there is an increasing sense that gaining a better understanding of attention deficits in aphasia is not only theoretically important but also clinically relevant, in terms of both the assessment and treatment of aphasia.

Notably, a number of studies have provided evidence that the attention deficits in aphasia are domain general in nature—in other words, attention deficits in aphasia are evident not just on linguistic tasks but also on nonlinguistic tasks (e.g., Erickson et al., 1996; Hunting-Pompon et al., 2011; Kreindler & Fradis, 1968; Laures et al., 2003; Peach et al., 1993; Robin & Rizzo, 1989; Villard

& Kiran, 2015). An important point in studying attention in aphasia is that if an attention task that involves linguistic stimuli is administered to a patient with known language deficits, it will be difficult to conclude that impaired performance is necessarily due to deficits in attention. The above-referenced studies all removed this confound through the use of nonlinguistic tasks. Their findings demonstrate that persons with aphasia exhibit attentional impairments in situations where no language is required, suggesting that the attention impairment in aphasia is, at least to some extent, domain general.

An interesting feature of aphasia —possibly connected to attention impairments in this population—is that substantial within-person, or **intraindividual**, variability has been observed on a variety of different types of language tasks (Cameron et al., 2010; Caplan et al., 2007; Freed et al., 1996; Howard et al., 1985; Kreindler & Fradis, 1968). It is not unusual to observe an individual with aphasia correctly name a picture or answer a question one moment but then be unable to repeat this behavior a few moments later—even if shown the exact same picture or asked the exact same question. This variability has been observed not only from moment to moment but also from day to day. Work by McNeil and colleagues (Hula & McNeil, 2008; McNeil, 1982, 1983; McNeil et al., 1991) has suggested that this variability in performance, along with several other features of aphasia such as stimulability and preserved metalinguistic knowledge, indicates that individuals with aphasia have not lost their representations of language in the brain, as is often assumed. Rather, McNeil and colleagues argue, these individuals experience a fluctuating ability to access these representations due to a failure to effectively and efficiently **allocate** attentional resources (see McNeil et al., 2011, for a review). On a related note, other work has shown that individuals with aphasia demonstrate not only variability on language tasks but also elevated variability on attention tasks relative to controls and that this variability is evident when measured not only from moment to moment (Villard & Kiran, 2018) but also from day to day (Villard & Kiran, 2015).

Evidence supporting the existence of divided attention deficits and/or attention allocation deficits in aphasia has been presented in a number of studies. One study implemented a nonlinguistic dual-task experiment using an auditory tone discrimination task and the Wisconsin Card Sorting Task (WISC) (Grant & Berg, 1981), a test of set-shifting involving visual categorization of colored symbols (Erickson et al., 1996). Results showed that while patients and controls performed similarly while focusing on only one task, patient performance was significantly worse than that of controls during the dual-task condition, suggesting that these patients exhibited deficits in attention allocation and/or differences in capacity limitations. Another study by Murray and colleagues (1997) also found evidence of divided attention deficits in aphasia using a primary linguistic listening task combined in one condition with a secondary linguistic task and in another condition with a secondary nonlinguistic task. When a secondary task was added, patient performance decreased more than control performance, suggesting that patients had more difficulty allocating attention between the two tasks. Additionally, patient performance was worse when the secondary task was linguistic. More recently, Heuer and Hallowell (2015) used eye tracking during a dual-task paradigm in which participants were asked to complete two tasks: One was an auditory sentence comprehension task, and one was a visual search task. Murray (2018) also found evidence of reduced resource allocation in patients with aphasia during a divided attention task involving sentence comprehension as well as tone discrimination. Results suggested that while all participants experienced more difficulty in a dual-task relative to a single-task condition, participants with aphasia experienced additional difficulty allocating attention between the two tasks.

The question of whether language deficits in aphasia could be driven or exacerbated by underlying attention deficits, or if these two impairments simply co-occur, is still under discussion in the literature. The view put forth by McNeil and colleagues (described above) implies a relatively strong influence of attention on language performance in aphasia, such that impaired attention is at the root of language deficits in aphasia. Others, such as Murray (1999), Villard and Kiran (2017), and Varkanitsa and colleagues (2023), have suggested a somewhat weaker view, in which attention deficits influence language performance in aphasia to some extent but can only partially explain the linguistic deficit. Some studies have examined this question by looking at the relationship between attention severity and language severity in aphasia. If attention deficits do in fact drive language deficits in apha-

sia, we would expect poorer attention skills to be associated with poorer language skills. One study by Murray (2012) reported significant associations between scores on standardized attention tests and standardized language tests in patients with aphasia. Another, however, found connections between lesion location and performance on an experimental attention task, but did not see associations between performance on that same attention task and overall severity of aphasia (Murray et al., 1997). Recent work has begun to look more closely at lesion characteristics as a means of better understanding how attention deficits and language deficits manifest in individual patients (e.g., Meier et al., 2022; Schumacher et al., 2019; Spaccavento et al., 2019; Varkanitsa et al., 2023).

Additionally, a number of studies have investigated visuospatial attention in aphasia; findings from these studies have suggested that individuals with aphasia may orient or respond to objects in their visual field differently than healthy controls. Generally, severe visuospatial deficits in the form of visual neglect are associated with damage to the right hemisphere (refer to Chapter 4 for more on this topic); however, there is also evidence that left hemisphere stroke can cause visual neglect. In a recent study on 117 patients with acute left hemisphere stroke, 17.4% were found to have symptoms of visual neglect (Beume et al., 2017). An earlier study by Petry and colleagues found that patients with aphasia following left hemisphere stroke demonstrated slowed reaction times responding to stimuli in their right visual field when they were given a misleading, or invalid, cue prior to the stimulus, whereas controls did not show this difficulty (Petry et al., 1994).

Other recent research on visuospatial attention in patients with aphasia has used eye tracking to examine eye gaze patterns of individuals with aphasia while attending to visual stimuli. Thiessen and colleagues used eye tracking to examine visual attention patterns in individuals with aphasia and healthy individuals while looking at visual scenes (Thiessen et al., 2016). Results suggested that the visual attention exhibited by patients with aphasia differed from that exhibited by healthy controls in several ways, including a higher tendency to look at background images in a scene, as well as a lower degree of responsiveness to engagement cues. Additionally, a study by Heuer and colleagues (2017) found evidence that when looking at multiple-choice image displays, physical stimulus characteristics had a notable influence on visual attention in patients with aphasia. Such findings may prove relevant to the development and optimization of visual displays in augmentative-alternative communication (AAC) devices for persons with aphasia.

Finally, a recent line of research has begun to examine selective auditory attention in persons with aphasia, using paradigms where listeners are asked to attend to speech that is presented simultaneously with other, distracting speech (or with unintelligible noise). These studies have revealed that listeners with aphasia particularly struggle in multitalker environments where they must ignore some intelligible speech streams in order to attend to others (Rankin, 2014; Villard & Kidd, 2019, 2020). While the mechanisms underlying this finding are yet to be uncovered, it seems very likely that performance by persons with aphasia (PWA) in these listening situations is caused by a breakdown in selective attention as well as in receptive language processing.

Dementia

With the most recent update to the *DSM*, the terminology referring to the various types of dementia has been reconfigured. Specifically, the diagnostic category that had previously been labeled **delirium**, **dementia**, **amnestic**, and **other cognitive disorders** has been renamed major/minor neurocognitive disorders. This category includes a number of more specific etiologies, including neurocognitive disorder due to Alzheimer's disease, dementia with Lewy bodies, vascular neurocognitive disorder, and frontotemporal neurocognitive disorder. Despite these official changes to the diagnostic nomenclature, the more familiar terms Alzheimer's disease, dementia with Lewy bodies, vascular dementia, and frontotemporal dementia continue to be widely used in clinical and research settings and will therefore be employed here as well.

Research suggests that attention impairments are common in dementia and that deficits in different domains of attention may be helpful in differentiating certain types of dementia (Foldi et al., 2002; Harciarek & Jodzio, 2005). However, dementia with Lewy bodies (DLB) is the only subtype of progressive neurocognitive disorders for which attention deficits are a key diagnostic feature. In the fourth consensus report of the Dementia with Lewy Bodies Consortium (McKeith et al., 2017), one of the core features of DLB is listed as "fluctuating cognition with pronounced variations in attention and alertness" (p. 90). Importantly, these fluctuations manifest early on in patients with DLB, which may aid in differentiating this cognitive disorder from others in which marked deficits in attention appear only later, after the disease has progressed further. Variability in processes such as attention may cause patients with DLB to appear to lose focus during ordinary activities or to "zone out." This variability during everyday situations is typically brief and is not related to specific task demands (Metzler-Baddeley, 2007).

In other types of dementia, such as Alzheimer's disease, vascular dementia, and frontotemporal dementia, attention is not considered to be a diagnostic criterion and is therefore not typically the main focus of assessment or management of the disease. However, even in these types of dementia, information about patients' attention skills may prove valuable during the diagnostic process and may also be relevant when designing plans of treatment or care. In Alzheimer's disease (AD), attentional abilities certainly decline as the disease progresses and are notably impaired during the later stages (Foldi et al., 2002; McGuinness et al., 2010; Perry & Hodges, 1999). Different subtypes of attention, however, may begin to decline at different stages. Patients with AD have been found to have relatively preserved sustained attention abilities until the later stages of the disease (Calderon et al., 2001), whereas higher-level forms of attention, such as executive control and divided attention, have

been shown to be impaired even in early AD (Baddeley et al., 2001; Foldi et al., 2002; Perry & Hodges, 1999). There is also some evidence that AD patients and DLB patients demonstrate similar deficits in selective attention (Calderon et al., 2001).

Additionally, several recent studies suggest that small changes in attention may be associated with preclinical AD biomarkers such as increased levels of amyloid in the brain (Gordon et al., 2015; Lim et al., 2016). Gaining a better understanding of preclinical AD and mild cognitive impairment (MCI) is a major of focus in AD research today, as improving early detection of AD could lead to the development of treatments for individuals whose abilities have not yet been substantially impaired by the disease. There is also evidence that visual selective attention abilities may be helpful in predicting the progression of AD in individual patients (Chau et al., 2017).

Regarding frontotemporal dementia, researchers have suggested that selective attention, as measured by subtests of the Test of Everyday Attention (TEA) (Robertson et al., 1994), described in the Assessment section of this chapter, is more impaired in the frontal variant of FTD than in the temporal variant or in AD (Perry & Hodges, 2000). Patients with vascular dementia have been found to have attention deficits as well (Akanuma et al., 2016).

Assessment of Attention

This section will describe some widely available tests of attention that may be used in clinical and/or research settings to evaluate attention in individuals with cognitive communication disorders. Before jumping into the details of these tests, however, it may be helpful to begin by outlining some important considerations in approaching an assessment of attention and choosing appropriate tools.

As discussed in the previous section, attention comprises a variety of subtypes. While these subtypes may overlap in some respects (e.g., basic sustained attention is necessary in order for successful selective attention to occur), they are often assessed separately. It is essential, therefore, to choose attention measures that assess the subtype or subtypes of attention that are most relevant to the patient being assessed. To begin with, this should involve considering the patient's current abilities. For example, it would probably not be appropriate to administer a challenging dual-task assessment to a patient known to have inconsistent alertness or difficulty focusing on a simple task for more than a few seconds. Similarly, a basic sustained attention measure might not be sensitive enough to detect subtler attention deficits in a higher-level patient hoping to return to work.

Next, when selecting a test of attention—or a test of any cognitive-linguistic skill, for that matter—test validity should be carefully examined. Test validity can be defined as the extent to which a test measures what it claims to measure (Thorndike, 1997). It includes several subcomponents, two of which—construct validity and ecological validity—will be discussed here. The first, construct validity, is whether the results of a test are really a reflection of the construct it purports to assess. Theoretically, anyone could cre-

ate a new test and name it "My New Test of Selective Attention"; however, this would not necessarily mean that the test-takers' scores on this measure were at all indicative of their selective attention abilities. A published test should provide specific information about construct validity, including a research-based description of the theoretical construct that the test aims to measure, as well as an explanation of how the developed test relates to this construct. A comprehensive analysis of construct validity will involve statistical testing (e.g., a factor analysis conducted on test data from a normative sample), comparison of scores on the test in question with scores on other established tests believed to measure the same construct, and/or other quantitative procedures.

The second type of validity that is important to consider is ecological validity, which is how well an individual's performance on a test of a given skill reflects the way they are able to apply that skill in a functional, real-world context (Sbordone, 2001). Ecological validity is particularly important to think about when selecting tests of attention, as many available tests of attention involve repetitive listening or computer-based tasks that may differ considerably from most real-world situations. It is important to consider to what extent such tests are—or are not—reflective of patients' attention abilities in everyday contexts (Bate et al., 2001a; Kim et al., 2005). The concept of ecological validity, along with related principles of treatment (e.g., generalizability of trained skills), is one we will return to again later in this chapter. Note that there can often be somewhat of a trade-off between construct validity and ecological validity. A highly structured, repetitive, computer-based attention test may have high construct validity but low ecological validity. A patient or caregiver questionnaire about attentional lapses in everyday situations, on the other hand, could have high ecological validity but limited construct validity.

Another complication in selecting tests of attention is the fact that attention can be difficult to tease apart from other cognitive communicative abilities such as executive function, language processing, and visual/auditory processing. After all, most real-world activities requiring attention require other skills as well. For example, a child listening to a bedtime story is attending to the story, but they are also processing the language they hear. Similarly, a teenager playing a video game is attending to the game, but they are also visually processing what they see on the screen. The same principle holds true for the clinical assessment of attention, and for many patients, this point can introduce complications. An attention task requiring the patient to attend to written words or letters, for example, could be problematic if administered to a patient with aphasia, alexia, or visual impairment, as these other impairments would cloud interpretation of the resulting scores. On a somewhat different note, the patient's native language or bilingual/multilingual status should also be considered, as administering a test in English to a patient who is nonnative speaker of English could impact results. Additionally, many tests of attention may require additional cognitive abilities of the patient: Short-term and/or working memory may be required to retain and apply the task instructions, or executive function may be required to plan and execute a response. The full range of processes required for a particular task should therefore be identified when choosing a test of attention, with potentially confounding issues considered.

Other factors that should be considered when selecting test materials include the purpose and goals of assessment. In some cases, the purpose of assessing attention may be to demonstrate that the individual has an attention deficit that warrants rehabilitative treatment. In these cases, a norm-referenced test with high validity and sufficient guidance for thorough interpretation of results would be appropriate. In other cases, the purpose might be to track improvement in attention over time, perhaps in relation to the implementation of an attention treatment program. (For situations in which the test is expected to be administered again following treatment, issues such as test-retest reliability and practice effects should be taken into account.) Test selection should also be related to the goals and concerns of the patient or family. Depending on the setting, these goals may be centered around safety, independence, discharge to a lower level of care, improvement of maintenance of functional abilities, or personal factors. Finally, as is true when evaluating any cognitive-linguistic skills, the presence or absence of impairment should never be based on the results of a single measure. Instead, several complementary methods of assessment should be used to paint a full picture of the patient's ability in a given domain.

With these considerations in mind, let us now look at some of the available tests of attention that may be used by speech-language pathologists in clinical or research settings. This list is intended to be representative, but it is by no means exhaustive. Many of the tests described below were designed for use in clinical settings (Table 1–2 presents a summary of these); however, some descriptions of well-known tests that have been used in research settings are also included. As noted earlier, the

Table 1–2. Selected Assessment Tasks and Instruments for Evaluating Attention in Clinical Settings

Test	Component(s) of Attention and Related Processes Assessed
Test of Everyday Attention	
Map Search	Selective attention
Telephone Search	Sustained and selective attention
Telephone Search With Counting	Divided attention
Elevator Counting	Sustained attention
Elevator Counting With Distraction	Working memory, alternating attention
Visual Elevator	Alternating and sustained attention
Auditory Elevator With Reversal	Alternating attention, working memory
Lottery	Sustained attention
Attention Process Training–Test	Sustained, selective, alternating, and divided attention
WAIS-IV	
Digit Span Forward	Sustained attention
Digit Span Backward	Sustained attention, working memory
Digit Sequencing	Sustained attention, working memory
Brief Test of Attention	Divided attention, working memory
Symbol Digit Modalities Test	Divided attention, visual scanning and tracking, perceptual motor speed
Paced Auditory Serial Addition Task	Sustained and divided attention, speed of processing
Conners' Continuous Performance Test	Sustained, selective, and divided attention
Moss Attention Rating Scale	Restlessness/distractibility, initiation, sustained attention
Rating Scale of Attentional Behavior	General attention, ability to focus

Source: Hula and Biel (2014).

evaluation of attention overlaps with the evaluation of other cognitive processes; therefore, some tests that may often be considered to measure attention are described in other chapters of this book.

Test of Everyday Attention

One widely used and fairly comprehensive tool designed to assess a number of different subtypes of attention is The Test of Everyday Attention (TEA) (Robertson et al., 1994). This measure was designed for adults aged 18 to 80 and is intended to take approximately 60 minutes to administer. Initial validation performed by the developers involved analysis of scores from 154 unimpaired individuals, as well as 80 unilateral stroke patients, as well as comparison of these scores with performance on previously existing tests of attention. Brief descriptions of the eight TEA subtests are provided below. All subtests were designed around the theme of an imagined trip to Philadelphia.

- **Map Search:** The test-taker is given a map of Philadelphia and asked to find and circle as many restaurant symbols (a knife and fork) as they can in 2 minutes. Two scores are taken from this task: the number of symbols circled in 1 minute and the number of symbols circled in 2 minutes.
- **Telephone Search:** The test-taker is given a telephone directory and asked to cross out specific symbols.
- **Telephone Search Dual Task:** As in the Telephone Search, the test-taker is asked to cross out specific symbols in a telephone directory;

however, they are also asked to simultaneously count auditory tones. Scores on Telephone Search and Telephone Search Dual Task can be compared to determine the decrement in performance when a second task is added.

- **Elevator Counting:** In this auditory task, the test-taker is instructed to pretend they are in an elevator in which the visual floor number indicator is not working. They are presented with a series of tones and asked to count these tones to determine what floor they are "on."
- **Elevator Counting With Distraction:** This task is identical to Elevator Counting, except that two types of tones (medium-pitched and high-pitched) are presented. The test-taker is asked to count the medium tones and ignore the high ones.
- **Visual Elevator:** In a visual version of the elevator task, the test-taker is presented with a series of pictured stimuli including elevator doors and arrows pointing up or down and is asked to keep track of what floor they are on (with the arrows indicating a switch in the up/down direction).
- **Auditory Elevator With Reversal:** The final elevator task is an auditory version of the visual elevator task, in which the test-taker is asked to keep track of what floor they are on by counting medium auditory tones. In this task, high and low tones indicate a change in direction.
- **Lottery:** The test-taker is presented with series of spoken letters and numbers. They are instructed to listen for a target number and, each time they hear it, to write down the preceding two letters.

Analysis of the TEA subtests provides a good illustration of how the constructs of specific attentional subtypes can be difficult to identify, separate, and measure. Available analyses of TEA results have yielded differing results about which TEA subtests measure which attentional subtypes. For example, the authors' principal components analysis of their normative sample data during development and validation of the test suggested that the TEA subtests load on four factors: visual selective attention/speed, attentional switching, sustained attention, and auditory-verbal working memory. However, more recent studies of a Cantonese version of the TEA in individuals with and without TBI (Chan & Lai, 2006; Chan et al., 2006) found evidence for a three-factor structure consistent with Posner and Petersen's (1990) model, including sustained attention, visual selection, and attentional switching. These differing structures have included conflicting interpretations of specific tasks. For example, the authors' original analysis found that the Visual Elevator task loaded onto the attentional switching factor. However, a different study found that while accuracy on this task loaded onto an attentional switching factor, the timing score loaded onto a sustained attention factor (Chan & Lai, 2006), and another study found the task overall to load onto a sustained attention factor (Bate et al., 2001a).

The TEA has several key advantages. To begin with, it is theory based and is considered to have high construct validity. It also includes instructions for three different administrations (where each includes slight variations in stimuli), which increases the validity of multiple administrations. It may

also be useful, in situations where time for testing may be limited, to selectively administer one or several subtests of the TEA (although this approach may not provide a full picture of the patient's attention skills).

However, there are also limitations to administering the TEA. As a structured test, it is considered to have only moderate ecological validity. Additionally, the evidence on the sensitivity of the TEA to differences between healthy individuals and individuals with neurological impairment is somewhat mixed. The authors of the test found differences in performance between healthy individuals and those with brain injury (Robertson et al., 1996). However, a later study examined performance on the TEA in 35 patients recovering from severe TBI and 35 age- and education-matched controls and found significant group differences in scores on only two of the eight subtests (Map Search and Telephone Search) (Bate et al., 2001a). Finally, the authors note that the TEA should be used with caution in individuals who have known sensory deficits such as reduced visual or auditory acuity and that ceiling or floor effects may be an issue for some subtests.

Attention Process Training Test

The Attention Process Training Test (APT-Test; Sohlberg & Mateer, 2001a) was designed based on the authors' original theoretical framework of attentional subtypes, with the goal of providing clinicians with a tool to systematically assess attention deficits in sustained attention, selective attention, alternating attention, and divided attention. The APT-Test tasks are highly structured and involve both visual and audio-recorded stimuli. This test was originally designed for use with the APT-I and APT-II attention treatment programs; the more recently released APT-III program (see the Treatment portion of this chapter for additional information on this) was not designed to be used with the APT-Test. Nevertheless, the APT-Test is still available and may be useful in contexts where highly structured assessment of specific attentional types is desirable.

Digit Span

A simple and common attention task is the digit span task, versions of which are included in many comprehensive cognitive and neuropsychological batteries, such as the Wechsler Adult Intelligence Scale (WAIS-IV) (Wechsler, 2008). In the digit span task, the test administrator reads aloud a sequence of digits at the rate of one digit per second while the test-taker listens. When the sequence is finished, the test-taker repeats the digits in either forward or backward order (as instructed prior to the task). In other forms of the digit span task, the test-taker may be instructed to manipulate the digits in some way, such as sequencing them into ascending order. Typically, the test begins with a span of two digits, with subsequent items increasing the span, up to eight or nine digits. Two sequences of each length are presented, progressing to longer sequences until the patient misses both sequences at a given level. The length of the longest repeated sequence is the digit span score.

Although digit span is a relatively straightforward task, it also provides another example of overlapping constructs. While forward digit span certainly requires attention to the presented sequences, it can also be considered a test of short-term verbal memory (Lezak et al., 2012). Similarly, the backward and sequencing digit span tasks likely recruit working memory, as well as, possibly, visuospatial processing (Black, 1986; Larrabee & Kane, 1986; Rapport et al., 1994). It should also be recognized that while a digit span task may be appropriate for an individual who has no known difficulty with speech or numbers, it may not be the best choice for patients with aphasia, apraxia, acalculia, or other deficits that could complicate the interpretation of performance. Additionally, there is somewhat conflicting information about the how digit span scores should be understood and about the sensitivity and specificity of digit span scores in differentiating performance in healthy individuals versus a variety of patient populations (see Schroeder et al., 2012, for a review). Notably, some studies have found no reliable difference between backward digit span scores in healthy individuals and individuals with TBI in the chronic stage of recovery (Bate et al., 2001a; Vallat-Azouvi et al., 2007).

Brief Test of Attention

The Brief Test of Attention (BTA) (Schretlen et al., 1996) was developed to be a quick test of auditory divided attention. This measure includes two parts. In the first part, the test-taker listens to sequences of letters and numbers read aloud at the rate of one per second (e.g., "M-6-3-R-2"); after each sequence, they are expected to report how many numbers they heard. In the second part, the test-taker listens to the same sequences of letters and numbers; this time, after each sequence, they are expected to report how many letters they heard. In each of the two parts, the sequences start with 4 items and increase to 18 items. Psychometric testing and validation conducted by the developers of the BTA, involving 926 patients and healthy individuals, suggest that the BTA has good construct validity (Schretlen et al., 1996). However, like many tests of attention, it may also recruit other processes such as auditory working memory and language comprehension.

Symbol Digit Modalities Test

In the Symbol Digit Modalities Test (SDMT) (Smith, 1991), the test-taker is presented with a sheet of paper containing a sequence of symbols, as well as a symbol-digit coding key, in which each digit 1 to 9 is paired with a symbol. The test-taker is asked to provide the digit corresponding to each symbol in the sequence and is given 90 seconds to do so. The SDMT has been considered by some studies to be a measure of visual selective attention (Bate et al., 2001a; Chan, 2000) and by others to be a measure of divided attention (Ponsford & Kinsella, 1992). In addition to requiring attention, the successful completion of this task requires complex visual scanning abilities, processing speed, and memory (Bate et al., 2001a). It has been shown to be sensitive in differentiating individuals with TBI from healthy individuals (Ponsford & Kinsella, 1992). Although the SDMT is traditionally a pencil-and-paper test, computerized

versions have also been developed and used in research settings (e.g., Forn et al., 2009; Tung et al., 2016).

Flanker Inhibitory Control and Attention Test (NIH Toolbox)

The Flanker Inhibitory Control and Attention (FICA) Test from the NIH Toolbox (Gershon et al., 2013) is an assessment of attention, along with inhibitory control. It can be considered to have a strong selective attention component, as it requires the test-taker to respond to some stimuli while ignoring (and inhibiting a response to) others. It contains the classic "flanker" element of distractor symbols that are either congruent or incongruent (i.e., pointing in the same or a different direction as the target). This test has the advantage of being very quick to administer (~3 minutes).

Paced Auditory Serial Addition Test

The Paced Auditory Serial Addition Test (PASAT), originally developed by Gronwall and Sampson (1974) for the purpose of detecting minor cognitive impairments in concussion patients, measures sustained attention, divided attention, and processing speed and likely recruits working memory as well. The PASAT is a challenging task in which a series of random digits (usually 50 or 60) are presented auditorily to the test-taker. Each time a digit is presented (with the exception of the first digit), the test-taker is expected to add that digit to the previous digit and provide the response (a number between

2 and 18). Divided attention is required to add the new number with the previous one while also holding the new number in mind so it can be added to the following number. Research on this test in patients with TBI suggests that it is sensitive to mild deficits. However, it may also be sensitive to factors not related to neurological impairment, such as age, IQ, and mathematical ability; notable practice effects have also been observed (Tombaugh, 2006).

Conners' Continuous Performance Test

Conners' Continuous Performance Test, Second Edition (CPT II) (Conners, 2000) was originally designed for use in children and adolescents with attention-deficit/hyperactivity disorder; however, it may be useful for assessing attention deficits in other populations and ages as well. Studies examining clinical utility of the CPT-II in TBI have found group differences between moderate-to-severe TBI patients and age-matched controls (Zane et al., 2016). Like the SART, the CPT-II asks test-takers to respond to all presented items *except* a specific target; in this case, a series of letters are presented on the screen and test-takers are instructed to respond to all letters except "X." The CPT II provides several indices of performance, including attentiveness, impulsivity, sustained attention, and consistency of response time.

Covert Orienting of Visual Attention

The Covert Orienting of Visual Attention (COVAT) task (Posner & Cohen, 1980) was designed to assess an individual's ability to disengage, move, and engage attention. In this computerized task, the test-taker is seated in front of a computer and instructed to keep their eyes focused on a fixation located at the center of the screen during the entire task. For each item, a spatial cue (right or left) appears, followed by a target (also on the right or left). The subject is expected to then press a button indicating the location of the target. In some of the trials, the target appears on the cued side (congruent trials); in other trials, the target appears on the noncued side (incongruent trials). The ratio of congruent to incongruent trials can be varied in the COVAT, but typically 50% or more of the targets appear in the location designated by the cue. In order to respond to incongruent trials, the test-taker needs to disengage their attention from the cue, move their attention to the side of the screen opposite the visual cue, and then reengage their focus on the target. One study comparing performance on the COVAT in severe TBI patients and age-matched controls found no differences in the two groups' ability to disengage, move, and engage during incongruent trials, though they did find that the patients were significantly slower than the controls in responding (Bate et al., 2001b). Another TBI study on the COVAT revealed that participants with TBI demonstrated an impaired ability to use correct cues (Cremona-Meteyard et al., 1992). One study also found the COVAT to be sensitive to attention deficits in Alzheimer's disease (Wright et al., 1994). The COVAT has primarily been used for research purposes and is seldom seen in clinical settings.

Sustained Attention to Response Test

The Sustained Attention to Response Test (SART) (Robertson et al., 1997) is a computerized task designed to assess sustained attention. The test-tasker is presented with a series of 225 random digits on a screen at unpredictable intervals. They are instructed to press a button as quickly as possible each time they see a digit, unless the digit is a 3, in which case they are told they should not press the button. This type of task is categorized as a go/no-go task and relies on the ability of the subject to remain vigilant toward an infrequently occurring target stimulus and to inhibit an accustomed response when that target appears; such inhibition is thought to require attentional control. SART scores have been shown to differ between healthy individuals and TBI patients, especially those with damage to the frontal lobes (Manly et al., 1999, 2000, 2003; Robertson et al., 1997). The SART was originally designed for use in research settings and is not frequently used in clinical evaluations.

Visual Search Tasks

When the goal is to assess visual attention specifically, paper-and-pencil visual search tasks are often used. In these tasks, the patient is typically given a large piece of paper with many different types of symbols on it (the exact symbol can vary from test to test). They are asked to search for and circle (or cross out) all exemplars of a specific symbol in a given amount of time, while ignoring all other symbols. Some examples of this type of task are the TEA Map Search task (Robertson et al., 1994; see also the discussion of the full TEA earlier in this section) and the WAIS Symbol Search subtest (Wechsler, 2008). While visual search tasks—also sometimes called visual cancellation tasks—are quite different from computerized tasks in which symbols are presented one at a time, they can provide valuable information about a patient's ability to selectively attend to target visual stimuli.

Clinician-Completed Rating Scales of Attention

In addition to the measures listed above, all of which require the patient to sit and complete specific tasks in a controlled testing environment, there are also a number of attention rating scales available. An attention rating scale takes a markedly different approach to the assessment of a patient's attention. The patient is not asked to sit and take a test; instead, a clinician rates the patient on a variety of behaviors related to attention. In order for such scales to be used effectively, the clinician must be familiar with the patient's behavior and must have had substantial opportunity to interact with the patient in everyday situations, usually over the course of 2 or more days. Rating scales tend to have high ecological validity due to their focus on patient behavior and capabilities in everyday environments; however, they can also have disadvantages, such as subjectivity of clinician judgments or application to limited settings.

One such scale is the Moss Attention Rating Scale (MARS) (Hart et al., 2006; Whyte et al., 2003, 2008). This measure includes 22 scales, including "initiates communication with others," "performs better on tasks when directions are given slowly," and "sustains conversation without interjecting irrelevant or off-topic comments." Analysis of the MARS provided by the authors suggests that it measures three factors (restlessness/distraction, initiation, and sustained/consistent attention) (Hart et al., 2006). The authors of the MARS have provided evidence that it has good construct validity and interrater reliability and that it is sensitive to change over time (Hart et al., 2009; Whyte et al., 2008). It has also been shown to be predictive of 1-year outcomes of disability in TBI patients (Hart et al., 2009). Disadvantages of the MARS include a somewhat limited scope of validation—it was designed for use mainly with moderate-to-severe TBI patients and has been evaluated only in inpatient (acute and subacute rehab) settings.

Another example of an attention rating scale is the Rating Scale of Attentional Behavior (Ponsford & Kinsella, 1991), a tool that includes 14 specific scales, such as "performed slowly on mental tasks" and "unable to pay attention to more than one task at a time." Initial validation of the Rating Scale of Attentional Behavior noted that it demonstrated good interrater reliability between professionals from the same discipline but weaker interrater reliability between professionals from different disciplines. It was also found to correlate moderately with scores on other, more impairment-based tests of attention. Like the MARS, the Rating Scale of Attentional Behavior may most useful in a limited population and setting (in this case, patients with severe TBI in a rehabilitation setting).

Quick Attention Screenings and Informal Observation

We turn our focus now to yet another approach to the assessment of attention. While the neuropsychological tests and behavior scales detailed above can provide valuable and, in some cases, relatively comprehensive information about patients' attention abilities, it should be recognized that an in-depth assessment of attention skills is ambitious and may not be feasible in all clinical settings, especially when a clinician is tasked with assessing and treating a variety of cognitive-linguistic skills in a limited period of time. Additionally, some inpatient facilities may have guidelines designed to standardize or streamline screening procedures, and depending on the setting, the available testing materials may be limited. For these reasons, extensive attention testing may not always be realistic.

In such cases, attention can still be examined to some extent through the use of standard cognitive screening/ evaluation tools that assess a variety of domains of cognitive functioning. A few examples of cognitive tests that are not specific to attention but may be encountered in rehabilitation or skilled nursing settings include the Montreal Cognitive Assessment (MoCA; Nasreddine et al., 2005), the Brief Cognitive Assessment Tool (BCAT) (Mansbach et al., 2012), the Cognitive Log (Cog-Log) (Alderson & Novack, 2003), the Cognitive-Linguistic Quick Test (CLQT) (Helm-Estabrooks, 2001), and the Mini-Mental State Examination (MMSE) (Folstein et al., 1975). While none of these tests are specific to attention, they may provide an opportunity to learn something about the patient's attention skills, either through the administration of specific items or through informal observation of the patient and their overall performance. Note, however, that many of the tasks included in these shorter cognitive screening tools may recruit multiple processes, such as working memory, attention, and problem solving, and are no substitute for a fine-grained assessment of attention. If attention impairments are suspected, a more in-depth assessment would ideally follow.

To give an example, the MoCA includes a short "Attention" section, including one forward digit span item, one backward digit span item, a short vigilance task, and a serial subtraction task. Additionally, the MoCA includes a clock drawing task, which is not considered to be a task that specifically evaluates attention; however, informal observation of the patient during the clock drawing may provide some basic information about their ability to attend to a task for several minutes. While these tasks would not provide specific, in-depth, or definitive information about the patient's attention abilities, they may allow the clinician to gain some basic insight, which may then guide further assessment. Observing the patient's language and behavior during informal conversation can also be valuable, as it may reveal more about their ability to attend to a task or conversation for a sustained period of time.

patients with TBI, with another moderately sized group of studies examining attention treatment in stroke. Interestingly, a somewhat separate line of research investigating possible attention treatments in patients with aphasia has also evolved. Attention is typically not a primary focus of treatment for most types of dementia. For a review of how attention may be taken into consideration when designing treatment plans for patients with dementia, see Choi and Twamley (2013).

Approaches used to treat attention in neurogenically impaired populations can be divided into several groups, including direct training of attention, training of specific everyday skills requiring attention, training in self-management of attention deficits, environmental modifications, self-management strategies, and the implementation of external aids. The first two approaches listed, direct training and training of specific skills, can be considered restorative approaches, meaning that they are intended to improve function. The other approaches listed are considered to be more compensatory in nature, meaning that they are strategies to help compensate for, or accommodate, the deficit. This section includes a discussion of each of these approaches, followed by an overview of the literature specifically on treatment of attention in aphasia.

Attention and Treatment

A sizable amount of the available literature on cognitive-behavioral attention treatment in patients with acquired neurological deficits has focused on

Direct Training

The goal of direct training is to treat the underlying attention impairment, usually through the use of repetitive, decontextualized tasks. There is substantial evidence in the literature suggesting that direct training in attention does result in improved performance on trained tasks, on tasks similar to the trained tasks, and on neuropsychological measures (e.g., Sohlberg & Mateer, 1987; Sohlberg et al., 2000; Sturm et al., 1997). However, it is essential to recognize that improvements on repetitive attention tasks may not necessarily generalize to improved attention function in everyday, real-world situations. Several reviews have concluded that there is insufficient evidence that direct training of attention is effective (e.g., Cicerone et al., 2011; Michel & Mateer, 2006; Park & Ingles, 2001; Ponsford et al., 2014). One systematic review examining the efficacy of computerized cognitive rehabilitation of attention and executive function in acquired brain injury did find evidence that these types of direct training methods may be effective; however, the authors acknowledge that many of the studies reviewed had notable methodological limitations such as small sample size or inadequate control groups (Bogdanova et al., 2016). More research on this topic is therefore needed.

Attention Process Training (APT-III) (Sohlberg & Mateer, 2010) is an example of a widely utilized program that uses the direct training approach. APT-III is the most updated version of the program; the second edition (APT-II) (Sohlberg et al., 2001) continues to be widely used in clinical settings as well. APT-II is based on Sohlberg and Mateer's original attention framework and involves a series of tasks that build upon one another, starting with sustained attention, then moving to selective, alternating, and divided attention. Auditory tasks include listening for target words in presented strings, either in quiet or in the presence of competing background noise; visual tasks include search tasks or reading, with or without visual distractions. Tasks are adapted as difficulty levels increase from sustained attention up through divided attention. The updated APT-III is aligned with Sohlberg and Mateer's (2010) revised attention model. It also includes additional training in metacognitive strategies and self-monitoring, is computer based, and supports home practice. There is evidence that APT-II may be effective in treating attention deficits following stroke (Barker-Collo et al., 2009), and there is promising evidence for the effectiveness of APT-III as well (Lee et al., 2018).

Over the past decade or so, there has been a notable increase in the appearance and popularity of computer-based and tablet-based training programs targeting attention and other cognitive skills. These programs, which in many cases are marketed to the general public, can be considered a form of direct training of attention and are worth discussing here for several reasons. For one thing, there is literature suggesting that some of these programs could be able to help facilitate improvements in attention. For example, one study on the use of the program CogMed (Pearson Company, Scandinavia, Sweden) in TBI patients suggested that it may be able to help patients improve attention and working memory (Westerberg et al., 2007), and another study suggested that training in CogMed may result in fewer cognitive failures in everyday life (Lundqvist et al., 2010). Another widely available cognitive training program, Lumosity (Lumos Lab, San Francisco, CA), has been shown in at least one study to facilitate improvements on an untrained measure of visual attention (Finn & McDonald, 2011). Another study found that a combination of Lumosity and APT-III resulted in a small amount of generalization to standardized measures (Zickefoose et al., 2013). The reader is referred to Sigmundsdottir and colleagues (2016) for a more in-depth review of a wide variety of computer- and tablet-based programs.

However, while it is true that there is some preliminary evidence suggesting the potential utility of computer- and tablet-based cognitive training programs, there is still insufficient evidence to definitively support the effectiveness of these methods in facilitating real improvements in everyday functioning for patients with TBI (Sigmundsdottir et al., 2016). It is important to keep in mind that cognitive training programs should be subjected to the same scrutiny and held to the same scientific, evidence-based standards as any other potential treatment method. Additionally, since many cognitive training programs are available on the Internet for potential independent use by patients, the role of clinician-guided training versus independent home practice should be considered before implementing or recommending this type of treatment approach (Cicerone et al., 2011; Connor & Shaw, 2016). For further discussion of the issues and questions surrounding cognitive training programs in a variety of populations, see also Rabipour and Raz (2012).

Training of Specific Functional Skills Requiring Attention

A second approach to attention treatment attempts to narrow the gap be-tween impairment-based training and generalization to everyday situations by treating attention in the context of real-world activities of daily living. A notable review by Park and Ingles (2001) found that specific skills treatments showed greater effects than direct, impairment-based treatments, particularly when control conditions were taken into account. This finding led them to suggest that rehabilitation efforts will be most effective when they focus on skills of functional importance to patients. Park and Ingles also emphasize the role of "neuropsychological scaffolding" in training specific skills. Neuropsychological scaffolding refers to the ways in which a clinician may identify the simpler component parts involved in a more complex task and break these parts down so the patient can practice each one individually—a step that may be necessary for successful practice of the task but that the patient may not be able to take on their own. Specific skills trained may include ADLs such as preparing food, bathing, or dressing. In these cases, collaboration with other disciplines such as occupational therapy or physical therapy can be valuable.

Self-Management Strategies, External Aids, and Environmental Modifications

Finally, attention may be treated through the use of compensatory techniques such as self-management strategies, external aids, and/or environmental modifications. These approaches can be implemented in somewhat overlapping ways and therefore will be discussed here as a group.

The self-management approach to treating attention consists of instructing and training the patient in strategies for self-management of attentional difficulties in everyday functional settings. A self-management strategy could be specific to a particular routine. For example, an individual who has difficulty maintaining consistent attention throughout their entire morning routine might be instructed to post a list next to the bathroom mirror that includes each of the tasks they need to complete (e.g., wash face, brush teeth, floss, brush hair). Note that this strategy could be considered to be a self-management tool that addresses not only attention but also memory and executive function. Self-management strategies can also be more general, making them potentially applicable to many situations—for instance, a patient could be taught to verbally mediate their actions (i.e., describe each step of a task while completing it) or to verbally rehearse important information. There also exist self-management strategies designed specifically to improve attention, comprehension, and memory while reading, such as the PQRST (preview, question, read, summarize, test) method and the SQ3R (survey, question, read, recite, review) method.

Some self-management strategies may also involve the use of external aids, including timed electronic reminders. One example is Goal Management Training (GMT) (Levine et al., 2011), a metacognitive approach that trains patients to pause periodically during a task to monitor performance and define goal hierarchies, sometimes using audible tones as cues. Another strategy suggested by Sohlberg and Mateer (2001b),

which targets self-management of orientation, memory, and attention, is to set a watch to beep at the top of each hour and to ask oneself the following questions whenever it beeps: "What am I currently doing? What was I doing before this? What am I supposed to do next?" as a way to help manage orienting, attention, and memory. Other examples of self-management/strategy training combined with external aids that have been piloted include content-free cueing (Fish et al., 2007) and NeuroPage (Wilson et al., 2001, 2005). In a recent systematic review, Gillespie and colleagues (2012) found strong evidence supporting the use of devices that provide alerts to individuals with cognitive impairments, drawing their attention to stimuli that are either external (e.g., bringing one's attention back to a current task) or internal (e.g., shifting one's attention to a goal in memory).

Environmental modifications, while typically designed to help with memory or executive function (Gillespie et al., 2012), can also help compensate for the effects of attention impairments. Environmental modifications are often designed and implemented by the clinician and then carried over by the patient, possibly with some degree of assistance from family members or other caregivers. Examples could include a computer system or app designed to help with organization or time-based reminders, the implementation of filing systems, or the modification of the home environment to reduce visual or auditory distractions (Sohlberg & Mateer, 2001b).

As with any treatment method, self-management strategies, external aids, and environmental modifications should be carefully selected or designed, tailored for the individual patient, and customized to evolve with patients' needs over time (Lopresti et al., 2004). Ideally, patients themselves should be actively involved in choosing and developing these kinds of strategies, and implementation should involve adequate training and practice time, social and/or environmental supports, and a maintenance program to assess outcomes (Sohlberg & Mateer, 2001b).

Notes on Selecting, Combining, and Implementing Treatment Approaches

A number of reviews and meta-analyses have compared the different types of approaches discussed above, and while recommendation are somewhat mixed, several commonalities emerge. In general, findings from these reviews have recommended a combination of two or more approaches in treating attention, such as direct attention training combined with instruction in metacognitive strategies, or strategy training combined with environmental modifications (Cicerone et al., 2011; Michel & Mateer, 2006; Ponsford et al., 2014).

The *Cognitive Rehabilitation Manual* (Haskins, 2012), developed by the American Congress of Rehabilitation Medicine, recommends several principles that are applicable for both self-management strategies and direct attention training. These principles are to select theory-based treatment approaches; to organize treatment in a hierarchical way, beginning with simpler forms of attention and building upon them; to base treatment decisions on ongoing patient performance data; to help patients work toward generalization of treatment tasks to real-world situations; and to flexibly adapt treatment according to patients' changing needs.

Attention Treatments Designed for Patients With Aphasia

Treating attention in aphasia is often conceptualized differently than treating attention in other neurologically impaired populations. Although attention deficits are common in aphasia, they are usually not as salient as language deficits. As a result, improving attention is typically not the primary goal of treatment for either the patient or the clinician. Research on attention and treatment in aphasia has therefore been motivated by slightly different questions than research on attention treatment in TBI. Some of the work on attention in aphasia has examined whether attention and other cognitive abilities may be able to predict language treatment outcomes in aphasia and have generally found that better nonlinguistic cognitive skills such as attention do help predict better treatment outcomes (Diedrichs et al., 2022; Gilmore et al., 2019; Lambon Ralph et al., 2010). Other studies have investigated the possible utility of using treatment that incorporates—or consists of—attention training to try to address language deficits.

Several studies have examined the effects of direct, impairment-level treatment of attention in patients with aphasia. The APT-II program (Sohlberg et al., 2001) has been used to target attention in patients with aphasia in a number of studies. For example, two case studies examined whether APT-II training would be effective in facilitating mild reading impairments secondary to aphasia (Coelho, 2005; Sinotte & Coelho, 2007). Differences observed from pre- to posttreatment included improved reading comprehension and decreased reading effort (Coelho, 2005), as well as decreased variability in the comprehension of longer reading passages, which the authors theorized could be due to improved attention allocation (Sinotte & Coelho, 2007). Another case study found that APT-II training facilitated some degree of improvement on standardized testing of cognitive abilities, but no changes in everyday attention or communication abilities were noted (Murray et al., 2006). Several other small studies piloting the use of other direct attention training programs have been conducted (e.g., Helm-Estabrooks, 2011; Helm-Estabrooks et al., 2000), with one utilizing a combined direct training and metacognitive facilitation method (Lee & Sohlberg, 2013). In general, findings from these studies have provided only modest support for the potential of direct attention training in remediating linguistic or cognitive deficits in aphasia. Additional evidence, including studies with larger sample sizes, would be necessary before direct attention training could be clinically recommended for patients with aphasia.

More recently, Peach and colleagues have developed a different type of approach for patients with aphasia, called language-specific attention treatment (L-SAT) (Peach et al., 2017, 2018), in which sustained attention, attentional switching, and auditory-verbal working memory are implicitly incorporated into a systematic, skill-based language treatment program targeting lexical and sentence processing. L-SAT is based upon the idea that treating attention within the language domain may be of greater use than direct training of attention in patients with aphasia and that language treatment can be structured in such a way that attentional processes are heavily recruited. This approach could perhaps be considered a specific skills training approach tailored to the specific skill of communication. Preliminary results from a small study suggest that L-SAT may be successful in facilitating language recovery and auditory-verbal working memory in patients with aphasia whose attention deficits are not severe (Peach et al., 2018, 2019). Another study has also found promising results combining language training and gradual attention training, in which attention training was introduced slowly throughout language treatment (Zhang et al., 2019).

Finally, there are also a growing number of tablet-based apps designed specifically for use by persons with aphasia (for reviews, see Cassarino et al., 2022; Des Roches & Kiran, 2017; Kurland, 2014; Nikolaev et al., 2022; Swales et al., 2016). Some of these apps target attention and other cognitive skills in addition to language. One example is Constant Therapy (The Learning Corp, Newton, MA), a tablet-based program created to remediate a variety of cognitive-linguistic skills in patients with aphasia. The creators of Constant Therapy have provided evidence suggesting that consistent use of the app (involving individualized programs targeting a variety of cognitive-linguistic skills) may facilitate improved performance on standardized tests of various language and cognitive abilities, including improvements in attention (Des Roches et al., 2015; Godlove et al., 2019).

Finally, it is worth briefly mentioning that in recent years, several studies have investigated mindfulness meditation as a possible tool for remediation of attention and/or language in individuals with aphasia (e.g., Bislick et al., 2022; Laures-Gore & Marshall, 2016; Marshall et al., 2018; Orenstein et al., 2012; Wang et al., 2022), as well as TBI (McMillan et al., 2002). Though small positive effects have been reported in some cases, there is currently insufficient evidence that mindfulness meditation is effective in remediating attention skills in neurologically impaired populations.

Case Study

The following case study is intended to provide an example of how the principles of assessment and treatment of attention discussed in this chapter might be applied in a specific clinical case. This case study is based on a composite of several patients encountered by the author in clinical settings.

A 69-year-old patient, KW, has just been admitted to the rehabilitation unit of a skilled nursing facility following a head injury sustained during a fall at home. KW spent 2 weeks in acute care following the injury, prior to being transferred to this facility for continued recovery and possible discharge to home, depending on progress. KW also has a history of right hemisphere stroke (2 years prior to this admission). Fol-

lowing her stroke 2 years ago, she was diagnosed with a mild cognitive communication disorder; however, due to steady progress, she was subsequently determined to be safe to return to an independent living situation with regular help from nearby family.

Notes from the acute facility from the current admission suggest that KW demonstrates reduced insight, reduced short-term memory, reduced attention, and perseveration on specific topics. KW lives alone in a first-floor apartment; her niece visits her once a day after work to bring over groceries and to do a little cooking and cleaning. The patient also cooks light meals for herself, manages her medications with supervision from her niece, and spends much of the day watching TV or chatting on the phone with friends or relatives. She does not drive. The patient's niece is concerned that the patient may fall again.

An initial brief cognitive screening in this facility indicates that the patient can name the month (but not the date) and can state that she is here because of a fall. However, she is unconvinced that use of her walker is necessary (though she has been instructed consistently by nursing staff to use it), and she has difficulty maintaining a conversational topic, often jumping from topic to topic and continually perseverating on several specific topics, such as stories about her next-door neighbor in the apartment complex where she lives at home.

As the facility's speech-language pathologist, you are tasked with evaluating KW's cognitive communication skills and, if appropriate, designing a treatment plan. Your facility recommends administration of the MoCA as an initial evaluation procedure for all patients with a suspected or diagnosed cognitive communication disorder. With this information in mind, some clinical questions going forward may include:

1. Is additional attention-related testing appropriate for KW?
2. How does attention relate to the goals of KW and her family?
3. Should attention be incorporated into treatment for KW, and if so, how?

One of the primary issues at stake is whether or not KW can safely return to her previous living environment. Questions involved in this issue include whether she can continue to manage her medications and cook, whether she can complete ADLs independently, and how likely she is to sustain another fall.

Attention Testing

Since your facility recommends use of the MoCA, you begin with this test. KW has notable difficulty with the items under the Attention subheading. She also requires occasional redirection to the task throughout the 15-minute assessment. Her clock drawing is missing both hands, as well as the numbers "4" and "11." Based on this testing, as well as other observations of the patient such as her difficulty in maintaining a conversational topic, you decide to complete additional attention testing.

Since KW is new to you and to the facility, you conclude that an attention rating scale is not appropriate at this time, as you would need to have in-depth knowledge of her daily functioning in order to complete one. Because you have limited evaluation time and also want to assess some other domains of cognitive functioning, you decide to

administer the Map Search, Telephone Search, Elevator Counting, and Elevator Counting With Distraction subtests of the TEA in order to assess KW's sustained and selective attention abilities. Impairments are noted on all subtests. You also speak with the occupational therapist and physical therapist to find out more about KW's functioning during ADLs and learn that she needs frequent cueing to stay on task and to sequence steps of ADLs.

Goals and Treatment

Because KW appears to exhibit a variety of cognitive deficits, including not only impaired attention but also reduced insight, impaired orientation, and impaired short-term memory, you as the clinician will likely need to make decisions about how to target multiple skills in treatment. With this in mind, however, initial short-term objectives for this patient specifically targeting attention could include one or more of the following:

- The patient will successfully use a written external aid for medication management, given a once-per-day check-in, in 80% of measured opportunities.
- The patient will sustain a single conversational topic for 3 minutes in a structured conversational setting, given a visual cue and no more than two verbal reminders to stay on topic, in 80% of measured opportunities.
- The patient will complete three steps of an activity of daily living, given a written external aid and training in a verbal mediation

strategy, in 80% of measured opportunities.

- The patient will state two personally relevant strategies learned via metacognitive training, such as verbal mediation of the steps involved in an ADL and use of a written external aid, in 80% of measured opportunities.

Treatment will be guided by the final objectives chosen and will combine specific skills training with training in metacognitive strategies and use of compensatory external aids, which may include posted reminders and lists with check-off boxes. The treatment program will also include strategies and practice in topic maintenance during structured conversation. Additionally, cotreatment sessions with occupational therapy are planned in order to determine implementation of strategies and aids during ADLs. Finally, KW's niece will be educated on how to assist with these strategies. Treatment will include ongoing monitoring of progress toward objectives, and treatment data and observations will be presented at interdisciplinary meetings to help track KW's progress and determine a safe and appropriate discharge setting.

dual-task situations. Attention comprises a number of different subtypes, including sustained attention, selective attention, and divided attention; the specifics of these subtypes are under debate and can differ from model to model. Attention processing overlaps substantially with other skills such as executive function, working memory, and communication. Patients with acquired and degenerative neurological conditions—including brain injury, aphasia, and dementia—often exhibit attention deficits along with deficits in other, related skill areas. Key responsibilities of clinicians treating patients with suspected attention impairments include identifying whether an attention impairment is indeed present, determining if attention treatment is warranted, and designing appropriate treatment programs. Tools for assessing attention should be carefully and specifically selected, and results of assessments should be considered within the context of the patient's overall profile, as well as within relevant theoretical frameworks. Treatment for attention should be based on patient characteristics, abilities, and goals.

References

Abdelrahman, Y., Khan, A. A., Newn, J., Velloso, E., Safwat, S. A., Bailey, J., . . . Schmidt, A. (2019). Classifying attention types with thermal imaging and eye tracking. *Proceedings of the ACM on Interactive, Mobile, Wearable and Ubiquitous Technologies*, 3(3), 1–27.

Akanuma, K., Meguro, K., Kato, Y., Takahashi, Y., Nakamura, K., & Yamaguchi, S. (2016). Impaired attention function based on the Montreal Cognitive Assessment

Summary

Attention is both a fundamental cognitive skill essential for many simple tasks and a complex neuropsychological construct. Key dimensions of the human attention system include capacity limitations, selection of relevant stimuli to attend to, and allocation of attentional resources during in vascular dementia patients with frontal hypoperfusion: The Osaki-Tajiri project. *Journal of Clinical Neuroscience, 28,* 128–132.

Alderson, A. L., & Novack, T. A. (2003). Reliable serial measurement of cognitive processes in rehabilitation: The Cognitive Log. *Archives of Physical Medicine and Rehabilitation, 84*(5), 668–672.

Arbogast, T. L., Mason, C. R., & Kidd, G., Jr. (2002). The effect of spatial separation on informational and energetic masking of speech. *The Journal of the Acoustical Society of America, 112*(5), 2086–2098.

Baddeley, A. D., Baddeley, H. A., Bucks, R. S., & Wilcock, G. K. (2001). Attentional control in Alzheimer's disease. *Brain, 124,* 1492–1508.

Barker-Collo, S. L., Feigin, V. L., Lawes, C. M., Parag, V., Senior, H., & Rodgers, A. (2009). Reducing attention deficits after stroke using attention process training: A randomized controlled trial. *Stroke, 40*(10), 3293–3298.

Bate, A. J., Mathias, J. L., & Crawford, J. R. (2001a). Performance on the Test of Everyday Attention and standard tests of attention following severe traumatic brain injury. *Clinical Neuropsychologist, 15,* 405–422.

Bate, A. J., Mathias, J. L., & Crawford, J. R. (2001b). The covert orienting of visual attention following severe traumatic brain injury. *Journal of Clinical and Experimental Neuropsychology, 23,* 386–398.

Ben-David, B. M., Nguyen, L. L., & van Lieshout, P. H. (2011). Stroop effects in persons with traumatic brain injury: Selective attention, speed of processing, or color-naming? A meta-analysis. *Journal of the International Neuropsychological Society, 17*(2), 354–363.

Beume, L.-A., Martin, M., Kaller, C. P., Klöppel, S., Schmidt, C. S. M., Urbach, H., . . . Umarova, R. M. (2017). Visual neglect after left-hemispheric lesions: A voxel-based lesion–symptom mapping study in 121 acute stroke patients. *Experimental Brain Research, 235*(1), 83–95.

Bislick, L., Dietz, A., Duncan, E. S., Garza, P., Gleason, R., Harley, D., . . . Van Allan, S. (2022). Finding "Zen" in Aphasia: The benefits of yoga as described by key stakeholders. *American Journal of Speech-Language Pathology, 31*(1), 133–147.

Black, F. W. (1986). Digit repetition in brain-damaged adults: Clinical and theoretical implications. *Journal of Clinical Psychology, 42,* 770–782.

Bleiberg, J., Garmoe, W. S., Halpern, E. L., Reeves, D. L., & Nadler, J. D. (1997). Consistency of within-day and across-day performance after mild brain injury. *Neuropsychiatry, Neuropsychology, & Behavioral Neurology, 10*(4), 247–253.

Bloomfield, I. L., Espie, C. A., & Evans, J. J. (2010). Do sleep difficulties exacerbate deficits in sustained attention following traumatic brain injury? *Journal of the International Neuropsychological Society, 16*(1), 17–25.

Bogdanova, Y., Yee, M. K., Ho, V. T., & Cicerone, K. D. (2016). Computerized cognitive rehabilitation of attention and executive function in acquired brain injury: A systematic review. *The Journal of Head Trauma Rehabilitation, 31*(6), 419–433.

Bonnelle, V., Leech, R., Kinnunen, K. M., Ham, T. E., Beckmann, C. F., De Boissezon, X., . . . Sharp, D. J. (2011). Default mode network connectivity predicts sustained attention deficits after traumatic brain injury. *Journal of Neuroscience, 31*(38), 13442–13451.

Broadbent, D. E. (1952). Failures of attention in selective listening. *Journal of Experimental Psychology, 44*(6), 428.

Broadbent, D. E. (1958). *Perception and Communication.* Pergamon Press.

Bronkhorst, A. W. (2015). The cocktail-party problem revisited: Early processing and selection of multi-talker speech. *Attention, Perception, & Psychophysics, 77*(5), 1465–1487.

Brouwer, W. H., Ponds, R. W., Van Wolffelaar, P. C., & Van Zomeren, A. H. (1989). Divided attention 5 to 10 years after severe closed head injury. *Cortex, 25*(2), 219–230.

Brouwer, S., Van Engen, K. J., Calandruccio, L., & Bradlow, A. R. (2012). Linguistic contributions to speech-on-speech masking for native and non-native listeners: Language familiarity and semantic content. *The Journal of the Acoustical Society of America*, *131*(2), 1449–1464.

Brouwer, W. H., Withaar, F. K., Tant, M. L., & van Zomeren, A. H. (2002). Attention and driving in traumatic brain injury: A question of coping with time-pressure. *The Journal of Head Trauma Rehabilitation*, *17*(1), 1–15.

Brungart, D. S., Chang, P. S., Simpson, B. D., & Wang, D. (2006). Isolating the energetic component of speech-on-speech masking with ideal time-frequency segregation. *The Journal of the Acoustical Society of America*, *120*(6), 4007–4018.

Bruya, B., & Tang, Y. Y. (2018). Is attention really effort? Revisiting Daniel Kahneman's influential 1973 book Attention and Effort. *Frontiers in Psychology*, *9*, 1133.

Calderon, J., Perry, R. J., Erzinclioglu, S. W., Berrios, G. E., Dening, T. R., & Hodges, J. R. (2001). Perception, attention, and working memory are disproportionately impaired in dementia with Lewy bodies compared with Alzheimer's disease. *Journal of Neurology, Neurosurgery, and Psychiatry*, *70*, 157–164.

Cameron, R. M., Wambaugh, J. L., & Mauszycki, S. C. (2010). Individual variability on discourse measures over repeated sampling times in persons with aphasia. *Aphasiology*, *24*(6–8), 671–684.

Caplan, D., Waters, G., DeDe, G., Michaud, J., & Reddy, A. (2007). A study of syntactic processing in aphasia I: Behavioral (psycholinguistic) aspects. *Brain and Language*, *101*(2), 103–150.

Cassarino, L., Santoro, F., Gelardi, D., Panerai, S., Papotto, M., Tripodi, M., . . . Lanza, G. (2022). Post-stroke aphasia at the time of COVID-19 pandemic: A telerehabilitation perspective. *Journal of Integrative Neuroscience*, *21*(1), 8.

Castriotta, R. J., Wilde, M. C., Lai, J. M., Atanasov, S., Masel, B. E., & Kuna, S. T. (2007).

Prevalence and consequences of sleep disorders in traumatic brain injury. *Journal of Clinical Sleep Medicine*, *3*(4), 349–356.

Chan, R. C. (2000). Attentional deficits in patients with closed head injury: A further study to the discriminative validity of the test of everyday attention. *Brain Injury*, *14*, 227–236.

Chan, R. C. K. (2002). Attention deficits in patients with persisting postconcussive complaints: A general deficit or specific component deficit? *Journal of Clinical and Experimental Neuropsychology*, *24*, 1081–1093.

Chan, R. C., & Lai, M. K. (2006). Latent structure of the Test of Everyday Attention: Convergent evidence from patients with traumatic brain injury. *Brain Injury*, *20*, 653–659.

Chan, R. C., Lai, M. K., & Robertson, I. H. (2006). Latent structure of the Test of Everyday Attention in a non-clinical Chinese sample. *Archives of Clinical Neuropsychology*, *21*, 477–485.

Chau, S. A., Herrmann, N., Sherman, C., Chung, J., Eizenman, M., Kiss, A., & Lanctot, K. L. (2017). Visual selective attention toward novel stimuli predicts cognitive decline in Alzheimer's disease patients. *Journal of Alzheimer's Disease*, *55*(4), 1339–1349.

Cherry, E. C. (1953). Some experiments on the recognition of speech, with one and two ears. *Journal of the Acoustical Society of America*, *25*, 975–979.

Choi, J., & Twamley, E. W. (2013). Cognitive rehabilitation therapies for Alzheimer's disease: A review of methods to improve treatment engagement and self-efficacy. *Neuropsychology Review*, *23*(1), 48–62.

Cicerone, K. D., Langenbahn, D. M., Braden, C., Malec, J. F., Kalmar, K., Fraas, M., . . . Azulay, J. (2011). Evidence-based cognitive rehabilitation: Updated review of the literature from 2003 through 2008. *Archives of Physical Medicine and Rehabilitation*, *92*(4), 519–530.

Coelho, C. (2005). Direct attention training as a treatment for reading impairment in mild aphasia. *Aphasiology, 19*(3–5), 275–283.

Conners, C. K. (2000). *Conners' Continuous Performance Test II.* Multi-Health Systems.

Connor, B. B., & Shaw, C. (2016). Case study series using brain-training games to treat attention and memory following brain injury. *Journal of Pain Management, 9*(3), 217–226.

Corbetta, M., & Shulman, G. L. (2002). Control of goal-directed and stimulus-driven attention in the brain. *Nature Reviews Neuroscience, 3,* 201–215.

Cowan, N. (1997). *Attention and memory.* Oxford University Press.

Cremona-Meteyard, S. L., Clark, C. R., Wright, M. J., & Geffen, G. M. (1992). Covert orientation of visual attention after closed head injury. *Neuropsychologia, 30*(2), 123–132.

Cyr, A. A., Stinchcombe, A., Gagnon, S., Marshall, S., Hing, M. M., & Finestone, H. (2009). Driving difficulties of brain-injured drivers in reaction to high-crash-risk simulated road events: A question of impaired divided attention? *Journal of Clinical and Experimental Neuropsychology, 31*(4), 472–482.

Des Roches, C. A., Balachandran, I., Ascenso, E. M., Tripodis, Y., & Kiran, S. (2015). Effectiveness of an impairment-based individualized rehabilitation program using an iPad-based software platform. *Frontiers in Human Neuroscience, 8,* 1015.

Des Roches, C. A., & Kiran, S. (2017). Technology-based rehabilitation to improve communication after acquired brain injury. *Frontiers in Neuroscience, 11,* 382.

Desimone, R., & Duncan, J. (1995). Neural mechanisms of selective visual attention. *Annual Review of Neuroscience, 18*(1), 193–222.

Deutsch, J. A., & Deutsch, D. (1963). Attention: Some theoretical considerations. *Psychological Review, 70*(1), 80–90.

Diedrichs, V. A., Jewell, C. C., & Harnish, S. M. (2022). A scoping review of the relationship between nonlinguistic cognitive factors and aphasia treatment response. *Topics in Language Disorders, 42*(3), 212–235.

Dockree, P. M., Bellgrove, M. A., O'Keeffe, F. M., Moloney, P., Aimola, L., Carton, S., & Robertson, I. H. (2006). Sustained attention in traumatic brain injury (TBI) and healthy controls: Enhanced sensitivity with dual-task load. *Experimental Brain Research, 168*(1–2), 218–229.

Driver, J. (2001). A selective review of selective attention research from the past century. *British Journal of Psychology, 92*(1), 53–78.

Driver, J., & Baylis, G. C. (1989). Movement and visual attention: The spotlight metaphor breaks down. *Journal of Experimental Psychology: Human Perception and Performance, 15*(3), 448.

Dykiert, D., Der, G., Starr, J. M., & Deary, I. J. (2012). Age differences in intra-individual variability in simple and choice reaction time: Systematic review and meta-analysis. *PLoS One, 7*(10), e45759.

Dymowski, A. R., Owens, J. A., Ponsford, J. L., & Willmott, C. (2015). Speed of processing and strategic control of attention after traumatic brain injury. *Journal of Clinical and Experimental Neuropsychology, 37*(10), 1024–1035.

Egan, J. P., & Wiener, F. M. (1946). On the intelligibility of bands of speech in noise. *The Journal of the Acoustical Society of America, 18*(2), 435–441.

Erickson, R. J., Goldinger, S. D., & LaPointe, L. L. (1996). Auditory vigilance in aphasic individuals: Detecting nonlinguistic stimuli with full or divided attention. *Brain and Cognition, 30*(2), 244–253.

Finn, M., & McDonald, S. (2011). Computerised cognitive training for older persons with mild cognitive impairment: A pilot study using a randomised controlled trial design. *Brain Impairment, 12*(3), 187–199.

Fish, J., Evans, J. J., Nimmo, M., Martin, E., Kersel, D., Bateman, A., . . . Manly, T. (2007). Rehabilitation of executive dysfunction following brain injury: "Content-free" cueing improves everyday prospective memory performance. *Neuropsychologia, 45*, 1318–1330.

Foldi, N. S., Lobosco, J. J., & Schaefer, L. A. (2002). The effect of attentional dysfunction in Alzheimer's disease: Theoretical and practical implications. *Seminars in Speech and Language, 23*, 139–150.

Folstein, M. F., Folstein, S. E., & McHugh, P. R. (1975). "Mini-Mental State": A practical method for grading the cognitive state of patients for the clinician. *Journal of Psychiatric Research, 12*(3), 189–198.

Forn, C., Belloch, V., Bustamante, J. C., Garbin, G., Parcet-Ibars, M. À., Sanjuan, A., . . . Ávila, C. (2009). A symbol digit modalities test version suitable for functional MRI studies. *Neuroscience Letters, 456*(1), 11–14.

Freed, D. B., Marshall, R. C., & Chuhlantseff, E. A. (1996). Picture naming variability: A methodological consideration of inconsistent naming responses in fluent and nonfluent aphasia. *Clinical Aphasiology, 24*, 193–205.

Freyman, R. L., Balakrishnan, U., & Helfer, K. S. (2001). Spatial release from informational masking in speech recognition. *The Journal of the Acoustical Society of America, 109*(5), 2112–2122.

Fritz, J. B., Elhilali, M., David, S. V., & Shamma, S. A. (2007). Auditory attention—focusing the searchlight on sound. *Current Opinion in Neurobiology, 17*(4), 437–455.

Gershon, R. C., Wagster, M. V., Hendrie, H. C., Fox, N. A., Cook, K. F., & Nowinski, C. J. (2013). NIH toolbox for assessment of neurological and behavioral function. *Neurology, 80*(11, Suppl. 3), S2–S6.

Gillespie, A., Best, C., & O'Neill, B. (2012). Cognitive function and assistive technology for cognition: A systematic review. *Journal of the International Neuropsychological Society, 18*(1), 1–19.

Gilmore, N., Meier, E. L., Johnson, J. P., & Kiran, S. (2019). Nonlinguistic cognitive factors predict treatment-induced recovery in chronic poststroke aphasia. *Archives of Physical Medicine and Rehabilitation, 100*(7), 1251–1258.

Godlove, J., Anantha, V., Advani, M., Des Roches, C., & Kiran, S. (2019). Comparison of therapy practice at home and in the clinic: A retrospective analysis of the constant therapy platform data set. *Frontiers in Neurology, 10*, 140.

Gopher, D., Brickner, M., & Navon, D. (1982). Different difficulty manipulations interact differently with task emphasis: Evidence for multiple resources. *Journal of Experimental Psychology: Human Perception and Performance, 8*, 146–157.

Gordon, B. A., Zacks, J. M., Blazey, T., Benzinger, T. L., Morris, J. C., Fagan, A. M., . . . Balota, D. A. (2015). Task-evoked fMRI changes in attention networks are associated with preclinical Alzheimer's disease biomarkers. *Neurobiology of Aging, 36*(5), 1771–1779.

Grant, D. A., & Berg, E. A. (1981). *Wisconsin Card Sorting Test*. Psychological Assessment Resources Inc.

Gronwall, D., & Sampson, H. (1974). *The psychological effects of concussion*. Auckland University Press.

Harciarek, M., & Jodzio, K. (2005). Neuropsychological differences between frontotemporal dementia and Alzheimer's disease: A review. *Neuropsychology Review, 15*(3), 131–145.

Hart, T., Whyte, J., Ellis, C., & Chervoneva, I. (2009). Construct validity of an attention rating scale for traumatic brain injury. *Neuropsychology, 23*, 729–735.

Hart, T., Whyte, J., Millis, S., Bode, R., Malec, J., Richardson, R. N., & Hammond, F. (2006). Dimensions of disordered attention in traumatic brain injury: Further validation of the Moss Attention Rating Scale. *Archives of Physical Medicine and Rehabilitation, 87*, 647–655.

Haskins, E. C. (2012). *Cognitive rehabilitation manual: Translating evidence-based recommendations into practice*. ACRM Publishing.

Helm-Estabrooks, N. (2001). *Cognitive Linguistic Quick Test*. The Psychological Corporation.

Helm-Estabrooks, N. (2011). Treating attention to improve auditory comprehension deficits associated with aphasia. *Perspectives on Neurophysiology and Neurogenic Speech and Language Disorders, 21*(2), 64–71.

Helm-Estabrooks, N., Connor, L. T., & Albert, M. L. (2000). Treating attention to improve auditory comprehension in aphasia. *Brain and Language, 74*(3), 469–472.

Hervais-Adelman, A. G., Carlyon, R. P., Johnsrude, I. S., & Davis, M. H. (2012). Brain regions recruited for the effortful comprehension of noise-vocoded words. *Language and Cognitive Processes, 27*(7–8), 1145–1166.

Heuer, S., & Hallowell, B. (2015). A novel eye-tracking method to assess attention allocation in individuals with and without aphasia using a dual-task paradigm. *Journal of Communication Disorders, 55*, 15–30.

Heuer, S., Ivanova, M. V., & Hallowell, B. (2017). More than the verbal stimulus matters: Visual attention in language assessment for people with aphasia using multiple-choice image displays. *Journal of Speech, Language, and Hearing Research, 60*(5), 1348–1361.

Howard, D., Patterson, K., Franklin, S., Orchard-Lisle, V., & Morton, J. (1985). Treatment of word retrieval deficits in aphasia. *Brain, 108*(8), 17–29.

Hula, W., & Biel, M. (2014). Attention. In M. L. Kimbarow (Ed.), *Cognitive-communication disorders* (2nd ed., pp. 1–48). Plural Publishing.

Hula, W. D., & McNeil, M. R. (2008). Models of attention and dual-task performance as explanatory constructs in aphasia. *Seminars in Speech and Language, 29*(3), 169–187.

Hultsch, D. F., MacDonald, S. W., Hunter, M. A., Levy-Bencheton, J., & Strauss, E.

(2000). Intraindividual variability in cognitive performance in older adults: Comparison of adults with mild dementia, adults with arthritis, and healthy adults. *Neuropsychology, 14*(4), 588.

Hunting-Pompon, R., Kendall, D., & Bacon Moore, A. (2011). Examining attention and cognitive processing in participants with self-reported mild anomia. *Aphasiology, 25*(6–7), 800–812.

Itti, L., & Koch, C. (2001). Computational modeling of visual attention. *Nature Reviews Neuroscience, 2*(3), 194–203.

James, W. (1950). *The principles of psychology*. Dover. (Original work published 1890)

Kahneman, D. (1973). *Attention and effort*. Prentice-Hall.

Kahneman, D., & Beatty, J. (1966). Pupil diameter and load on memory. *Science, 154*(3756), 1583–1585.

Kahneman, D., & Tresiman, A. (1984). Changing views of attention and automaticity. In R. Parasuraman & D. A. Davies (Eds.), *Varieties of attention* (pp. 29–61). Academic Press.

Kidd, G., & Colburn, H. S. (2017). Informational masking in speech recognition. In J. C. Middlebrooks, J. Z. Simon, A. N. Popper, & R. R. Fay (Eds.), *The auditory system at the cocktail party* (pp. 75–109). Springer.

Kim, J., Whyte, J., Hart, T., Vaccaro, M., Polansky, M., & Coslett, H. B. (2005). Executive function as a predictor of inattentive behavior after traumatic brain injury. *Journal of the International Neuropsychological Society, 11*, 434–445.

Kreindler, A., & Fradis, A. (1968). *Performances in aphasia: A neurodynamical diagnostic and psychological study*. Gauthier-Villars.

Künstler, E. C., Penning, M. D., Napiórkowski, N., Klingner, C. M., Witte, O. W., Müller, H. J., . . . Finke, K. (2018). Dual task effects on visual attention capacity in normal aging. *Frontiers in Psychology, 9*, 1564.

Kurland, J. (2011). The role that attention plays in language processing. *Perspectives* on *Neurophysiology and Neurogenic Speech and Language Disorders, 21*(2), 47–54.

Kurland, J. (2014). iRehab in aphasia treatment. *Seminars in Speech and Language, 35*(1), 003–004.

Laeng, B., Sirois, S., & Gredebäck, G. (2012). Pupillometry: A window to the preconscious? *Perspectives on Psychological Science, 7*(1), 18–27.

Lambon Ralph, M. A., Snell, C., Fillingham, J. K., Conroy, P., & Sage, K. (2010). Predicting the outcome of anomia therapy for people with aphasia post CVA: Both language and cognitive status are key predictors. *Neuropsychological Rehabilitation, 20*(2), 289–305.

Larrabee, G. J., & Kane, R. L. (1986). Reversed digit repetition involves visual and verbal processes. *International Journal of Neuroscience, 30,* 11–15.

Laures, J., Odell, K., & Coe, C. (2003). Arousal and auditory vigilance in individuals with aphasia during a linguistic and nonlinguistic task. *Aphasiology, 17*(12), 1133–1152.

Laures-Gore, J., & Marshall, R. S. (2016). Mindfulness meditation in aphasia: A case report. *NeuroRehabilitation, 38*(4), 321–329.

Lee, J. B., & Sohlberg, M. M. (2013). Evaluation of attention training and metacognitive facilitation to improve reading comprehension in aphasia. *American Journal of Speech-Language Pathology, 22*(2), S318–S333.

Lee, J. B., Sohlberg, M. M., Harn, B., Horner, R., & Cherney, L. R. (2018). Attention Process Training-3 to improve reading comprehension in mild aphasia: A single-case experimental design study. *Neuropsychological Rehabilitation, 30*(3), 430–461.

Levine, B., Schweizer, T. A., O'Connor, C., Turner, G., Gillingham, S., Stuss, D. T., . . . Robertson, I. H. (2011). Rehabilitation of executive functioning in patients with frontal lobe brain damage with goal management training. *Frontiers in Human Neuroscience, 5,* 9.

Lezak, M. D., Howieson, D. B., Bigler, E. D., & Tranel, D. (2012). *Neuropsychological Assessment* (5th ed.). Oxford University Press.

Lim, Y. Y., Snyder, P. J., Pietrzak, R. H., Ukiqi, A., Villemagne, V. L., Ames, D., . . . Rowe, C. C. (2016). Sensitivity of composite scores to amyloid burden in preclinical Alzheimer's disease: Introducing the Z-scores of Attention, Verbal fluency, and Episodic memory for Nondemented older adults composite score. *Alzheimer's & Dementia: Diagnosis, Assessment & Disease Monitoring, 2,* 19–26.

Lopresti, F, E., Mihailidis, A., & Kirsch, N. (2004). Assistive technology for cognitive rehabilitation: State of the art. *Neuropsychological Rehabilitation, 14*(1–2), 5–39.

Lundqvist, A., Grundström, K., Samuelsson, K., & Rönnberg, J. (2010). Computerized training of working memory in a group of patients suffering from acquired brain injury. *Brain Injury, 24*(10), 1173–1183.

MacDonald, S. W., Li, S. C., & Bäckman, L. (2009). Neural underpinnings of within-person variability in cognitive functioning. *Psychology and Aging, 24*(4), 792.

Manly, T., Davison, B., Heutink, J., Galloway, M., & Robertson, I. H. (2000). Not enough time or not enough attention? Speed, error and self-maintained control in the Sustained Attention to Response Test (SART). *Clinical Neuropsychological Assessment, 3*(10), 1–12.

Manly, T., Owen, A. M., McAvinue, L., Datta, A., Lewis, G. H., Scott, S. K., . . . Robertson, I. H. (2003). Enhancing the sensitivity of a sustained attention task to frontal damage: Convergent clinical and functional imaging evidence. *Neurocase, 9,* 340–349.

Manly, T., Robertson, I. H., Galloway, M., & Hawkins, K. (1999). The absent mind: Further investigations of sustained attention to response. *Neuropsychologia, 37*(6), 661–670.

Mansbach, W. E., MacDougall, E. E., & Rosenzweig, A. S. (2012). The Brief Cognitive

Assessment Tool (BCAT): A new test emphasizing contextual memory, executive functions, attentional capacity, and the prediction of instrumental activities of daily living. *Journal of Clinical and Experimental Neuropsychology, 34*(2), 183–194.

Marshall, R. S., Laures-Gore, J., & Love, K. (2018). Brief mindfulness meditation group training in aphasia: Exploring attention, language and psychophysiological outcomes. *International Journal of Language & Communication Disorders, 53*(1), 40–54.

Mathias, J. L., & Wheaton, P. (2007). Changes in attention and information-processing speed following severe traumatic brain injury: A meta-analytic review. *Neuropsychology, 21*, 212–223.

McDowd, J. M., & Craik, F. I. (1988). Effects of aging and task difficulty on divided attention performance. *Journal of Experimental Psychology: Human Perception and Performance, 14*(2), 267.

McGuinness, B., Barrett, S. L., Craig, D., Lawson, J., & Passmore, A. P. (2010). Attention deficits in Alzheimer's disease and vascular dementia. *Journal of Neurology, Neurosurgery & Psychiatry, 81*, 157–159.

McKeith, I. G., Boeve, B. F., Dickson, D. W., Halliday, G., Taylor, J. P., Weintraub, D., . . . Bayston, A. (2017). Diagnosis and management of dementia with Lewy bodies: Fourth consensus report of the DLB Consortium. *Neurology, 89*(1), 88–100.

McMillan, T., Robertson, I. H., Brock, D., & Chorlton, L. (2002). Brief mindfulness training for attentional problems after traumatic brain injury: A randomised control treatment trial. *Neuropsychological Rehabilitation, 12*(2), 117–125.

McNeil, M. R. (1982). The nature of aphasia in adults. In N. J. Lass, L. V. McReynolds, J. L. Northern, & D. E. Yoder (Eds.), *Speech, language, and hearing: Vol. II. Pathologies of speech and language* (pp. 692–740). Saunders.

McNeil, M. R. (1983). Aphasia: Neurological considerations. *Topics in Language Disorders, 3*, 1–19.

McNeil, M., Hula, W., & Sung, J. E. (2011). The role of memory and attention in aphasic language performance. In J. Guendouzi, F. Loncke, & M. J. Williams (Eds.), *The handbook of psycholinguistic and cognitive processes: Perspectives in communication disorders* (pp. 551–578). Psychology Press.

McNeil, M. R., Odell, K., & Tseng, C. H. (1991). Toward the integration of resource allocation into a general theory of aphasia. *Clinical Aphasiology, 20*, 21–40.

Meier, E. L., Kelly, C. R., & Hillis, A. E. (2022). Dissociable language and executive control deficits and recovery in post-stroke aphasia: An exploratory observational and case series study. *Neuropsychologia, 172*, 108270.

Metzler-Baddeley, C. (2007). A review of cognitive impairments in dementia with Lewy bodies relative to Alzheimer's disease and Parkinson's disease with dementia. *Cortex, 43*, 583–600.

Michel, J. A., & Mateer, C. A. (2006). Attention rehabilitation following stroke and traumatic brain injury: A review. *Europa Medicophysica, 42*, 59–67.

Mirsky, A. F., Anthony, B. J., Duncan, C. C., Ahearn, M. B., & Kellam, S. G. (1991). Analysis of the elements of attention: A neuropsychological approach. *Neuropsychology Review, 2*(2), 109–145.

Moray, N. (1959). Attention in dichotic listening: Affective cues and the influence of instructions. *Quarterly Journal of Experimental Psychology, 11*, 56–60.

Murray, L. L. (1999). Review attention and aphasia: Theory, research and clinical implications. *Aphasiology, 13*(2), 91–111.

Murray, L. L. (2012). Attention and other cognitive deficits in aphasia: Presence and relation to language and communication measures. *American Journal of Speech-Language Pathology, 21*, S51–S64.

Murray, L. L. (2018). Sentence processing in aphasia: An examination of material-specific and general cognitive factors. *Journal of Neurolinguistics, 48*, 26–46.

Murray, L. L., Holland, A. L., & Beeson, P. M. (1997). Auditory processing in individuals with mild aphasia: A study of resource allocation. *Journal of Speech, Language, and Hearing Research, 40,* 792–808.

Murray, L. L., Keeton, R. J., & Karcher, L. (2006). Treating attention in mild aphasia: Evaluation of Attention Process Training-II. *Journal of Communication Disorders, 39*(1), 37–61.

Murtha, S., Cismaru, R., Waechter, R., & Chertkow, H. (2002). Increased variability accompanies frontal lobe damage in dementia. *Journal of the International Neuropsychological Society, 8*(3), 360–372.

Nasreddine, Z. S., Phillips, N. A., Bédirian, V., Charbonneau, S., Whitehead, V., Collin, I., . . . Chertkow, H. (2005). The Montreal Cognitive Assessment, MoCA: A brief screening tool for mild cognitive impairment. *Journal of the American Geriatrics Society, 53*(4), 695–699.

Naveh-Benjamin, M., Craik, F. I., Guez, J., & Kreuger, S. (2005). Divided attention in younger and older adults: Effects of strategy and relatedness on memory performance and secondary task costs. *Journal of Experimental Psychology: Learning, Memory, and Cognition, 31*(3), 520.

Navon, D., & Gopher, D. (1979). On the economy of the human-processing system. *Psychological Review, 86,* 214–255.

Nikolaev, V. A., Safonicheva, O. G., & Nikolaev, A. A. (2022). A review of international experience for telerehabilitation of post-stroke patients with aphasia and cognitive problems. *Bulletin of Rehabilitation Medicine, 21*(1), 64–69.

Niogi, S. N., Mukherjee, P., Ghajar, J., Johnson, C. E., Kolster, R., Lee, H., . . . McCandliss, B. D. (2008). Structural dissociation of attentional control and memory in adults with and without mild traumatic brain injury. *Brain, 131*(12), 3209–3221.

Oberauer, K. (2019). Working memory and attention—A conceptual analysis and review. *Journal of Cognition, 2*(1), 36.

Orenstein, E., Basilakos, A., & Marshall, R. S. (2012). Effects of mindfulness meditation on three individuals with aphasia.

International Journal of Language & Communication Disorders, 47(6), 673–684.

Ortoleva, C., Brugger, C., Van der Linden, M., & Walder, B. (2012). Prediction of driving capacity after traumatic brain injury: A systematic review. *The Journal of Head Trauma Rehabilitation, 27*(4), 302–313.

Park, N. W., & Ingles, J. L. (2001). Effectiveness of attention rehabilitation after an acquired brain injury: A meta-analysis. *Neuropsychology, 15,* 199–210.

Park, N. W., Moscovitch, M., & Robertson, I. H. (1999). Divided attention impairments after traumatic brain injury. *Neuropsychologia, 37,* 1119–1133.

Pashler, H. (1994). Dual-task interference in simple tasks: Data and theory. *Psychological Bulletin, 116,* 220–244.

Peach, R. K., Beck, K. M., Gorman, M., & Fisher, C. (2019). Clinical outcomes following language-specific attention treatment versus direct attention training for aphasia: A comparative effectiveness study. *Journal of Speech, Language, and Hearing Research, 62*(8), 2785–2811.

Peach, R. K., Nathan, M. R., & Beck, K. M. (2017). Language-specific attention treatment for aphasia: Description and preliminary findings. *Seminars in Speech and Language, 38*(1), 005–016.

Peach, R. K., Newhoff, M., & Rubin, S. S. (1993). Attention in aphasia as revealed by event-related potentials: A preliminary investigation. *Clinical Aphasiology, 21,* 323–333.

Peach, R. K., Schenk, K. A., Nathan, M. R., & Beck, K. M. (2018). Construct validity, external validity, and reliability for a battery of language-specific attention tasks. *Aphasiology, 32*(6), 618–645.

Perry, R. J., & Hodges, J. R. (1999). Attention and executive deficits in Alzheimer's disease: A critical review. *Brain, 122*(3), 383–404.

Perry, R. J., & Hodges, J. R. (2000). Differentiating frontal and temporal variant frontotemporal dementia from Alzheimer's disease. *Neurology, 54,* 2277–2284.

Petersen, S. E., & Posner, M. I. (2012). The attention system of the human brain: 20 years after. *Annual Review of Neuroscience, 35*, 73–89.

Petry, M. C., Crosson, B., Rothi, L. J. G., Bauer, R. M., & Schauer, C. A. (1994). Selective attention and aphasia in adults: Preliminary findings. *Neuropsychologia, 32*(11), 1397–1408.

Ponsford, J., & Kinsella, G. (1991). The use of a rating scale of attentional behavior. *Neuropsychological Rehabilitation, 1*(4), 241–257.

Ponsford, J., & Kinsella, G. (1992). Attentional deficits following closed-head injury. *Journal of Clinical and Experimental Neuropsychology, 14*(5), 822–838.

Ponsford, J. L., Downing, M. G., Olver, J., Ponsford, M., Acher, R., Carty, M., & Spitz, G. (2014). Longitudinal follow-up of patients with traumatic brain injury: Outcome at two, five, and ten years post-injury. *Journal of Neurotrauma, 31*(1), 64–77.

Posner, M. I., & Cohen, Y. (1980). Covert orienting of visuospatial attention task. In G. G. Stelmach & J. Requin (Eds.), *Tutorials in motor behaviour* (pp. 243–258). North-Holland.

Posner, M. I., Inhoff, A. W., Friedrich, F. J., & Cohen, A. (1987). Isolating attentional systems: A cognitive-anatomical analysis. *Psychobiology, 15*, 107–121.

Posner, M. I., & Petersen, S. E. (1990). The attention system of the human brain. *Annual Review of Neuroscience, 13*(1), 25–42.

Posner, M. I., Snyder, C. R., & Davidson, B. J. (1980). Attention and the detection of signals. *Journal of Experimental Psychology: General, 109*(2), 160.

Posner, M. I., Walker, J. A., Friedrich, F. J., & Rafal, R. D. (1984). Effects of parietal injury on covert orienting of attention. *Journal of Neuroscience, 4*(7), 1863–1874.

Rabipour, S., & Raz, A. (2012). Training the brain: Fact and fad in cognitive and behavioral remediation. *Brain and Cognition, 79*(2), 159–179.

Rankin, E., Newton, C., Parker, A., & Bruce, C. (2014). Hearing loss and auditory processing ability in people with aphasia. *Aphasiology, 28*(5), 576–595.

Rapport, L. J., Webster, J. S., & Dutra, R. L. (1994). Digit span performance and unilateral neglect. *Neuropsychologia, 32*, 517–525.

Ríos, M., Periáñez, J. A., & Muñoz-Céspedes, J. M. (2004). Attentional control and slowness of information processing after severe traumatic brain injury. *Brain Injury, 18*(3), 257–272.

Robertson, I. H., Manly, T., Andrade, J., Baddeley, B. T., & Yiend, J. (1997). "Oops!": Performance correlates of everyday attentional failures in traumatic brain injured and normal subjects. *Neuropsychologia, 35*, 747–758.

Robertson, I. H., Ward, T., Ridgeway, V., & Nimmo-Smith, I. (1994). *The Test of Everyday Attention (TEA)*. Thames Valley Test Company.

Robertson, I. H., Ward, T., Ridgeway, V., & Nimmo-Smith, I. (1996). The structure of normal human attention: The Test of Everyday Attention. *Journal of the International Neuropsychological Society, 2*(6), 525–534.

Robin, D. A., & Rizzo, M. (1989). The effect of focal cerebral lesions on intramodal and cross-modal orienting of attention. *Clinical Aphasiology, 18*(1), 61–74.

Rosenberg, M. D., Scheinost, D., Greene, A. S., Avery, E. W., Kwon, Y. H., Finn, E. S., . . . Chun, M. M. (2020). Functional connectivity predicts changes in attention observed across minutes, days, and months. *Proceedings of the National Academy of Sciences, 117*(7), 3797–3807.

Sarter, M., Givens, B., & Bruno, J. P. (2001). The cognitive neuroscience of sustained attention: Where top-down meets bottom-up. *Brain Research Reviews, 35*(2), 146–160.

Sbordone, R. J. (2001). Limitations of neuropsychological testing to predict the cognitive and behavioral functioning of persons with brain injury in real-world settings. *NeuroRehabilitation, 16*, 199–201.

Schepker, H., Haeder, K., Rennies, J., & Holube, I. (2016). Perceived listening effort and speech intelligibility in reverberation and noise for hearing-impaired listeners. *International Journal of Audiology, 55*(12), 738–747.

Schnabel, R., & Kydd, R. (2012). Neuropsychological assessment of distractibility in mild traumatic brain injury and depression. *The Clinical Neuropsychologist, 26,* 769–789.

Schneider, W., & Shiffrin, R. A. (1977). Controlled and automatic human information processing: I. Detection, search, and attention. *Psychological Review, 84,* 1–66.

Schretlen, D., Bobholz, J. H., & Brandt, J. (1996). Development and psychometric properties of the Brief Test of Attention. *The Clinical Neuropsychologist, 10*(1), 80–89.

Schroeder, R. W., Twumasi-Ankrah, P., Baade, L. E., & Marshall, P. S. (2012). Reliable Digit Span: A systematic review and cross-validation study. *Assessment, 19*(1), 21–30.

Schumacher, R., Halai, A. D., & Lambon Ralph, M. A. (2019). Assessing and mapping language, attention and executive multidimensional deficits in stroke aphasia. *Brain, 142*(10), 3202–3216.

Shiffrin, R. A., & Schneider, W. (1977). Controlled and automatic human information processing: II. Perceptual learning, automatic attending, and a general theory. *Psychological Review, 84,* 127–190.

Shinn-Cunningham, B. G. (2008). Object-based auditory and visual attention. *Trends in Cognitive Sciences, 12*(5), 182–186.

Shulman, G. L., & Corbetta, M. (2012). Two attentional networks. In M. I. Posner (Ed.), *Cognitive neuroscience of attention* (2nd ed., pp. 113–128). Guilford.

Sigmundsdottir, L., Longley, W. A., & Tate, R. L. (2016). Computerised cognitive training in acquired brain injury: A systematic review of outcomes using the International Classification of Functioning (ICF). *Neuropsychological Rehabilitation, 26*(5–6), 673–741.

Sinotte, M. P., & Coelho, C. A. (2007). Attention training for reading impairment in mild aphasia: A follow-up study. *NeuroRehabilitation, 22*(4), 303–310.

Smith, A. (1991). *Symbol Digit Modalities Test.* Western Psychological Services.

Sohlberg, M. M., Johnson, L., Paule, L., Raskin, S. A., & Mateer, C. A. (2001). *Attention Process Training-II: A program to address attentional deficits for persons with mild cognitive dysfunction* (2nd ed.). Lash & Associates.

Sohlberg, M. M., & Mateer, C. A. (1987). Effectiveness of an attention-training program. *Journal of Clinical and Experimental Neuropsychology, 9,* 117–130.

Sohlberg, M. M., & Mateer, C. A. (2001a). *Attention Process Training* (2nd ed.). Lash & Associates.

Sohlberg, M. M., & Mateer, C. A. (2001b). *Cognitive rehabilitation: An integrative neuropsychological approach.* Guilford.

Sohlberg, M. M., & Mateer, C. A. (2010). *APT-III: Attention Process Training: A direct attention training program for persons with acquired brain injury.* Lash & Associates Publishing/Training Incorporated.

Sohlberg, M. M., McLaughlin, K. A., Pavese, A., Heidrich, A., & Posner, M. I. (2000). Evaluation of Attention Process Training and brain injury education in persons with acquired brain injury. *Journal of Clinical and Experimental Neuropsychology, 22,* 656–676.

Spaccavento, S., Marinelli, C. V., Nardulli, R., Macchitella, L., Bivona, U., Piccardi, L., . . . Angelelli, P. (2019). Attention deficits in stroke patients: The role of lesion characteristics, time from stroke, and concomitant neuropsychological deficits. *Behavioural Neurology, 2019.*

Strauch, C., Wang, C. A., Einhäuser, W., Van der Stigchel, S., & Naber, M. (2022). Pupillometry as an integrated readout of distinct attentional networks. *Trends in Neurosciences, 45*(8), 635–647.

Sturm, W., Willmes, K., Orgass, B., & Hartje, W. (1997). Do specific attention deficits need specific training? *Neuropsychological Rehabilitation, 7,* 81–103.

Stuss, D. T., Pogue, J., Buckle, L., & Bondar, J. (1994). Characterization of stability of performance in patients with traumatic brain injury: Variability and consistency on reaction time tests. *Neuropsychology, 8*(3), 316.

Swales, M. A., Hill, A. J., & Finch, E. (2016). Feature rich, but user-friendly: Speech pathologists' preferences for computer-based aphasia therapy. *International Journal of Speech-Language Pathology, 18*(4), 315–328.

Thiessen, A., Beukelman, D., Hux, K., & Longenecker, M. (2016). A comparison of the visual attention patterns of people with aphasia and adults without neurological conditions for camera-engaged and task-engaged visual scenes. *Journal of Speech, Language, and Hearing Research, 59*(2), 290–301.

Thorndike, R. M. (1997). *Measurement and evaluation in psychology and education.* Prentice-Hall.

Tombaugh, T. N. (2006). A comprehensive review of the Paced Auditory Serial Addition Test (PASAT). *Archives of Clinical Neuropsychology, 21*, 53–76.

Treisman, A. (1960). Contextual cues in selective listening. *Quarterly Journal of Experimental Psychology, 12*, 242–248.

Tung, L. C., Yu, W. H., Lin, G. H., Yu, T. Y., Wu, C. T., Tsai, C. Y., . . . Hsieh, C. L. (2016). Development of a Tablet-based symbol digit modalities test for reliably assessing information processing speed in patients with stroke. *Disability and Rehabilitation, 38*(19), 1952–1960.

Vallat-Azouvi, C., Weber, T., Legrand, L., & Azouvi, P. (2007). Working memory after severe traumatic brain injury. *Journal of the International Neuropsychological Society, 13*(5), 770–780.

Van Engen, K. J., & Bradlow, A. R. (2007). Sentence recognition in native-and foreign-language multi-talker background noise. *The Journal of the Acoustical Society of America, 121*(1), 519–526.

Varkanitsa, M., Godecke, E., & Kiran, S. (2023). How much attention do we pay to attention deficits in poststroke aphasia? *Stroke, 54*(1), 55–66.

Villard, S., & Kidd, G., Jr. (2019). Effects of acquired aphasia on the recognition of speech under energetic and informational masking conditions. *Trends in Hearing, 23*, 2331216519884480.

Villard, S., & Kidd, G., Jr. (2020). Assessing the benefit of acoustic beamforming for listeners with aphasia using modified psychoacoustic methods. *The Journal of the Acoustical Society of America, 148*(5), 2894–2911.

Villard, S., & Kiran, S. (2015). Between-session intra-individual variability in sustained, selective, and integrational non-linguistic attention in aphasia. *Neuropsychologia, 66*, 204–212.

Villard, S., & Kiran, S. (2017). To what extent does attention underlie language in aphasia? *Aphasiology, 31*(10), 1226–1245.

Villard, S., & Kiran, S. (2018). Between-session and within-session intra-individual variability in attention in aphasia. *Neuropsychologia, 109*, 95–106.

Vossel, S., Geng, J. J., & Fink, G. R. (2014). Dorsal and ventral attention systems: Distinct neural circuits but collaborative roles. *The Neuroscientist, 20*(2), 150–159.

Wagner, A. E., Nagels, L., Toffanin, P., Opie, J. M., & Başkent, D. (2019). Individual variations in effort: Assessing pupillometry for the hearing impaired. *Trends in Hearing, 23*, 2331216519845596.

Wang, X., Thiel, L., & Graff, N. D. (2022). Mindfulness and relaxation techniques for stroke survivors with aphasia: A feasibility and acceptability study. *Healthcare, 10*(8), 1409.

Wechsler, D. (2008). *Wechsler Adult Intelligence Scale-IV*. Pearson.

Westerberg, H., Jacobaeus, H., Hirvikoski, T., Clevberger, P., Östensson, M-L., Bartfai, A., & Klingberg, T. (2007). Computerized working memory training after stroke: A pilot study. *Brain Injury, 21*(1), 21–29.

Whyte, J., Fleming, M., Polansky, M., Cavallucci, C., & Coslett, H. B. (1998).

The effects of visual distraction following traumatic brain injury. *Journal of the International Neuropsychological Society, 4,* 127–136.

Whyte, J., Grieb-Neff, P., Gantz, C., & Polansky, M. (2006). Measuring sustained attention after traumatic brain injury: Differences in key findings from the sustained attention to response task (SART). *Neuropsychologia, 44,* 2007–2014.

Whyte, J., Hart, T., Bode, R. K., & Malec, J. F. (2003). The Moss Attention Rating Scale for traumatic brain injury: Initial psychometric assessment. *Archives of Physical Medicine and Rehabilitation, 84,* 268–276.

Whyte, J., Hart, T., Ellis, C. A., & Chervoneva, I. (2008). The Moss Attention Rating Scale for traumatic brain injury: Further explorations of reliability and sensitivity to change. *Archives of Physical Medicine and Rehabilitation, 89,* 966–973.

Whyte, J., Polansky, M., Fleming, M., Coslett, H. B., & Cavallucci, C. (1995). Sustained arousal and attention after traumatic brain injury. *Neuropsychologia, 33*(7), 797–813.

Whyte, J., Schuster, K., Polansky, M., Adams, J., & Coslett, H. B. (2000). Frequency and duration of inattentive behavior after traumatic brain injury: Effects of distraction, task, and practice. *Journal of the International Neuropsychological Society, 6,* 1–11.

Wickens, C. D. (1980). The structure of attentional resources. In R. S. Nickerson (Ed.), *Attention and performance VIII* (pp. 239–258). Erlbaum.

Wijayasiri, P., Hartley, D. E., & Wiggins, I. M. (2017). Brain activity underlying the recovery of meaning from degraded speech: A functional near-infrared spectroscopy (fNIRS) study. *Hearing Research, 351,* 55–67.

Willmott, C., Ponsford, J., Hocking, C., & Schönberger, M. (2009). Factors contributing to attentional impairments after traumatic brain injury. *Neuropsychology, 23*(4), 424.

Wilson, B. A., Emslie, H. C., Quirk, K., & Evans, J. J. (2001). Reducing everyday memory and planning problems by means of a paging system: A randomized control crossover study. *Journal of Neurology, Neurosurgery, and Psychiatry, 70,* 477–482.

Wilson, B. A., Emslie, H., Quirk, K., Evans, J., & Watson, P. (2005). A randomized control trial to evaluate a paging system for people with traumatic brain injury. *Brain Injury, 19,* 891–894.

Wright, M. J., Cremona-Meteyard, S. L., Geffen, L. B., & Geffen, G. M. (1994). The effects of closed head injury, senile dementia of the Alzheimer's type, and Parkinson's disease on covert orientation of visual attention. *Australian Journal of Psychology, 46*(2), 63–72.

Zane, K. L., Gfeller, J. D., Roskos, P. T., & Bucholz, R. D. (2016). The clinical utility of the Conners' Continuous Performance Test-II in traumatic brain injury. *Archives of Clinical Neuropsychology, 31*(8), 996–1005.

Zhang, H., Li, H., Li, R., Xu, G., & Li, Z. (2019). Therapeutic effect of gradual attention training on language function in patients with post-stroke aphasia: A pilot study. *Clinical Rehabilitation, 33*(11), 1767–1774.

Zickefoose, S., Hux, K., Brown, J., & Wulf, K. (2013). Let the games begin: A preliminary study using Attention Process Training-3 and Lumosity™ brain games to remediate attention deficits following traumatic brain injury. *Brain Injury, 27*(6), 707–716.

Ziino, C., & Ponsford, J. (2006). Selective attention deficits and subjective fatigue following traumatic brain injury. *Neuropsychology, 20*(3), 383.

2

Principles of Human Memory: An Integrative Clinical Neuroscience Perspective

Fofi Constantinidou and
Marianna Christodoulou Devledian

After reading this chapter you will be able to:

1. Define the key concepts related to memory, including the concept of multiple memory systems, encoding, storage, and retrieval.
2. Identify the different types of memory, such as short-term memory and long-term memory.
3. Describe the process of information processing in memory, including attention, encoding, storage, and retrieval.
4. Describe the process of consolidation and how memories are transferred from short-term memory to long-term memory and identify anatomical structures involved in these processes.
5. Understand the different types of memory impairments resulting from different types of acquired brain conditions and describe their impact on daily living.
6. Understand the importance of individualized assessment and intervention in the context of the WHO-ICF model.
7. Describe the different assessment tools and techniques that can be used to evaluate memory, including screening measures and neuropsychological tests.
8. Understand the principles of memory rehabilitation and the different strategies that can be used to improve memory abilities.

Introduction

Memory is probably the most studied cognitive system in both human and animal behavioral literature. Researchers from various theoretical and philosophical backgrounds, including cognitive psychology, neuropsychology, education, neurolinguistics, neurobiology, cognitive science, nuclear medicine, neurology, neuroscience, psychiatry, and computer science, have contributed to different aspects of the memory literature and to our conceptualization of animal and human memory mechanisms. Perhaps the fascination with memory results from our understanding that memory is adaptive in two perspectives. One perspective relates to the survival processing effect (Forester et al., 2020). Individuals need to accurately remember situations that were potentially threatening to them in the past so that they can avoid them in the future. In evolutionary terms, an organism that was able to remember where food sources were located or how dangerous potential predators were, were far more likely to survive.

The other perspective, in addition to survival, is that memory is critical for learning. Conceptual knowledge development and language acquisition, higher reasoning abilities, and effective decision-making are all possible because of a phenomenon known as anticipation or obtainment of reward (Shohamy & Adcock, 2010). Specifically, learning and memory allow for progression through various levels of problem solving and are essential for generating responses and modifying responses following feedback/reward. For instance, someone is reading this book chapter to gain a more in-depth knowledge of memory for personal growth, career growth, and so on.

Memory is conceptualized as being divided into multiple memory systems. The broadest classification of memory distinguishes long-term memory (i.e., permanent memory, such as where you were born or what the word firefly refers to) from short-term memory (i.e., what sort of coffee you had with your breakfast this morning). Long-term memories are of different types. We consciously recall explicit (declarative) memories for facts (semantic knowledge), events (episodic memory), and delayed intentions (prospective memory). We recall unconsciously or prompted (through priming, classical conditioning), implicit (nondeclarative) memories of procedural skills, actions, and emotional responses. See Table 2–1 for more detail.

Given that memory is an integral part of most daily activities, children learn how to develop strategies to reduce the demands on memory. Working memory capacity and the ability to incorporate encoding, organization, and retrieval strategies improve during elementary school years, as there is significant improvement in verbal learning performance between older and younger children (Constantinidou et al., 2011). These abilities continue to develop and peak through early adulthood. There is a subtle (but statistically significant) decline in working memory capacity for each decade past 30 (Constantinidou et al., 2014). Formal education and life experiences contribute to a great extent in the development of strategies that facilitate working memory capacity, and it is the most robust predictor of memory performance in adults (Chadjikyprianou et al., 2021; Constantinidou et al., 2012).

Table 2–1. Multiple Memory Systems—The Broad Classification of Memory Distinguishes Relatively Permanent, Long-Term Memory From Short-Term/Working Memory

Long-Term Memory							Working Memory
Explicit Declarative/Conscious			Implicit Nondeclarative/Unconscious				
Episodic	Semantic	Prospective Memory	Skills (Procedural Knowledge)	Priming	Conditioning	Emotional	Working Memory
Autobiographical (i.e., the night you graduated from college)	Factual knowledge (i.e., George Washington was the first president of the United States)	Delayed intentions. (i.e., pick up milk after work today)	Riding a bike or playing a game of checkers	Responding faster to "butter" when you hear the word "bread"	Associating the sound of a fire siren with a fire emergency	Physical attraction or fear	Repeating a number until you can dial it

Memory impairment is probably the most commonly observable clinical symptom in a variety of acquired brain conditions. In fact, memory decline is the hallmark of neurodegenerative disorders, such as pathologic aging (i.e., mild cognitive impairment and dementia), and is a common disorder in acquired brain injury, epilepsy disorders, and psychiatric conditions such as major depression and psychosis. Since the COVID-19 pandemic, long-COVID has been added to the list of etiologies (Altuna et al., 2021). However, memory disorders are not uniformed, and their presentation and severity are dependent on the disrupted brain networks. In addition, memory networks are facilitated by other cognitive systems such as attention and executive networks; hence, damage to these systems can compound the memory impairment.

The purpose of this chapter is to apply cognitive theory, as well as current findings in cognitive neuroscience and brain research, and present contemporary theoretical models of memory processes with a focus on adult acquired memory disorders. Consistent with the previous editions, the chapter uses an integrative life span approach to present information on the organization of memory systems and discusses assessment methodologies, types of memory disorders, and treatment planning principles for the management of memory disorders.

Cognitive Theory and Memory

Cognitive theory organizes human cognition into a hierarchy of basic and complex processes and systems. Basic processes such as sensory perception, attention, and memory underlie more complex systems, including language, abstract thought, reasoning, categorization, and executive functioning. Neurobiological research in humans and animals provides support for the cognitive systems generated by cognitive theory. When these systems are disrupted, the cognitive deficits could manifest in predictable, observable outcomes. Neurologic disorders may produce focal brain damage (e.g., resulting from a stroke or a contained neoplastic lesion) or complex diffuse lesions as in the case of traumatic brain injury (TBI) and degenerative disorders such as multiple sclerosis and Alzheimer's disease (AD). Neuropsychiatric conditions, such as major depression, bipolar disorder, and psychosis, interfere with normal functioning of cognitive networks, leading to cognitive and thought dysfunction. These complex conditions can result in both focal and diffuse cortical and subcortical disruptions and a cascade of neurobiological changes that can be bilateral and extensive. The challenge of rehabilitation is first to assess the patient's abilities and then implement effective and efficient treatment modalities that will enable the person to maximize their level of functioning.

Theoretical Framework for Human Memory: Multiple System Model

In the past 50 years, several models of memory functioning have been proposed. The model of memory implemented in this chapter combines Baddeley's theory of working memory (Baddeley, 1986, 2000, 2001, 2003; Baddeley et al., 2011; Baddeley & Hitch, 1974) and subsequent updates (Baddeley et al., 2011; Doherty & Logie, 2016) with Tulving's and Squire's models of long-term memory and subsequent updates (Schacter & Tulving, 1994; Squire, 1992). This framework has considerable utility in populations with memory disorders.

As described earlier, memory is organized with respect to both time and contents (Markowitsch, 1995). On the basis of behavioral evidence (Brown, 1958; Peterson & Peterson, 1959) and neuropsychological data (Milner, 1966), the distinction between a short-term and a long-term retention system was the first to be made (e.g., Atkinson & Shiffrin, 1968). Atkinson and Shiffrin (1968) distinguished between short- and long-term memory stores. The short-term store was considered to be temporary and of limited capacity, whereas the long-term store was considered to be permanent.

Initially, the nature of the information handled within these time-delineated systems was thought to be unitary, and earlier models influenced by cognitive science and computer science conceptualized memory as a single system consisting of several stages or processes (Atkinson & Shiffrin, 1968; Sohlberg & Mateer, 2001). Concepts such as encoding, consolidation, storage, and retrieval were coined to explain the various stages of information processing. While the stage model has been replaced by a content-based subdivision incorporating multiple memory systems and subsystems, certain terminology from the stage models of memory has been retained and can be useful for understanding memory per-

formance when working with patients with memory impairments (Constantinidou & Thomas, 2017; Sanders et al., 2007).

Encoding, a process that starts with perception and attention, refers to the early processing of the material, during which information is transformed so that it can be stored. How well information is encoded can contribute to how well it is stored for later use and eventually recalled. Encoding encompasses a variety of operations that can be performed on material to be learned, including simple repetition through rehearsal and organizing material in a way that is meaningful (e.g., creating an acronym to assist with recall of word lists) (Sanders et al., 2007). Findings indicate that this sort of organizational structure, which employs executive processes in order to be successful, is a key function of left dorsolateral prefrontal cortex (Constantinidou et al., 2012; Ezzyat et al., 2017; Fletcher et al., 1998). Therefore, encoding is highly dependent on frontal lobe mechanisms and networks.

Consolidation refers to the process via which recently encoded information is transferred into permanent storage. Consolidation is more efficient after successful encoding. Recent events in comparison to past events are more vulnerable to forgetting as a result of trauma or disease because their consolidation process was not complete (Lechner et al., 1999). During the consolidation stage, information is susceptible to proactive and retroactive interference. That is, recently learned information can hamper the storage and recall of newly learned material (proactive interference), whereas retroactive interference implies that competing information can hamper the successful storage and recall of recently learned material. Once the consolidation process is complete, then information has entered permanent storage. For this to occur, memories initially dependent on the hippocampus are reorganized as time passes.

According to Squire and colleagues (2015), by this process, the hippocampus gradually becomes less important for storage and retrieval, and a more permanent memory develops in distributed regions of the neocortex. The idea is not that memory is literally transferred from the hippocampus to the neocortex, for information is encoded in the neocortex as well as in hippocampus at the time of learning. The idea is that gradual changes in the neocortex, beginning at the time of learning, establish stable long-term memory, by increasing the complexity, distribution, and connectivity among multiple cortical regions. (p. 2)

Prior knowledge regarding the material to be learned will influence the rate of consolidation (van Kesteren et al., 2012). Given the involvement of the hippocampus in this process, the medial temporal lobe networks and structures are important for effective consolidation.

Storage refers to the way that information is held in memory for future use. Encoding and storage are interactive processes because the quality of the encoding process can affect the way that information is stored. Once a memory is placed in the long-term store, it is considered permanent unless disrupted by a pathologic process. In addition, stored information is vulnerable to time and not all information entered in the permanent storage system is available for spontaneous retrieval (Constantini-

dou, 1998). For example, TBI commonly produces time-dependent retrograde amnesia. Retrograde amnesia is defined as the inability to access memories that were accessible to someone before a brain injury. The severity of the injury will determine how far back in time the amnesia will extend. It is possible, for instance, that older memories can be accessed, whereas more recent memories cannot. Opportunities for rehearsal, or reconsolidation, as described by Tronson and Taylor (2007), will increase the likelihood of successful future recall of stored information (Tulving, 1966).

Retrieval refers to the act of pulling information from storage, typically from the long-term store. On most memory tests, this is measured via delayed recall paradigms consisting of free recall and recognition tasks. Immediate recall presumably does not necessitate retrieval of information from long-term memory because the material is still being held in working memory system and may be undergoing encoding processes, such as rehearsal. For example, on a story recall task, recall of the information immediately after presentation relies on the short-term store. Recall of the information 30 minutes after presentation relies on the long-term store. Persons with retrieval deficits often benefit from presentation of information in a recognition format, such as a multiple-choice or yes/no format. Improved recognition over free recall performance points to the fact that information was not lost due to storage or rapid forgetting difficulties; decline in free recall could be due to inability to access the information successfully, resulting from retrieval deficits or impaired or unsuccessful encoding. During information retrieval, the individual can monitor the success of the process and individuals with strong memories, and meta-memories can delineate whether the retrieved information is correct. Cortical, cortical-subcortical structures and networks support the retrieval process, including the hippocampus prefrontal cortex. The frontal lobes are activated during the retrieval process to implement strategies and search in the correct schemas; the hippocampi are activated as they may need to hold multiple pieces of information for brief periods of time during the retrieval process (Constantinidou, 1998).

Encoding, storage, and retrieval are interactive processes and require mediation by the executive network. Disruptions in frontal-subcortical networks can interfere with these memory processes. Specifically, the way information is encoded can affect the form in which it is stored, which can later affect its retrieval. The ability of the individual to implement active memory strategies and organize information meaningfully into already existing schemas increases the likelihood for successful retrieval later. For example, word lists are more likely to be recalled when they can be organized by semantic category such as foods, animals, colors, and so on. Similarly, a new mathematical formula is more likely to be remembered if students can build on existing knowledge (e.g., the formula for calculating a standard deviation is built on the formula used to calculate averages). Persons with frontal lobe damage and executive functioning deficits may perform better on story recall tasks when compared to list-learning paradigms because their impaired ability to impose structure on material is more obvious with the unstructured word list.

There is also evidence to support that the act of retrieving information can strengthen its representation in long-term storage. For example, it has been shown that repeated retrieval of information from long-term store strengthens memories, increasing the probability that information will be accurately retrieved later (Tulving, 1966). Furthermore, the strength of representations is influenced by how the information is initially learned, including the frequency and spacing of stimulus presentation at encoding (Sohlberg et al., 2005), the depth of semantic encoding (Craik & Lockhart, 1972), and the type of stimulus presentation (Christoforou et al., 2013; Constantinidou et al., 2011; Constantinidou & Evripidou, 2012). Our discussion of the human memory systems integrates the aforementioned terms as they assist in our understanding of memory performance in adults with neurologic disorders.

Working Memory.

The term "short-term memory," which was coined in the 1950s (refer to the "modal model" by Atkinson & Shiffrin, 1968), gave way to the more contemporary concept of "working memory" in recent decades. Contemporary views of working memory incorporate the initial concepts of short-term memory, which is limited in both capacity and function but consists of multiple components that require the coordination of multiple cognitive resources (Baddeley et al., 2019).

An original version of this multicomponent model of working memory was proposed by Baddeley and Hitch (1974). This was a three-component model comprising the central executive, an attentional control system, aided by two temporary storage systems: the phonological loop (which relates to verbally presented stimuli) and the visuospatial sketchpad (the visual equivalent of the phonological loop). Baddeley revised this model to include a fourth component, called the "episodic buffer," in 2000.

When information arrives via the sense organs, that is, perceptually encoded, it is deposited into an immediate working memory system that is divided into three subsystems specialized for different functions (Baddeley et al., 2011): a control system, the executive network of attention (please refer to Chapter 1 on Attention), and two subsystems, each handling different types of information: (a) the visuospatial sketchpad and (b) the phonological, or articulatory, loop. Visual (e.g., color and shape), spatial (i.e., location and orientation), and haptic (e.g., kinesthetic, tactile) information is held and manipulated in the visuospatial sketchpad. Recent evidence suggests that visual working memory is not unitary, and during maintenance, the brain segregates visual information depending on the physical attributes of each piece of information (e.g., shape, orientation, color, motion, spatial location; Baddeley et al., 2011; Doherty & Logie, 2016; Konstantinou et al., 2017). Cortical areas that are involved in visual perception (the occipital lobe) and spatial orienting (the parietal areas, especially the right parietal lobe) subserve the operations of the visuospatial sketchpad (Baddeley et al., 2011; Doherty & Logie, 2016; Farah, 1988; Jonides et al., 1993; Konstantinou et al., 2017).

Sounds (e.g., phonological and music) as well as linguistically encoded information (e.g., sign and lip reading) are stored and processed by the phonological or articulatory loop, a term that emphasizes its prototypical activity of recycling acoustic and linguistic information to keep it in conscious awareness. The episodic buffer proposed by Baddeley is responsible for receiving information directly through perception (the phonological loop or the visuospatial system) or indirectly from long-term memory (Baddeley, 2021; Baddeley et al., 2019, 2020) and allows storing information that exceeds the span capacities of the two subsystems. The neuroanatomic correlates of this additional system have not been confirmed, but it seems that its functions might be dependent on the frontal lobe. This working memory buffer deploys effective organization strategies (such as chunking) and pulls information from long-term memory stores that will assist with semantic processing and information manipulation and organization into already known schemata or create new schemata. Demanding working memory tasks that exceed the typical span of 7 ± 2 items and tasks that require delayed recall after presentation will require active engagement of the buffer for successful task completion (Figure 2–1).

Studies of the capacity of auditory working memory often use a task in which a sequence of items (e.g., letters or digits) is presented to a person who must reproduce them immediately from memory in the correct order. The length of the longest sequence (in terms of number of digits/letters) correctly produced, termed the letter or digit span, indicates the capacity of the phonological loop and is an indication of attention, rather than a reflection of the entire working memory system. The

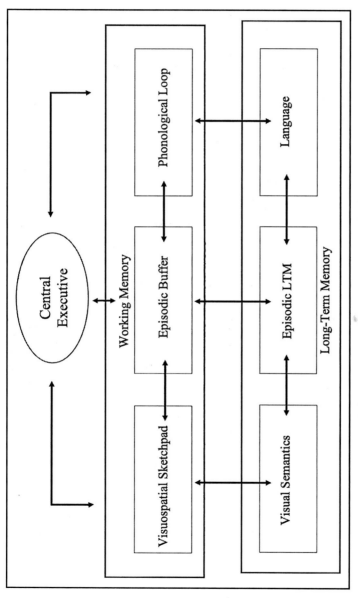

Figure 2–1. Schematic of Baddeley's memory model and its four key components, the central executive, the visuospatial loop, the episodic buffer, and the phonological loop. Here is an example of how the model works. Someone just gave you their phone number. First, the sound of the phone number is processed by your auditory cortex and sent to your phonological loop. The phonological loop is responsible for temporarily storing and processing verbal information, like speech sounds. As you're trying to hold onto the phone number, you note it down on a piece of paper in front of you. The sight of the phone number is processed by your visual cortex and sent to your visuospatial sketchpad. The visuospatial sketchpad is responsible for briefly storing and processing visual information, like images and spatial relationships. While this processing is going on, you also remember that the person who gave you the phone number asked you to meet at a particular location. This entire process is monitored by the central executive unit, which uses the incoming information from the fluid systems (i.e., visuospatial sketchpad, phonological loop) to integrate it with crystalized knowledge (i.e., semantic and episodic memory) in order to create a single integrated memory in episodic buffer.

role of the phonological loop in general cognitive function has been called into question (Baddeley, 1995; Conway et al., 2005; Unsworth & Engle, 2007). The phonological loop appears to be necessary, however, for language acquisition, either the early childhood learning of a native language or multiple languages (Gathercole & Baddeley, 1990), or in adult learning of foreign languages (Baddeley et al., 1988; Papagno et al., 1991).

True working memory capacity of the executive network that has been shown to relate to higher cognitive functioning (Salthouse, 2005) is better measured by tasks that require either dual processing or inhibiting prepotent responses, both activities that are the hallmark of flexible control of attention (Colfesh & Conway, 2007; Conway et al., 2005; Kane & Engle, 2002, 2003). Tests that measure static spans (e.g., forward span of the Wechsler Adult Intelligence Scale–IV [WAIS-IV] or the Wechsler Memory Scale–IV [WMS-IV]) are dissociable from those that measure the more active processes involved in attentional control such as digit span backward and verbal learning paradigms like the Rey Auditory Verbal Learning Test or the California Verbal Learning Test (Conway et al., 2005; Kane et al., 2004; Sanders et al., 2007).

Doherty and Logie (2016) demonstrated that processing accuracy is affected during dual-task processing when task demands exceed the measured memory span. Furthermore, in the case of visual memory, capacity limits in visual short-term memory (VSTM) are correlated with sustained activity in the dorsal and ventral visual streams responsible for perception of spatial and object information, respectively. Voxel-based morphometry (VBM) analyses revealed dissociable neuroanatomical correlates of spatial versus object VSTM reflected in interindividual variability in the gray matter density of the inferior parietal lobule and the left insula, respectively (Konstantinou et al., 2017). Furthermore, deficits in visual memory capacity were associated with reduced white matter integrity of the corpus collosum in chronic TBI (Yiannakkaras et al., 2019).

Patients with significant disruptions in the executive and attentional control systems, such as patients who sustained moderate to severe brain injury or patients with amnestic mild cognitive impairment, typically demonstrate difficulty in allocating resources and actively organizing (and encoding) incoming information (Kennedy et al., 2009; Konstantinou et al., 2017; Metzler-Baddeley et al., 2012). However, research indicates that these patients can learn how to implement strategies or to follow external organizational schemes (Constantinidou, 2019; Constantinidou et al., 2008; Crosson et al., 1993; Goldstein et al., 1990; Kennedy & Krause, 2011).

As mentioned earlier in this chapter, developmentally, working memory capacity and the ability to incorporate encoding, organization, and retrieval strategies improve during elementary school years (Constantinidou et al., 2011). Working memory and episodic memory performance can be frequently affected in patients with neurologic and psychiatric conditions because of focal and diffuse brain lesions or due to a functional disruption of working memory and executive functioning networks hampering the deployment of memory strategies (Behnken et al., 2010; Constantinidou, 1999; Voss et al.,

2011). Additionally, changes are also seen as part of the healthy aging process and are associated with changes in brain structure that affect working memory and executive functioning mechanisms (Giogkaraki et al., 2013; Pettemeridou et al., 2021).

Long-Term Memory.

Some incoming information undergoes the process known as consolidation, which results in it being stored in various long-term retention systems. The different routes to storage, together with the distinctions among the kinds of information permanently stored, define the various hierarchical subsystems of long-term memory. At the top level of the taxonomy adopted by many cognitive neuroscientists (e.g., Schacter & Tulving, 1994; Squire & Zola-Morgan, 1991) is the divide between information that can be consciously declared to have been learned or experienced (explicit, or declarative, memory) and information whose learning is reflected only by changes in future behavior as a result of the prior experience without conscious remembrance (implicit, or nondeclarative, memory). The kinds of items deemed declarative include general knowledge or facts about the world, termed semantic memory, and personal, autobiographical recollection of experiences, termed episodic memory. The exact locus of stored memories is not known (Thompson & Krupa, 1994), but it has been suggested that various cortical sites involved in perception may hold perceptual memories regarding events, whereas general factual knowledge is likely to be represented at least in the temporal cortex (Gazzaniga et al., 1998).

Explicit or Declarative Memory. Based on animal and human studies, researchers propose a temporal–frontal lobe neural representation for explicit memory. Provided many connections between the prefrontal cortex and the temporal cortex are made through the thalamus, nuclei in the thalamus are also involved. Both semantic and episodic memories are thought to require a functioning medial temporal lobe system (hippocampus, amygdala, and adjacent cortex but especially the hippocampus) for their learning (Smith et al., 2014; Squire & Knowlton, 1995; Squire & Zola-Morgan, 1991). Lesions in the medial temporal lobe structures result in pronounced anterograde amnesia in comparison to retrograde amnesia. That is, patients will have trouble recalling new events that occur after the injury (anterograde amnesia). They perform poorly on the standard measures of declarative memory such as free recall and recognition of newly studied material such as word lists, paragraphs, and figures. The patients can recall a new experience for a few seconds, before it fades, reflecting an intact immediate recall or span performance. In contrast, their ability to recall events prior to the injury (retrograde amnesia) is largely intact, except for events immediately preceding insult, perhaps because the injury process interrupted the consolidation process. The role of the medial temporal system appears to be one of storage or consolidation of short-term memories rather than one of retrieval given that individuals with amnesia can retrieve remote memories with little difficulty.

There has been some debate in the literature regarding the role of the hippocampus in semantic memories (Tulving et al., 1991; Vargha-Khadem et al.,

1997). A prevailing position states that hippocampal damage will affect the episodic memory system to a greater extent than the semantic system. However, a study by Manns and colleagues (2003) demonstrated that hippocampal damage interferes with the acquisition of new semantic/factual knowledge. This difficulty continues in years postinjury and is associated with temporal lobe networks (Konstantinou et al., 2019). In addition, patients experienced retrograde amnesia for semantic information, but that span was limited to a few years. Hence, the authors concluded, the hippocampus supports both episodic and semantic knowledge, but it has a time-limited role in the acquisition and storage of semantic knowledge (Manns et al., 2003).

Evidence from the developmental literature also supports the involvement of the hippocampus in explicit memory. Cases in which hippocampal damage was incurred prenatally or early in life resulted in children having difficulties with developing or remembering solutions to problems and having difficulties with spatial memory (Cimadevilla et al., 2014). Other resulting difficulties reported include having difficulty with language skills (Lee et al., 2015), grammar learning (Kepinska et al., 2018), and linking objects to places and making face-voice associations (Vargha-Khadem et al., 1997).

Explicit memories not only are vulnerable to disruption following prefrontal and medial temporal brain lesions and TBI but also are relatively vulnerable in healthy individuals, and episodic memories typically are more vulnerable than semantic memories. Most people could not remember the event or moment during which they learned that 1 meter equals 100 centimeters,

unless this information was associated with an event of emotional significance. Although semantic or factual memory appears to be strengthened by repeated exposure (especially in the presence of interfering or distracting information), episodic memory by its nature cannot undergo repeated exposure. It appears that most episodic memories fade unless they include or are accompanied by some emotionally significant experience or there is a systematic and accurate recount of the events, that is, rehearsal of information (McGaugh, 2000). Furthermore, bilateral cortical injuries in the parietal, posterior temporal, and possibly occipital cortices can lead to specific long-term memory difficulties affecting semantic and episodic memory (i.e., anomia, prosopagnosia). Memory impairments also result from diffuse cortical damage, such as in the case of dementia or brain infections like herpes encephalitis.

Similar to episodic memory, prospective memory is also vulnerable to brain pathology and to interference. Prospective memory refers to delayed intentions. Test paradigms typically design tasks that require an intention (e.g., an act) to be carried out at a later time. The time between the assigned intention and the time to act (retention interval) is filled with an ongoing activity that typically prevents rehearsal (Gonen-Yaacovi & Burgess, 2012). Imaging studies indicate that during prospective memory paradigms, the rostral prefrontal cortex (Brodmann's 10) is a key area of activation during the creation, maintenance, and execution of intentions.

Implicit or Nondeclarative Memory. Implicit memory consists of a heterogeneous collection of different types of memories that are generally preserved in the loss of declarative memory ability. These implicit memory systems are quite distinct from one another and rely on entirely different brain structures. They include procedural memory, priming, and classical conditioning. The development of procedural memory is independent of the hippocampal formation and medial temporal lobe structures but appears to depend on the basal ganglia, especially the caudate nucleus (Ashby & Waldron, 2000; Ewert et al., 1989). Procedural memory typically is divided into two major subtypes, which, on their surface, appear to be quite different but appear to depend on the integrity of similar brain systems. One of the major categories is motor skill memory; the other is cognitive skill or reference memory. If an individual learned how to skip rope today, and their episodic memory is intact, tomorrow they will report having remembered the experience. However, even if they have no explicit memory of the experience (due to hippocampal damage), they will demonstrate intact motor skill memory as manifested by their improved ability to skip rope. Subjects with lesions invading the motor and premotor areas of the frontal cortex frequently display difficulty in motor skill learning. Yet, if their hippocampus is intact, they will recall the experience of attempting to skip rope.

Reference or cognitive skill memory (i.e., the memory of the procedures that are necessary to win a game or solve a problem) constitutes the second kind of procedural memory. This form of memory does not refer to explicit declarative memory for the rules of the game but refers to the acquisition of successful strategies (Gathercole et al., 2019). An individual with a medial temporal lobe lesion could improve their skill at board games, such as checkers, without recalling ever playing the game before. Thus, the solution of some complex cognitive tasks does not require explicit memory but rather repeated exposure to a specific situation and rules for solutions. Quite possibly, the learned strategies are a collection of observations of cause and effects that are reinforced according to the principles of operant or instrumental conditioning. Consequently, patients with medial temporal lobe lesions may benefit from the repetitive nature of certain activities in cognitive rehabilitation (Squire et al., 2004) and become more adapted and independent without necessarily demonstrating improvement in explicit memory tasks. Domain-specific memory training capitalizes on procedural memory. The patient receives training for specific tasks relating to their work demands or daily activities. Although functional performance on these tasks typically does not translate to generalization to new tasks (Schnider & Ptak, 2023), the patient's level of functioning and independence (on the specific activities) may improve. Both forms of procedural learning (motor skill and cognitive skill) involve the basal ganglia; however, motor skill learning appears to be dependent on the integrity of the motor areas of the neocortex, including the premotor strip, and cognitive skill learning appears to be more dependent on sensory cortices in the parietal and occipital lobes (Ewert et al., 1989; Schnider & Ptak, 2023).

Another type of implicit memory relates to priming phenomena. Priming refers to the facilitation in the processing, detection, or identification of an item because of its prior exposure in tasks not requiring conscious recollection

(Schacter, 1992). Classic research paradigms of priming involve an initial study of items, such as a list of words, under the disguise of some ruse instructions, followed with a nonmemory task such as lexical decision ("is this letter string a word or nonword?"), word identification ("what is this word?"), or word-stem completion ("wo_ _"). The typical finding is that lexical decisions and word identifications occur more quickly or require less stimulus energy to achieve a given level of performance for words previously seen. In the word-stem completion task, subjects tend to supply words seen from the earlier list to complete the partial words (Schacter, 1987). Other, nonverbal paradigms implemented include dot patterns and geometric paradigms. Several studies have demonstrated that priming is dependent on a different anatomical system than explicit memory. Individuals with amnesia who fail traditional tests of explicit memory exhibit normal priming (Graf & Mandler, 1984; Jacoby & Witherspoon, 1982; Schacter, 1985; Shimamura & Squire, 1984). Individuals with damage to perceptual areas such as the occipital lobe show normal performance on explicit measures of memory but do not evidence priming (Gabrieli et al., 1995), and performance on standard recognition and recall tasks can be dissociated from priming tasks in normal subjects (Graf & Mandler, 1984; Graf et al., 1982; Jacoby & Dallas, 1981; Tulving et al., 1982). Priming appears to be perceptual in nature as any surface change of the stimulus (e.g., font changes for word stimuli or changes in picture orientation for visual stimuli), from prior exposure to test, can reduce its effect (Biederman & Cooper, 1991; Cave & Squire, 1992; Graf & Ryan, 1990; Jacoby & Hayman, 1987; Roediger

& Blaxton, 1987). Priming is mediated by the corresponding sensory cortices (e.g., visual priming in visual cortex, auditory priming in auditory cortex). This system responsible for priming is referred to as the perceptual representation system in Schacter's framework (e.g., Schacter, 1990) and is the system involved in the initial perception and encoding of a stimulus (Constantinidou & Thomas, 2017).

Although research studies provide evidence that priming is supported by nontemporal lobe structures, brain imaging studies suggest that the medial temporal lobe may also have a role in implicit learning as well as for information relating to meaningful implicit tasks (Beauregard et al., 1998; Smith et al., 2014). Koenig et al. (2008) implemented a prototype extraction task during an fMRI task to assess implicit learning of a meaningful novel visual category in young adults, in healthy older adults, and in adults with AD. As expected, occipital deactivation was observed consistent with perceptually based implicit learning and lateral temporal cortex deactivation reflecting implicit acquisition of the category's semantic nature. In addition, young adults showed medial temporal lobe (MTL) activation during the exposure and test period, suggesting involvement of explicit memory as well. In contrast, adults with AD who had significant MTL atrophy did not show MTL activation, and their performance on the implicit memory task was not as strong as their healthy counterparts. The other patterns of cortical activation/deactivation associated with implicit learning were similar to the healthy controls. The authors concluded that patients with AD appear to engage a cortically based implicit memory mechanism, whereas their relative deficit on this task may reflect their MTL disease. These findings suggest that implicit and explicit memory systems collaborate in neurologically intact individuals performing a seemingly implicit memory task.

A final category of implicit memory includes simple classical conditioning and associative learning of the sort often studied in animal learning research. These simple forms of learning, evidenced even in invertebrates, may reflect principles of neuronal plasticity in general such as Hebbian learning or long-term potentiation. That is, repeated stimulation of a postsynaptic neuron by a presynaptic neuron results in synaptic efficiency. There is evidence for the special role of the cerebellum in classical conditioning of discrete motor responses, such as eye blinks in the presence of air puffs (Lee & Thompson, 2006; Thompson & Krupa, 1994). Most neurologic disorders do not disrupt this form of learning provided that the patient is conscious and not in a coma or vegetative state and has preserved basic cognitive functioning. This type of memory is mentioned here to provide a complete picture of what is known regarding memory systems (Constantinidou et al., 2004).

Assessment of Memory Functions

The above sections describe different categories of memories emphasizing the nature of the memory content, as revealed by dissociations of the effects of variables on performance using different types of tasks and materials. Most forms of memory assessment, especially in clinical neuropsychological contexts, rely heavily on explicit measures (Lezak, 1995; Lezak et al., 2004) as this type of memory is most characteristic of human cognitive performance and seems to be most influenced by brain pathology. Table 2–2 depicts common tests that assess memory in relationship to the systems model of memory. Table 2–3 depicts testing paradigms relating to the systems model.

Assessment of memory abilities needs to follow an integrative multidisciplinary approach. In most rehabilitation settings, memory assessment is part of the cognitive assessment process and conducted by speech-language pathologists and neuropsychologists. These professionals have an array of formal and informal tools designed to test different aspects of memory. To select the appropriate tools, the goals of assessment need to be taken into consideration (Vakil, 2012). Answers to the following questions could provide guidance for appropriate test selection:

- What is the goal of the assessment? Is the goal to obtain a global indication of cognitive function or to provide a thorough memory assessment to develop treatment goals? For instance, most global tests of cognition will assess certain aspects of memory; however, they are not designed to provide a thorough assessment of memory. Hence, the clinician needs to be aware of this limitation when administering a general cognitive test. If the test results suggest a memory decline, or if the purpose of assessment is to evaluate memory functions, testing should be followed up with a comprehensive memory assessment.

Table 2–2. Commonly Administered Tests and Their Relationship to the Systems Memory Model

Testing Task	Batteries/Screens					Memory Assessment				
	Test	Immediate Recall	Delayed Recall	Recognition	Forced Choice	Test	Immediate Recall	Delayed Recall	Recognition	Forced Choice
List Learning Memory	RBANS	+	+	+		CVLT3	+	+	+	+
Supraspan Lists (>9 items per list)	NAB	+	+	+		HVLT-R	+	+	+	
	WJ-IV	+				RAVLT	+	+	+	
						WMS-IV	+	+	+	
						TOMAL-2	+	+		
						DTLA-A	+			
Subspan Lists (<7 items per list; typically single presentation)	ABCD	+		+						
	COGNISTA	+	+	+						
	RIPA-II	+	+							
	SCATBI	+	+							
Paragraph Memory	ABCD	+	+			RBMT-3	+	+		
	ADP	+				TOMAL-2	+			
	NAB	+	+	+		WMS-IV	+	+	+	
	SCATBI	+		+						
	RBANS	+		+						

	Batteries/Screens				Memory Assessment				
Testing Task		**Immediate Recall**	**Delayed Recall**	**Recog-nition**	**Forced Choice**		**Immediate Recall**	**Delayed Recall**	**Recog-nition**	**Forced Choice**
Paired Associates Learning						TOMAL-2	+			
						WMS-IV	+	+		
Digit Span Task or Serial Recall	WAIS-IV	+				DTLA-A	+			
Task–Backward (verbal)	WJ-IV	+				TOMAL-2	+			
						WMS-IV	+			
Picture Recall	WJ-IV			+		BVRT	+			
	NAB	+	+	+	+	CVMT	+	+	+	
						RMT	+			
						TOMAL-2	+			
						WMS-IV	+	+	+	
Figure Recall	RBANS	+	+			DTLA-A	+			
						WMS-IV	+	+		
						RCFT	+	+	+	
						TOMAL-2			+	

continues

Table 2–2. *continued*

Testing Task	Batteries/Screens				Memory Assessment			
	Immediate Recall	Delayed Recall	Recognition	Forced Choice	Immediate Recall	Delayed Recall	Recognition	Forced Choice
Visual Span Task or Serial Recall Task–Backward					WMS-IV + TOMAL-2 +			
Visual-Auditory Learning	WJ-IV +	+			TOMAL-2 +			

Note: The above list is not intended as an exhaustive list of tests, and a test's inclusion in the table does not imply endorsement by the author. Furthermore, some categorization of the aforementioned "testing tasks" stimulates debate. It is important to keep in mind that the individual's approach to a task may lead to the use of a variety of cognitive functions. As an example, if a patient approaches the task passively, there may not be a demand on executive functioning. However, if a participant chooses to semantically organize the words on a list-learning task, the use of executive functions will ensue. Moreover, one needs to keep in mind the potential of a test to tap into multiple cognitive functions. BVRT = Benton Visual Retention Test; COGNISTAT = Cognitive Status Examination; CVLT3 = California Verbal Learning Test-3; CVMT = Continuous Visual Memory Test; HVLT-R = Hopkins Verbal Learning Test-Revised; NAB = Neuropsychological Assessment Battery; RAVLT = Rey Auditory Verbal Learning Test; RBANS = Repeatable Battery for the Assessment of Neuropsychological Status; RCFT = Rey Complex Figure Test; RMT = Warrington's Recognition Memory Test; WAIS-IV = Wechsler Adult Intelligence Scale-IV; WMS-IV = Wechsler Memory Scale-IV; ADP = Aphasia Diagnostic Profiles; ABCD = Arizona Battery for Communication Disorders of Dementia; RIPA-II = Ross Information Processing Ability-II; SCATBI = Scales of Cognitive Ability for Traumatic Brain Injury; RBMT-3 = Rivermead Behavioural Memory Test-3; TOMAL-2 = Test of Memory and Learning-2; DTLA-A = Detroit Test of Learning Aptitude–Adult; WJ-IV= Woodcock Johnson–IV PsychoEducational Battery-Tests of Cognitive Abilities.

Table 2–3. Testing Paradigms and their Relationship to the Systems Memory Model

| Testing Task | Short Term Store (Working Memory) | | | Long-Term Store | |
	Visual	Phono-logical	Central Executive	Declarative Memory	Non-Declarative Memory
List Learning Memory					
Supraspan Lists (>9 items per list)					
Immediate Recall (IR)		+	+		
Delayed Recall (DR)			+	+	
Recognition (Rec)			+	+	
Forced Choice (FC)			+	+	
Subspan Lists (<7 items per list; typically single presentation)					
Immediate Recall		+	+		
Delayed Recall			+	+	
Recognition			+	+	
Paragraph Memory					
Immediate Recall		+	+		
Delayed Recall			+	+	
Recognition			+	+	
Paired Associates Learning					
Immediate Recall		+	+		
Delayed Recall			+	+	
Recognition			+	+	

continues

Table 2–3. *continued*

Testing Task	Short Term Store (Working Memory)			Long-Term Store	
	Visual	Phono-logical	Central Executive	Declarative Memory	Non-Declarative Memory
Digit Span Task or Serial Recall Task—Backward (verbal)					
Immediate Recall		+	+		
Prospective Task		+	+	+	
Visual-Auditory Learning					
Immediate Recall	+	+	+		
Delayed Recall			+	+	
Picture Recall					
Immediate Recall	+		+		
Delayed Recall			+	+	
Recognition			+	+	
Figure Recall					
Immediate Recall	+		+		
Delayed Recall			+	+	
Recognition			+	+	
Visual Span Task or Serial Recall Task—Backward					
Immediate Recall	+		+		
Procedural Memory Tasks (e.g., pursuit rotor)			+		+

■ Is the patient able to participate in standardized testing procedures? For instance, patients in the acute recovery process post-TBI, who are experiencing posttraumatic amnesia and are disoriented, agitated, and unable to engage in sustained attention tasks, as a general rule, cannot participate in thorough formal working memory testing. Results from such testing are not considered clinically reliable. Assessments should focus on testing orientation skills (such as the Galveston Orientation and Amnesia Test; Levin et al., 1979) and obtaining informal measures of memory and cognitive function. Once posttraumatic amnesia (PTA) is resolved, and the patient can sustain attention to complete test tasks, then formal memory testing can be implemented.

■ What is the theoretical framework of memory adopted by the test, and how does it relate to contemporary theoretical models of memory?

■ What aspects of memory does the test assess? How do these aspects relate to the patient's neurological disease or condition?

■ What are the psychometric properties of the test? Content validity, interitem reliability, test-retest reliability, and standardization process (including population demographics)? Are the patient's cultural, linguistic, educational, and socioeconomic strata represented in the normative sample?

■ How does the assessment relate to the model of International Classification of Functioning Disability and Health (ICF) (World Health Organization [WHO], 2001)?

Assessment of Verbal Memory

The following types of stimuli typically are implemented in the assessment of verbal memory (auditory or visual) memory:

■ Letters in Words and Names
■ Numbers
■ Paragraphs
■ Pictures of familiar objects and faces

Photos of familiar objects and people are considered verbal (even though they are visual stimuli) because most people will assign verbal labels to pictorial stimuli. Pictorial stimuli need to be abstract to escape verbal labeling (Lezak, 1983). The most common verbal working memory paradigms include one of the following activities:

■ Verbal Learning Tasks (e.g., serial presentation of words that may or may not be related). Stimulus words may be presented in three to five learning trials. Multiple scores may be generated from this type of task representing the examinee's ability to benefit from repetition and other cognitive constructs such as attention.
Formal verbal list learning tasks often have recall of stimulus materials at various delay intervals. During subspan learning tasks, typically, the words are only presented once and then the patient is asked to recall the items from the list.

■ Paragraph/Story Recall (e.g., a story that incorporates meaningful material along with episodic information). Most paragraph recall paradigms incorporate immediate and delayed recall conditions.

- Paired Associates Learning (e.g., presenting pairs of words together and later on presenting one of the pair items and requesting the patient to recall the other item)
- Digit Span or Serial Recall Task (e.g., presenting a series of digits or letters to be remembered and gradually increasing the number of items)
- Prospective Memory Tasks (e.g., requesting to carry out an intention at a later time)

Comprehensive memory assessment typically incorporates all the above tasks because patient performance may vary across them. For example, patients who have difficulty implementing organization and encoding strategies may perform poorly on multitrial verbal learning paradigms consisting of word lists that exceed the normal span of seven to nine items. Their recognition performance may be better than their free recall abilities (Constantinidou, 1998). During paragraph/story recall, the patients may perform comparatively better (than their free recall performance on list learning tasks) because stories provide contextual support and inherent organization as they follow a logical sequence. Hence, story recall facilitates encoding for patients who have a more passive learning style.

Patients with normal auditory attention span may perform well on digit span tasks by remembering five to nine items. In order for digit or serial recall tasks to engage working memory mechanisms, they need to involve manipulation of information (which involves the central executive system) or exceed the capacity of the human span (e.g., nine items or chunks of information). Therefore, in addition to the digit forward span serving as a mere short-term memory (STM) test as its storage component requires no manipulation (Egeland, 2015), even the digit backward task cannot be considered a test for working memory (WM) but rather a load on STM as it does not engage higher-order interference and manipulation when the patient is asked to reorder digits (Wells et al., 2018).

Prospective memory tasks also have gained popularity in the recent years because they resemble real-life situations. The patient is asked to remember and carry on a task or intention at a later time (e.g., to turn off the radio in 15 minutes). Therefore, the integrative work of attention, episodic buffer, and executive abilities are needed to complete the task successfully.

Assessment of Nonverbal Memory

Problems can arise when using linguistic stimuli with adults with neurologically based disorders as such might prove to be challenging for these patients. Subtests in standardized assessment batteries, which include letters and words, might impose such linguistic demands on a patient that could ultimately deplete cognitive resources resulting in a breakdown in WM (Mayer & Murray, 2012). With this admission, multiple presentation modalities of test stimuli must be utilized. The suggestion to use the visual modality when assessing patients with auditory and perceptual deficits, as well as linguistic and speech motor deficits and eye-hand motor coordination and vice versa, has been proposed (Ettenhofer et al., 2020; Ivanova et al., 2018).

The following types of stimuli typically are implemented in the assessment of nonverbal memory:

- Abstract designs
- Complex figures
- Unfamiliar melodies
- Spatial positions
- Unfamiliar faces

The most common nonverbal working memory paradigms include one of the following activities:

- Complex Figure Test (copy, immediate, delayed, and recognition conditions)
- Picture Recall of unfamiliar faces (immediate and delayed condition)
- Spatial Span Tasks (forward and backward)
- Spatial Navigation paradigms

Like its verbal memory counterpart, visual-spatial memory assessment needs to incorporate a variety of paradigms that test visual organization abilities, learning, recall, and recognition of information. Complex (abstract) figure recall tasks have considerable clinical utility for the assessment of visual-spatial skills. Most tasks require an initial copy of the figure followed by immediate, delayed, and recognition conditions. During the copy administration, the clinician can observe the patient's ability to organize visual information and their visual construction skills. Patients who, during the copy administration, demonstrate difficulty grasping the general organizational theme of the figure predictably

will have difficulty recalling information during the immediate and recall conditions. Patients with TBI often copy figures using a piecemeal approach because of difficulty processing complex multiple pieces of information at once (Lezak, 1995).

Most patients will demonstrate similar immediate and delayed recall performance of abstract figures unless they experience pronounced forgetting (Lezak et al., 2004). Furthermore, subgroups of patients with perceptual problems may perform better during the recall conditions than the copy administration because of delayed perceptual organization skills.

As mentioned previously, pictorial stimuli of familiar objects are considered verbal tasks because humans assign verbal labels to photos. However, presentation and subsequent recall of unfamiliar faces have a higher probability of escaping verbal encoding and are typically used in visual-spatial memory testing. It has been demonstrated that some individuals will use verbal encoding strategies to organize perceptual features of objects (Constantinidou & Kreimer, 2004) and unfamiliar faces. However, damage in the posterior right hemispheres can result in difficulty in remembering faces, and this difficulty is characteristic of patients with right hemisphere focal lesions.

Spatial span tasks typically incorporate memory for location in a two- or three-dimensional space. The number of items to recall gradually increases until the spatial span capacity is reached (typically five to nine items). Like its verbal counterpart (i.e., the digit span), spatial paradigms should incorporate backward recall because it requires manipulation of information and engages the executive mechanisms of working memory. Spatial navigation paradigms involve route finding or mental rotation paradigms in a three-dimensional space.

Memory assessment typically includes immediate recall to determine span capacity and learning performance. A 20- to 30-minute delayed recall will provide information about the patient's ability to transfer newly acquired information into long-term memory, thus making predictions regarding learning and storage capacity. Delayed recall paradigms typically involve free recall and recognition performance. Patients with difficulty in actively retrieving information have poorer free recall scores than recognition scores. However, if information has not been transferred into long-term storage, then recognition performance will also be affected.

Contextual Assessment of Memory.

In addition to test performance on the aforementioned formal tasks, clinicians should consider the WHO-ICF framework and obtain information on how the patient performs in different contexts. Central to the WHO-ICF model is the interaction between the health condition that results in impairment in certain body functions and structures and how that condition and impairment can affect the execution of activity required for participation in meaningful tasks and roles. The model stresses the contribution of contextual factors, such as the environment (i.e., support services, environmental adaptations) and personal factors (i.e., patient motivation, coping mechanisms, and psychosocial functioning) that can contribute to the individual's ability to engage in social, educational, and vocational activities. The intimate interplay between contextual and health factors contributes to differences among patients in levels of activity and participation and resulting disability (Constantinidou & Kennedy, 2022; WHO, 2001).

Structured questionnaires such as the Everyday Memory Questionnaire–Revised (EMQ-R; Royle & Lincoln, 2008) with good psychometric properties provide a liable tool of subjective memory deficits and can complement formal clinical tests. Results from above testing should be interpreted in relation to the patient's sensory difficulties (i.e., visual acuity, hearing adequacy) (Shaughnessy, 2019), influences by intellectual level and educational effects (Brooks et al., 2011), but also effects from deficits in other cognitive functions such as attention and executive function. Specifically considering the interplay between memory and executive functions, questionnaires such as the Dysexecutive Questionnaire–Revised (DEX-R; Simblett et al., 2017) and the Behavior Rating Inventory of Executive Function (BRIEF; Gioia et al., 2000) can provide information about the patient's functioning and goal-directed behavior during everyday activities. The latter provide the opportunity for an informant to provide information regarding the patient's performance. Discrepancies between the informant rating and the patient ratings offer information on self-awareness deficits. Using the DEX, self-awareness deficits were evident in young adults with chronic TBI at 5.5 years postinjury in the Social and Self-Regulation and Motivation and Attention domains (Pettemeridou et al., 2020).

Screening Tools

A final consideration in regards to memory testing is recognizing that long testing times might contribute further to attentional difficulties. Intercorrelations between sustained attention and WM have been reported (Kapa et al., 2017; Smolak et al., 2020). Long testing times have also been reported to affect patient motivation and increase fatigue and frustration in adults with neurogenic disorders (Mohapatra & Laures-Gore, 2021). Hence, screening tests can be used to obtain a global estimate of performance (Bulzacka et al., 2016; Fan et al., 2019; van Ool et al., 2018).

For these and other reasons, screenings have several advantages:

a. Brief and time efficient
b. Often tap on a wide array of cognitive processes
c. Easy to administer
d. Typically have good face validity
e. Often known to many disciplines such as the Folstein Mini Mental State Examination (MMSE; Folstein et al., 1975), the Montreal Cognitive Assessment (Nasreddine et al., 2005), the Ross Information Processing Assessment II (RIPA-II; Ross-Swain, 1996), or the Repeatable Battery of Assessment of Neuropsychological Status (RBANS; Randolph et al., 1998)

Clinicians should be cautioned that often patients with mild memory decline (as in the case of patients with amnestic mild cognitive impairment or mild TBI) may perform well on screening tests because these tools assess memory only crudely. Therefore, screening tools should not be used exclusively to make clinical decisions, and any interpretations should be made with caution (Mohapatra & Laures-Gore, 2021). The sensitivity of screening tools such as the MMSE improve when contextual information in the form of informant input is incorporated (Demetriou & Constantinidou, 2018). Patients who fail the screening or who are suspected of having memory decline should be administered comprehensive memory tests designed to assess and diagnose memory deficits.

Relating Memory Models to Memory Assessment

Memory assessment can be organized according to the systems of memory processes such as working memory versus long-term memory and types of memory, such as verbal versus nonverbal, declarative versus nondeclarative. Testing tasks may incorporate the following types of activities:

- Immediate Recall: The examinee is asked to spontaneously (i.e., without hints/cues) recall stimulus material immediately following presentation.
- Delayed Recall: The examinee is asked to spontaneously recall stimulus materials presented at an earlier time interval (i.e., 20 to 30 minutes).
- Recognition: Performance of examinee when asked to recognize target stimuli among distracter materials.
- Forced-Choice Recall: The examinee is read pairs of words and asked to choose the word from each pair that was from a specific list read previously. This task is helpful

in identifying those who simulate memory deficits.

Reiterating what was earlier stated, immediate recall should incorporate manipulation of information versus mere repetition of information to be considered a working memory task. Manipulation of information requires the involvement of the central executive system, which is an integral component of working memory. The type of stimulus (i.e., verbal or nonverbal) will determine as to whether the phonological or visual-spatial sketchpad is activated in the immediate recall task. Each of the above testing tasks assesses a different aspect of memory. Hence, memory assessment should incorporate all of them.

Specific Types of Memory Disorders

There are several types of memory disorders associated with different neuropathologies. Therefore, it is important for the clinician and the rehabilitation team in general to have a thorough understanding of how the brain pathology can affect cognition and memory abilities. Papanicolaou (2006) in the book, *The Amnesias*, discusses extensively the most common types of memory disorders associated with normal aging, dementia, limbic system damage, brain injury, acute confusional state, epilepsy, and psychiatric disorders. Most of these conditions involve anterograde and/or retrograde memory loss.

Anterograde amnesia (AA) refers to the difficulty learning and remembering new information/events after the onset of the memory loss. Most memory assessment procedures discussed in this chapter address anterograde memory. In contrast, retrograde amnesia (RA) refers to loss of information that occurred prior to the onset of the memory impairment. The length of RA typically decreases in patients with nondegenerative acquired brain conditions and prior memories fill the gaps. However, the most recent events (such as what happened minutes prior to the incident that caused brain injury) are vulnerable to RA effects in comparison to older events. The vulnerability of the events might be because their consolidation process was disrupted and information was not transferred into long-term memory. In contrast, patients with degenerative conditions such as AD initially don't demonstrate RA during the early phases of the disease. However, as the disease progresses, their RA worsens and patients have significant difficulty with autobiographical memory, remembering previous events, and recalling previously acquired knowledge.

Acquired brain injury often results in PTA. PTA includes the period of RA plus AA. The onset of RA is the last memory remembered prior to the injury; the end of AA is the point of complete return to continuous memory after the injury. The Galveston Orientation and Amnesia Test (GOAT; Levin et al., 1979) can be used to assess a patient's orientation during the acute and subacute stage. This can be administered several times during the day until recovery of orientation and PTA resolution is demonstrated (Levin et al., 1979). The duration of PTA is used as an indicator of brain injury severity along with other critical variables such as length of impaired conscious-ness, initial Glasgow Coma Scale score, presence of focal neurologic signs, and neuroimaging results.

The Role of Processes and Strategies in Memory Performance

The current view of the organization of memory and its processes has been developed in part from studies investigating focal lesions in humans and animals. However, certain neuropathologies such as TBI and AD cause diffuse neuronal disruption. Subsequently, multiple memory systems may be affected (Barak et al., 2013; Pettemeridou & Constantinidou, 2021).

Standardized memory testing provides quantitative information regarding the patient's memory performance. To interpret this information in a meaningful manner, clinicians should examine and consider memory strategies implemented by the patient during the various memory tasks. For example, early cognitive studies of memory formation focusing on the stage model argued that certain ways of organizing the to-be-remembered material led to more durable memory traces (Craik & Lockhart, 1972). Consequently, if the individual elaborated on the deeper meaning of items, emphasizing connections to already learned material or involving visual imagery (Paivio, 1971, 1976), those items would be less likely to be forgotten than items merely rehearsed by being recycled in the phonological loop. This idea of (elaboration) has been exploited in various prescriptions of strategies to improve memory

performance in cognitive rehabilitation (Crosson & Buenning, 1984; Goldstein et al., 1990; Levin, 1989; Wilson, 1987; Yubero et al., 2011).

Active elaboration clearly places demands on working memory, especially on executive control mechanisms (of the frontal lobes) responsible for the planning and sequencing of currently active mental operations. Patients with TBI may present normal immediate recall (suggesting an intact auditory span), but a passive learning style can interfere with their ability to implement effective strategies and acquire new words during supraspan tasks like the Auditory Verbal Learning Test (AVLT) (Constantinidou, 1998).

Studies incorporating demanding multitrial tasks such as the AVLT and the California Verbal Learning Test (CVLT) also demonstrated a decline in active memory processes secondary to brain injury (Constantinidou & Neils, 1995; Konstantinou et al., 2019; Lezak, 1995; Millis & Ricker, 1994). Furthermore, research with the CVLT and AVLT indicates that decreased memory performance could be due to inefficiency in guiding the retrieval process (Constantinidou, 1999), especially in the presence of right frontal lobe damage (Konstantinou et al., 2019; Nyberg et al., 1996) or due to aging (Blachstein et al., 2012). Difficulty in transferring of information from working memory to long-term memory (i.e., consolidation) can be disrupted by the appearance of distracting or interfering material (Waugh & Norman, 1965) as well as by failure to appropriately organize information. Patients with TBI seem to be most vulnerable to the debilitating effects of interference possibly due to insult to the frontal lobes, especially the left frontal (Konstantinou et al., 2016; Nyberg et al., 1996) or the medial temporal lobe areas (Konstantinou et al., 2016, 2019). Studies following TBI suggest that immediate recall (measured by span tasks) appears to be intact (Brooks, 1975; O'Donnell et al., 1988). However, when interference is imposed, memory performance is significantly affected, indicating difficulties in consolidating declarative information into long-term memory (Brooks, 1975; Constantinidou, 1999). Interference can be introduced in the form of a delay or in the form of a competing stimulus (O'Donnell et al., 1988). Even a 10-second delay between stimulus presentation and response has been reported to affect recall performance (Constantinidou & Prechel, 1996).

Research demonstrates that patients who don't apply active memory strategies tend to have a decreased rate of learning compared to normal subjects, and their ability to recognize information is superior to their free recall performance. In contrast, subgroups of patients who apply active memory typically show improvements in their working memory capacity (Constantinidou, 1999; Constantinidou & Neils, 1995; Spikman et al., 1995). Consequently, teaching patients how to implement active memory strategies may be a useful therapy approach to memory rehabilitation.

The ability to apply strategies that guide learning and recall of information has also been associated with the "cognitive reserve" (CR) hypothesis. According to the CR hypothesis, individuals with higher reserve can cope with brain pathology through some form of active compensatory strategy better than those with lower reserve. Thus, greater CR could allow indi-

viduals to cope better with the cognitive changes associated with aging or brain injury, by promoting more flexible usage of cognitive processes and implementation of new strategies (Brickman et al., 2011; Singh-Manoux et al., 2011). CR is not a unitary theoretical construct, and variables such as education, social and cognitive engagement, vocabulary knowledge, and reading abilities have been incorporated in latent model analyses in order to define it and determine its prognostic utility in rehabilitation (Giogkaraki et al., 2013; Levi et al., 2013). Giogkaraki et al. (2013) reported that higher levels of CR have a moderating role in reducing the direct negative effect of age on verbal episodic memory and on executive function in healthy aging. Consequently, in addition to injury or disease-specific characteristics, CR could be another parameter for consideration during patient rehabilitation.

Implications for Rehabilitation

To decide how to plan therapy goals and organize memory rehabilitation, the clinician needs to have a thorough understanding of the underlying brain pathology and its impact on overall cognition and health status. Most patients with neurologic conditions, who experience memory deficits, also demonstrate difficulties in other cognitive domains such as executive function, attention, categorization, and language. Furthermore, psychosocial functioning and psychological well-being needs to be taken into consideration as symptoms of anxiety and depression can be evident in a variety of patients with chronic brain conditions (Stavrinides et al., 2012). Patients with documented memory decline report feelings of anxiety and frustration during social encounters (Radford et al., 2012). Hence, it is imperative to obtain complete information regarding the patient's history and neuropsychological status for effective management and treatment planning.

Memory rehabilitation and, more extensively, cognitive rehabilitation fall under two primary categories: restorative and compensatory (Cumming et al., 2013). Restorative rehabilitation is based on neuroanatomic and neurophysiologic models of learning, suggesting that neuronal growth and synaptogenesis result directly from repeated exposure and repetition of stimulation through experience (Squire, 1987), underpinned by the notions of neuroplasticity (Spreij et al., 2014). Consequently, cognitive training potentially could lead to the development of new neuronal networks, which could facilitate reorganization of partially damaged systems, reduce cognitive impairment, and improve function (Constantinidou et al., 2004).

An increasing body of evidence supports the use of memory retraining (see systematic reviews by Cicerone et al., 2005, 2011, 2019). Memory therapy focusing on restorative principles incorporates a variety of methodologies such as attention training, semantic organization and association, rehearsal techniques, chunking and rhyming strategies, and organization strategies such as wh-questions. Studies with patients who sustained moderate severe brain injuries and had difficulty organizing incoming information demonstrated that participants were able to learn how to implement strategies or to follow external organizational schemes. Training activities that incorporate self-regulation, organize incoming information, and require allocation of attentional resources to a task train the central executive system of working memory (Crosson et al., 1993; Goldstein et al., 1990; Kennedy & Krause, 2011).

Such restorative approaches can be delivered in the form of computerized cognitive training (CCT). CCT can be easily accessible and convenient for home use (Sigmundsdottir et al., 2016). However, the ability to generalize to new skills and the overly repetitive nature of the tasks can limit their ecological validity. The use of complex virtual reality (VR) presented using immersive devices has also offered promise. However, there is not enough evidence yet to draw definite conclusions as to the advantages of immersive VR over nonimmersive technology (Plechata et al., 2021) or to its generalization effectiveness. Finally, the use of noninvasive brain stimulation methodologies using transcranial magnetic stimulation (TMS) or transcranial direct current stimulation (tDCS) as add-on methodologies have some promising results (Lofitou et al., 2023; Traikapi et al., 2022). We expect that in the next 5 years, there will be a proliferation of research demonstrating their effectiveness and utility in conjunction with more conventional neurobehavioral treatments.

Further, recent reviews of the literature support that semantic processing supports episodic memory (Lepping et al., 2015; Nelson et al., 2013; Paterno et al., 2017). The Intensive Semantic Memory Treatment (ISMT) (D'Angelo et al., 2021) involves asking participants to find meaningful connections among diverse concepts represented by sets of two to three words. The researchers provided this focused semantic treatment in addition to the traditional episodic memory intervention and reported significant differences between pre- and posttest performance on cognitive domains such as episodic and semantic memory but also attention.

On the other side of the spectrum, the compensatory rehabilitation approach operates under the assumption that some functions cannot be recovered or restored completely. Therefore, the patient needs to use specific strategies to improve functional performance and reduce the impact of this impairment without relying on the restoration of the damaged neurocognitive systems (Coelho et al., 1996; Kennedy & Coelho, 2005). Specific strategies may include internal (O'Neil-Pirozzi et al., 2016) and/or external (de Joode et al., 2010) strategies. The restorative and compensatory approaches, where appropriate, could be used together in memory rehabilitation to maximize performance (Constantinidou & Thomas, 2017). Compensatory strategies, including environmental modifications, are also implemented in the acute management of sports concussion, where formal cognitive treatment is typically not warranted for the majority of the cases. The acute phases of the injury, concentration, learning, and retention deficits are prominent for several days, and the patient's improvement is closely monitored by an interdisciplinary team (Knollman-Porter et al., 2019). Environmental modifications and use of external memory aids are especially useful during the first weeks of the recovery process. They are also useful in facilitating memory functioning in healthy older adults and in adults with Mild Cognitive

Impairment (MCI) as part of a multidimensional group program (Chadjikyprianou & Constantinidou, 2022).

Patients with severe memory impairment benefit more from external memory aids and alerting devices for activities of daily living, if they receive extensive training for the use of the strategy/device (Cicerone et al., 2005, 2011). Specific external memory strategies such as the implementation of a memory notebook or a smartphone may be beneficial for everyday (or prospective) memory functions such as remembering important dates and appointments (McDonald et al., 2011; Sohlberg & Mateer, 1989; Wilson et al., 2013). Furthermore, patients with moderate severe TBI, as well as normal older adults with memory decline due to normal aging, benefit from pictorial presentation of verbal material rather than auditory presentation of information alone (Constantinidou & Baker, 2002; Constantinidou et al., 1996). Hence, the type of stimulus presentation modality may affect learning and recall, with the pictorial modality resulting in better recall and recognition performance.

Regardless of the method used, a key component to establishing consistent and effective use of compensatory strategies includes self-awareness training and the use of strategies to solve functional problems. In other words, the patient needs to "buy in" to the functional utility of the strategy (Armstrong et al., 2012). Patients with extensive neurologic involvement and executive functioning deficits demonstrate difficulty transferring new knowledge acquired in therapy to novel situations. In these patients, domain-specific treatment of memory may be a successful therapy method. Domain-specific therapy is designed to meet the needs of a given task or activity (hence the term "domain"). Its success may be attributed to the fact that it incorporates procedural memory, repetition, and routine building (Glisky, 1992; Parente & Anderson-Parente, 1989), which is less affected by cortical disease or injury. The following case study illustrates this approach to managing difficulties associated with memory decline.

Nondeclarative memory tends to be more resistive to several types of cortical brain pathology as compared to declarative memory. However, the application of newly learned skills to novel situations and problems likely will be unsuccessful as it requires declarative knowledge of strategies, as well as intact executive abilities (Malec, 1996), frequently impaired in the dementias, TBI, and frontal lobe pathology (Stuss, 2011).

There has been a great deal of emphasis in recent years, for the early and timely diagnosis of pathologic aging (i.e., mild cognitive impairment) and dementia. Interestingly, in a large cohort study, older adults were aware of their memory deficits before their informants, as evidenced by significant differences in the memory factor of the DEX (Demetriadou et al., 2018). The benefit of early detection relates to the notion that, during the early stages of the disease, therapy can benefit from the relatively intact nondeclarative system and help the patient implement strategies to maximize independence. Furthermore, in a small unpublished study, patients with MCI were able to learn new strategies to support categorization abilities (Constantinidou & Nikou, 2014). Through the Categorization Program, which was originally designed to remediate cognitive deficits in patients with TBI (Constantini-

dou et al., 2008), patients were able to demonstrate learning as measured by improvement on a variety of hierarchical categorization tasks. Strategies such as repetition, errorless learning, and cued recall were instrumental to the learning process, and outcomes indicate that declarative learning is possible even during amnestic MCI.

Compensatory strategies, in order to be effective, require sufficient self-awareness. Metacognitive skills training can facilitate self-awareness and strategy use (Fleming et al., 2022). Concepts such as metacognition and metamemory are used in the rehabilitation literature referring to the individual's ability for self-awareness regarding their cognitive and memory abilities. These functions are developed through experience and rely heavily on executive abilities and frontal lobe networks. Patients who have difficulty in this area may not be aware of their deficits and subsequently may see no need for rehabilitation or implementation of strategies discussed during therapy. Patients who are able to benefit from increased self-awareness training can learn about the nature of their memory problem and how specific strategies implemented in therapy can improve memory functioning. Furthermore, therapy may incorporate metamemory training to help patients predict their performance on certain tasks (Sohlberg & Mateer, 2001). Improvement of self-awareness has been linked to rehabilitation success (Armstrong et al., 2012; Kennedy & Coehlo, 2005; Kennedy & Krause, 2011), improved psychosocial integration (Fleming et al., 2022), and quality of life (Pettemeridou & Constantinidou, 2021). It is based on the expectation that the patient assumes greater responsibility for their deficits and implements strategies to facilitate effective performance (Constantinidou & Kennedy, 2022).

A final remark regarding interventions relating to memory is to pay attention and not disregard the systemic factors that affect this ability. An abundance of research increasingly highlights the importance of sleep quality and quantity as it relates to patients' memory and learning abilities (Antony & Paller, 2017; Batterink & Paller, 2017; Morrow & Duff, 2020) but also in general the role of sleep in health and wellness (McAlpine et al., 2019; Tall & Jelic, 2019).

Case Study: Patient With Mild Cognitive Impairment

Mr. SS is a retired 78-year-old engineer with 18 years of education (BA and MSc degrees). He is a native of Cyprus and attended university in Greece. He worked for 40 years in a private company as a survey engineer and retired at age 65. About 3 years prior to the evaluation, he began noticing "memory lapses." He described them as episodes of forgetting various events during the day (including conversations) and misplacing things or forgetting to do important tasks to the extent that he was feeling worried. Forgetting names of familiar people and word-finding problems during conversation were also frequent phenomena. He was a veteran of the Cypriot independence struggle (1955–1959) and enjoyed reading history books and attending various lectures on the same matter. He reported having trouble retaining information he read and found himself rereading information to retain it. These difficulties affected his quality of life, but he

attributed them to getting older. Mr. SS belongs to a retirement club whose members participate in the Neurocognitive Study for Aging (NEUROAGE). NEUROAGE is a longitudinal study on aging in Cyprus, established in 2009 to examine health, demographic, and biological factors contributing to cognitive aging in Greek Cypriot participants (Constantinidou et al., 2012). The study has a rolling admission process (e.g., participants can enter the study at any time), and NEUROAGE participants are assessed at baseline and subsequently followed every 2 years. Participants whose performance deviates from the expected ranges for age and education are followed up further and are referred for medical and rehabilitation services.

Assessment Battery and Procedures

Mr. SS volunteered to participate in the NEUROAGE project. Testing was conducted at the Center for Applied Neuroscience, University of Cyprus, which is the host organization for the project. The project incorporates the following battery of tests to assess key areas of impairment and function following the WHO-ICF model. All tests have been adapted in Greek and have been used in prior research by our team. Following are the measures organized in domains.

1. Cognitive screening: MMSE (Fountoulakis et al., 2000)
2. Attention/concentration: The Greek version of Trail Making Test A (also processing speed), Digit Span Forward and Backward (Wechsler Memory Scale III [WMS-III]), and Visual Span

Forward and Backward (WMS-III)
(Wechsler, 1997)

3. Working memory: Rey Complex
Figure Test—recall and recognition (Myers & Myers, 1995), Greek
version of the Hopkins

4. Verbal learning test (HVLT; Benedict et al., 1998; adapted in Greek,
see Giogkaraki et al., 2013) and
Greek Story Recall (Immediate
and Delayed) (Constantinidou &
Ioannou, 2008)

5. Executive function: Copy administration of the Rey Complex
Figure, Symbol Digits Modalities Test (Smith, 1982), Control
Oral Word Association (COWAT;
Kosmidis et al., 2004), Greek
version of the Trail Making Test
B (Zalonis et al., 2008), and Greek
version of the Dysexecutive
Questionnaire from the Behavioral Assessment of Dysexecutive

Syndrome (BADS) (Demetriadou
et al., 2018)

6. Language: Greek version of the
Boston Naming Test (Simos et
al., 2011), short version of the
Peabody Picture Vocabulary Test
(Simos et al., 2011), and word
reading and pseudowords (Simos
et al., 2013)

7. Greek version of Quality of Life &
Outcome Measures: WHOQOL-
BREF (Ginieri-Coccossis et al., 2011)

8. Psychosocial measures: Geriatric
Depression Scale (Fountoulakis
et al., 1999)

Test Results

Raw scores were converted to z scores
according to age and years of education. As indicated in Figure 2–2, Mr.
SS performed at the mean or above the

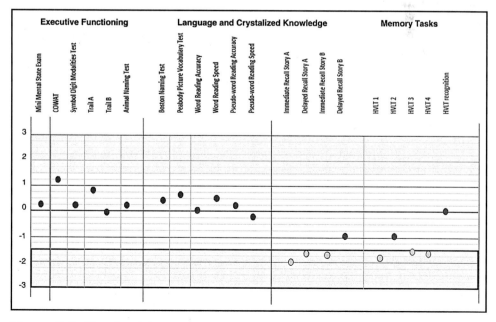

Figure 2–2. The plot of the test scores converted as z scores. Performance on the MMSE and on executive, language, and memory domains. Fluctuations between + or – 1 z score is considered within the average range for age and educational level.

mean on all measures, with the exception of the learning trials and delayed recall on the HVLT and the immediate and delayed recall of the story recall tasks. Notably, his performance (score of 28) on the general screening test (MMSE) was well within the normal range. From a psychosocial perspective, he did not report elevated depression symptomatology that could explain the presenting cognitive symptoms. Performance on the DEX did not indicate discrepancies with the scores assigned by his informant, and no meaningful changes were noted in executive functioning. Notably, the patient noticed more cognitive changes than his son, who provided the informant rating. The objective measures of the test battery in conjunction with his subjective measures of memory difficulties indicate that Mr. SS's performance is consistent with amnestic MCI. Figure 2–2 is the plot of the test scores converted as z scores.

Recommendations

The patient was referred to the collaborating neurologist for a medical evaluation, which included a clinical examination, an imaging study, and laboratory workup. Medical etiologies for cognitive decline were excluded. MRI findings were negative other than mild hyperintensities in the deep white matter (classification: Fazekas grade 1, punctuate foci of ischemic nature), associated with vascular changes, a finding that is not uncommon in older adults. Fazekas grade of 2 or 3 is associated with pathological aging or vascular dementia. Furthermore, the patient had no history of cardiovascular risk

factors, including hyperlipidemia or diabetes. Family history was negative for dementia. The confirmed diagnosis was amnestic MCI.

Neurocognitive Treatment

The short-term goals of treatment were (a) to implement the systematic use of compensatory strategies to facilitate memory performance and (b) to improve neurocognitive functioning through systematic remedial neurocognitive training with the Categorization Program. The long-term objective was to help the patient remain at a high functioning level and delay further neurocognitive decline through the use of strategies that would maintain instrumental activities of daily living and participation.

The patient was enrolled in neurocognitive treatment two times per week, which included psychoeducational training on cognitive decline and the implementation of memory strategies in order to help Mr. SS compensate for his deficits. Memory strategies included the use of a planner and smartphone for prospective memory tasks with reminders and establishment of procedures that could ensure successful implementation of the strategies. For example, the patient would generate a daily "to-do" list before dinnertime and would review the information every morning at breakfast. In addition, he was trained on the use of wh-questions during reading as well as implementing note taking of important names and characters for longer text. Domain-specific strategies were also implemented to manage memory difficulties and improve recall for content relevant to his hobby, reading and attending lectures about history.

Hierarchical neurocognitive training was implemented with the Categorization Program (CP; Constantinidou et al., 2008). The CP is a rigorous systematic, hierarchical, eight-level program initially designed as a restorative cognitive rehabilitation program in adults with acquired brain injury. Initial research findings (Constantinidou et al., 2005) and a subsequent randomized controlled trial (Constantinidou et al., 2008) indicate that the CP is an effective therapy tool for adults with brain injury who exhibit categorization deficits. In a small unpublished study with older adults with MCI, the CP was also found effective in improving cognitive performance. The CP was found effective in healthy older adults, who were also able to maintain their gains for up to 4 months posttraining (Constantinidou, 2019). Following are the active ingredients of the CP:

- The CP addresses both aspects of categorization, novel category learning, and categorization of established concepts or categories. It incorporates concrete visual stimuli and gradually progresses into abstract concepts through the use of repetition, cueing, and strategy building that facilitate learning.
- The CP was built using a very systematic hierarchical structure that corresponds to the neurodevelopmental categorization and cognitive processes hierarchy.
- Tasks gradually increase in difficulty and cognitive abstraction. CP tasks begin with basic feature identification and feature extraction (such as color, shape, and size) and

progress to higher levels of concept formation and abstraction (such as rule-based decision-making).
- The program integrates cognitive processes such as executive skills, attention, organization, conceptual reasoning, linguistic flexibility, and explicit memory for the completion of the categorization tasks.
- The redundancy and the repetition integrated in each level, along with the extensive cueing systems and errorless learning principles, provide support and organization for participants with more passive learning styles. The program provides a standardized approach to categorization training, yet it incorporates mastery criteria for each level in order to account for individual differences.

Treatment Duration

Twelve weeks per three times per week at 60 minutes. One time was devoted to memory strategies and other two times to the CP training.

Treatment Outcome Measures

Memory log of memory difficulties prior to treatment and during treatment. Log of use of strategies during targeted activities (e.g., reading, attending lectures). In addition, the CP training included three tests measuring change in skills learning during the training administered at baseline and at the end of the 12-week training and four probe tasks designed to test generalizability of performance. For a more in-depth discussion of the training and dependent measures, the reader is referred to Constantinidou et al. (2008).

Treatment Results

Mr. SS demonstrated systematic usage of memory strategies on 80% of targeted tasks. In addition, he reported reduction in daily memory difficulties by 30%. He completed the CP training and demonstrated gains in the three CP tests by 30%. In addition, his performance on the CP probe tasks consistently improved from baseline (score 18/30) to 20/30, 24/30, and 26/30 for the subsequent administrations.

Conclusions

Neurocognitive treatment for Mr. SS incorporated compensatory memory strategies and hierarchical cognitive retraining. Treatment captured intact procedural memory to establish routines that incorporated the memory strategies. The patient was highly motivated and aware of his deficits as demonstrated by performance on the tests and during treatment. Consequently, his engagement and eagerness to improve was a significant key ingredient to treatment success. This case also illustrates the value of including domain-specific tests in our assessment strategy. In relationship with the memory model incorporated in this chapter, had we relied on the cognitive screening of the MMSE, we would have missed the memory impairment demonstrated by performance on verbal learning (HVLT) and story recall tasks.

for the acquisition of important cognitive functions such as language, reasoning, and problem solving. Research and clinical experience indicate that most brain pathologies will disrupt the efficiency of memory networks. The extent of disruption and its impact on social and professional activities will depend on the severity of the memory impairment and how this impairment can interfere with participation in social, educational, and vocational activities (see ICF model; WHO, 2001).

Memory abilities are interdependent with other cognitive skills such as attention and executive functioning. In fact, the multiple systems model of memory incorporates a central executive control system that coordinates the function of two subslave systems (phonological loop and visuospatial sketchpad). Hence, disruption in the efficiency of this multiple-system network can result in difficulty acquiring new information as in anterograde amnesia.

Comprehensive memory assessment is an integral component of cognitive and neuropsychological assessment. Test results along with information regarding the patient's overall cognitive and psychosocial status, personal/professional goals, and overall health should be taken into consideration to make an accurate diagnosis, determine prognosis, and develop an effective management plan to maximize the patient's level of functioning and participation.

Chapter Conclusions

The ability to acquire new information and recall it later is an important cognitive ability necessary for survival and

References

Altuna, M., Sánchez-Saudinós, M. B., & Lleó, A. (2021). Cognitive symptoms after COVID-19. *Neurology Perspectives,* *1,* S16–S24.

Antony, J. W., & Paller, K. A. (2017). Hippocampal contributions to declarative memory consolidation during sleep. In D. E. Hannula & M. C. Duff (Eds.), *The hippocampus from cells to systems* (pp. 245–280). Springer.

Armstrong, J., McPherson, K., & Nayar, S. (2012). External memory aid training after traumatic brain injury: 'Making it real.' *British Journal of Occupational Therapy,* *75*(12), 541–548.

Ashby, F. G., & Waldron, F. G. (2000). The neuropsychological basis of category learning. *Current Directions in Psychological Science,* *9,* 10–14.

Atkinson, R. C., & Shiffrin, R. M. (1968). Human memory: A proposed system and its control processes. In K. W. Spence & J. T. Spence (Eds.), *The psychology of learning and motivation* (Vol. 2, pp. 89–195). Academic Press.

Baddeley, A. D. (1986). *Working memory.* Oxford University Press.

Baddeley, A. D. (1995). Working memory. In M. S. Gazzaniga (Ed.), *The cognitive neurosciences* (pp. 755–764). MIT Press.

Baddeley, A. D. (2000). The episodic buffer: A new component of working memory? *Trends in Cognitive Sciences,* *4,* 417–423.

Baddeley, A. D. (2001). Is working memory still working? *American Psychologist,* *56*(11), 851–864.

Baddeley, A. D. (2003). Working memory and language: An overview. *Journal of Communication Disorders,* *36,* 189–208.

Baddeley, A. D. (2021). Developing the concept of working memory: The role of neuropsychology. *Archives of Clinical Neuropsychology,* *36,* 861–873.

Baddeley, A. D., Allen, R. J., & Hitch, G. J. (2011). Binding in visual working memory: The role of the episodic buffer. *Neuropsychologia,* *49*(6), 1393–1400.

Baddeley, A. D., & Hitch, G. (1974). Working memory. In G. A. Bower (Ed.), *The psychology of learning and motivation* (Vol. 18, pp. 47–89). Academic Press.

Baddeley, A. D., Hitch, G. J., & Allen, R. J. (2019). From short-term store to multicomponent working memory: The role of the modal model. *Memory & Cognition,* *47,* 575–588.

Baddeley, A. D., Hitch, G. J., & Allen, R. J. (2020). A multicomponent model of working memory. In R. H. Logie, V. Camos, & N. Cowan (Eds.), *Working memory: State of the science* (pp. 10–240). Oxford University Press.

Baddeley, A. D., Papagno, C., & Vallar, C. (1988). When long-term learning depends on short-term storage. *Journal of Memory and Language,* *27,* 586–595.

Barak, O., Vakil, E., & Levy, D. A. (2013). Environmental context effects on episodic memory are dependent on retrieval mode and modulated by neuropsychological status. *Quarterly Journal of Experimental Psychology,* *66*(10), 2008–2022.

Batterink, L. J., & Paller, K. A. (2017). Sleep-based memory processing facilitates grammatical generalization: Evidence from targeted memory reactivation. *Brain and Language,* *167,* 83–93.

Beauregard, M., Gold, D., Evans, A. C., & Chertkow, H. (1998). A role for the hippocampal formation in implicit memory: A 3-D PET study. *NeuroReport,* *9,* 1867–1873.

Behnken, A., Schöning, S., Gerß, J., Konrad, C., de Jong-Meyer, R., Zwanzger, P., & Arolt, V. (2010). Persistent non-verbal memory impairment in remitted major depression—Caused by encoding deficits? *Journal of Affective Disorders,* *122*(1), 144–148.

Benedict, R. H. B., Schretlen, D., Groninger, L., & Brandt, J. (1998). Hopkins Verbal Learning Test–Revised: Normative data and analysis of inter-form and test-retest reliability. *Clinical Neuropsychologist,* *12,* 43–55.

Biederman, I., & Cooper, E. E. (1991). Priming contour-deleted images: Evidence for intermediate representations in visual object recognition. *Cognitive Psychology,* *23,* 393–419.

Blachstein, H., Greenstein, Y., & Vakil, E. (2012). Aging and temporal order memory: A comparison of direct and indirect measures. *Journal of Clinical and Experimental Neuropsychology, 34*(1), 107–112.

Brickman, A. M., Siedlecki, K. L., Muraskin, J., Manly, J. J., Luchsinger, J. A., Yeung, L. K., . . . Stern, Y. (2011). White matter hyperintensities and cognition: Testing the reserve hypothesis. *Neurobiology of Aging, 32*(9), 1588–1598.

Brooks, B. L., Holdnack, J. A., & Iverson, G. L. (2011). Advanced clinical interpretation of the WAIS-IV and WMS-IV: Revalence of low scores varies by level of intelligence and years of education. *Assessment, 18*, 156–167.

Brooks, D. N. (1975). Long-term and short-term memory in head injured patients. *Cortex, 11*, 329–340.

Brown, J. A. (1958). Some tests of the decay theory of immediate memory. *Quarterly Journal of Experimental Psychology, 10*, 12–21.

Bulzacka, E., Meyers, J. E., Boyer, L., Le Gloaec, T., Fond, G., Szoke, A., Leboyer, M., & Schurhoff, F. (2016). WAIS-IV seven-subtest short form: Validity and clinical use in schizophrenia. *Archives of Clinical Neuropsychology, 31*, 915–925.

Cave, C. B., & Squire, L. S. (1992). Intact and long-lasting repetition priming in amnesia. *Journal of Experimental Psychology: Learning, Memory, and Cognition, 18*, 509–520.

Chadjikyprianou, A., & Constantinidou, F. (2022). Results from the "Healthy Mind" Intervention Program. *Archives of Physical Medicine and Rehabilitation, 103*, e79–e80.

Chadjikyprianou, A., Hadjivassiliou, M., Papacostas, S., & Constantinidou, F. (2021). The neurocognitive study for the aging: Longitudinal analysis on the contribution of sex, age, education and APOE ε4 on cognitive performance. *Frontiers in Genetics, 12*, 1179.

Christoforou, C., Constantinidou, F., Shoshilou, P., & Simos, P. G. (2013). Single-trial linear correlation analysis: Application to characterization of stimulus modality effects. *Frontiers in Computational Neuroscience, 7*, 15.

Cicerone, K. D., Dahlberg, C., Malec, J. F., Langenbahn, D. M., Felicetti, T., Kneipp, S., . . . Catanese, J. (2005). Evidence-based cognitive rehabilitation: Updated review of the literature from 1998 through 2002. *Archives of Physical Medicine and Rehabilitation, 86*, 1681–1692.

Cicerone, K. D., Goldin, Y., Ganci, K., Rosenbaum, A., Wethe, J. V., Langenbahn, D. M., . . . Trexler, L. (2019). Evidence-based cognitive rehabilitation: Systematic review of the literature from 2009 through 2014. *Archives of Physical Medicine and Rehabilitation, 100*(8), 1515–1533.

Cicerone, K. D., Langenbahn, D. M., Braden, C., Malec, J. F., Kalmar, K., Fraas, M., . . . Ashman, T. (2011). Evidence-based cognitive rehabilitation: Updated review of the literature from 2003 through 2008. *Archives of Physical Medicine and Rehabilitation, 92*(4), 519–530.

Cimadevilla, J. M., Roldan, L., Paris, M., Arnedo, M., & Roldan, S. (2014). Spatial learning in a virtual reality-based task is altered in very preterm children. *Journal of Clinical and Epxerimental Neuropsychology, 36*, 1002–1008.

Coelho, C. A., DeRuyter, F., & Stein, M. (1996). Treatment efficacy: Cognitive communicative disorders resulting from traumatic brain injury in adults. *Journal of Speech and Hearing Research, 39*, 5–17.

Colfesh, G. J. H., & Conway, A. R. A. (2007). Individual differences in working memory capacity and divided attention in dichotic listening. *Psychonomic Bulletin and Review, 14*, 699–703.

Constantinidou, F. (1998). Active memory strategies following moderate-to-severe head injury: In search of important components. *Hearsay, 12*(1), 20–26.

Constantinidou, F. (1999). The effects of stimulus modality on interference and recognition performance following brain injury. *Journal of Medical Speech-Language Pathology, 7*(4), 283–295.

Constantinidou, F. (2019). Effects of systematic categorization training on cognitive performance in healthy older adults and in adults with traumatic brain injury. *Behavioral Neurology, 2019*, 1–17, https://doi.org/10.1155/2019/9785319

Constantinidou, F., & Baker, S. (2002). Stimulus modality and verbal learning performance in normal aging. *Brain and Language, 82*(3), 296–311.

Constantinidou, F., Christodoulou, M., & Prokopiou, J. (2012). The effects of age and education on executive functioning and oral naming performance in Greek Cypriot adults: The Neurocognitive Study for the Aging. *Folia Phoniatrica et Logopaedica, 64*(4), 187–198.

Constantinidou, F., Danos, M. A., Nelson, D., & Baker, S. (2011). Effects of modality presentation on working memory in school-age children: Evidence for the pictorial superiority hypothesis. *Child Neuropsychology, 17*(2), 173–196.

Constantinidou, F., & Evripidou, C. (2012). Stimulus modality and working memory performance in Greek children with reading disabilities: Additional evidence for the pictorial superiority hypothesis. *Child Neuropsychology, 18*(3), 256–280.

Constantinidou, F., & Ioannou, M. (2008). The effects of age and language on paragraph recall performance: Findings from a preliminary cross-sectional study. *Psychologia, 15*, 342–361.

Constantinidou, F., & Kennedy, M. (2022). Traumatic brain injury. In P. Coppens & I. Papathanasiou (Eds.), *Aphasia and neurogenic communication disorders* (3rd ed., pp. 465–502). Jones & Bartlett Publishers.

Constantinidou, F., & Kreimer, L. T. (2004). Feature description and categorization of common objects after traumatic brain injury: The effects of a multi-trial paradigm. *Brain and Language, 89*(1), 216–225.

Constantinidou, F., & Neils, J. (1995). Stimulus modality and verbal learning in moderate to severe closed head injury. *Journal of Head Trauma Rehabilitation, 10*, 90–100.

Constantinidou, F., Neils, J., Bouman, D., Lee, L., & Shuren, J. (1996). Pictorial superiority during verbal learning tasks in moderate to severe closed head injury: Additional evidence. *Journal of General Psychology, 123*(3), 173–184.

Constantinidou, F., & Nikou, M. (2014, July). *Categorization training for persons with mild cognitive impairment: A feasibility study*. Oral presentation at the 11th Neuropsychological Rehabilitation Satellite Meeting, Limassol, Cyprus.

Constantinidou, F., & Prechel, D. (1996). *Is the initial memory span recovered following moderate to severe brain injury?* Unpublished manuscript, Miami University, Oxford, OH.

Constantinidou, F., & Thomas, R. D. (2017). Principles of cognitive rehabilitation in TBI: An integrative neuroscience approach. In M. Ashley & D. Hovda (Eds.), *Traumatic brain injury: Rehabilitation, treatment, and case management* (4th ed., pp. 513–540). Taylor & Francis: CRC Press.

Constantinidou, F., Thomas, R. D., & Best, P. (2004). Principles of cognitive rehabilitation: An integrative approach. In M. J. Ashley (Ed.), *Traumatic brain injury rehabilitation: Rehabilitative treatment and case management* (2nd ed., pp. 337–366). CRC Press.

Constantinidou, F., Thomas, R. D., & Robinson, L. (2008). Benefits of categorization training in patients with traumatic brain injury during post–acute rehabilitation: Additional evidence from a randomized controlled trial. *Journal of Head Trauma Rehabilitation, 23*(5), 312–328.

Constantinidou, F., Thomas, R. D., Scharp, V. L., Laske, K. M., Hammerly, M. D., & Guitonde, S. (2005). Effects of categorization training in patients with TBI during post acute rehabilitation: Preliminary findings. *Journal of Head Trauma Rehabilitation, 20*(2), 143–157.

Constantinidou, F., Wertheimer, J., Evans, C., Tsanadis, J., & Brown, D. (2012). Assessment of executive functioning in brain injury: Collaboration between speech-language pathology and neuropsychology for an integrative neuropsychological perspective. *Brain Injury*, 26(13–14), 1549–1563.

Constantinidou, F., Zaganas, I., Papastefanakis, E., Kasselimis, D., Nidos, A., & Simos, P. G. (2014). Age-related decline in verbal learning is moderated by demographic factors, working memory capacity, and presence of amnestic mild cognitive impairment. *Journal of the International Neuropsychological Society, 20*(8), 822–835. https://doi.org/10.1017/S1355 617714000678

Conway, A. R. A., Kane, M. J., Bunting, M. F., Hambrick, D. Z., Wilhelm, O., & Engle, R. V. (2005). Working memory span tasks: A methodological review and user's guide. Psychonomic. *Bulletin and Review, 12*, 769–786.

Craik, F. I. M., & Lockhart, R. S. (1972). Levels of processing: A framework for memory research. *Journal of Verbal Learning and Verbal Behavior, 11*, 671–684.

Crosson, B., & Buenning, W. (1984). An individualized memory retraining program after closed-head injury: A single-case study. *Journal of Clinical Neuropsychology, 6*(3), 287–301.

Crosson, B., Cooper, P. V., Lincoln, R. K., Bauer, R. M., & Velozo, C. A. (1993). Relationship between verbal memory and language performance after blunt head injury. *Clinical Neuropsychologist, 7*(3), 250–267.

Cumming, T. B., Marshall, R. S., & Lazar, R. M. (2013). Stroke, cognitive deficits, and rehabilitation: Still an incomplete picture. *International Journal of Stroke, 8*, 38–45.

D'Angelo, E. C., Ober, B. A., & Shenaut, G. K. (2021). Combined memory training: An approach for episodic memory deficits in traumatic brain injury. *American Journal of Speech-Language Pathology, 30*, 920–932.

de Joode, E., van Heugten, C., Verhey, F., & van Boxtel, M. (2010). Efficacy and usability of assistive technology for patients with cognitive deficits: A systematic review. *Clinical Rehabilitation, 24*, 701–714.

Demetriadou, M., Michaelides, M., Bateman, A., & Constantinidou, F. (2018). Measurement of everyday dysexecutive symptoms in normal aging with the Greek version of the Dysexecutive Questionnaire–Revised. *Neuropsychological Rehabilitation, 30*(6), 1024–1043. https://doi.org/10.1080/09602011.2018.1543127

Demetriou, F., & Constantinidou, F. (2018). The Greek version of AD8 informant interview: Data from the Neurocognitive Study on Aging (NEUROAGE). *Dialogues in Clinical Neuroscience & Mental Health, 1*(2), 31–35.

Doherty, J. M., & Logie, R. H. (2016). Resource-sharing in multiple-component working memory. *Memory & Cognition, 44*(8), 1157–1167.

Egeland, J. (2015). Measuring working memory with Digit Span and the Letter-Number Sequencing subtests from the WAIS-IV: Too low manipulation load and risk for underestimating modality effects. *Applied Neuropsychology: Adult, 22*(6), 445–451.

Ettenhofer, M. L., Gimbel, S. I., & Cordero, E. (2020). Clinical validation of an optimized multimodal neurocognitive assessment of chronic mild TBI. *Annals of Clinical and Translational Neurology, 7*, 507–516.

Ewert, J., Levin, H. S., Watson, M. G., & Kalisky, Z. (1989). Procedural memory during posttraumatic amnesia in survivors of severe closed head injury. *Archives of Neurology, 46*, 911–916.

Ezzyat, Y., Kragel, J. E., Burke, J. F., Levy, D. F., Lyalenko, A., Wanda, P., . . . Kahana, M. J. (2017). Direct brain stimulation modulates encoding states and memory performance in humans. *Current Biology, 27*, 1251–1258.

Fan, H. Z., Zhu, J. J., Wang, J., Cui, J. F., Chen, N., Yao, J., . . . Zou, Y. Z. (2019). Four subtest index based short form of WAIS-IV: Psychometric properties and clinical utility. *Archives of Clinical Neuropsychology, 34*, 81–88.

Farah, M. J. (1988). Is visual imagery really visual? Overlooked evidence from neuropsychology. *Psychological Review, 95*, 307–317.

Fleming, J., Ownsworth, T., Doig, E., Hogan, C., Hamilton, C., Swan, S., . . . Shum, D. (2022). Efficacy of prospective memory rehabilitation plus metacognitive skills training for adults with traumatic brain injury: A randomized controlled trial. *Neurorehabilitation and Neural Repair, 36*, 487–499.

Fletcher, P. C., Shallice, T., & Dolan, R. J. (1998). The functional roles of prefrontal cortex in episodic memory. I. Encoding. *Brain, 121*, 1239–1248.

Folstein, M. F., Folstein, S. E., & McHugh, P. R. (1975). "Mini-Mental Status": A practical method for grading the cognitive state of patients for the clinician. *Journal of Psychiatric Research, 12*(3), 189–198.

Forester, G., Kroneisen, M., Erdfelder, E., & Kamp, S.-M. (2020). Adaptive memory: Independent effects of survival processing and reward motivation on memory. *Frontiers in Human Neuroscience, 14*, 1–13.

Fountoulakis, K. N., Tsolaki, M., Chantzi, H., & Kazis, A. (2000). Mini Mental State Examination (MMSE): A validation study in Greece. *American Journal of Alzheimer's Disease and Other Dementias, 15*, 342–345.

Fountoulakis, K. N., Tsolaki, M., Iacovides, A., Yesavage, J., O'Hara, R., Kazis, A., & Ierodiakonou, C. (1999). The validation of the short form of Geriatric Depression Scale (GDS) in Greece. *Aging Clinical and Experimental Research, 11*, 367–372.

Gabrieli, J. D. E., Fleischman, D. A., Keane, M. M., Reminger, S. L., & Morel, F. (1995). Double dissociation between memory systems underlying explicit and implicit memory in the human brain. *Psychological Science, 6*, 76–82.

Gathercole, S., & Baddeley, A. D. (1990). Phonological memory deficits in language-disordered children: Is there a causal connection? *Journal of Memory and Language, 29*, 336–360.

Gathercole, S. E., Dunning, D. L., Holmes, J., & Norris, D. (2019). Working memory training involves learning new skills. *Journal of Memory and Language, 105*, 19–42.

Gazzaniga, M. S., Ivry, R. B., & Mangun, G. R. (1998). *Cognitive neuroscience: The biology of the mind*. W. W. Norton.

Ginieri-Coccossis, M., Triantafillou, E., Tomaras, V., Soldatos, C., Mavreas, V., & Christodoulou, G. (2011). Psychometric properties of WHOQOL-BREF in clinical and health Greek populations: Incorporating new culture-relevant items. *Psychiatrike, 23*(2), 130–142.

Giogkaraki, E., Michaelides, M., & Constantinidou, F. (2013). The role of cognitive reserve in cognitive aging: Results from the Neurocognitive Study on Aging. *Journal of Clinical and Experimental Neuropsychology, 35*(10), 1024–1035.

Gioia, G. A., Isquith, P. K., Guy, S. C., & Kenworthy, L. (2000). Test review behavior rating inventory of executive function. *Child Neuropsychology, 6*(3), 235–238.

Glisky, E. L. (1992). Computer-assisted instruction for patients with traumatic brain injury: Teaching of domain-specific knowledge. *Journal of Head Trauma Rehabilitation, 7*(3), 1–12.

Goldstein, F. C., Levin, H. S., Boake, C., & Lohrey, J. H. (1990). Facilitation of memory performance through induced semantic processing in survivors of severe closed-head injury. *Journal of Clinical and Experimental Neuropsychology, 12*(2), 286–300.

Gonen-Yaacovi, G., & Burgess, P. (2012). Prospective memory: The future for future intentions. *Psychologica Belgica, 52*, 2–3.

Graf, P., & Mandler, G. (1984). Activation makes words more accessible, but not necessarily more retrievable. *Journal of Verbal Learning and Verbal Behavior, 23*, 553–568.

Graf, P., Mandler, G., & Haden, P. (1982). Simulating amnesic symptoms in normal subjects. *Science, 218*, 1243–1244.

Graf, P., & Ryan, L. (1990). Transfer-appropriate processing for implicit and explicit memory. *Journal of Experimental Psychology: Learning, Memory, and Cognition, 16*, 978–992.

Ivanova, M. V., Dragoy, O., Kuptsova, S., Akinina, S. Y., Petrushevskii, A., Fedina, O., . . . Dronkers, N. (2018). Neural mechanisms of two different verbal working memory tasks: A VLSM study. *Neuropschologia, 115*, 25–41.

Jacoby, L. L., & Dallas, M. (1981). On the relationship between autobiographical memory and perceptual learning. *Journal of Experimental Psychology: General, 110*, 306–340.

Jacoby, L. L., & Hayman, C. A. G. (1987). Specific visual transfer in word identification. *Journal of Experimental Psychology: Learning, Memory and Cognition, 13*, 456–463.

Jacoby, L. L., & Witherspoon, D. (1982). Remembering without awareness. *Canadian Journal of Psychology, 32*, 300–324.

Jonides, J., Smith, E. E., Koeppe, R. A., Awh, E., Minoshima, S., & Mintun, M. A. (1993). Spatial working memory in humans as revealed by PET. *Nature, 363*, 623–625.

Kane, M. J., & Engle, R. W. (2002). The role of prefrontal cortex in working-memory capacity, executive attention, and general fluid intelligence: An individual-differences perspective. *Psychonomic Bulletin and Review, 9*, 637–671.

Kane, M. J., & Engle, R. W. (2003). Working-memory capacity and the control of attention: The contributions of goal neglect, response competition, and task set to Stroop interference. *Journal of Experimental Psychology: General, 132*, 47–70.

Kane, M. J., Hambrick, D. Z., Tuholski, S. W., Wilhelm, O., Payne, T. W., & Engle, R. W. (2004). The generality of working memory capacity: A latent variable approach to verbal and visuospatial memory span and reasoning. *Journal of Experimental Psychology: General, 133*, 189–217.

Kapa, L. L., Plante, E., & Doubleday, K. (2017). Applying an integrative framework of executive function to preschoolers with specific language impairment. *Journal of Speech, Language, and Hearing Research, 60*, 2170–2184.

Kennedy, M. R., & Coelho, C. (2005). Self-regulation after traumatic brain injury: A framework for intervention of memory and problem solving. *Strategies, Seminars in Speech and Language, 26*(4), 242–255.

Kennedy, M. R., & Krause, M. O. (2011). Self-regulated learning in a dynamic coaching model for supporting college students with traumatic brain injury: Two case reports. *Journal of Head Trauma Rehabilitation, 26*(3), 212–223.

Kennedy, M. R., Wozniak, J. R., Muetzel, R. L., Mueller, B. A., Chiou, H. H., Pantekoek, K., & Lim, K. O. (2009). White matter and neurocognitive changes in adults with chronic traumatic brain injury. *Journal of the International Neuropsychological Society, 15*(1), 130–136.

Kepinska, O., de Rover, M., & Caspers, J. (2018). Connectivity of the hippocampus and Broca's area during acquisition of a novel grammar. *Neuroimage, 165*, 1–10.

Knollman-Porter, K., Constantinidou, F., Beardslee, J., & Dailey, S. (2019). Multidisciplinary management of collegiate sports-related concussions. *Seminars in Speech & Language, 40*(1), 3–12.

Koenig, P., Smith, E. E., Troiani, V., Anderson, C., Moore, M., & Grossman, M. (2008). Medial temporal lobe involvement in an implicit memory task: Evidence of collaborating implicit and explicit memory systems from fMRI and Alzheimer's disease. *Cerebral Cortex, 18*(12), 2831–2843.

Konstantinou, N., Constantinidou, F., & Kanai, R. (2017). Discrete capacity limits and neuroanatomical correlates of visual short-term memory for objects and spatial locations. *Human Brain Mapping, 38*(2), 767–778.

Konstantinou, N., Pettemeridou, E., Seimenis, I., Eracleous, E., Papacostas, S. S., Papanicolaou, A. C., & Constantinidou, F. (2016). Assessing the relationship between neurocognitive performance and brain volume in chronic moderate-severe traumatic brain injury. *Frontiers in Neurology, 7*, 29.

Konstantinou, N., Pettemeridou, E., Stamatakis, E. A., Seimenis, I., & Constantinidou, F. (2019). Altered resting functional connectivity is related to cognitive outcome in males with moderate-severe TBI. *Frontiers in Neurology, 9*, 1163.

Kosmidis, M. C., Vlahou, C. H., Panagiotaki, P., & Kiosseoglou, G. (2004). The verbal fluency task in the Greek population: Normative data and clustering and switching strategies. *Journal of the International Neuropsychology Society, 10*, 164–172.

Lechner, H. A., Squire, L. R., & Byrne, J. H. (1999). 100 years of consolidation— Remembering Müller and Pilzecker. *Learning and Memory, 6*, 77–87.

Lee, J. K., Nordahl, C. W., Amaral, D. G., Lee, A., Solomon, M., & Ghetti, S. (2015). Assessing hippocampal development and language in early childhood: Evidence from a new application of the automatic segmentation adapter tool. *Human Brain Mapping, 36*, 4483–4496.

Lee, K. H., & Thompson, R. R. (2006). Multiple memory mechanisms in the cerebellum? *Neuron, 51*, 680–682.

Lepping, R. J., Brooks, W. M., Kirchhoff, B. A., Martin, L. E., Kurylo, M., Ladesich, L., . . . Savage, C. R. (2015). Effectiveness of semantic encoding strategy training after traumatic brain injury is correlated with frontal brain activation change. *International Journal of Physical Medicine & Rehabilitation, 3*, Article 254.

Levi, Y., Rassovsky, Y., Agranov, E., SelaKaufman, M., & Vakil, E. (2013). Cognitive reserve components as expressed in traumatic brain injury. *Journal of the International Neuropsychological Society, 19*(6), 664–671.

Levin, H. S. (1989). Memory deficit after closed-head injury. *Journal of Experimental Psychology, 12*(1), 95–103.

Levin, H. S., O'Donnell, V. M., & Grossman, R. G. (1979). The Galveston Orientation and Amnesia Test: A practical scale to assess cognition after head injury. *Journal of Nervous and Mental Disease, 167*, 675–684.

Lezak, M. D. (1983). *Neuropsychological assessment* (2nd ed.). Oxford University Press.

Lezak, M. D. (1995). *Neuropsychological assessment* (3rd ed.). Oxford University Press.

Lezak, M. D., Howieson, D. B., & Loring, D.W. (2004). *Neuropsychological assessment* (4th ed.). Oxford University Press.

Lofitou, K., Pettemeridou, E., & Constantinidou, F. (2023). Treatment of Awareness Deficits (ACESO): The application of tDCS on individuals with TBI and stroke. *Archives of Physical Medicine and Rehabilitation, 104*(3), e58.

Malec, J. F. (1996). Cognitive rehabilitation. In R. W. Evans (Ed.), *Neurology and trauma* (pp. 231–248). W. B. Saunders.

Manns, J. R., Hopkins, R. O., & Squire, L. (2003). Semantic memory and the human hippocampus. *Neuron, 38*, 127–133.

Markowitsch, H. J. (1995). Anatomical basis of memory disorders. In M. S. Gazzaniga (Ed.), *The cognitive neurosciences* (pp. 765–779). MIT Press.

Mayer, J. F., & Murray, L. L. (2012). Measuring working memory deficits in aphasia. *Journal of Communication Disorders, 45*, 325–339.

McAlpine, C. S., Kiss, M. G., Rattik, S., He, S., Vassalli, A., Valet, C., . . . Swirski, F. K. (2019). Sleep modulates hematopoiesis and protects against atherosclerosis. *Nature, 566*(7744), 383–387.

McDonald, A., Haslam, C., Yates, P., Gurr, B., Leeder, G., & Sayers, A. (2011). Google calendar: A new memory aid to compensate for prospective memory deficits following acquired brain injury. *Neuropsychological Rehabilitation, 21*(6), 784–807.

McGaugh, J. L. (2000). Memory: A century of consolidation. *Science, 287*, 248–251.

Metzler-Baddeley, C., Hunt, S., Jones, D. K., Leemans, A., Aggleton, J. P., & O'Sullivan, M. J. (2012). Temporal association tracts and the breakdown of episodic memory in mild cognitive impairment. *Neurology, 79*(23), 2233–2240.

Milner, B. (1966). Amnesia following operation on the temporal lobes. In C. W. M. Whitty & O. L. Zangwill (Eds.), *Amnesia* (pp. 109–133). Butterworth.

Millis, S. R., & Ricker, J. H. (1994). Verbal learning patterns in moderate and severe traumatic brain injury. *Journal of Clinical and Experimental Neuropsychology, 16,* 498–507.

Mohapatra, B., & Laures-Gore, J. (2021). Moving toward accurate assessment of working memory in adults with neurogenically based communication disorders. *American Journal of Speech-Language Pathology, 1044,* 1–9.

Morrow, E. L., & Duff, M. C. (2020). Sleep supports memory and learning: Implications for clinical practice in speech language pathology. *American Journal of Speech-Language Pathology, 29,* 577–585.

Myers, J. E., & Meyers, K. R. (1995). *Rey Complex Figure Test and Recognition Trial.* Psychological Assessment Resources.

Nasreddine, Z. S., Phillips, N. A., Bédirian, V., Charbonneau, S., Whitehead, V., Collin, I., & Chertkow, H. (2005). The Montreal Cognitive Assessment, MoCA: A brief screening tool for mild cognitive impairment. *Journal of the American Geriatrics Society, 53*(4), 695–699.

Nelson, D. L., Kitto, K., Galea, D., McEvoy, C. L., & Bruza, P. D. (2013). How activation, entanglement, and searching a semantic network contribute to event memory. *Memory & Cognition, 41,* 797–819.

Nyberg, L., Cabeza, R., & Tulving, E. (1996). PET studies of encoding and retrieval: The HERA model. *Psychonomic Bulletin and Review, 3,* 135–148.

O'Donnell, J. P., Radtke, R. C., Leicht, D. J., & Caesar, R. (1988). Encoding and retrieval processes in learning-disabled, head-injured, and nondisabled young adults. *Journal of General Psychology, 115,* 335–368.

O'Neil-Pirozzi, T. M., Kennedy, M. T., & Sohlberg, M. M. (2016). Evidence-based practice for the use of internal strategies as a memory compensation technique after brain injury: A systematic review. *The Journal of Head Trauma Rehabilitation, 31,* E1–E11.

Paivio, A. (1971). *Imagery and verbal processes.* Holt, Rinehart, & Winston.

Paivio, A. (1976). Imagery in recall and recognition. In J. Brown (Ed.), *Recall and recognition.* John Wiley & Sons.

Papagno, C., Valentine, T., & Baddeley, A. D. (1991). Phonological short-term memory and foreign language vocabulary learning. *Journal of Memory and Language, 30,* 331–347.

Papanicolaou, A. (2006). *The amnesias: A clinical textbook of memory disorders.* Oxford University Press.

Parente, R., & Anderson-Parente, J. K. (1989). Retraining memory: Theory and application. *Journal of Head Trauma Rehabilitation, 4*(3), 55–65.

Paterno, R., Folweiler, K. A., & Cohen, A. S. (2017). Pathophysiology and treatment of memory dysfunction after traumatic brain injury. *Current Neurology & Neuroscience Reports, 17,* Article 52.

Peterson, L. R., & Peterson, M. J. (1959). Short-term retention of individual verbal items. *Journal of Experimental Psychology, 58,* 193–198.

Pettemeridou, E., & Constantinidou, F. (2021). The association between brain reserve, cognitive reserve, and neuropsychological and functional outcomes in males with chronic moderate-to-severe traumatic brain injury. *American Journal of Speech-Language Pathology, 30*(2S), 883–893.

Pettemeridou, E., Kallousia, E., & Constantinidou, F. (2021). Regional brain volume, brain reserve and MMSE performance in healthy aging from the NEUROAGE cohort: Contributions of sex, education, and depression symptoms. *Frontiers in Aging Neuroscience, 13,* 711301.

Pettemeridou, E., Kennedy, M. R. T., & Constantinidou, F. (2020). Self-awareness and quality of life in chronic moderate-to-severe TBI. *NeuroRehabilitation, 46,* 109–118.

Plechata, A., Nekovarova, T., & Fajnerova, I. (2021). What is the future immersive virtual reality in memory rehabilitation? A systematic review. *NeuroRehabilitation, 48,* 389–412.

Radford, K., Lah, S., Thayer, Z., Say, M. J., & Miller, L. A. (2012). Improving memory in outpatients with neurological disorders using a group-based training program. *Journal of the International Neuropsychological Society, 18,* 738–748.

Randolph, C., Tierney, M. C., Mohr, E., & Chase, T. N. (1998). The Repeatable Battery for the Assessment of Neuropsychological Status (RBANS): Preliminary clinical validity. *Journal of Clinical and Experimental Neuropsychology, 20*(3), 310–319.

Roediger, H. L., & Blaxton, T. A. (1987). Retrieval modes produce dissociations in memory for surface information. In D. S. Gorfein & R. R. Hoffman (Eds.), *The Ebbinghous Centennial Conference* (pp. 349–379). Erlbaum.

Ross-Swain, D. (1996). *Ross Information Processing Assessment, 2nd ed. (RIPA-2).* Pro-Ed.

Royle, J., & Lincoln, N. B. (2008). The Everyday Memory Questionnaire–Revised: Development of a 13-item scale. *Disability and Rehabilitation, 30*(2), 114–121.

Salthouse, T. A. (2005). Relations between cognitive abilities and measures of executive functioning. *Neuropsychology, 19,* 532–545.

Sanders, A., Nakase-Thomson, R., Constantinidou, F., Wertheimer, J., & Paul, D. (2007). Memory assessment on an interdisciplinary rehabilitation team: A theoretically based framework. *American Journal of Speech-Language Pathology, 16,* 316–330.

Schacter, D. L. (1985). Priming of old and new knowledge in amnesic patients and normal subjects. *Annals of the New York Academy of Sciences, 444,* 44–53.

Schacter, D. L. (1987). Implicit memory: History and current status. *Journal of Experimental Psychology: Learning, Memory and Cognition, 13,* 501–518.

Schacter, D. L. (1990). Perceptual representation systems and implicit memory: Toward a resolution of the multiple memory systems debate. In A. Diamond (Ed.), *Development and neural bases of higher cognitive functions* (pp. 543–571). New York Academy of Sciences.

Schacter, D. L. (1992). Understanding implicit memory: A cognitive neuroscience approach. *American Psychologist, 47,* 559–569.

Schacter, D. L., & Tulving, E. (1994). *Memory systems.* MIT Press.

Schnider, A. & Ptak, R. (2023). Rehabilitation of memory disorders. *Clinical and Translational Neuroscience, 7,* 1–8.

Shaughnessy, M. F. (2019). The Wechsler Intelligence Scale for Adults and the Bender Gestalt-2: Two revised instruments foundational to the neurological examination. *EC Neurology, 11,* 156–161.

Shimamura, A. P., & Squire, L. R. (1984). Paired-associate learning and priming effects in amnesia—A neuropsychological study. *Journal of Experimental Psychology–General, 113,* 556–570.

Shohamy, R., & Adcock, A. (2010). Dopamine and adaptive memory. *Trends in Cognitive Sciences, 10,* 464–472.

Sigmundsdottir, L., Longley, W. A., & Tate, R. L. (2016). Computerised cognitive training in acquired brain injury: A systematic review of outcomes using the international classification of functioning (ICF). *Neuropsychological Rehabilitation, 26,* 673–741.

Simblett, S. K., Ring, H., & Bateman, A. (2017). The Dysexecutive Questionnaire Revised (DEX-R): An extended measure of everyday dysexecutive problems after acquired brain injury. *Neuropsychological Rehabilitation, 27*(8), 1124–1141.

Simos, P. G., Kasselimis, D., & Mouzaki, A. (2011). Age, gender, and education effects on vocabulary measures in Greek. *Aphasiology, 25,* 475–491.

Simos, P., Sideridis, G. D., Kasselimis, D., & Mouzaki, A. (2013). Reading fluency estimates of current intellectual function: Demographic factors and effects of type of stimuli. *Journal of the International Neuropsychological Society, 19*, 1–7.

Singh-Manoux, A., Marmot, M. G., Glymour, M., Sabia, S., Kivimäki, M., & Dugravot, A. (2011). Does cognitive reserve shape cognitive decline? *Annals of Neurology, 70*(2), 296–304.

Smith, A. (1982). *Symbol Digit Modalities Test (SDMT) manual (revised)*. Western Psychological Services.

Smith, N. C., Urgolites, J. Z., Hopkins, O. R., & Squire, R. L. (2014). Comparison of explicit and incidental learning strategies in memory-impaired patients. *Proceedings of the National Academy of Sciences, 111*, 475–479.

Smolak, E., McGregor, K. K., Arbisi-Kelm, T., & Eden, N. (2020). Sustained attention in developmental language disorder and its relation to working memory and language. *Journal of Speech, Language, and Hearing Research, 63*, 4096–4108.

Sohlberg, M. M., Ehlhardt, L., & Kennedy, M. (2005). Instructional techniques in cognitive rehabilitation: A preliminary report. *Seminars in Speech and Language, 26*(4), 268–279.

Sohlberg, M. M., & Mateer, C. A. (1989). *Introduction to cognitive rehabilitation*. Guilford.

Sohlberg, M. M., & Mateer, C. A. (2001). *Cognitive rehabilitation: An integrative neuropsychological approach*. Guilford.

Spikman, J. M., Berg, I. J., & Deelman, B. G. (1995). Spared recognition capacity in elderly and closed-head injury subjects with clinical memory deficits. *Journal of Clinical and Experimental Neuropsychology, 17*, 29–34.

Spreij, L. A., Visser-Meily, J. M. A., van Hengten, C. M., & Nijboer, T. C. (2014). Novel insights into the rehabilitation of memory post acquired brain injury: A systematic review. *Frontiers in Human Neuroscience, 8*, 1–19.

Squire, L. R. (1987). *Memory and brain*. Oxford University Press.

Squire, L. R. (1992). Memory and the hippocampus: A synthesis from findings with rats, monkeys, and humans. *Psychological Review, 99*, 195–231.

Squire, L. R., Genzel, L., Wixted, J. T., & Morris, R. G. (2015). Memory consolidation. *Perspectives in Biology, 7*, 1–21.

Squire, L. R., & Knowlton, B. J. (1995). Learning about categories in the absence of memory. *Proceedings of the National Academy of Sciences of the United States of America, 92*, 12470–12474.

Squire, L. R., Stark, C. E., & Clark, R. E. (2004). The medial temporal lobe. *Annual Review of Neuroscience, 27*, 279–306.

Squire, L. R., & Zola-Morgan, S. (1991). The medial temporal lobe memory system. *Science, 253*, 1380–1386.

Stavrinides, P., Constantinidou, F., Anastassiou, I., Malikides, A., & Papacostas, S. (2012). Psychosocial adjustment of patients with epilepsy in Cyprus. *Epilepsy and Behavior, 25*, 98–104.

Stuss, D. T. (2011). Functions of the frontal lobes: Relation to executive functions. *Journal of the International Neuropsychological Society, 17*(5), 759–765.

Tall, A. R., & Jelic, S. (2019). How broken sleep harms blood vessels. *Nature, 566*, 329–330.

Thompson, R. F., & Krupa, D. J. (1994). Organization of memory traces in the mammalian brain. *Annual Review of Neuroscience, 17*, 519–550.

Traikapi, A., Kalli, I., Kyriakou, A., Stylianou, E., Symeou, R. T., Kardama, A., . . . Konstantinou, N. (2022). Episodic memory effects of gamma frequency precuneus transcranial magnetic stimulation in Alzheimer's disease: A randomized multiple baseline study. *Journal of Neuropsychology, 17*(2), 279–301.

Tronson, N. C., & Taylor, J. R. (2007). Molecular mechanisms of memory reconsolidation. *Nature Reviews Neuroscience, 8*, 262–275.

Tulving, E. (1966). Subjective organization and effects of repetition in multi-trial free-recall learning. *Journal of Verbal Learning and Verbal Behavior, 5,* 193–197.

Tulving, E., Hayman, C. A. G., & MacDonald, C. A. (1991). Long-lasting perceptual priming and semantic learning in amnesia: A case experiment. *Journal of Experimental Psychology: Learning, Memory, and Cognition, 17,* 595–617.

Tulving, E., Schacter, D. L., & Stark, H. A. (1982). Priming effects in word-fragment completion are independent of recognition memory. *Journal of Experimental Psychology: Learning, Memory, and Cognition, 8,* 352–373.

Unsworth, N., & Engle, R. W. (2007). On the division of short-term and working memory: An examination of simple and complex span and their relations to higher order abilities. *Psychological Bulletin, 133,* 1038–1066.

Vakil, E. (2012). Neuropsychological assessment: Principles, rationale, and challenges. *Journal of Clinical and Experimental Neuropsychology, 34*(2), 135–150.

van Kesteren, M. T. R., Ruiter, D. J., Fernández, G., & Henson, R. N. (2012). How schema and novelty augment memory formation. *Trends in Neurosciences, 35,* 211–219.

van Ool, J. S., Hurks, P. P., Snoeijen-Schouwenaars, F. M., Tan, I. Y., Schelhaas, H. J., Klinkenberg, S., . . . Hendriksen, J. G. (2018). Accuracy of WISC-III and WAIS-IV short forms in patients with neurological disorders. *Developmenta Neurorehabilitation, 21,* 101–107.

Vargha-Khadem, F., Gadian, D. G., Watkins, K. E., Connelly, A., Van Paesschen, W., & Mishkin, M. (1997). Differential effects of early hippocampal pathology on episodic and semantic memory. *Science, 277,* 376–380.

Voss, J. L., Galvan, A., & Gonsalves, B. D. (2011). Cortical regions recruited for complex active-learning strategies and action planning exhibit rapid reactivation during memory retrieval. *Neuropsychologia, 49*(14), 3956–3966.

Waugh, N. C., & Norman, D. A. (1965). Primary memory. *Psychological Review, 72,* 89–104.

Wechsler, D. (1997). *Wechsler Memory Scale®– Third edition (WMS-III).* Harcourt Assessment.

Wells, E. L., Kofler, M. J., Soto, E. F., Schaefer, H. S., & Sarver, D. E. (2018). Assessing working memory in children with ADHD: Minor administration and scoring changes may improve digit span backward's construct validity. *Research in Developmental Disabilities, 72,* 166–178.

Wilson, B. A. (1987). *Rehabilitation of memory.* Guilford.

Wilson, B. A., Emslie, H. C., Quirk, K., & Evans, J. J. (2013). Reducing everyday memory and planning problems by means of a paging system. In B. A. Wilson (Ed.), *The assessment, evaluation, and rehabilitation of everyday memory problems: Selected papers of Barbara A. Wilson* (pp. 96–107). Psychology Press.

World Health Organization. (2001). *International classification of functioning, disability and health.*

Yiannakkaras, C., Konstantinou, N., Constantinidou, F., Pettemeridou, E., Eracleous, E., Papacostas, S. S., & Seimenis, I. (2019). Whole brain and corpus callosum diffusion tensor metrics: How do they correlate with visual and verbal memory performance in chronic traumatic brain injury. *Journal of Integrative Neuroscience, 18*(2), 95–105.

Yubero, R., Gil, P., & Paul, N., & Maestú, F. (2011). Influence of memory strategies on memory test performance: A study in healthy and pathological aging. *Aging, Neuropsychology, and Cognition, 18,* 497–515.

Zalonis, I., Kararizou, E., Triantafyllou, N. I., Kapaki, E., Papageorgiou, S., Sgouropoulos, P., & Vassilopoulos, D. (2008). A normative study of the Trail Making Test A and B in Greek adults. *Clinical Neuropsychologist, 22*(5), 842–850.

3

Executive Functions: Theory, Assessment, and Treatment

Mary H. Purdy and Katy H. O'Brien

Chapter Learning Objectives

After reading this chapter you will be able to:

1. Describe a model of executive functioning, including the core and higher-order executive function processes and the role of metacognition.
2. Identify the neuroanatomical correlates of executive functioning.
3. Explain the challenges associated with assessment of executive functioning.
4. Describe specific assessment tools and the executive function processes they measure.
5. Summarize the general treatment categories for management of executive function disorders.
6. Apply the Rehabilitation Treatment Specification System (RTSS) framework to identify the treatment targets and ingredients of executive function interventions.

Introduction

Executive functioning is a complex neuropsychological construct that overlaps with, yet is distinct from, attention and memory as described in the previous chapters. Executive function processes play a critical role in goal-directed and purposeful behavior and assist in planning, organizing, initiating, and adapting effectively and flexibly as the situation demands (Lezak et al., 2012). Consider the following example: As the speech-language pathologist (SLP) on the brain injury unit of the rehabilitation hospital, you are about to begin a 45-minute talk on communication disorders following traumatic brain injury (TBI) for a Family Education Series. The program director pulls you aside right before you begin and says you have 30 minutes. Your executive function processes engage, and you immediately determine the change in expectations (15 minutes less time), consider your options (cut down on several sections or eliminate an entire section), identify pros and cons of each option, and then select the best option and execute your plan. As you move through your talk, you simultaneously monitor the time and adjust the content as needed.

When executive functioning is disrupted, everyday activities become challenging. This is demonstrated through the following cases (all names have been changed): Brian, a 56-year-old self-employed salesman who also sustained a TBI, cannot schedule appointments and plan travel routes efficiently or adequately describe his products to his customers; Carmi, a 21-year-old college student studying medicine, cannot complete projects or meet deadlines and is struggling to participate in class discussions since she sustained a TBI after being hit by a car while crossing the street. Both individuals demonstrated preservation of basic cognitive skills, yet could not regulate these skills to carry out more complex tasks. Because executive functions are required in virtually all daily life activities, it is critical for SLPs to understand the nature of executive functions and their relation to cognitive and communicative behavior.

This chapter reviews the theoretical basis of executive functioning, its neuroanatomical correlates, its impact on communication, assessment tools, and management approaches. The cases of Brian and Carmi mentioned above will be embedded throughout the chapter to illustrate specific concepts.

Defining Executive Functions

Many models and definitions of executive function exist, and the components and nomenclature vary, often depending on the specific field of study (e.g., cognitive psychology, educational psychology, neuropsychology). The construct of executive function, sometimes referred to as cognitive control, is typically defined in terms of its relationship with goal-directed behavior versus habits and controlled versus automatic responding (Friedman & Robbins, 2022). There is general agreement that the term executive function refers to a set of cognitive processes that guide goal-directed actions and behaviors essential to performing everyday tasks and contribute to the monitoring or regulation of task performance (Baggetta & Alexander, 2016). These self-regulatory (controlled) actions allow people to manage time, plan, focus attention, and handle multiple tasks to successfully achieve a goal. In the absence of executive functioning, behavior is automatic or habitual.

In a sense, executive functions help people to be more efficient, developing routines around familiar activities that can be deployed with very little effort (thus reducing cognitive load when encountering a common day-to-day situation) and managing responses to novel or unfamiliar situations as these arise (Norman & Shallice, 1986). Here, executive functions help to identify the goal, along with behaviors that may be effective (or ineffective, as the case may be) in meeting that goal. In both cases—standard, well-known routines and newly developed responses to novel circumstances—executive function also monitors progress throughout to determine when the plan may be deviating from meeting the goal and deploying strategies or adjustments to get back on track (Kennedy & Coelho,

2005). As an example, you may recall the first few times that you worked with a real client in a therapy session or completed a first evaluation. You likely planned your approach carefully, identifying goals for the session, determining activities and cueing hierarchies that would align with those goals, perhaps even planning out specific greetings and where everyone would sit in the room. All of this was very novel, and each activity required great effort in both planning and execution. Over time and with repeated practice, you likely have lots of routines now in place around your clinical practice. You may have data collection routines, correction versus reinforcement routines, routines for summarizing and closing out a session, and maybe even routines around your documentation. Because of your repeated experiences, those initially novel situations became familiar, and you became more efficient, resulting in your sessions probably feeling less effortful now. Your executive functions allowed you to manage novel situations until new routines could be formed, while also supporting flexible in-the-moment deviations when things did not go according to plan.

Executive function processes may be divided into core processes and higher-order processes (Baggetta & Alexander, 2016; Diamond, 2013; Friedman & Robbins, 2022; Miyake & Friedman, 2012), which are integrated as well as monitored and controlled through self-regulation and the use of metacognitive strategies (Kennedy & Coelho, 2005; Stuss, 2011). Figure 3–1 presents this model of executive functioning. It is important to recognize that executive function processes are not mutually exclusive; rather, they interact and overlap. That is, they correlate with one another, thus tapping a common underlying ability, yet they also show some separability (Miyake & Friedman, 2012).

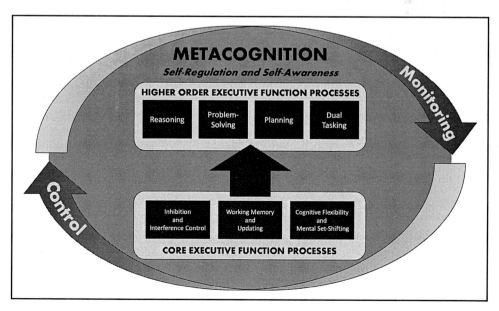

Figure 3–1. Model of executive functions.

Core Executive Function Processes

An extensive literature review found that researchers identified 39 different processes as executive functions, which illustrates the complexity of the concept (Baggetta & Alexander, 2016). However, there is general agreement that there are three core executive function processes: (a) inhibitory control/response inhibition, (b) working memory/updating, and (c) cognitive flexibility/set shifting (Baggetta & Alexander, 2016; Diamond, 2013; Friedman & Robbins, 2022; Miyake & Friedman, 2012).

The first core executive function process is **inhibitory control**, or response inhibition. This is the ability to deliberately control or inhibit an automatic response, behavior, or thought and instead do what is more appropriate or needed in a given situation (Diamond, 2013). Without inhibitory control, impulses or conditioned responses take over our behavior. Inhibitory control of attention helps us selectively attend to or focus on what we choose and suppress attention to other stimuli, such as attending to a specific conversation in a noisy environment. Inhibitory control also allows us to have control over our emotions and resist temptations (e.g., self-control), as well as have the discipline to stay on task despite the temptation to give up (Diamond, 2013).

A second core executive function process is **working memory**, which is the ability to maintain a task or idea in mind and mentally manipulate it. Working memory has a limited capacity for short-term storage of information, and controlled attention processes permit the volitional manipulation of this information (Heinz-Martin et al.,

2002; Otermans et al., 2022). Working memory is constantly being updated, which involves replacing old, irrelevant information with new, more relevant information that is related to the task at hand (Strobach et al., 2014). Working memory is critical for understanding anything that occurs over time, which requires holding in mind what happened earlier and relating that to what comes later. Many everyday tasks are dependent on working memory, such as comprehending spoken or written language, following directions, weighing pros and cons, sequencing activities, or performing calculations in our heads.

The third core executive function process is **cognitive flexibility**, or set shifting, which is the ability to intentionally move between tasks, mental sets, or goals as well as reacting to changing circumstances (Baggetta & Alexander, 2016). Cognitive flexibility requires and builds on inhibitory control and working memory (Diamond, 2013). Shifting involves the disengagement of irrelevant information (e.g., a previous task) and activating relevant information (the upcoming task) (Strobach et al., 2014). For example, to change your perspective and see something from another's point of view, you need to inhibit your previous perspective and activate (e.g., load into working memory) a different perspective. As with the example at the start of this chapter, cognitive flexibility was also necessary when your planned 45-minute talk became a 30-minute talk. This change in the parameters of the task meant that you had to let go of the previous plan to allow for a new, now more appropriate plan to be put in place. Cognitive flexibility is also required for verbal fluency and creative thinking. For example, if you were asked to list all the possible uses of a knife, your first response is likely to be the most common— you cut with a knife. However, more flexible and creative responses may include using it to undo a screw, open the lid of a paint can, or scrape off a price sticker on a recently purchased item.

Higher-Order Executive Function Processes

Higher-order executive function processes are built from the core processes. Frequently reported higher-order processes include reasoning, problem solving, planning, and dual-tasking (Collins & Koechlin, 2012; Diamond, 2013; Otermans et al., 2022; Strobach et al., 2014). As with the core executive function processes, higher-order executive processes are highly interrelated. When reviewing each of these below, you may also see where the core processes of inhibitory control, working memory, and cognitive flexibility all play a role in successful execution of these more complex activities. In addition, as with the core processes, remember that each of these may be regulated and monitored through metacognition.

Reasoning is the process of using existing knowledge to draw conclusions, make predictions, or construct explanations. There are several methods of reasoning, including deductive, inductive, analogical, and abstract. In deductive reasoning, information is analyzed to prove or refute a theory or hypothesis. It begins with a general rule and leads to a specific conclusion (e.g., Mary's favorite color is purple. Lucinda's jacket is Mary's favorite color.

Therefore, Lucinda's jacket is purple). Inductive reasoning begins with specific observations and moves to a general conclusion. Evidence is gathered and analyzed to explain what was observed (e.g., if a bag contained 10 coins and the first 8 coins you pulled out of the bag were pennies, you may logically conclude that all coins in the bag were pennies). Analogical reasoning involves identifying similarities/differences between concepts to gain a deeper understanding of the concepts (e.g., sky is to blue as sun is to yellow). Abstract reasoning allows us to move beyond concrete, observable facts and make connections across information sources, including integration of contextual, pragmatic, or other cues (e.g., when reading a story, understanding a character's motivation or making reasonable predictions about future events). All types of reasoning require constant organization, synthesis, and updating of information and are therefore highly dependent on working memory (Diamond, 2013). Reasoning also plays a critical role in problem solving and decision-making (Collins & Koechlin, 2012).

Problem solving involves determining whether there is a problem, identifying the specific problem, generating potential solutions, choosing a solution, evaluating the outcome, and trying another solution if the expected outcome is not achieved (Cantor et al., 2014). This complex task relies on working memory to hold relevant information in mind as an individual considers a potential solution and its outcome. Additionally, cognitive flexibility is required to generate an alternative solution if the first attempt to solve the problem was unsuccessful.

Planning involves thinking about an end goal and determining a course of action, or a "road map" to achieve that goal (Lezak et al., 2012). To plan effectively, an individual needs to regulate and anticipate situations, break larger tasks into smaller parts, and self-monitor performance while holding an overall goal in memory (Brown & Hux, 2017). This process requires time management and organizational skills, as well as relying heavily on working memory and cognitive flexibility. Good planners are sensitive to potential problems and negative stimuli, demonstrate cognitive control to regulate behavior, and put forth effort (Krpan et al., 2011).

Dual-tasking or **multitasking** involves performing two or more tasks at the same time, which results in decreased working memory capacity (Otermans et al., 2022). Fluent integration of all three core executive processes is necessary to manage multiple tasks, allowing for maintenance of multiple goals, shifting between these, and inhibition of distractions or competing goals to maintain focus on the tasks. Attentional resources used to process the information in working memory may be shared, or they can be volitionally controlled, that is, consciously devoted to one task at a time. Simple, habituated tasks require fewer attentional resources and may be performed automatically. Automatic processing is effortless and is conducted unconsciously due to permanent connections that are developed over repeated practice, resulting in routinized sets of behaviors or scripts. Complex tasks are completed with controlled processing, which is slow, effortful, and completely conscious. Controlled processing may become automatic with repeated prac-

tice (Otermans et al., 2022; Schneider & Chein, 2003). The more automatic a task is, the fewer resources it requires, thereby leaving more resources available for other tasks. For example, when you are driving to school with a friend, you can most likely simultaneously listen to the radio and have a conversation without really thinking about where you are going because you have driven the route numerous times. However, if you are driving in a new city and trying to follow directions to a place you have never been before, the radio may need to be turned off and the conversation ceased so you can devote your attention to where you are going. Just as executive function supports greater efficiency in general, the more well learned a routine is, the more successfully other tasks may be added. As the situation becomes more novel (in this case, navigating in a new city), the switch to developing a new set of behaviors strains available cognitive resources, reducing the ability to manage other tasks or incoming stimuli.

Metacognition

In general, metacognition is the act of thinking about thinking. This includes the awareness and regulation of one's cognitive functioning, including task-related self-evaluation, self-regulation, and prediction and anticipation of performance and outcomes (Yeo et al., 2021). Metacognitive knowledge is a subset of metacognition and is defined as a systematic fund of information and beliefs about one's cognition (Flavell, 1979; Schraw & Moshman, 1995). Metacognitive knowledge is not related to any specific task; rather, it is considered a dynamic process that is built from prior experiences that affects future actions (Toglia & Kirk, 2000). Metacognition is required for the execution of novel or complex behaviors but also monitors to ensure that more basic routines are meeting established goals. That is, to successfully perform a task that is novel, one must be able to detect what is different, monitor performance, make a strategy decision, and execute the strategy (Kennedy & Coelho, 2005). Importantly, though, that metacognitive knowledge can be separate from active, online metacognitive monitoring and self-regulation during activities (Fischer et al., 2004; Toglia & Kirk, 2000). For example, you may have developed metacognitive knowledge about yourself that you are often rushed or late for appointments. This knowledge is likely based on many previous experiences of feeling stressed while driving to appointments, experiencing others' annoyance at your tardiness, or rescheduling or missing important events when you arrive too late. Ideally, now that you have that hard-acquired knowledge, it will then impact how you approach future situations, for example, by setting alarms to leave earlier or ensuring that you do not schedule meetings back-to-back. Because you know that this is a difficult task for you, you are more likely to use strategies to prevent failure.

Metacognitive knowledge then also underlies a more general sense of intellectual awareness (Toglia & Kirk, 2000), in which a person knows their strengths and weaknesses along with when it may be particularly important to use specific strategies (O'Keeffe et al., 2007). In contrast, during tasks, self-regulation allows for ongoing in-the-moment monitoring (comparing performance to the desired outcome or goal) and controlling (strategy use) behaviors. Understanding the relationship between these two—metacognitive knowledge and ongoing, active self-regulation—is particularly important for people with acquired neurological disorders, as metacognitive knowledge is based on years of experiences accrued before their brain injury or disease process occurred (Hart & Evans, 2006; Kennedy & Coehlo, 2005). While some people after brain injury experience a severe form of unawareness known as anosognosia, particularly after right hemisphere injury (Orfei et al., 2009; Steward & Kretzmer, 2022), more common is the experience of unawareness related to postinjury skillsets no longer matching with preinjury established metacognitive beliefs. Adjusting those metacognitive beliefs or knowledge requires repeated experience over time, which perhaps explains why awareness improves over time in many people with brain injury (Dirette & Plaisier, 2007; Pagulayan et al., 2007; Powell et al., 2001; Richardson et al., 2015; Robertson & Schmitter-Edgecombe, 2015). Even so, given that the self-regulation system that monitors performance is often impacted by brain injury, building in concrete feedback that allows the person to observe their own performance and make judgments about it is often a key aspect of executive function and awareness treatment (Cicerone et al., 2019; Tate et al., 2014).

There is a dynamic relationship between metacognition and executive functions. Executive function processes support learning while metacognition is considered the behavioral output of executive functions. For example, the executive function process of working memory helps us understand what we read by maintaining and updating information in our mind from the beginning to the end of a passage. Metacognition allows us to be aware of our own learning and improve it by self-regulating and applying metacognitive strategies, for example, recognizing we did not fully process a sentence and rereading it.

Table 3–1 provides examples of cognitive and communicative problems that correspond to deficits in each of the executive function processes.

Neuroanatomy of Executive Functions

Executive functions have been associated with the frontal lobes as far back as 1840, when the case of Phineas Gage was presented (see Ratiulon et al., 2004). While working on the railroad, Phineas Gage was pierced through his frontal lobe with a large iron rod. Although the majority of his left frontal lobe was destroyed, Phineas survived. However, significant changes in his behavior and personality became apparent, behaviors currently associated with executive functioning.

The frontal lobes are the largest of the four human lobes and are dramatically larger than those of animals lower on the phylogenetic scale. The prefrontal area is divided into subsections (dorsolateral, dorsomedial, ventrolateral, ventromedial, and orbitofrontal), each subserving different neurobehavioral functions. The dorsolateral prefrontal cortex is associated with working memory and the manipulation of information held "on line." The dorso-medial area plays a significant role in social cognition, specifically integrating several sources of information to form social judgments. The ventrolateral prefrontal cortex assists with vigilance, inhibition, and shifting of attention. The ventromedial prefrontal cortex is interconnected with limbic structures such as the amygdala and is related to emotional control. The orbitofrontal cortex is associated with personality, the maintenance of appropriate social behavior, and decision-making (Martin et al., 2017; Smolker et al., 2015; Vanderah et al., 2021).

However, there is clear evidence that the symptoms attributed to executive dysfunction are not restricted to damage to frontal areas. In fact, the independent role of the prefrontal lobe volumes on executive functions markedly diminishes when considering the contribution from temporal, parietal, and occipital lobe effects (Bettcher et al., 2016). A broad range of gray and white matter structures and networks subserve executive functions, and persistent deficits in mental flexibility, set shifting, planning, and other executive function processes result from damage to the integrity of these white matter tracts that connect brain regions (Bettcher et al., 2016; Caeyenberghs et al., 2014; Friedman & Robbins, 2022). See Table 3–2 for a summary of these neuroanatomical correlates.

Diffusion tensor imaging (DTI) has been used to examine neural networks and structural connectivity to more specifically identify the impact of injury to white matter tracts on cognitive functioning. Studies have found that greater white matter pathology, or diffuse axonal injury (DAI), led to greater cognitive deficits due to weak integration of

Table 3–1. Executive Function Processes and Related Problems

Executive Function Processes	Example of Cognitive Deficit	Example of Communication Deficit
Core Executive Function Processes		
Inhibition	A waitress poured Susan a cup of coffee and warned Susan it was hot. Susan took a drink and burned her tongue.	Mary met her friend for lunch and told her that her new haircut makes her look like a poodle.
Working memory	Cho and Maya were trying to figure out a time to meet. Maya gave Cho three possible dates, but Cho could not hold the dates in her head long enough to compare her schedule to Maya's.	Luis was sharing a story from a family vacation with his friend Daniel. Daniel could not hold all of the different family members in his head well enough to keep track of who was doing what.
Cognitive flexibility	Max tried to turn on the TV with the remote but the TV did not turn on. He kept pointing the remote at the screen and pressing buttons, becoming increasingly agitated when the TV failed to turn on—he attempted the same solution over and over again despite its ineffectiveness.	Kaitlyn and Whitney were talking about upcoming vacation plans. Kaitlyn moved on to talking about her work schedule and Whitney became confused and continued to talk about the vacation dates.
Higher-Order Processes		
Reasoning	Jerome wants to ask Tasha to the movies on Friday. She told him she could after 7:30 when she gets off work. Jerome bought tickets for a 7:15 movie.	Mark was excited that his wife was home from work. When his wife got home, she threw her bag on the table and buried her head in her hands. Mark asked how work had gone and she groaned, "Great." Mark was pleased and told her he was happy she had such a good day.

continues

Table 3–1. *continued*

Executive Function Processes	Example of Cognitive Deficit	Example of Communication Deficit
Problem-solving	Denzel was invited away for the weekend. He had an appointment scheduled for the Saturday he'd be away. He did not attempt to reschedule the appointment and had to pay a "no show" fee.	Lauren was listening to her boss explain how to take apart the ice machine to clean the chute when it got jammed, but didn't understand what she was supposed to do. She decided just to nod along and not ask questions.
Planning	Juanita invited friends for dinner at 6:30. She started to cook the arroz con pollo after they finished some appetizers. She did not consider how long it would take to prepare and cook everything and they ended up eating at 9:30.	Kwame was excited to tell his coworkers about his new job, but told them without explaining that he had been looking for a new position, who would take his current responsibilities, or when his last day would be.
Dual-tasking	Bruno was paying bills online while watching TV. Later, he received two messages that the wrong amount had been paid.	Frank was listening to his coworker Michael while he was trying to write an email and kept accidentally writing what Michael was saying.
Metacognition	George regularly attended class but didn't study for his exam, and he failed. His next exam was coming up. He figured that because he went to every class since the last exam, he would do well, but he failed again.	Chris was invited to give a talk on cryptocurrency and the financial markets. He was informed ahead of time that the audience did not know much on the topic. He began his talk at too high a level, asking people what they thought about particular currencies and was surprised when they looked at him with confused expressions.

Table 3–2. Neurobehavioral Correlates of the Prefrontal Cortex

	Connections	General Functions	Consequences of Lesions
Dorsolateral	Parietal cortex Caudate nucleus Global pallidus Substantia nigra Thalamus	Monitors and adjusts behavior using working memory and executive functions	Executive function deficit Disinterest/ emotional reactivity Decreased attention to relevant stimuli
Dorsomedial	Temporal, parietal Caudate nucleus Global pallidus Substantia nigra Cingulate Thalamus	Arousal Motivation Initiation of activity	Apathy Decreased drive/ awareness Akinetic-abulic syndrome Mutism
Ventrolateral	Temporal cortex Amygdala Posterior cingulate Parahippocampal gyrus Inferior parietal lobe	Response inhibition Goal appropriate response selection Attentional control Vigilance	Emotional dysregulation Poor attention and vigilance
Ventromedial	Amygdala Temporal lobe Prelimbic cortex	Emotional control, empathy	Impaired judgment Inappropriate social behavior
Orbitofrontal	Temporal, parietal Insula Globus pallidus Caudate nucleus Substantia nigra Amygdala Thalamus Cerebrocerebellar circuit	Personality Emotional input Social behavior Suppression of distracting signals	Emotional lability Disinhibition Distractibility Social inappropriateness

networks related to executive functioning and a limited capacity to integrate information across brain regions (Caeyenberghs et al., 2014; Kinnunen et al., 2011). The frontal lobes rely on high-quality information being supplied rapidly from more posterior areas and, in turn, directing those more posterior areas in accordance with goals (Stuss & Levine, 2005). Thus, white matter volume loss can be a superior predictor of recovery and a crucial factor driving clinical outcomes. White matter damage may place an additional burden on recovery by deteriorating signal transmission between cortical areas within a functional network (Caeyenberghs et al., 2014; Cristofori et al., 2015).

Executive Dysfunction in Clinical Populations

Executive dysfunction has been identified in almost all neurologic conditions due to the disruption of complex neuroanatomical networks. Although the specific pathophysiology may differ among neurologic conditions, symptoms of executive dysfunction may be similar.

Acquired Brain Injury

Traumatic Brain Injury

Perhaps because the frontal lobes and white matter connections are particularly susceptible to damage from TBI, and that executive function relies on robust connections and communication across areas of the brain, impairments of executive functions are among the most enduring cognitive deficits seen following TBI (Bedard et al., 2020; Marsh et al., 2016). A wide range of deficits have been documented in this population, including difficulties with problem solving, reasoning, planning, and emotional self-regulation (Spitz et al., 2012). These problems have a significant impact on functional outcome

after injury, including return to work (Hart et al., 2019; Weber et al., 2018) and quality of life (Pettemeridou et al., 2020). Persistent deficits in executive functioning have also been identified in individuals who sustained a single or multiple concussions (Belanger et al., 2010; McInnes et al., 2017).

Stroke

Executive dysfunction following a stroke has been well documented (Shao et al., 2020). Different presentations may be observed based on where in the brain the stroke occurred.

Right Hemisphere Stroke. Individuals who suffer a stroke in the right hemisphere may also present with executive dysfunction. Following right hemisphere stroke, individuals may exhibit problems with planning, problem solving, cognitive flexibility, inhibition, and/or less cohesive and coherent connected speech (Barker et al., 2017; Lehman-Blake et al., 2002). In addition, many individuals with right hemisphere brain damage may display an unawareness of their problems, referred to as anosognosia (Hartman-Maeir et al., 2002). Common cognitive and communication consequences of right hemisphere stroke are described in detail in Chapter 4 of this text but should not be overlooked when there are more apparent disorders such as left neglect.

Left Hemisphere Stroke. Left hemisphere stroke can also lead to executive dysfunction. Individuals with aphasia have been found to demonstrate problems in several executive control processes, including problem solving, self-monitoring, and cognitive flexibility, and these deficits may exacerbate language difficulties (Keil & Kaszniak, 2002; Murray, 2012; Nicholas & Connor, 2017; Purdy, 2002). Higher levels of executive control in people with aphasia have been linked to better functional communication (Fridriksson et al., 2006) and conversational skills (Frankel et al., 2007). Furthermore, greater cognitive flexibility has been significantly correlated with better strategy use in functional communication tasks (Purdy & Koch, 2006). A recent systematic review examining the relationships among executive functions, language, and response to treatment concluded that although both baseline executive functioning and language skills were correlated with treatment gains, executive functioning may be a more robust indicator of treatment gains than baseline language ability (Simic et al., 2019). Thus, assessment of executive functioning ability is a crucial step in the diagnostic characterization of aphasia (Simic et al., 2019).

Progressive Neurologic Diseases

Dementia

Dementia is not a specific disease but rather a syndrome that leads to a progressive deterioration in cognitive functioning beyond what might be expected from typical biological aging (World Health Organization, 2022). It results from a variety of diseases that affect brain function. Executive dysfunction is a prominent clinical feature of many dementing diseases (Ramanan et al., 2017), although memory impairments may present earlier and be the primary

complaint leading to evaluation. It should be noted that tools often used to screen for signs of dementia, such as the Mini Mental State Examination, are not sensitive to executive dysfunction, potentially allowing an important diagnostic characteristic to be overlooked (Royall et al., 2002).

Executive dysfunction has been well documented in Alzheimer's disease (AD) and has been correlated with impaired autonomy, decision-making, instrumental activities of daily living, and increased caregiver burden (Gaubert & Chainay, 2021; Godefroy et al., 2016). Executive dysfunction may occur throughout the course of AD and is frequently associated with other neuropsychiatric features (Ramanan et al., 2017).

Vascular dementia (VaD) is the second most common form of dementia after AD (Schneck, 2008). VaD may occur as a consequence of a larger stroke but is also associated with other diseases or conditions that may impact the circulatory system, such as diabetes mellitus, hypertension, and hypercholesterolemia. Unlike AD, VaD is often observable with standard neuroimaging techniques, which may show small subcortical infarcts or white matter lesions (Román, 2003). Executive dysfunction is common in VaD, particularly when lesions are in the anterior cerebral artery distribution (Bhat & Biswas, 2022). Memory and language deficits also frequently occur in VaD, though to a milder degree.

Early and prominent deficits in executive functioning, particularly verbal fluency and set shifting, are critical diagnostic features of frontotemporal dementia (FTD) (Kiselica & Benge, 2021; Rascovsky et al., 2011). Marked behavioral changes—including disinhibition, apathy, perseveration, and cognitive inflexibility—are also evident in this population (Rascovsky et al., 2011). For those with behavioral variant FTD, these executive impairments extend to social cognition as well, with empathy and perspective-taking commonly impaired, straining caregiver relationships (Eslinger et al., 2011).

Parkinson's Disease

Parkinson's disease (PD) is a neurodegenerative disease that results in the progressive loss of dopaminergic cells in the substantia nigra that produces numerous motor symptoms, including bradykinesia, rigidity, resting tremor, and posture and balance disturbance (Simon et al., 2020). Cognitive deficits, including executive dysfunction, have been consistently identified in individuals with PD (Kudlicka et al., 2011; Ravizza et al., 2012). Some people will eventually develop Parkinson's disease dementia (PDD), while others may remain in a transitional state between normal aging and dementia, referred to as Parkinson's disease mild cognitive impairment (PD-MCI). Impaired executive functioning is the most significant predictor of future transition from PD-MCI to PDD (Wallace et al., 2022).

Motor Neuron Diseases

Motor neuron diseases are a group of progressive neurological disorders that destroy motor neurons, the cells that control skeletal muscle activities such as breathing, speaking, swallowing, and walking (National Institute of Neurological Disorders and Stroke [NINDS], 2019). Two of the most common motor neuron diseases include amyotrophic lateral sclerosis (ALS) and primary lateral sclerosis (PLS). ALS involves deterioration of both upper and lower motor neurons while PLS affects only the upper motor neurons. In addition to motor symptoms, cognitive and behavioral impairments occur frequently, and research has found a genetic link between motor neuron disease and dementia, specifically, ALS and FTD (Ng et al., 2015).

Cognitive deficits have been reported in up to 45% of individuals diagnosed with ALS (Pender et al., 2020). Cognitive change most commonly manifests as executive dysfunction, specifically deficits in verbal fluency, set shifting, initiation, and/or cognitive inhibition, and are an indicator of more rapid decline (Kasper et al., 2015). Approximately 14% of people with ALS present with significant cognitive deficits that meet the diagnostic criteria for FTD (Pender et al., 2020). Agarwal et al. (2018) identified distinct cognitive/behavioral profiles of people diagnosed with PLS, ALS, and ALS plus FTD. Individuals with ALS primarily demonstrated problems with executive functions, while those diagnosed with PLS showed executive dysfunction along with changes in memory, language, and visuospatial skills. Individuals with ALS plus FTD showed a cognitive profile similar to those with PLS but with the addition of significant behavioral changes, particularly disinhibition and apathy.

Multiple Sclerosis

Multiple sclerosis (MS) is a progressive demyelinating and neurogenerative disease that presents with two variants: relapsing-remitting multiple sclerosis (RRMS) and primary or secondary progressive multiple sclerosis (PPMS) (Borkowska et al., 2021). Cognitive impairment, including executive dysfunction, has been reported in 25% to 70% of individuals at all stages of the disease process (Trenova et al., 2016). A meta-analysis of 47 studies established that patients with PPMS present slightly more severe impairments in all cognitive domains than patients with RRMS (Johnen et al., 2017). However, Borkowska et al. (2021) found that all patients with RRMS in the remitting stage presented cognitive deficits in at least one domain of executive functioning such as fluency, interference suppression, planning, and the ability to modify activity in response to feedback. Because cognitive deficits interfere with quality of life, Borkowska et al. (2021) recommended assessment and implementation of rehabilitation services early in the course of the disease.

Cognitive Communication Consequences of Executive Dysfunction

Models describing communication impairments following brain injury tend to fall into one of three categories: cognitive, social competence, or pragmatic (Academy of Neurologic Communication Disorders and Sciences [ANCDS] et al., 2020). Cognitive models explain communication failures through changes to the underlying cognitive systems that support communication, for example, poorly organized discourse as a result of executive function impairments. In contrast, social competence models consider deficits related to social cognition, including aspects such as emotional processing and theory of mind. Finally, pragmatic models take a more rules-based approach to understanding how communication breakdowns may violate assumptions about particular communication contexts, with the goal of adjusting a person's communication style to more closely fit the model. MacDonald (2017) proposed a model of cognitive communication competence that captures the complexity of understanding communication in context—describing the influence of cognitive, emotional and physical domains—all of which may be regulated by executive functions but which are also context dependent.

Cognitive communication disorders addressed in this chapter will largely follow cognitive models, with a focus on the manifestation of communication deficits as a result of executive dysfunction (Figure 3–2).[1] Social communication is an umbrella term that encompasses a wide range of skills that allow for expression and understanding across modalities and contexts (Sohlberg et al., 2019). Components of social

---

[1]Because a complete discussion of cognitive and social communication deficits, particularly those related to social cognition deficits, is beyond the scope of the current chapter, interested readers are directed toward the Academy of Neurologic Communication Disorders and Sciences (ANCDS) Traumatic Brain Injury Writing Committee documents, the INCOG Writing Committee's guidelines on cognitive-communication disorders (Togher et al., 2023), and texts such as McDonald et al.'s (2013) *Social and Communication Disorders Following Traumatic Brain Injury*.

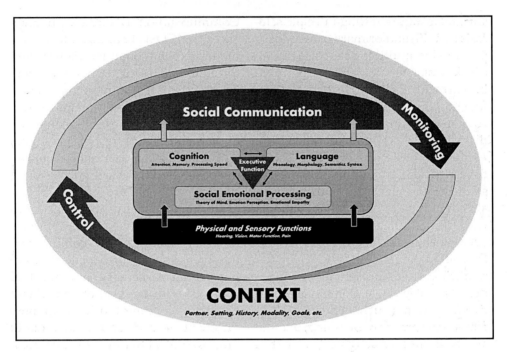

Figure 3–2. Model of social communication and executive function.

communication include both language and cognition, as well as social emotional processing or **social cognition skills**—such as theory of mind, emotion recognition, and emotional empathy—all of which are underpinned by sensory and motor functions (ANCDS et al., 2020; MacDonald, 2017; Togher et al., 2023). As described by Figure 3–2, executive function may be central to managing the interactive nature of these cognitive, linguistic, and social components. In addition, as with the model of executive function presented in Figure 3–1, self-regulatory monitoring and control functions similarly assess communication effectiveness relative to contextual demands and make adjustments as needed for communicative success. Although communication problems may occur due to breakdowns in any component of this

model (see Hill et al., 2018, for review) (and practically, most clients experience changes to more than one component or subcomponent), successful communication requires individuals to plan and use language flexibly across contexts, inhibit inappropriate responses, and continuously update information in working memory as context and social cues change over time (Byom & Turkstra, 2017).

It follows then that cognitive communication deficits following brain injury occur primarily from a breakdown in the interactional use of language and cognitive functions and are typically evident at the level of discourse rather than at the linguistic word or sentence level (Steel & Togher, 2018). In addition, executive function is often associated with communication problems (e.g., Brookshire et al., 2000;

Coelho, 2002, 2007; Coelho et al., 2013; Lê et al., 2014; Mozeiko et al., 2011). Conversely, for those who may have breakdowns in other domains, intact or relatively preserved executive function may be leveraged to maximize communication. Overall, communication is cognitively challenging and places high demands on executive functions, even though it can be difficult to tease apart the contribution of executive functions versus other domains in this model (Byom & Turkstra, 2017).

Zimmermann et al. (2011) examined the relationship between pragmatic behavior and executive function skills and found that individuals with TBI exhibited difficulty in conversational and narrative discourse tasks, which was associated with a general profile of executive dysfunction affecting mainly working memory, initiation, inhibition, planning, and switching. In contrast, the conversational and narrative discourse problems of individuals with right brain damage were predominantly related to working memory and verbal initiation impairments. McDonald et al. (2014) reported speakers with TBI failed to address the perspective of others on a variety of high- and low-cognitive flexibility tasks, which was due to problems with executive control. Impaired executive function has also been associated with poor comprehension of social implications (Channon & Watts, 2003) and inaccurate or poorly structured discourse (Coelho, 1995; Coelho et al., 2005; Lê et al., 2014; Marini et al., 2014). Pearce and colleagues (2016) reported that reduced inhibition speed contributed to disinhibited communication behaviors. Poor control of inhibition has been linked to significant social implications and poor vocational

outcomes for individuals with brain injury (McDonald et al., 2013).

Though not explicitly documented as the result of executive dysfunction, additional observations of individuals with TBI showed that their conversational skills may be characterized by difficulty responding to open-ended questions, presenting new information, organizing discourse, and adapting to interlocutor knowledge (Rousseaux et al., 2010). Discourse production has been described as lacking in macrostructure (e.g., omission or sequencing errors of essential steps or story components), cohesion (e.g., inaccurate or nonspecific use of pronouns and other referents), and informativeness (e.g., omission of important units of information, or inclusion of inaccurate information) (Coelho, 2002; Davis & Coelho, 2004). As described in greater detail in Chapter 4 of this text, pragmatic and social communication deficits following right brain damage may be rooted more centrally in social cognition and emotional processing deficits, along with difficulty comprehending abstract language and humor, making inferences, differentiating between relevant and irrelevant information, and interpreting extralinguistic or contextual information (Bryan & Hale; 2001; Lehman-Blake et al., 2002; Purdy et al., 1993; Tompkins et al., 1994).

World Health Organization's International Classification of Functioning Framework

The American Speech-Language-Hearing Association (ASHA) promotes the use of the World Health Organization's

International Classification of Functioning Framework (WHO-ICF; WHO, 2001) to guide assessment and treatment decisions (ASHA, 2004). This classification system was developed to supplement the International Classification of Diseases (ICD), in recognition of the fact that a person's disease process (e.g., stroke) does not predict function (e.g., functional communication). There are two primary components of the ICF: (a) Functioning and Disability and (b) Contextual Factors (Environmental and Personal). Functioning and Disability includes Body Function/Structure Impairment, which describes the specific changes in the anatomy or physiology of the body and resulting impairment (e.g., brain damage resulting in cognitive communication impairment). Activity and participation describe the impact of impairment on a person's ability to complete functional tasks and changes in life roles. Both completion of activities and life participation may be impacted by Environmental and/or Personal Factors. Environmental Factors are things that are not within the person's control, such as support from family or employer and access to technological aids. Personal Factors include things such as age, motivation, coping styles, and culture. Figure 3–3 provides an example of how this framework may be applied to Brian.

Assessment

General Assessment Issues

Decision-making regarding assessment will depend on a range of factors related to the clinical setting, the patient's stage of recovery, the purpose of the assessment, and resources available (Steel & Togher, 2018).

It is very difficult to assess executive functioning in the acute care hospital very soon after neurologic injury. The patient is often overwhelmed with medical testing and visits from doctors, nurses, and rehabilitation therapists. Fatigue and pain medication may decrease the patient's level of alertness. As the patient moves through the continuum of care and becomes less dependent on caregivers, there is more potential for executive function deficits to present themselves, and the therapist is more likely to obtain reliable results from executive function tests.

For individuals with TBI, the Ranchos Los Amigos (RLA) Scale of Cognitive Functioning–Revised (Hagen, 1997; Hagen et al., 1972) may help guide assessment decisions for evaluation of executive functioning. In general, patients at RLA Levels I through IV are not appropriate for executive function testing due to their overall low level of functioning and/or agitation. Patients at RLA Levels V and VI may demonstrate generalized confusion and global cognitive deficits, and administration of a brief assessment of general cognitive functioning may be appropriate. As the patient progresses through these stages of confusion, the clinician may observe behaviors associated with executive dysfunction, such as reduced error awareness, self-monitoring, initiation, and planning, but at this stage, it is difficult to differentiate between specific executive function deficits versus underlying global cognitive dysfunction. By the time patients reach RLA VII–X, the general confusion has subsided and executive dysfunction

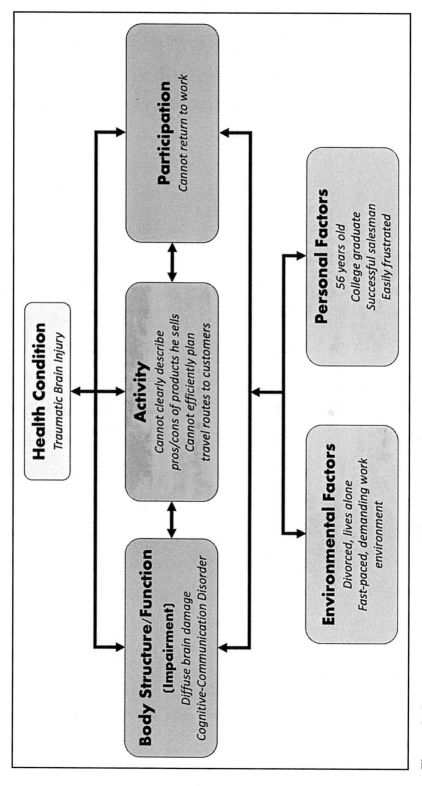

Figure 3–3. World Health Organization framework applied to Brian.

can be more reliably diagnosed. The clinician can do a task analysis of the specific troublesome activities, hypothesize about the executive function processes needed to successfully perform the activities, and select a test battery that addresses those specific executive function processes. At these stages, individuals are more aware of their deficits and can often describe specific activities that are challenging. In fact, as people progress through the higher Rancho levels, self-reflection and problem-based interviews are key to understanding executive function needs and developing intervention plans that are both person centered and foster development or deepening of insight and awareness (Figure 3–4).

There are some unique challenges related to assessment of executive functions. One issue relates to the task-impurity problem (Friedman & Robbins, 2022). Because any target executive function process must be embedded within a specific task context so the target executive process has something to work upon, it is difficult to separate errors related to the target executive function process versus other cognitive skills required to perform the task. For example, the Stroop task addresses the executive function process of inhibition by asking the person to name the ink color of a color word when the word and ink color are incongruent (e.g., say "blue" when presented with the word RED printed in

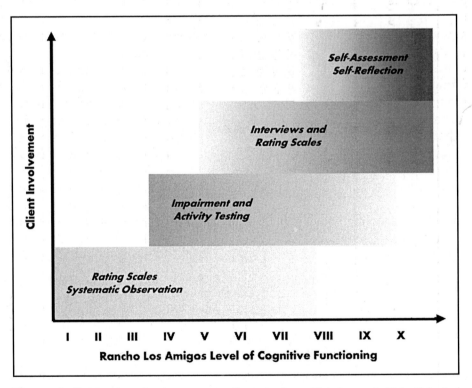

Figure 3–4. Mapping of assessment to client needs and involvement. *Note:* Adapted from Kennedy (2010) with the permission of the author.

blue ink). This task requires the ability to discriminate colors and read single words; therefore, the ability to inhibit a response cannot be determined if the person is color-blind or cannot read. Additionally, many assessments address multiple executive functions simultaneously, particularly assessments of higher-order executive functions, making it difficult to determine the impact of a specific executive function process on test performance. Ideally, task triangulation would allow for targeted understanding of needs—for example, if a person scores well on tests of attention and memory but poorly on tests of executive function, then it may be that the person's needs are more specific to executive function—but many people with neurogenic disorders have complex needs across cognitive domains, requiring careful consideration of strengths and weaknesses.

Another challenge of executive function assessment is the paradox between testing in a structured environment and the need to observe self-directed goal setting, planning and organization of behavior, monitoring and evaluation of performance, and flexible shifting in strategy use. Testing protocols typically provide structure and cues for initiation, maintenance of on-task behavior, and explicit goals, reducing the likelihood of exposing executive dysfunction (Lezak et al., 2012). Inadequate concurrent and predictive validity have also been cited as a weakness of most executive function tests (Mueller & Dollaghan, 2013).

To increase the reliability of the results and make an accurate diagnosis of executive dysfunction, it is important to use a variety of tests and measures. Results from a single test may over- or underestimate a client's executive abilities. A client with executive dysfunction may do well if their problematic components were not tapped by the measure used, causing the clinician to overestimate the client's skills. Conversely, a client may do poorly, not because of impaired executive skills, but due to a problem with a more fundamental process such as visual perception, language, or attention. For example, people who have survived a right hemisphere stroke may have significant visual perceptual problems, and clinicians should select tests that do not rely heavily on visual perception. Likewise, for people with left brain damage and aphasia, selected tests should not have a heavy linguistic load. For this reason, it is important for the clinician to be aware of more basic cognitive-linguistic deficits before administering executive function batteries so tests may be interpreted appropriately.

In an ideal world, the clinician would select both impairment and activity/ participation assessment measures that help identify strengths and challenges related to executive functioning. Impairment-based measures may provide information on the specific executive function processes affected, as well as the severity of the disorder. These measures may also be useful in determining which particular cognitive functions underlie failures in more complex functional activities. Activity/ participation-based tools are helpful in determining the impact of the executive function impairment on the person's ability to carry out daily tasks at home and the prognosis for returning to work or school. Activity/participation-based tools are also useful in setting person-centered goals so that treatment reflects needs directly applicable to the person's daily life and contexts. This not only increases a person's motivation toward goal achievement but supports generalization and carryover of skills learned in the therapy room to real-world activities. However, the current health care environment does not permit clinicians to perform extensive evaluations, so they must design their assessment protocols to gather as much information as possible in as little time as possible. Consultation with other team members (e.g., psychology, occupational therapy, physical therapy) will help provide a more complete picture of the person's executive function profile and prevent redundancy in testing. In fact, the need for increased efficiency and accountability in service delivery necessitates the integration of findings and the reduction of overlap among disciplines (Joint Commission on Interprofessional Relations, 2007).

In addition, not all assessments may be available to the treating SLP due to either publishing or facility policies. For example, publishers often limit the availability of assessments to those who can demonstrate specific qualifications, including formal training in the specific domain of interest, as well as test administration, scoring, and interpretation. While core speech and language tests are generally accessible to SLPs, cognitive tests may or may not be available, and specific qualification requirements may vary by publisher. Because other disciplines, particularly neuropsychology, may administer similar assessments, facilities often have specific guidance around which tests may be given when (e.g., inpatient rehabilitation vs. outpatient) by each discipline. Discussion with colleagues and supervisors at clinical sites regarding clinical use of the tools described below is encouraged.

Case History

Assessment of executive functions should begin with a detailed case history. Information can be obtained through a medical record review and interviews with the patient and a reliable contact person. Additionally, screening for visual or hearing changes is critical, as these may be present either premorbidly or as a result of the neurological injury.

Medical Record Review

Information related to the person's acute medical history—such as type, location, and extent of brain damage; presence/length of coma; and medical complications (WHO Body Structure/Function)—provides information relevant to recovery and prognosis. Information on the client's level of education and occupation (e.g., WHO Personal Factors) is important for the clinician to know to estimate the type and extent of demands previously placed on the executive function system. This information also helps with interpretation of test results. Knowledge of the person's residential setting, marital status, and support system (WHO Environmental Factors) will help the clinician plan for discharge.

Information regarding the person's current cognitive status should be obtained if available. Behaviors associated with executive dysfunction (e.g., impulsivity, disinhibition, lack of awareness of cognitive problems, off-target or disorganized responses to questions) may be documented by other health professionals. If the person has been evaluated previously, reports should be reviewed prior to additional testing of executive functioning. Having a general idea of the potential severity of a problem will assist the clinician in developing an assessment protocol. For example, if it is known that a person has a significant attentional problem, testing will need to be brief. Likewise, if a client has a concurrent aphasia, executive functioning tests with a high linguistic load should be avoided.

Interview

Interviewing people regarding their medical history, perception of the cognitive and situational changes since the injury, and the personal goals they wish to achieve through rehabilitation provides the clinician with information on the patient's awareness and insight, attitude regarding the injury, and ability to cope with the changes (WHO Personal Factors). Interviewing a reliable informant regarding any changes in behavior, communication, or cognitive function can aid in establishing hypotheses regarding potential executive function problems and help with identifying potential assessment tools. Refer to Tables 3–3 and 3–4 for a summary of Brian's and Carmi's case history.

A common therapeutic framework that bridges both assessment and treatment is motivational interviewing. Motivational interviewing is structured both for information gathering as well as engendering self-reflection, making it particularly well suited for individuals with executive function impairments (Sohlberg & Turkstra, 2011). At its most basic level, motivational interviewing provides guidance about the kinds of questions that support information sharing. Specifically, motivational interviewing uses the OARS model of open questions, affirmations, reflections, and summaries to encourage information exchange (Miller & Rollnick, 2012). Table 3–5 provides a summary of these strategies, as well as examples from Carmi's assessment. Motivational interviewing can be an important component of assessment because asking meaningful questions and demonstrating engagement with the client through affirmations, reflections, and summaries allows for information gathering while also building rapport, thereby supporting development of the therapeutic alliance between client and clinician (Medley & Powel, 2010). It also allows for early tailoring of treatment to the individual's self-identified needs and goals (which, in turn, supports engagement with therapy in the longer term). However, as described below under treatment, motivational interviewing can also be an important tool toward self-reflection and insight building and so should not be set aside once an assessment session is complete.

Table 3–3. Brian's Case History

Category	Information	Relevance to Assessment
Medical History	• 56-year-old male • MVC 3 months ago • Upon admission to ER was confused and agitated (RLA IV) • Initial CT scan = negative • Follow-up MRI = evidence of diffuse axonal injury (DAI) • Improved to RLA VI by discharge 2 weeks postadmission	• Still relatively early in recovery • Good progress in 2 weeks • DAI = likelihood of executive function problems
Rehabilitation History	• Inpatient rehabilitation for 4 weeks • Transitional living program for 6 weeks • Safe for discharge home independently • Given medical clearance to drive • Received outpatient rehab for persistent moderate executive function deficits and mild memory problems	• Made good progress during rehab • Safe at home • Need more information regarding completion of daily activities at home such as managing his son's schedule, meal planning, and paying bills
Sensory and Motor Status	• No difficulty hearing • Wears glasses for distance only (driving) • No upper or lower extremity deficits	• No restrictions/limitations for participating in assessment
Educational and Vocational History	• College graduate • Successful self-employed salesman of office equipment	• Likely had good executive function skills prior to injury since he was skillful in planning and managing his time and persuading customers to purchase expensive equipment
Psychosocial Background	• Divorced • 19-year-old son living at home, going to community college • Speaks English	• Limited support system

Table 3–3. *continued*

Category	Information	Relevance to Assessment
Interview: Patient	• Attempted to go back to work (against medical advice) • Was late for his appointment with customer • Couldn't answer customer's questions regarding differences/ pros/cons of newer copier and fax machines • Became flustered and "mind went blank" • Complained that everything takes longer to do than it used to	• Questionable judgment • Acknowledges problems when they occur • Potential deficits in working memory, verbal reasoning, organization, time management
Interview: Son	• Mostly still acts like Dad but "flakey" at times • Forgets items at grocery store • Dinner is usually later than planned • Takes him longer to do the usual things around the house—gets frustrated when he can't get everything done • Son can't always follow what Dad is trying to tell him	• Problems identified are consistent with patient report • Son may need education on TBI

Note: MVC = motor vehicle collision; ER = emergency room; RLA = Rancho Los Amigos; CT = computerized tomography; MRI = magnetic resonance imaging; DAI = diffuse axonal injury; TBI = traumatic brain injury.

Table 3–4. Carmi's Case History

Category	Information	Relevance to Assessment
Medical History	• 21-year-old female • Pedestrian hit by vehicle 10 months ago • Upon admission to ER was comatose (GCS 3) • Initial CT scan = right subdural frontal hematoma requiring emergency surgical evacuation • Follow-up MRI = evidence of DAI, hematoma resolving • Improved to RLA VI by discharge 6 weeks postadmission	• Far enough into recovery that return to school is a reasonable goal • Young, otherwise healthy, athletic • DAI, frontal injury = likelihood of executive function problems
Rehabilitation History	• Inpatient rehabilitation for 6 weeks • Transitional living program for 8 weeks • Safe for discharge home with parental supervision • Not yet given medical clearance to drive and does not have an interest in driving • Received weekly outpatient rehab for persistent moderate executive function deficits as well as milder attention, memory problems • Returning for new episode of care as she transitions back to school	• Made good progress during rehab • Safe at home, continuing to improve, but how does she return to school away from family support?
Sensory and Motor Status	• No difficulty hearing • No upper or lower extremity deficits • Some balance problems • Frequent headaches	• No restrictions/limitations for participating in assessment
Educational and Vocational History	• Current undergraduate student • Studying biochemistry as premed major • Worked in campus fundraising 2 days a week calling alumni	• Likely had good executive function and communication skills prior to injury since she was a scholarship student in a difficult major, juggling part-time work and volunteering with a local animal rescue nonprofit

Table 3–4. *continued*

Category	Information	Relevance to Assessment
Psychosocial Background	• Had lived in sorority house • University is about 2 hours from home • Bilingual, speaks English, Spanish with extended family • Some PTSD from accident, fearful of cars and traffic	• Good familial support system, campus support system is less clear • Receiving ongoing support from behavioral health related to PTSD
Interview: Patient	• Has done some practice with free online courses and watching video lectures • Sometimes watches videos repeatedly in online courses or completes the reading multiple times and still doesn't "get it" • Reports particular concerns about the amount of reading required by her studies • Frustrated by how slowly she feels she learns • Really wants to be back with her friends and to be back in school • Isn't sure if premed is still the best major for her but hasn't come up with any better ideas • Is sometimes short with her parents but says that she doesn't do that with her friends	• Does have good intellectual awareness that things have changed, but not yet anticipating when she may encounter difficulties • Can be somewhat rigid in managing problems when she does encounter them; unclear if she has too few strategies or doesn't know when to apply them • Question of communication deficits, unclear if she is able to be flexible to needs of conversational partner and organize extended responses • Potential deficits in cognitive flexibility, planning, problem solving, and metacognition
Interview: mother	• Carmi still has very high goals for herself, becomes very frustrated when she encounters her limitations • Often creates lots of plans around returning to school, but they are poorly formed or she doesn't see them through (e.g., doesn't finish her online courses)	• Parent reports slightly more problems than daughter; caretaking may impact mother's judgment of daughter's needs, but daughter also may not have considered the extent of the independence that will be required of her when she returns to university

continues

Table 3–4. *continued*

Category	Information	Relevance to Assessment
Interview: mother *continued*	• Likely needs some help coming up with alternative plans for what comes next—mother is supportive of school, but agrees that another major might suit her better, or that it would be better if Carmi could return just part-time to school at first	
	• Carmi can be very short with her parents, frequently snapping at them when she feels like they don't understand. Mother reports that "the longer she talks, the less it makes sense," which is usually when Carmi gets frustrated.	
	• Few friends at home, most are away at college. She connects with friends on social media, but mother can tell how much she misses being around friends on campus.	

Note: ER = emergency room; GCS = Glasgow Coma Scale; CT = computerized tomography; MRI = magnetic resonance imaging; DAI = diffuse axonal injury; RLA = Rancho Los Amigos; PTSD = posttraumatic stress disorder.

Table 3–5. Motivational Interviewing Question Types From Carmi's Case History Interview

Question Type	Demonstrates the Interviewer	Example
Open (O)		
Questions framed to allow for rich description rather than closed-ended yes/no or either/or responses, sometimes framed as statements ("tell me . . . ").	Is interested in hearing the person's story and perspective.	"What brings you in to see me today?" "Where would you like to see yourself in a year?" "Tell me more about your goals in school." "You mentioned that you have been doing some online classes. Tell me more about how that has been going."
Affirmation (A)		
Nonjudgmental statements that show understanding or respond positively to the effort the person is putting toward sharing their story or the rehabilitation process. These can also build client self-efficacy through affirming their strengths and abilities.	Sees and supports the work the person is doing to understand and share their experience.	"You've really put a lot of thought into this." "Thanks for taking the time to come in and talk through all this with me." "You've got a lot of ideas for where to go from here."
Reflection (R)		
These statements can reflect words, emotions, or behaviors, allowing the person to "hear" their own experience shared back with them. These can allow for clarity around specific reactions or emotions as well as deeper understanding of what is being shared.	Is listening carefully not just to the person's words, but to their overall self.	"I heard you talking a lot about your friends and how much you miss them. It sounds like you are really missing your friends at school. It makes sense that you want to be closer to them." "When we started talking about choosing a major, you seemed really unsure about what you want to do from here." "You smiled when I mentioned the Disability Resource Office. Can you tell me more about that?"

continues

Table 3–5. *continued*

Question Type	Demonstrates the Interviewer	Example
Summary (S)		
Statements that confirm understanding and also help move through the interview topics, providing closure as need be. These may link ideas, summarize a particular topic, or transition to closure.	Has been listening and is able to recap what has been covered to confirm understanding and can also be used to shift to a new topic.	"I think what I heard you say is that you are open to a new major, but you aren't sure yet what that might look like. It also sounded like something that was really important to you that we get figured out. Does that sound right?"

Impairment-Based Assessment of Executive Functioning (WHO-ICF Body Structure and Function)

Table 3–6 contains a list of commonly used impairment-based tests of executive functioning and examples of the specific core and higher-order executive process(es) addressed by each test. Where available, assessments with alternate norms allowing for greater cultural and linguistic specificity in either normative scores or test administration are provided in Table 3–7.

Delis-Kaplan Executive Function System

The Delis-Kaplan Executive Function System (D-KEFS; Delis et al., 2001) was the most commonly used assessment battery identified in the literature (Baggetta & Alexander, 2016). It measures a wide spectrum of verbal and nonverbal executive function processes. The national standardization study of the test included over 1,700 neurologically normal participants, ages 8 to 89 years, carefully selected to match the demographic characteristics of the population in the United States. A unique feature of this test battery is that each subtest contains conditional tasks to rule out fundamental cognitive problems (e.g., word-level reading, numerical or alphabetic sequencing, task comprehension) and a primary task that addresses executive function processes (e.g., cognitive flexibility). There are nine subtests (refer to Table 3–6), and each subtest is designed to be a standalone instrument that can be administered individually or along with other subtests.

Wisconsin Card Sorting Test

The Wisconsin Card Sorting Test (WCST; Grant & Berg, 1948) examines the client's ability to identify abstract categories and shift cognitive set. It contains 128 cards depicting one to four colored shapes. People must determine a sorting strategy according to a criterion

Table 3–6. Executive Function Processes Addressed in Impairment-Based Executive Function Assessments

Impairment-Based Test	Core Executive Function Process			Higher-Order Executive Process			
	Inhibition	Working Memory	Flexibility/ Set-Shifting	Reasoning	Planning	Problem Solving	Dual-Tasking
D-KEFS							
Trail-Making Test		X	X		X		
Verbal Fluency Test		X	X	X			
Design Fluency Test	X		X				
Color-Word Interference	X		X				
Sorting Test			X	X		X	
Twenty Questions				X		X	
Word Context Test			X	X			
Tower Test	X		X		X		
Proverb Test				X		X	
WCST							
WCST			X	X			
CLQT							
Generative Naming		X					
Design Generation		X	X				
Symbol Trails		X	X		X		
Mazes	X		X		X		
COWAT							
COWAT		X					

Note: D-KEFS = Delis-Kaplan Executive Function System (Delis et al., 2001); WCST = Wisconsin Card Sorting Test (Grant & Berg, 1948); CLQT = Cognitive-Linguistic Quick Test (Helm-Estabrooks, 2001); COWAT = Controlled Oral Word Association Test (Benton et al., 1994).

Table 3–7. Cultural Linguistic Diversity References for Executive Function Assessments

Assessment	References
Delis-Kaplan Executive Function System	• Sri Lankan adults (Dassanayake et al., 2021) • Turkish Capa adult speakers (Emek-Savas et al., 2019) • Spanish-speaking adult norms (García-Escobar et al., 2021) • Persian-speaking adults (Ghasemian-Shirvan et al., 2018) • Indian adults (Indorewalla et al., 2022) • Korean adults (Kim et al., 2017) • Chinese adults (Ruan et al., 2020) • Iranian adults (Tavakoli et al., 2015)
Wisconsin Card Sorting Test	• African American norms (Norman et al., 2011) • Spanish-speaking adult norms (Yassai-Gonzalez et al., 2019) • Portuguese-speaking adult norms (Faustino et al., 2022) • Argentinian-speaking adult norms (Miranda et al., 2020) • Setswana-speaking university student norms (Gadd & Phipps, 2012) • Farsi-speaking Iranian norms (Avila et al., 2019; Kohli & Kaur, 2006; Marquine et al., 2021; Zimmermann et al., 2015) • Taiwanese adult norms (Shan et al., 2008)
Modified Wisconsin Card Sorting Test	• Lebanese norms (Rammal et al., 2019)
Cognitive-Linguistic Quick Test	• Published Spanish version
Functional Assessment of Verbal Reasoning and Executive Strategies	• French Canadian–speaking norms (Marcotte et al., 2017)
Behavior Rating Inventory of Executive Function–Adult	• Iranian university student norms (Mohammadnia et al., 2022)

that an examiner has in mind (e.g., color, shape, or number) and that is deduced from the examiner's feedback (i.e., "right" or "wrong"). Once a client successfully completes 10 consecutive sorts, the examiner changes the criterion without alerting the individual, and the individual must determine the new rule for sorting.

Cognitive-Linguistic Quick Test–Plus

The Cognitive-Linguistic Quick Test–Plus (CLQT+; Helm-Estabrooks, 2001, 2017) may be used as a screening test for quick identification of strengths and weaknesses in five cognitive domains (attention, memory, executive functions, language, and visuospatial skills). Although population norms are not provided, cutoff scores were determined for two age groups (18–69 years and 70–89 years) based on two research studies involving 235 neurologically normal adults (Helm-Estabrooks, 2002). Four of the 10 tasks address executive functioning: Generative Naming, Design Generation, Symbol Trails, and Mazes. The newer edition (CLQT+, 2017) includes alternate administration and scoring guidelines for individuals with aphasia, as well as an optional semantic comprehension subtest.

Controlled Oral Word Association Test

The Controlled Oral Word Association Test (COWAT; Benton et al., 1994), a subtest of the Multilingual Aphasia Examination, is a measure of verbal fluency. It uses the three-letter set of C, F, and L to assess phonemic fluency. Individuals are given 1 minute to name as many words as possible beginning with the target letter.

Activity/Participation Assessments

Assessments that address activity/participation include both standardized tests (Table 3–8) and observational/performance-based tasks (Table 3–9).

Standardized Tests

Functional Assessment of Verbal Reasoning and Executive Strategies. The Functional Assessment of Verbal Reasoning and Executive Strategies (FAVRES; MacDonald, 2005) is an assessment tool particularly attractive to professionals interested in assessing the impact of executive dysfunction on a variety of real-life tasks dependent on communication skills. Performance on this test was positively associated with sustaining employment in skilled jobs after TBI (Meulenbroek & Turkstra, 2016). Each of the four tasks presents a novel problem that contains large amounts of information that must be comprehended and integrated prior to making a decision. Two tasks primarily examine planning (sequencing, organizing, and prioritizing tasks with time constraints), and two tasks primarily examine inhibition (examinee's ability to inhibit inappropriate remarks in response to conditions presented in the task). The tasks are scored in terms of efficiency of performance, accuracy of the solution, and quality of the rationale provided. Following administration

Table 3–8. Executive Function Processes Addressed in Activity/Participation Executive Function Assessments

Activity-Participation Test	Core Executive Function Process			Higher-Order Executive Process			
	Inhibition	Working Memory	Flexibility/ Set-Shifting	Reasoning	Planning	Problem Solving	Dual-Tasking
FAVRES							
Planning an Event			X	X	X		
Scheduling a Workday		X	X	X	X		
Making a Decision	X			X			
Building a Case	X			X	X		
BADS							
Rule Shift	X		X				
Action Program					X	X	
Key Search					X		
Temporal Judgment				X			
Zoo Map			X		X	X	
Modified Six Elements			X		X		X

Note: FAVRES = Functional Assessment of Verbal Reasoning and Executive Strategies (MacDonald, 2005); BADS = Behavioral Assessment of Dysexecutive Syndrome (Wilson et al., 1996).

Table 3–9. Observation/Performance-Based Measures

Behavior Rating Inventory of Executive Functions–Adult (BRIEF-A) (Roth et al., 2005)
The Dysexecutive Questionnaire (DEX) (Wilson et al., 1996)
Profile of Executive Control System (PRO-EX) (Braswell et al., 1992)
Executive Function Route Finding Task (Boyd et al., 1987; Lezak, 2012)
Cognitive Estimation Task (MacPherson et al., 2014)
American Multiple Errands Test (Aitken et al., 1993)

of each primary task, a variety of reasoning skills are assessed, including the client's ability to identify facts, eliminate irrelevant information, predict potential outcomes or consequences, generate alternative solutions, and provide a rationale for choices made. This information is helpful for treatment planning.

The normative sample for the FAVRES included 52 adults with acquired brain damage and 101 neurologically normal adults aged 18 to 79 years. The test was found to accurately differentiate individuals with acquired brain injury from neurologically normal peers (MacDonald & Johnson, 2005). Overall performance on the FAVRES is significantly related to cognitive measures of attention, speed of processing, memory, and executive functioning, establishing its concurrent validity (Avramović et al., 2017).

The Behavioral Assessment of Dysexecutive Syndrome. The Behavioral Assessment of Dysexecutive Syndrome (BADS; Wilson et al., 1996) was designed to assess a wide spectrum of executive function abilities and to predict everyday problems arising from dysexecutive syndrome. Normative data were obtained from 216 neurologically healthy control subjects aged between 16 and 87 years and 78 individuals who presented with a variety of neurological disorders (closed head injury, encephalitis, dementia, and stroke). The BADS demonstrates high discriminant validity and predictive validity (e.g., caregivers' ratings of executive problems were predicted by their brain-injured relatives' performance on the BADS). It also has high interrater reliability but only moderate test-retest reliability. This could be because repeated testing results in decreased novelty (Wilson et al., 1996).

The test contains six tasks, which yields a profile score ranging from 0 to 4 and incorporates both accuracy and time. Each task is designed to assess a specific component of executive functioning (refer to Table 3–8). The BADS also includes the Dysexecutive Questionnaire, as well as an observational assessment, which is described in the next section.

Observation/Performance-Based Measures of Executive Functioning

The true test of executive functioning is successful completion of daily life goals.

Observation of the client in a variety of contexts and under various conditions provides invaluable information on how the client performs independently without the structure that is often provided during formal testing. It may appear that a client knows what to do for a given task and may complete the task under structured conditions; however, when required to carry out the task spontaneously, performance may break down. Reliance on structured tests of executive functions may lead to underestimation of the difficulty individuals will have in real-world contexts (Ylvisaker & Feeney, 1998). Direct observation of functional behaviors also allows the clinician to assess the effect of corrective feedback with clients. Response to feedback often highlights the likelihood of a client's participation and success in rehabilitation (Manchester et al., 2004). For these reasons, observation of individuals in real settings, performing real activities, is encouraged.

Behavior Rating Inventory of Executive Function–Adult Version. The Behavior Rating Inventory of Executive Function–Adult Version (BRIEF-A; Roth et al., 2005) is a standardized measure that assesses executive functioning of individuals in their everyday environment. There are two formats: Self-Report and Informant. The assessment is composed of 75 items within nine scales that measure various aspects of executive functioning on the basis of frequency of occurrence (never, sometimes, often): Inhibit, Self-Monitor, Plan/Organize, Shift, Initiate, Task Monitor, Emotional Control, Working Memory, and Organization of Materials. The scales form two broad indexes: Behavior Regulation and Metacognition. It can be administered in approximately 10 to 15 minutes and has strong internal consistency, interrater reliability, construct validity, and concurrent validity.

The Dysexecutive Questionnaire. The Dysexecutive Questionnaire (DEX; Wilson et al., 1996) is part of the BADS. It is a 20-item questionnaire designed to sample emotional, motivational, behavioral, and cognitive changes in a person with suspected executive dysfunction. One version is designed for the subject to complete, and another version is designed for someone who is close to the individual, such as a relative or caregiver. Instructions are given to the participant to read 20 statements describing common problems of everyday life and to rate them according to their personal experience. Each item is scored on a 5-point scale according to its frequency from *never* (0 points) to *very often* (4 points). The total score may range from 0 to 80, with the higher score representing more significant deficits in executive functioning. A revised version of the DEX (DEX-R) includes four additional subtests (Simblett et al., 2017).

Profile of Executive Control System. The Profile of Executive Control System (PRO-EX; Braswell et al., 1992) is a tool that helps the clinician organize and interpret observational data. The PRO-EX is divided into seven scales delineating specific executive abilities, including Goal Selection, Planning/Sequencing, Initiation, Execution, Time Sense, Awareness of Deficits, and

Self-Monitoring. Ideally, the clinician observes the client performing several multistep activities (e.g., cooking and money management) in a variety of settings (e.g., clinic, home). At the completion of the task, the clinician rates performance on each scale from "able, only with physical prompting" to "independent."

Executive Function Route-Finding Task. In the Executive Function Route-Finding Task (EFRT; Boyd et al., 1987; Lezak et al., 2012), the client is faced with a novel problem to solve: finding a specific, but unfamiliar, location within the building where the testing takes place. No specific instructions are provided to the client regarding how the task may be completed. The task requires integration of several processes, including initiation, planning, and self-monitoring. Performance is rated on a 4-point scale in the areas of (a) Task Understanding, (b) Incorporation of Information Seeking, (c) Retaining Directions, (d) Error Detection, (e) Error Correction, and (f) On-Task Behavior. Additional problems that may contribute to performance are noted in emotional, communicative, interpersonal, and perceptual abilities.

Cognitive Estimation Test. The Cognitive Estimation Test (CET; MacPherson et al., 2014) requires people to mentally manipulate known facts to formulate reasonable answers to questions for which some relevant information may be known, but the exact answer is unknown (e.g., How many segments are there in an orange?). Participants are informed that there is no exact answer for most questions and that they should make a reasonable estima-

tion. All questions require numerical responses. This test provides information about a person's semantic memory, planning, working memory, and self-monitoring.

American Multiple Errands Test. The American Multiple Errands Test (AMET; Aitken et al., 1993) was modified from the original Multiple Errands Test (Shallice & Burgess, 1991). It allows the clinician to observe the client completing functional activities, including purchasing six items as quickly and cheaply as possible in a grocery store, sending a postcard with specific information to the clinician, and meeting the clinician at a certain time and place. The client's performance is rated in terms of successful task completion, rule breaks, and use of efficient strategies. McCue and colleagues (1995) compared the client's performance on this test to standardized tests of executive functioning and found that performance on the AMET was poorer than on standard executive function tests, and no strong associations were found among these measures. This suggests that the AMET is more sensitive in identification of executive dysfunction than standardized tests. More recently, a virtual reality version of the Multiple Errands Test (Raspelli et al., 2011) was developed for the assessment of executive functions. Raspelli and colleagues established ecological and construct validity when the measure was used with stroke patients.

Cognitive-Communication Assessment

Current guidelines for cognitive communication assessment after TBI recommend considering the communication needs of individuals, the communicative context, and the communication partner through use of both standardized and nonstandardized assessments (Togher et al., 2023). Although the tools below focus primarily on communication problems arising from cognitive deficits, thorough assessment is recommended for all domains, including screening of language, cognition, emotional processing, and sensory functions likely to impact communication (Togher et al., 2023). Numerous assessments and methods of analyses have been described in the literature; however, clinical use of these methods is infrequent (Frith et al., 2014; Riedeman & Turkstra, 2018). The ANCDS Traumatic Brain Injury Writing Committee recently evaluated tools used to assess cognitive and social communication, evaluating assessments based on the availability of normative data, reliability, validity, availability of the tool, administration and analytic feasibility, ecological validity, and person-centeredness of the tool (Sohlberg et al., 2019). A total of 15 communication measures were identified, but only 6 met the criteria of being readily available, designed for people with brain injury, and ecologically valid. Those measures and methods of assessment of cognitive communication are described below and listed in Table 3–10.

La Trobe Communication Questionnaire

The La Trobe Communication Questionnaire (LCQ; Douglas et al., 2000) is a measure of perceived communicative ability based on information gathered from the client and someone close to them (i.e., parent, significant other, sibling, child). It consists of two 30-question forms that assess how the individual with brain injury and their communication partner perceive communication quality. A sample item is "When talking to others do you [does your family member] say or do things others might consider rude or embarrassing?" Perceptions are recorded on a 4-point Likert scale ranging from *rarely/never* to *frequent/always*. However, since the LCQ is reliant on self and other awareness of communication changes, it may be less useful during the early stages of recovery, particularly in the hospital environment (Steel et al., 2017).

Although the LCQ has not been formally standardized, published normative data are often used for comparison purposes. Douglas et al. (2000) provide mean scores of healthy adult dyads, including individual items and subscale scores. Struchen et al. (2008) provide data on 276 adults with mixed-severity TBI, as well as a comparison between a subgroup of adults with TBI and healthy controls. The LCQ has also been used to identify cognitive communication problems in people with mild TBI, finding similar patterns in self-reported communicative needs to those with greater severity of injury (O'Brien et al., 2022). In general, though, as with many of the self-report tools that follow, the LCQ is most often used to identify particular areas of communication breakdown that the person reports experiencing and can therefore be useful for understanding needs and setting goals.

Table 3–10. Cognitive-Communication Measures

LaTrobe Communication Questionnaire (LCQ) (Douglas et al., 2000)

Pragmatic Profile of Impairments in Communication (PPIC) (Linscott et al., 2003)

The Adapted Kagan Scales (Kagan et al., 2004)

Montreal Evaluation of Communication (MEC) (Joanette et al., 2015)

Social Communication Skills Questionnaire–Adapted (SCSQ-A) (Dahlberg et al., 2006)

Socials Skills Questionnaire for Traumatic Brain Injury (SSQ-TBI) (Francis et al., 2017)

Discourse Analysis Measures

　Narrative

　　Macrolinguistic

　　Microstructural

　　Macrostructural

　　Story grammar

　Conversation

　　Obliges, comments, clarification

　　Exchange structure analysis

The Pragmatic Profile of Impairment in Communication

The Pragmatic Profile of Impairment in Communication (PPIC; Linscott et al., 2003; originally the PFIC, Linscott et al., 1996) is a clinician-rated assessment of videotaped interactions. It has 10 feature summary scales (Literal Content, General Participation, Quantity, Quality, Internal Relation, External Relation, Clarity of Expression, Social Style, Subject Matter, and Aesthetics), which assess the severity of the impairment, and 84 behavioral items rated by frequency of occurrence. The inclusion of both frequency of behaviors and severity ratings makes this instrument useful for measuring changes (Steel & Togher, 2018). Although the PPIC is commonly used in TBI research, this assessment is not yet available for commercial use, but it may be obtained by contacting the authors. Limitations also include that published norms are not available and that feasibility of administration may be challenging (Sohlberg et al., 2019).

The Adapted Kagan Scales

Kagan et al. (2004) developed two scales to assess the outcome of partner training for persons with aphasia: the Measure of Participation in Conversation (MPC) scale, which assesses how well the person with aphasia is able to engage in interactions, and the Measure of Support in Conversation (MSC), which evaluates the ability of the communication partner to acknowledge and reveal their partner's competence. Togher et al. (2010) modified the scales to incorporate supports identified as appropriate for individuals with cognitive communication deficits such as developing collaborative intent, cognitive support, emotional support, positive questioning style, and collaborative turn taking. This tool is both feasible and ecologically valid (Sohlberg et al., 2019), enabling examination of conversation as a mutual activity.

Montreal Evaluation of Communication

The Montreal Evaluation of Communication (MEC; Joanette et al., 2015) provides a battery of communication measures appropriate for adults with a range of neurological disorders, including TBI, right hemisphere disorder (RHD), and dementia. The MEC evaluates both production and comprehension of components of social communication, including emotional and linguistic prosody, metaphor, and indirect speech, along with conversational discourse. Self-awareness is assessed along with informant report. More recently, a brief version (MEC-B) has demonstrated similar psychometric properties to the full battery in adults with RHD (Casarin et al., 2020). Originally developed in French, English, Portuguese, and Persian versions have been developed and tested as well.

Social Communication Skills Questionnaire–Adapted

Among the 15 measures identified in the ANCDS review, the Social Communication Skills Questionnaire–Adapted (SCSQ-A; Dahlberg et al., 2006) was the only tool that specifically addressed personal relevance of communication breakdowns. Using a self-other comparison, the person with a communication disorder and a close other communication partner rate frequency of conversational performance ("I am able to initiate conversations about topics other than myself or my injury" or "I can follow and participate in an hour-long group discussion") on a 5-point scale (e.g., *never* to *always*). Despite limitations of self-other comparisons, the SCSQ-A has been shown to be sensitive to change following social communication treatment (Braden et al., 2010) and may be useful in documenting progress over time.

Social Skills Questionnaire for Traumatic Brain Injury

The Social Skills Questionnaire for Traumatic Brain Injury (SSQ-TBI; Francis et al., 2017) is designed for communication partners to assess communication competency of individuals with TBI using a 41-item tool. Items address specific skills related to social cognition and communication, such as empathy and emotion recognition.

Discourse Tasks and Measures

Discourse samples can be elicited using a variety of tasks, including picture descriptions, story retell, story generation, procedural descriptions, or conversation (see Table 3–10). Analysis may be conducted across different levels, including microlinguistic, microstructural, macrostructural, or superstructural (e.g., story grammar) (Coelho, 2007). For example, Cannizzaro and Coelho (2013) used a story retell task and segmented the narrative into T-units (a main clause and its subordinate clauses), then coded them into story grammar components (essential episodes consisting of initiating events, attempts, and direct consequences). Stubbs et al. (2018) used a simple procedural discourse task ("tell me how you would make a cheese and Vegemite sandwich") and examined productivity (number of meaningful words, total number of utterances, speaking time, speech rate, and words per minute) and macrostructure (number of essential steps, optional steps, and low content elements according to a checklist). Although these analyses are time-consuming, they can provide valuable information regarding communication strengths and weaknesses, which can inform the direction of treatment and document change over time (Stubbs et al., 2018).

Conversational discourse has been analyzed using an appropriateness paradigm that analyzed speaker initiations (obliges, comments, understanding, and clarification) and speaker responses (adequate: minimum response, adequate, adequate plus; inadequate: no response, partially unintelligible, completely unintelligible, delayed) (Youse et al., 2011). Bogart et al. (2012) used exchange structure analysis (Halliday, 1994) to analyze conversations between individuals with TBI and their friends. In exchange structure analysis, exchanges, or moves, are coded as syn-

optic (giving or requesting information) or dynamic negotiating meaning and assisting with communication breakdown and repair).

Brian's Assessment Results

Assessment began with an interview to hear Brian's story from his perspective using motivational interviewing strategies (refer to Table 3–5). Brian's goal was to return to work, so the assessment was designed to obtain information related to facilitating successful employment using activity/participation assessment tools. The FAVRES was selected because of its predictive validity and because it captures behaviors consistent with areas in which Brian reported difficulty. In addition, the Zoo Map subtest of the BADS was used to assess the benefit of structure on planning ability. Testing took place over two sessions. The interview was conducted and FAVRES Subtests 1, 3, and 4 were administered in the first session (60 minutes). FAVRES Subtest 2 and the BADS Zoo Map subtest were administered in the second session, and preliminary results were reviewed (45 minutes).

As can be seen in Table 3–11, Brian accurately completed Subtests 1 (Planning an Event) and 3 (Making a Decision) on the FAVRES. He provided a logical rationale for Subtest 3 but was a bit vague on Subtest 1. However, his performance on both subtests was inefficient, as it took longer than average to provide his responses. He had more difficulty with Subtests 2 (Scheduling) and 4 (Building a Case). It took a long time to successfully schedule 5 of the

Table 3–11. Brian's Assessment Results

Brian was assessed over two sessions
Session 1 (1 hour): Motivational interview, FAVRES Subtests 1, 3, 4   Session 2 (45 minutes): FAVRES Subtest 2, BADS–Zoo Maps

Tool	Rationale
FAVRES	Patient wants to return to work; high predictive validity; captures behaviors consistent with areas in which patient reported difficulty

	Planning an Event			Scheduling			Making a Decision			Building a Case		
	Raw	%ile	SS	Raw	%ile	SS	Raw	%ile	SS	Raw	%ile	SS
Accuracy	5	100	108	3	3	51	5	100	107	3	2	41
Rationale	4	15	69	0	6	58	5	100	103	4	29	59
Time (minutes)	10	11	79	27	3	72	11	9	86	18	11	77

	Planning an Event	Scheduling	Making a Decision	Building a Case	Total
Getting the facts	3/5	3/5	5/5	3/5	14/20
Eliminating irrelevant facts	1/1	1/1	1/1	1/1	4/4
Weighing the facts	0/1	0/1	1/1	1/2	2/5
Flexibility	1/1	0/1	0/1	0/1	1/4
Generating alternatives	9	9	8	7	33
Predicting consequences	4/4	3/4	4/4	2/2	13/14
TOTAL	18	16	19	14	67

<3 %ile, <70 SS

Tool	Rationale	
BADS	Has difficulty planning routes for work—determine benefit of structure	
	Zoo Map Subtest Version 1 (no structure)	Sequence Score = 1/8
	Zoo Map Subtest Version 2 (with structure)	Sequence Score = 8/8

Strengths	Weaknesses
Initiation	Efficiency
Attention	Organization
Comprehension	Strategy Use
Persistence	Flexibility
Insight	
Benefits from structure	

Note. FAVRES = Functional Assessment of Verbal Reasoning and Executive Strategies; BADS = Behavioral Assessment of Dysexecutive Syndrome.

12 tasks on the Scheduling subtest. He became overwhelmed ("I can't do this!"), omitted the remaining tasks, and did not provide a rationale for his responses. His written response on the Building a Case subtest identified three of seven problems, and he offered two potential solutions, though vague. Overall, his letter was disorganized and did not clearly define the problem.

On the reasoning questions following the primary FAVRES tasks, Brian performed relatively well with predicting outcomes, eliminating irrelevant information, getting the facts, and generating alternative solutions. Weighing the facts and flexibility of thinking were challenging.

On Version 1 of the BADS Zoo Map subtest, he achieved a sequence score of 1 out of a possible 8. He had difficulty determining alternate options when confronted with a problem and broke several rules in his attempts to create a route. In contrast, when provided with structure on Version 2, he achieved a sequence score of 8/8 and successfully completed the task.

Brian demonstrated several strengths during the assessment, including initiation, attention, comprehension, persistence, and insight. His challenges were in the areas of working memory, flexibility, organization/planning, efficiency, and strategy use. Overall, his test results were consistent with his subjective complaints and provided information needed to develop an effective treatment plan.

Carmi's Assessment Results

Carmi had a clear goal of returning to school, so the assessment focused both on general executive function as well as context-specific skills relevant to self-management and academics. As with Brian, the FAVRES was selected given its high applicability to functional activities likely to be encountered by Carmi, along with two impairment level assessments, the DKEFS Verbal Fluency and Tower Test. In addition, the BRIEF-A was administered to allow for a self-other comparison (with Carmi's mother providing the other report) of executive skills, providing an assessment of awareness as well as self-identified needs. Finally, the LCQ provided a similar self-other comparison of communication skills. The BRIEF-A and LCQ were mailed to Carmi for her and her mother to complete before arrival to the clinic; even so, the FAVRES took 83 minutes to complete, pushing the DKEFS testing to a second session. In the second session, testing was completed along with the clinical interview (using motivational interviewing), first with Carmi and then with her mother joining at the end with Carmi's permission. Test results were reviewed with both of them present (Table 3–12).

Across FAVRES tasks, Carmi's performance was markedly slow, although at times she was able to self-correct using that extra time and demonstrated high accuracy on Tasks 1 and 3. On Task 2, she attempted to use several strategies, creating several drafts of the schedule on scrap paper in order to try different ordering of events. Task 4 (Building a Case) provided a writing sample and revealed poor organization despite mechanics of writing being strong (good spelling, punctuation, syntax). In contrast, Carmi did well when providing her reasoning and eliminating irrelevant information.

Table 3–12. Carmi's Assessment Results

Carmi was assessed over two sessions
  Session 1 (100 minutes): Brief interview, FAVRES
  Session 2 (50 minutes): DKEFS, Motivational Interview (including complete case history, problem-based interview, test result review, general counseling about plan of care)

Tool	Rationale
FAVRES	Patient wants to return to school; high predictive validity; captures behaviors consistent with functional tasks that she will encounter

	Planning an Event			Scheduling			Making a Decision			Building a Case		
	Raw	%ile	SS	Raw	%ile	SS	Raw	%ile	SS	Raw	%ile	SS
Accuracy	5	100	108	4	17	79	5	100	107	4	15	74
Rationale	5	100	106	3	33	88	5	100	103	2	1	53
Time (minutes)	10	11	79	30	<1	64	18	<1	54	25	<1	48

	Planning an Event	Scheduling	Making a Decision	Building a Case	Total
Getting the facts	3/5	3/5	5/5	3/5	14/20
Eliminating irrelevant facts	1/1	1/1	1/1	1/1	4/4
Weighing the facts	0/1	0/1	1/1	1/2	2/5
Flexibility	1/1	0/1	0/1	0/1	1/4
Generating alternatives	9	8	6	7	30
Predicting consequences	4/4	2/4	4/4	2/2	12/14
TOTAL	18	14	17	14	63
					<3 %ile, <70 SS

continues

Table 3–12. *continued*

Tool	Rationale
DKEFS Verbal Fluency DKEFS Tower Test	Reports difficulty with planning, and noted difficulty with idea generation on FAVRES

	Raw	Scaled Score
Verbal Fluency		
Letter Fluency	29	8
Category Fluency	35	9
Category Switching Responses	11	7
Total Switching Accuracy	7	6
Letter vs. Category	−1	9
Category Switching vs. Fluency	−3	7
Tower Test		
Total Achievement	16	9
Mean First Move Time	7.7	7
Time Per Move Ratio	4.6	7

Tool	Rationale
BRIEF	Reports difficulty managing tasks, allows for self-other comparison

Scale/Index	Self			Informant		
	Raw Score	T Score	Percentile	Raw Score	T Score	Percentile
Inhibit	15	60	84	15	60	79
Shift	12	64	92	13	65	93
Emotional Control	19	58	76	18	54	67
Self-Monitor	11	59	83	12	58	80

Scale/Index	Self			Informant		
	Raw Score	T Score	Percentile	Raw Score	T Score	Percentile
Behavioral Regulation Index	57	62	81	58	59	80
Initiate	15	60	80	16	60	87
Working Memory	13	56	76	13	55	73
Plan/Organize	12	44	37	11	40	25
Task Monitor	9	50	56	9	49	56
Organization of Materials	11	45	38	11	44	32
Metacognitive Index	60	50	56	60	48	49
Global Executive Composite	117	56	72	118	53	67

Tool	Rationale
LCQ	Inconsistent reports of communication difficulty, allows for self-other comparison, will inform clinical interview

	Total Score Self	Mean Score Self	Total Score Other	Mean Score Other
Initiation/Conversation Flow	28	2.8	28	2.8
Disinhibition/Impulsivity	14	2.0	15	2.8
Conversational Effectiveness	14	2.3	17	2.83
Partner Sensitivity	8	2	9	2.25
Total LCQ	64	2.37	69	2.56

Strengths		Weaknesses	
Attention	Persistence	Initiation	Organization
Comprehension	Strategy Use	Working Memory	Flexibility/Idea Generation
		Efficiency	

Note: FAVRES = Functional Assessment of Verbal Reasoning and Executive Strategies; DKEFS = Delis Kaplan Executive Function System; BRIEF-A = Behavior Rating Inventory of Executive Function–Adults ; LCQ = La Trobe Communication Questionnaire.

Carmi struggled during switching tasks on the DKEFS Verbal Fluency subtest but did not perseverate, have off-target responses, or repeat previous responses. Instead, her performance was characterized by an overall paucity of output when challenged. On the Tower Test, she completed six out of nine towers with few errors; the final three towers she did not complete in the allowed time. Of note, she had a lengthy wait time before beginning to move pieces, showing that she was attempting to plan her moves in advance, but as the tasks became more complex, she had less success in doing so.

On the BRIEF-A, score patterns largely aligned between Carmi and her mother, with discrepancies most often occurring between frequency of problems occurring (e.g., rating items as "usually" vs. "sometimes," rather than disagreement about general problem areas). Self-reported deficits were greatest in the Metacognition subscale, with problems reported in initiation, working memory, planning, and organization. Finally, Carmi and her mother were overall well calibrated in total LCQ scores, with small discrepancies most apparent on the Conversational Effectiveness subscale; Carmi's mother reported that these problems were slightly more frequent. Overall, though, they were in alignment that both Conversational Effectiveness and Initiation/Conversational Flow were areas of need for Carmi.

Carmi's strengths included her persistence and willingness to engage with the tasks, even when they were clearly challenging for her. Her comprehension of the tasks and during conversation was good, and she attended to the tasks well. She attempted to use strategies on several occasions, and much of her inefficiency seemed to be around being unsure how she should adjust when something did not go right or the first repair attempt with a strategy failed. She demonstrated needs in initiation, cognitive flexibility, and idea generation, as well as difficulty with organization and planning. Overall, though, perhaps most notable was her inefficiency and slowness in completing all activities, which likely contributed to her reports of feeling like she could not get anything done and does not manage her schedule well.

Treatment

Selection of a specific treatment approach depends on many factors, including client preferences and goals, what behavior or task is the target of treatment, the executive function process(es) involved in performing the task, the person's awareness or understanding of the problem, and their response to feedback. In addition, as described in the other chapters in this text, their complete cognitive and linguistic profile will inform treatment selection and prioritization as well.

Rehabilitation Treatment Specification System

The Rehabilitation Treatment Specification System (RTSS) provides a framework for describing and categorizing interventions based on treatment theory—a prediction of how clinical actions impact patient functioning (Van Stan et al., 2021). Although the RTSS has its own terminology to learn, conceptually it well captures important aspects of decision-making when setting treatment plans (Turkstra et al., 2016). Specifically, the RTSS addresses treatment targets (aspect of functioning directly targeted for change), ingredients (what the therapist does), and mechanism of actions (why the treatment is expected to work) (Hamilton et al., 2022).

Treatment Targets

The treatment target is the specific aspect of function that the clinician hopes to change through direct intervention. Targets are described as being in one of three treatment groups: organ functions, skills and habits, and representations (knowledge, beliefs, and attitudes) (Hamilton et al., 2022; Hart et al., 2019). Cognitive rehabilitation is likely to be focused on training particular **skills and habits** to improve functional performance, and to change **mental representations** to better align with current skillsets following neurological injury and to support adjustment to cognitive changes and the need for compensatory strategies. The distinction between skills/habits versus representations is particularly important when working with individuals with executive dysfunction who often either know what to do (representation) but do not do it automatically (skill/habit), or develop an automatic routine with practice (skill/habit) but fail to anticipate or recognize when the routine will be useful (representation) (Hamilton et al., 2022).

Treatment targets should be distinguished from goals or aims, which are aspects of functioning that typically require more than one treatment target. For example, Brian set a goal to meet with two to three clients per week. To reach that goal, several targets needed to be attained (e.g., use a template to

plan and organize the meeting, schedule the meeting, accurately estimate time needed to drive to the meeting, remember to bring notes to the meeting). Therapy targets and goals should be easily observable and measurable, rather than being linked to standardized assessment results, and should be determined jointly by the clinician and client. Goal attainment scaling (GAS) is a collaborative technique used for developing individualized and meaningful goals (Grant & Ponsford, 2014) and has been associated with changes in functional outcomes (Churilov et al., 2020; Wallace et al., 2022). From a practical standpoint, Figure 3–5 provides a guide to collaborative goal attainment scaling. To begin the process, the clinician would support the client in providing a rich description of current performance, using motivational interviewing principles as needed (as described in the Assessment section). This provides an opportunity to build both personal insight as well as insight into the rehabilitative process. The client's current (baseline) performance is described as −1, and the goal is set for increasing performance to the level 0. Goals are then scaled into five levels of achievement ranging from −2 to +2. Typically, achievement of a +1 or +2 would be achievement beyond what might be expected during the treatment period, whereas a −2 would represent a decrease in performance. Once the anchors of "worst" (−2) and "best" (+2) performance have been established, discussion can move to what levels in between may represent. Again, this provides an opportunity not just to set goals but to describe specific behaviors associated with achievement at each level and to engage the client meaningfully in the therapeutic journey.

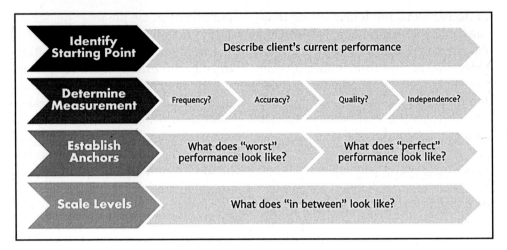

Figure 3–5. Collaborative goal attainment scaling guide.

Ingredients

Ingredients are what the clinician says, does, or provides when working toward achieving a target or goal (Van Stan et al., 2021). Clinician activity ingredients are often associated with specific treatment theories that hypothesize how the rehabilitation process results in change: behavioral activities (e.g., repeated practice, modeling, feedback, reinforcement, role-play), cognitive activities (e.g., cognitive drills, strategy instruction, self-regulation), educational activities, group process activities, or psychoemotional activities (Meulenbroek et al., 2019). Multiple ingredients are often embedded in a single intervention, and the specific ingredients used vary depending on the specific target.

Mechanism of Action

Least well defined in the RTSS is the mechanism of action (MoA). MoA is the reason by which we may anticipate ingredients to work toward a target. Consideration of the differing MoA demands of skill/habit acquisition versus representation change will allow for greater specification of treatment ingredients (Basilakos et al., 2021).

Skills and Habits. The most often cited example of an MoA related to developing skills and habits is "practice makes perfect." In deciding that this is the MoA, a clinician may then ensure that an included ingredient is sufficient practice so as to move the client's performance to more closely approximate "perfect." Particularly for acquisition of skills and habits, Kleim and Jones's (2008) tutorial on principles of neuroplasticity serves as a guide for possible MoAs to be considered when selecting ingredients. Rather than only practice makes perfect, these authors describe how aspects such as timing, intensity, salience, and transference of related skills may also be expected to effect change.

For example, if salience was thought to play a role in the MoA, then the clinician may focus on highlighting which skill is currently being exercised. Treatment may focus on training a person to execute a specific, discrete routine (such as sending and checking emails, or creating a grocery list by scanning items in the pantry), using a framework to structure the routines such as the Goal Management Training (GMT) approach described below. In this case, the person is being trained to **apply the framework** to a variety of scenarios, using it to guide management of novel situations. The clinician may need to ensure that flexible use of GMT is sufficiently salient as the target, rather than the routines employed as practice examples (e.g., "Here we are going to use GMT to choose a gift for your niece, but next, I want you to come up with two more examples of how you could use this strategy this week").

Representations. Cognitive or affective processing is thought to be the most prominent MoA for representational targets (e.g., increase knowledge or change in attitude). Change in knowledge representations may occur from ingredients such as providing education about a neurological disorder or component of executive function, whereas change in attitude representations (e.g., reformation and acceptance of the self-following brain injury) may benefit from ingredients such as self-reflection, group discussion, or observation of performance. Representations related to executive function may be particularly associated with elements of awareness, such as understanding of strengths and weaknesses, and the ability to implement strategies in anticipation of mitigating the impact of known areas of weakness.

Treatment Planning

The WHO-ICF framework and RTSS may also be used to guide treatment planning. The WHO-ICF provides a structure to help clinicians consider what should be addressed (e.g., specific impairment vs. an activity) and relevant factors that may impact response to treatment (e.g., personal, environmental; Hamilton et al., 2022). Treatment approaches for executive function typically address higher-order executive processes that are likely to interfere with activity/participation. The strongest research evidence favors treatments that train individuals to use metacognitive strategies to circumvent executive function impairments in daily activities (Raymer et al., 2018). The RTSS encourages the clinician to consider what specifically will be addressed (e.g., skills/habits, representations) and how the treatment will be delivered (e.g., which ingredients to be used). For example, acquisition of skills/habits may be trained using systematic instruction, while use of a skill may incorporate metacognitive strategies and thus change in representation.

In addition, motivational interviewing can be employed as a treatment approach to address change in mental representations. For example, clinicians can structure questions and listen for responses to encourage "change statements." These are statements that reflect the person's willingness to change, their motivation toward change, or barriers that they feel are preventing the change they are seeking. Table 3–13 provides a description and explanation of how clinicians can promote these kind of change statements, as well as what these sounded like for Carmi. In

Table 3–13. Sample Change Statements From Carmi's Intervention

Statement Type	Definition	Example of Clinician Questions to Evoke Change Talk	Example of Change Statement Responses
Desire	Expressing a desire for change, to reach a goal, or for things to be different	"What would you like to achieve in our time together?" "What is something that you really enjoy, or feel like is a strength for you?"	"I want to get back to school. I'm not sure what that will take. My mom is telling me to be patient, but I don't want to be patient. It has been almost a year and if I don't get back soon, all of my friends are going to graduate." "I started working with the social media team of the dog rescue I used to volunteer at. I get overwhelmed sometimes if I try to go into the shelter like I used to, but I downloaded one of those tools, kind of like PowerPoint, but it does graphics, but not like, a super fancy one. I make all kinds of graphics for them when they have events, or just to spotlight dogs or volunteers. It's low-key, but fun, and they seem to really appreciate it. I can get in a real zone with that."
Ability	Considering whether abilities or current skillsets are adequate for the change, and as with self-efficacy, reflecting on whether change feels possible	"What do you think needs to happen to get yourself ready to go back to school?"	"I need to be more organized. Like, I can't just randomly do stuff. Everything takes so much time. I get overwhelmed. I don't think I've figured out how to plan my time right yet. That's got to be something I figure out."
Reasons	Understanding reasons for actions or change, what is improved or gained by enacting change	"Why do you want to go back to school? What would you get from that?"	"I miss my friends so much. They just, they were everything to me. But also, I want to learn things again. I was good at school, and I want to think that my brain can still do that, learn things. Isn't that what all this is about, like, me getting back to doing what I was before? I want a good job too. I can't just live with my parents forever."
Need	Expressing an urgency toward the change	"How important is it for you to go back to your old school versus getting started here?"	"Like on a 10-point scale? It would be a 10, absolutely a 10. I mean, the goal is to go back to school—I want to be back and soon. It's why I am here. But I also need to figure out my major, and I can see taking some classes to figure that out. Like, maybe one semester, just to prove that I can do it and figure out my classes."

this way, motivational interviewing becomes a therapeutic tool, helping the person to identify their own motivators and barriers, and to problem-solve with the clinician to work toward their goals (Miller & Rollnick, 2012).

Treatment Approaches

A list of various treatment approaches and protocols is provided in Table 3–14, and the specific ingredients used in the treatments are listed in Table 3–15.

Table 3–14. Executive Function Treatments

Metacognitive Strategy Instruction
Goal Management Training
Goal-Oriented Attentional Self-Regulation (GOALS)
Implementation Intentions
Short-Term Executive Plus (STEP)
Interactive Strategy Modeling Training
Goal-Plan-Do-Review
Organizational Strategies
Self-Awareness Training
Reasoning Training
Strategic Memory and Reasoning Training (SMART)
Categorization Training
Systematic Instruction
Plan, Implement, Evaluate (PIE)
TEACH-M
Training Assistive Technology for Cognition (ACT/TATE)
Technology
Computer Cognitive Rehabilitation
Virtual Reality
Cognitive-Communication Treatment
Group Treatments
Group Interactive Structured Treatment (GIST)
Intervention for Metacognition and Social Participation (IMPACT)
Improving Natural Social Interaction: Group reHabilitation after Traumatic brain injury (INSIGHT)
Communication Partner Training
TBIconneCT
Joint Video Self-Monitoring
Individual and Discourse Treatments
The Communication-Specific Coping Intervention (CommCope-I)
Discourse Processing Treatment (DPT)

Table 3–15. Ingredients Used in Executive Function Treatments

Ingredients	Metacognitive Strategy Instruction												Reasoning Training			Systematic Instruction	
	GMT +EL: Bertens et al., 2015, 2016	STEP: Cantor et al., 2014	GMT + Tech: Elbogen et al., 2019	GMT + WM: Emmanouel et al., 2018	SA Tx: Goverover et al., 2007	GMT: Levine et al, 2011	ISMT: Marshall et al., 2004	GOALS: Novakovic-Agopian et al., 2011, 2018	II Tx: Radomski et al., 2018, 2022	GMT: Tomas et al., 2019	Return to Work tasks: Turkstra & Flora, 2002	GMT + Attn Tx: Waid-Ebbs, 2022	SMART: Cook et al. 2020	SMART: Vas et al., 2011, 2016	Cat Tx: Constantinidou et al., 2008	TEACH-M: Ehrhardt et al., 2005	ATC: Powell et al., 2015
Skills and Habits																	
Repeated trials/guided practice		X		X			X	X	X		X	X	X	X	X	X	X
Variable practice (settings/partners)								X	X		X						
Clinical model	X						X	X	X		X	X	X	X		X	X
Cueing hierarchy															X		
Feedback	X		X	X	X	X	X	X	X	X	X	X	X	X	X	X	X
Reinforcement	X		X	X	X	X	X	X	X	X	X	X	X	X	X	X	X
Role play											X						
Cognitive exercise/drill		X						X					X	X			
Task hierarchy															X		

154

Intervention component	GMT + EL	STEP	GMT + Tech	GMT + WM	GOALS	SA Tx	ISMT	II Tx	GMT + Attn Tx	SMART	Cat Tx	ATC
Task analysis	X	X	X		X					X		X
Error control	X	X							X			X
Cumulative review		X	X							X		X
Homework				X	X	X		X				
Technology training		X								X		X
Family/friend training		X										
Mental Representations												
Collaborative goal-setting	X	X			X	X				X		X
Organizational strategies		X		X	X	X		X		X		
Self-regulation/self-monitoring strategy instruction	X	X	X	X	X	X	X	X	X	X		X
Problem-solving strategies	X	X		X	X				X	X	X	
Educational/psychoeducational	X	X		X	X	X		X	X	X		X
Group process	X	X			X							

Note: GMT + EL = Goal Management Training plus errorless learning; STEP = Short-Term Executive Plus Intervention; GMT + Tech = Goal Management Training plus technology training; GMT + WM = Goal Management Training plus working memory training; SA Tx = Self-Awareness Training; ISMT = Interactive Strategy Modeling Training; GOALS = Goal-Oriented Attentional Self-Regulation; II Tx = Implementation Intentions Training; GMT + Attn Tx = Goal Management Training plus attention training; SMART = Strategic Memory Advanced Reasoning Training; Cat Tx = Categorization Training; ATC = Assistive Technology for Cognition.

Note that many treatment approaches incorporate the same ingredients. However, differences may be important in selecting an approach that will best fit a client's needs. Over time, skilled clinicians may be presumed to have a large pantry of ingredient options and refined decision-making trees or heuristics for matching and adapting sets of ingredients to client goals.

When reviewing the treatments that follow, it may be helpful to consider whether the intervention is targeting skills and habits (learning and practicing the steps in an executive function routine) versus representations (learning about executive function and what it looks like in everyday life), or if it perhaps has components addressing both (practicing an executive function routine both to learn the steps and to reflect on the results of that routine, or considering how to apply steps of an executive function routine in everyday life and why it might matter in their daily functioning and success). In addition, just as models of cognitive processes show attention and memory contributing to executive function, consider what other cognitive resources are necessary to train executive function. For example, whether training a discrete routine (e.g., ordering a latté at the coffee shop) or a self-management framework (e.g., using a problem-solving schema), both will need to be committed to memory for fluent recall at the appropriate time. In this way, executive function treatment rarely happens in isolation but builds on either previously learned skills or retained strengths in other cognitive domains. Therefore, the timing of executive function therapy must consider these other skills, providing complementary treatment or supports as necessary.

Metacognitive Strategy Instruction

Treatment of higher-order executive processes typically involves metacognitive strategy instruction (MSI) to teach individuals to self-regulate their behavior by breaking complex tasks into steps while thinking strategically (Kennedy et al., 2008). MSI does not emphasize training of a specific skill or task but rather guides the integration and internalization of self-regulation processes through direct instruction. This includes helping individuals identify an appropriate goal, predict their performance in advance of the activity, identify possible solutions based on their predictions, self-monitor or assess their performance during an activity, and change their behavior if the goal is not met (Kennedy et al., 2008). Metacognitive strategy training is recommended for with adults with TBI who demonstrate difficulty with problem solving, planning, and organization, with the caveat that the strategies should focus on everyday problems and functional outcomes (Jeffay et al., 2023; Tate et al., 2014). Protocols emphasizing MSI are briefly reviewed below.

Goal Management Training. Goal Management Training (GMT) is a standardized metacognitive training program based on the theory that executive function deficits arise from a disruption in the sustained attention system that maintains higher-order goals in mind while inhibiting automatic processes

(Robertson & Garavan, 2000). The main objective of GMT is to learn to regularly interrupt ongoing behavior to reflect on current behavior and intentions ("stop-and-think") and monitor performance (Levine et al., 2011). The intervention involves learning and practicing a self-instruction algorithm: *stop the behavior, state the current goal, compare ongoing behavior and goal, and adjust if necessary.* It combines education of key concepts such as the distinction between absent-mindedness and present-mindedness, slipups that occur in daily life, habitual responding (e.g., "auto-pilot"), stopping and thinking, task performance and feedback, and discussion of participants' own personal task failures and successes (Levine et al., 2011). Mindfulness exercises are also included to bring attention to the present moment to monitor the relationship between current circumstances and higher-order goals (Tornas et al., 2016; Tornas, Løvstad, et al., 2019; Tornas, Stubberud, et al., 2019). The current version of the program involves 20 hours of training (goalmanagementtraining.com); however, studies have reported training ranging from four to 23 hours (Stamenova & Levine, 2019).

Some studies have modified administration of the GMT program by including errorless learning (Bertens et al., 2015, 2016) or addressing specific cognitive skills such as working memory (Emmanouel et al., 2018) and attention (Waid-Ebbs et al., 2022). Bertens et al. (2015) found that preventing the occurrence of errors during executive strategy training enhanced the acquisition of self-chosen everyday activities. However, errorless learning did not generalize to improved performance on neuropsychological tests, subjective cognitive complaints, or quality of life (Bertens et al., 2016). Emmanouel et al. (2018) coached participants to systematically follow the instructions given at each step of GMT using a working memory strategy (visual image of a ladder with four substeps and key words for each GMT step). Participants receiving the GMT and working memory strategy treatment completed multistep tasks more accurately and efficiently than participants receiving only working memory treatment. Waid-Ebbs et al. (2022) supplemented GMT with Attention Process Training III and other attention tasks, finding that the combined training significantly improved overall executive functioning performance than GMT alone. The use of technology along with GMT has also optimized outcomes (Cuberos-Urbano et al., 2018; Elbogen et al., 2019).

A recent meta-analysis of GMT (Stamenova & Levine, 2019) found a significant beneficial effect on primary outcome measures (specific tests of executive functioning, everyday executive function tests, patient self-report questionnaires) immediately after training and at follow-up. Additionally, significant positive effects were found on secondary measures (tests of working memory and long-term memory, instrumental activities of daily living tasks, e.g., completion of tasks in everyday life situations) and mental health questionnaires immediately after training and at follow-up. No significant effect was found on speed of processing.

Goal-Oriented Attentional Self-Regulation. The Goal-Oriented Attentional Self-Regulation (GOALS) program

(Novakovic-Agopian et al., 2011, 2018) involves metacognitive goal management strategies as outlined in GMT, with special emphasis on mindfulness-based attention regulation strategies applied to progressively more challenging daily life situations and goals using the metacognitive strategy of "Stop-Relax-Refocus." Homework exercises involve practice planning and executing simple tasks and logging successes and failures in using strategies. Participants with brain injury significantly improved on tests of attention and executive function, complex task performance, and emotional regulation (Novakovic-Agopian et al., 2011, 2018).

Implementation Intentions. Implementation Intentions (II) are written pre-made decision statements that specify when, where, and how goal behaviors are to be enacted and accomplished (Gollwitzer, 1999, 2014; Radomski et al., 2022). In II, specific goals are identified and are written in an "if/when, then" format to develop an association between a specific situational trigger and desired behavior. For example, if a person's goal is to finish a book for book club, the II may be written as "when my husband sits down to watch TV after dinner (trigger), I will go to my room to read my book (goal-related action)." Radomski et al. (2017) used metacognitive strategy instruction to help individuals write and carry out IIs. Clinicians guided the participants in task prioritization and planning using worksheets, demonstrations, feedback, and self-reflection and practiced applying II in a variety of situations. Participants were required to write an II related to one of their goals each day and report it in a voicemail to their clinician each day, and the clinician provided feedback regarding homework follow through and II quality. In general, participants learned to generate IIs and reported improved attainment of their goals.

Short-Term Executive Plus. The goal of Short-Term Executive Plus (STEP) is to teach a core set of metacognitive skills for problem solving, emotional regulation, and attention that can be applied across a wide range of real-life activities (Cantor et al., 2014). Real-life problem situations were addressed using a five-step approach known by the acronym "SWAPS" (*Stop!* Is there a problem? *What* is the problem? *Alternatives* and options to solve the problem; *Pick and plan* the chosen option; and *Satisfied* with the outcome of the plan). Emotional self-regulation was addressed using classroom-style instruction regarding the impact of brain injury on behavior and practice applying strategies to identify emotional triggers and manage behavioral responses. Attention was addressed using Attention Process Training-II (Sohlberg et al., 2001). Following training, significant gains were made in problem-solving skills related to making life decisions and handling interpersonal difficulties. No significant gains were made in attention or emotional self-regulation following treatment targeting these areas. STEPS has also been adapted to a mobile health solution that replaces the paper-and-pencil activities with an interactive mobile application, but training is still provided by clinicians for the person to learn to use the SWAPS strategy (Wallace & Morris, 2020).

Interactive Strategy Modeling Training. The purpose of Interactive Strategy Modeling Training (ISMT) is to teach participants to use metacognitive strategies to solve verbal problems. In a study by Marshall et al. (2004), the participants and the examiner worked together to solve verbal problems through systematic question asking. The task was based on the Twenty Questions Task of Mosher and Hornsby (1966), and the training incorporated principles from educational psychology, including reciprocity (equal partnership/interactive) and exemplary modeling. Participants were presented with a grid containing 32 familiar words and had to determine a target word. The words could be grouped according to various semantic or perceptual categories. The examiner and participant exchanged roles of "problem solver" and "instructor." The examiner modeled strategies (i.e., constraint seeking questions) and provided the rationale for using the strategy (i.e., eliminated many of the options). Reinforcement was provided to the participant when appropriate questions were asked, and guessing was avoided. Results demonstrated improved problem solving, characterized by requiring fewer questions to solve the problem and use of more constraint-seeking questions.

Goal-Plan-Do-Review. Feeney and Ylvisaker (2003, 2006) implemented a metacognitive strategy (goal-plan-do-review) as part of a multicomponent cognitive, behavioral, and executive function intervention for reducing challenging behavior and increasing academic performance in young children with frontal lobe impairment following

TBI. The children were provided with a graphic outline of an executive function routine prior to initiating a task and were coached to identify the goal (i.e., What are you trying to accomplish?) and a plan (i.e., How do you plan to get this done?). Following completion of the task, they reviewed their performance (i.e., How did it work out?). Implementation of this routine, combined with positive behavior supports, resulted in a decrease in challenging behaviors and an increase in the quantity of work completed in the classroom. Kennedy and Krause (2011) also employed a similar plan-do-review technique with a college student with brain injury, finding that comparing predicted time to complete academic activities with actual time resulted in better planning and organization as time estimates became more accurate.

Organization Strategies. Turkstra and Flora (2002) provided treatment to a 49-year-old man with executive function problems following a TBI who was having difficulty returning to work as a social worker due to deficits related to organization of information. He reported difficulty with note-taking during interviews and writing reports; therefore, treatment addressed development of a report structure (e.g., S.O.A.P. format: Subjective, Objective, Assessment, Plan) that included carrier phrases to elicit and organize information (e.g., "The client talked about . . . " "I said to the client . . . "). He was provided with numerous opportunities to practice using the forms in a variety of role-play scenarios. Following 21 one-hour sessions over 10 weeks, he generated more accurate, detailed, and organized reports and became successfully employed.

Self-Awareness Training. MSI is optimized when the patient has awareness of the need to use a strategy and can identify contexts in which the strategy should be used (Tate et al., 2014). Described in terms of the RTSS, more accurate mental representation results in increased propensity to use strategies trained as new skills and habits. Self-awareness (SA) may be defined as one's ability to (a) recognize deficits, (b) understand and recognize the functional implications of deficits (i.e., task errors), and (c) anticipate possible future difficulties related to activity limitations and participation restrictions (Engel et al., 2019, p. 164). Because self-awareness is a complex, multidimensional cognitive process, there are multiple theories regarding the mechanisms of SA. Two prominent theories identify the mechanism as (a) neurological, which explains problems in SA as related to disruptions in brain function or cognitive processes, or (b) psychological, which proposes that premorbid personality, psychological coping methods, and defense mechanisms affect one's level of SA (Engel et al., 2019). In a clinical context, it may be difficult to differentiate between these elements of SA (Tate et al., 2014) and both may be present (Kennedy & Coelho, 2005).

Multiple intervention techniques have been found to be effective in improving SA at an activity and participation level (Engel et al., 2019). Many interventions include MSI such as training to anticipate obstacles, comparison of predicted performance and actual behavior, and tracking performance on tasks while using different strategies (Goverover et al., 2007; Sohlberg et al., 2005). A critical component of MSI is direct, corrective feedback, particularly when embedded in activities that include self-monitoring (verbal, audiovisual, experiential) (Cicerone et al., 2019; Engel et al., 2019; Jeffay et al., 2023).

Reasoning Training

Strategies to improve the capacity to analyze and synthesize information should be used with individuals who demonstrate impaired reasoning skills (Jeffay et al., 2023; Tate et al., 2014). Intervention approaches include strategies to analyze and synthesize complex information, training in categorization, applying past memories to plan and solve problems, and dual-task training (Tate et al., 2014).

Strategic Memory and Reasoning Training. The Strategic Memory and Reasoning Training (SMART) protocol (Vas et al., 2011) was developed to enhance the ability to abstract the gist of information presented in various formats. The program uses a top-down hierarchical strategy-based approach to train individuals to construct generalized meanings with no direct emphasis on recall of explicit facts. The program begins with strategies to strategically attend to incoming information and filter out less relevant details. The next stage focuses on integration of explicit content with preexisting knowledge to form gist-based representations. The final stage addresses generalization by evaluating information from different perspectives. Vas et al. (2011) examined the effects of SMART versus a general education program on 24 participants with TBI who engaged in 18 hours of training during 12 group sessions conducted over 8 weeks. Results showed that the SMART program resulted in improved gist-reasoning, with generalization to untrained tasks of working memory, and improvements were sustained over a 6-month period. These findings were replicated in a second study (Vas et al., 2016). Additionally, gains were evident in executive function and psychological health.

The SMART program has also been delivered via telepractice (tele-SMART) for adolescents with sports-related mild head injury (Cook et al., 2020). Results indicated significant improvement in abstract reasoning and recall of facts from complex information. In addition, parent ratings of real-life executive function behaviors showed significant improvement. Self-ratings suggested some improvement, though changes were not significant.

Categorization Training. Constantinidou et al. (2008) designed a categorization program that systematically trained participants through an eight-level hierarchical program that included identification of basic perceptual features, categorization and analogy tasks, abstract reasoning, and rule-based decision-making. Participants receiving the categorization treatment demonstrated significant improvement on neuropsychological tests and and functional outcome measures.

Systematic Instruction

While it is a common practice to introduce strategies to compensate for executive function deficits, use of these strategies may be unsuccessful due to lack of effective instruction and/or lack of instruction that targets maintenance and generalization of the strategies (Powell et al., 2012). However, it has been demonstrated that strategies can be successfully acquired and used in real-life situations when they are trained systematically (Ehlhardt et al., 2008; Powell et al., 2015; Sohlberg & Turkstra, 2011; Sohlberg et al., 2023). Systematic instruction is a method that focuses on how the instruction is designed and delivered. It emphasizes error control (e.g., errorless learning), particularly during the acquisition phase of an instructional target (Sohlberg & Turkstra, 2011). Several studies have found error control techniques to be helpful in teaching specific information to people with TBI (Cohen et al., 2010; Hunkin et al., 1998; Manly et al., 2002), as well as to persons with dementia (Jang et al., 2015; Kessels & Hensken, 2009). Systematic instruction also builds in factors influencing maintenance and generalization such as high amounts of correct practice, distributed practice spaced retrieval, effortful processing and self-generation, and use of metacognitive strategies (Sohlberg et al., 2005). Error control is not emphasized during generalization and maintenance stages because there is evidence that error-based learning (trial and error) may be more beneficial than errorless learning in transferring skills to new tasks or environments (Ownsworth et al., 2017).

Plan, Implement, Evaluate. Sohlberg and Turkstra (2011; Sohlberg et al., 2023) described a framework for systematic instruction that can be used when training specific targets: Plan, Implement, Evaluate (PIE). In the **planning stage**, the target is identified. To identify appropriate targets, the clinician needs to consider who the learner is, what type of information is to be trained (e.g., facts and concepts, multistep routines, or use of external aids), where the skill will be used (e.g., home, work, community), why is the skill being trained (e.g., increase independence, decrease caregiver burden), and how the outcome will be evaluated (e.g., direct observation, questionnaire).

During the **implementation stage**, the ingredients are applied. The specific ingredients used depend on the specific target (e.g., mental representations or skills/habits). When targeting skills/habits, ingredients may vary depending on whether the client is at the stage of initial acquisition, mastery and generalization, or maintenance. Acquisition of a skill is facilitated by use of error control techniques (e.g., spaced retrieval), massed and intensive practice, and specific and regular feedback, while generalization and maintenance are more likely to occur with use of distributed practice, trial and error, intermittent feedback, and increased level of cognitive engagement (e.g., metacognitive strategies such as prediction and reflection) (Ownsworth et al., 2017).

When **evaluating** the effectiveness of the instructional technique, the specific outcome needs to be identified (e.g., the client will independently use an electronic calendar to recall appointments). The data to be collected within the session should be planned in advance (e.g., how many steps were recalled; how many trials were needed to reach criteria), and generalization and maintenance probes should also be considered (e.g., if recording speech appointments in calendar was trained in treatment, probe whether patient spontaneously recorded PT appointments). Goal attainment scaling, as described previously, has been used frequently for evaluating the effectiveness of instructional techniques for individuals who have sustained a TBI (Keegan et al., 2020).

TEACH-M. Elhardt et al. (2005) used systematic instruction to facilitate learning and retention of steps needed for using an email program specifically designed for their study. The specific components, or ingredients, of program are represented by the acronym TEACH-M: *T*ask analysis (broke task into seven steps), *E*rrorless learning (modeled each step; patient practiced step one, then one and two, then one, two, three, etc.), *A*ssess performance (baseline performance, then probe before introducing a new step), *C*umulative review (regularly review previously learned skills), *H*igh rates of correct practice trials (e.g., spaced retrieval practice), and *M*etacognitive strategy training (e.g., patient predict performance). Using this technique, participants learned the seven-step email program in 7 to 15 treatment sessions. Participants reported the most helpful parts of learning the program were watching the instructor model and having the opportunity to practice the steps frequently.

Assistive Technology for Cognition. Assistive technology, defined as "any item, piece of equipment, or product that is used to increase, maintain, or improve the functional capabilities of individuals with disabilities" (Brunner et al., 2017, p. 1029), is often incorporated into rehabilitation to support individuals with cognitive deficits due to brain injury. There is evidence that electronic systems such as personal digital assistants (PDAs), electronic organizers, mobile or smartphones, and electronic voice memos can assist everyday functioning (Charters et al., 2015). Smartphones have been reported as being the most important technology used for simple functions such as texting and reminders; however, caregivers and survivors of TBI reported that many of the advanced apps that are available are often too complex (Chu et al., 2014). Successful use of technology requires tailoring the intervention to the needs and abilities of the individual (Brunner et al., 2017). Facilitators to successful use include motivation, consumer involvement in decisions, ease of use, training to use tech, good caregiver support, availability of tech support, and matching of technology to needs and preferences (Chu et al., 2014).

Powell et al. (2012) clearly summarized the components to include when designing instructional methods to train use of technology. First, conduct a detailed assessment of the learner's needs and abilities, including determining the environments in which the instructional targets will be used. Second, complete a task analysis by breaking the instructional targets into component parts. Third, carefully select and sequence examples. Delivery or implementation of instructional components includes (a) ongoing assessment of the learner's performance to gauge mastery; (b) preinstruction of component skills; (c) modeling of the skill by the instructor prior to learner practice; (d) carefully faded support; (e) frequent, correct, distributed practice and review; (f) immediate corrective feedback; (g) individualized instructional pacing to facilitate engagement; and (h) strategy instruction (p. 87). Powell et al. (2013) developed an instructional package detailing these instructional components to assist clinicians in train-

ing the use of assistive technology for cognition (TATE: Training Assistive Technology in the Environment). The TATE package includes training videos, needs assessment forms, sample scripts, and data tracking tools (available at https://cbirt.org/research/completed-projects/tate-training-assistive-technologyenvironment-toolkit).

Powell et al. (2012) conducted a randomized control study comparing this systematic instruction approach to "trial-and-error" learning on use of an electronic memory aid and found that both groups were more accurate in using the device immediately posttraining; however, only the systematic instruction group demonstrated generalization in using the device when interacting with other people immediately posttraining and maintained their skills at follow-up. This systematic instruction approach has also been successful in training use of assistive technology to compensate for executive function difficulties in the work environment (Powell et al., 2015).

Technology

Computer Cognitive Rehabilitation. Computer program interventions have been used in cognitive rehabilitation following TBI and stroke for many years (Cicerone et al., 2011). Bogdanova et al. (2016) conducted a systematic review of computerized cognitive rehabilitation for attention and executive functioning in acquired brain injury. A wide variety of interventions were used, and most of the studies used attention and executive function focused treatment programs specifically created or modified for the study. A large variety of standardized neuropsychological tests were used as the primary outcome variables, and approximately half the studies used subjective self-reports. The majority of studies reported significant gains on neuropsychological tests and on self-reports. It is important to note that there were no measures used that reflected functioning within a daily life context. Additionally, the role of supervision or clinician assistance in the administration of computer treatment programs was infrequently reported (Bogda-nova et al., 2016). There is evidence that computer programs for cognitive rehabilitation result in better outcomes when used in conjunction with other methods, particularly metacognitive strategy training (Fernández López & Antolí, 2020; Spikman et al., 2010; Tate et al., 2014).

Fernández López and Antolí (2020) completed a systematic review and meta-analysis of randomized control trials (RCTs) for computer cognitive rehabilitation. Six of the eight studies included used commercially available computer programs (i.e., RehaCom, Cog-med, BrainGymmer). Results showed improvement on neuropsychological tests of visual and verbal working memory; however, attention, process-ing speed, and executive functions did not benefit from the intervention. The authors concluded that this finding sup-ports previous studies indicating that if computerized cognitive training is used, metacognitive and compensatory strategies should be trained in conjunc-tion (e.g., Cicerone et al., 2019; McEwen et al., 2015).

Results of a systematic review on the effectiveness of computerized cognitive training for persons with PD indicated measurable gains in cognitive perfor-mance, including attention, memory,

executive functioning, and processing speed (Nousia et al., 2020). It was sug-gested that cognitive training programs that addressed multiple cognitive do-mains simultaneously were more effec-tive than programs addressing a single domain (Nousia et al., 2020). Of note, the impact of computerized cognitive retraining on neuropsychiatric symp-toms was conflicting, with some reports of improvements in depression and other reports of a negative impact on quality of life (Nousia et al., 2020).

There has been some suggestion that mental activity may serve as a protective mechanism for the brain and prevent the onset of dementia (Barnes & Yaffe, 2011). However, results of a system-atic review on computerized cognitive retraining for individuals diagnosed with MCI indicated there is not enough evidence to determine whether or not computerized cognitive training will prevent clinical dementia or improve or maintain cognitive function in those who already have evidence of cognitive impairment (Gates et al., 2019).

Virtual Reality. Virtual reality (VR) tech-nology may be a potentially useful tool for assessment and rehabilitation of executive functioning (Alashram et al., 2019; Jeffay et al., 2023). This technol-ogy creates computer-generated artifi-cial environments with specific sensory properties that allow users to interact with the environment in real time. VR training can provide active learning opportunities on motivating tasks. It allows repetitive practice on tasks that can be gradually increased in difficulty while gradually reducing the support given by a clinical therapist.

DeLuca et al. (2019) conducted a clinical trial to examine the effect of

VR training using the BTs-Nirvana system (https://www.btsbioengineering.com/nirvana/discover-nirvana-2/) compared to a traditional cognitive rehabilitation approach. Following 24 one-hour sessions, both groups demonstrated significant improvement in cognitive functioning and mood; however, only the VR group had a significant increase in selective attention and executive function skills of cognitive flexibility and shifting. Similar findings were reported from a systematic review examining the use of VR for cognitive rehabilitation (Alashram et al., 2019). The five studies that specifically examined executive function skills reported significant improvement in this cognitive domain. Overall, it is suggested that VR may be a useful and effective cognitive rehabilitation approach for individuals with acquired brain injury (e.g., stroke and TBI) (Alashram et al., 2019; DeLuca et al., 2019; Jeffay et al., 2023).

VR has also been explored as a form of cognitive rehabilitation for persons with mild-to-moderate dementia (Oliveira et al., 2021). The VR program comprised 12 simulations of instrumental activities of daily living. Results showed statistically significant improvement on a global measure of cognition; however, no significant changes were evident in specific cognitive domains, including executive functioning.

Cognitive Communication Treatment

Although cognitive communication disorders may occur as a result of wide range of cognitive changes (Cornis-Pop et al., 2012), many treatment ingredients mirror those of executive function, although some are unique to addressing communication as a shared activity. According to updated INCOG guidelines (Togher et al., 2023), cognitive communication treatment should include metacognitive awareness and strategy training, insight building, partner training, and, where possible and appropriate, group interventions. Project-based group therapy should also be considered, as it provides a structure around which many more complex communication activities can occur, such as shared problem solving, negotiating within a group, and rapid switching between listener and speaker roles, all while working toward a shared goal. High rates of contextualized practice are needed to effect change, and individualized, person-centered treatment should be in alignment with the person's gender, cultural, and linguistic identity.

In addition, goal attainment scaling is particularly well suited for measurement of change during cognitive communication treatment, capturing both individualized communication goals as well as encouraging self-monitoring of behaviors associated with progress toward goal achievement (Finch et al., 2018; Togher et al., 2023). Teletherapy is also an appropriate service delivery modality for cognitive communication treatment, allowing for delivery of key therapy ingredients including video feedback, role-play, clinician modeling, and rehearsal (Togher et al., 2023). Psychoeducation, adjustment to communication changes, and training in coping strategies are also recommended as important components of comprehensive cognitive communication treatments (Meulenbroek et al., 2019; Togher et al., 2023).

Although not addressed in the current chapter, as a reminder, social cognition should also be screened in individuals with cognitive communication disorders to determine if treatment should also address deficits in areas such as theory of mind, perception of emotions (e.g., facial expression, tone, prosody), and emotional empathy (Meulenbroek et al., 2019; Sohlberg et al., 2019; Togher et al., 2023). Such problems with social cognition are particularly common after right hemisphere injury (Blake, 2021; Minga et al., 2022; see Chapter 4) but may occur with other acquired brain injuries or neuropathological processes as well. Table 3–14 includes a list of cognitive communication treatments and Table 3–16 provides their ingredients.

Group Treatment for Cognitive Communication Disorders

Group Interactive Structured Treatment. Group Interactive Structured Treatment (GIST) is a program designed by Hawley and Newman (2010) to address cognitive, communication, and emotional contributors to communication success through a group intervention based on principles of cognitive-behavioral therapy. Key components include education around specific social competence skills, which are then modeled, practiced, and observed in the self and others, with feedback provided. In addition, mental representation changes are also addressed through cognitive restructuring and social reinforcement. Generalization is directly trained as part of the protocol, through involving family as well as weekly homework requiring practice in functional settings. Elements of effective group functioning are emphasized both to facilitate the group process and to provide explicit educational opportunities around implicit group communication rules. Modeling is emphasized over direct didactic instruction, with high rates of practice.

GIST proceeds through five stages across 13 weekly sessions. In the first, Engagement, participants are oriented to the group to address attentional and motivational factors and to ensure that they are prepared to play a role in the group and the treatment. In the second stage, Awareness, both general awareness (e.g., what makes a great communicator) and personal awareness are addressed through self-assessment and feedback from the facilitator and group. The third stage, Goal Setting, also includes feedback around specific therapeutic goals from the group, facilitator, and close communication partners to support development of achievable and meaningful outcomes. The fourth stage, Skill Mastery, provides more explicit discussion and practice of social routines and skills relevant to everyday communication success. Last, the fifth stage, Generalization, addresses use of learned skills in functional contexts and practice with family or close communication partners. Family and communication partner training supports continued carryover and consistency after program completion.

Studies examining outcomes following GIST suggest improvement to personal goal attainment scale goals, communication, and satisfaction with life (Braden et al., 2010). In a comparative efficacy study, similar gains in goal attainment scale goals and measures of communication competence were observed regardless of whether the intervention was delivered in an interactive group format or a traditional classroom setting (Harrison-Felix et al., 2018).

Intervention for Metacognition and Social Participation. In Intervention for Metacognition and Social Participation (IMPACT; Copley et al., 2015; Finch et al., 2017), individual and group sessions run twice weekly for 8 weeks. Sessions are typically 1 hour and move from an initial individual session that focuses on goal setting and understanding individualized needs to group sessions addressing use of metacognitive strategies and how these might be applied to communication contexts. Ingredients include feedback and modeling from both the therapist and the group members along with self-prediction, self-monitoring, and self-reflection. In group sessions, role-playing and group discussion around shared and unique needs are facilitated by the clinician. In a pilot trial, six out of eight participants with TBI met or exceeded their goal attainment scaling goals (Finch et al., 2017).

Improving Natural Social Interaction: Group Rehabilitation After Traumatic Brain Injury. Improving Natural Social Interaction: Group Rehabilitation After Traumatic Brain Injury (INSIGHT; Keegan et al., 2020) is an intervention based on positive behavioral supports (Ylvisaker & Feeney, 1998). INSIGHT is designed to (a) support naturalistic conversational practice, (b) maintain the value of authentic communication, (c) minimize environmental control or emphasis being placed on disabilities,

and (d) foster opportunities for expression of the individual's unique identity. Client-centeredness is promoted throughout, with clinicians facilitating and supporting rather than leading. In the pilot study, the ongoing group intervention was provided in weekly 2-hour group meetings facilitated by trained graduate students in a university clinic. For each session, participants first met at the clinic, then traveled to naturalistic settings for outings (e.g., parks, malls, coffee shops, museums). Collaborative goal setting using goal attainment scaling was based on The Aphasia: Framework for Outcome Measurement (A-FROM; Kagan et al., 2007), providing guidance toward a holistic understanding of the individual and their communication goals. The RTSS was used to frame the intervention, with clients establishing both aims and scaled targets (goals). Aims were longer-term goals that may or may not be achieved as a result of the intervention, but targets should map to these aims. In turn, ingredients were selected based on those client-centered goals and included many familiar ingredients from Table 3–16, including role-play, feedback, education, prompting, and modeling. Communication specific application of these included guidance on how to demonstrate listening or education, modeling of slowed rate and rephrasing for clarity, and environmental modification (removal of phone, management of background noise). Peer feedback and support were also encouraged in the group setting.

Results from the pilot study with six adults with moderate-to-severe TBI showed statistically significant gains in goal attainment scaling scores, along with improvements in communication

Table 3–16. Ingredients Used in Cognitive-Communication Treatments

Ingredients	Group Treatments			Communication Partner Trainings		Individual and Discourse Treatments		
	GIST (Hawley & Newman, 2010; Braden et al., 2010; Harrison-Felix et al., 2018)	IMPACT (Copley et al., 2015; Finch et al., 2017)	INSIGHT (Keegan et al., 2020; Keegan et al., 2022)	TBIconnecT (Rietdijk et al., 2019; Rietdijk et al., 2020)	Joint VSM (Hoepner & Olson, 2018; Hoepner et al., 2021)	CommCope-I (Douglas et al., 2014; Douglas et al., 2019)	DPT (Kintz et al., 2018)	NARNIA (Whitworth et al., 2015; Whitworth et al., 2020)
Skills and Habits								
Repeated trials/guided practice	X	X		X	X	X	X	X
Variable practice (settings/partners)	X	X	X	X	X	X		X
Clinical model	X	X	X	X				
Feedback	X	X	X	X	X			X
Reinforcement		X		X	X			
Role-play	X	X	X	X	X	X		
Error control	X			X	X			X
Cumulative review	X			X	X			X
Homework	X			X	X			

	GIST	IMPACT	INSIGHT	CommCope-I	VSM	DPT	NARNIA
Scaffolding				X		X	X
Direct instruction							X
Cueing/reminders	X	X	X	X		X	X
Scripts	X				X		
Visual stimuli	X					X	X
Environmental modification		X					
Alternative communication tools	X	X					
Mental Representations							
Imagery	X				X	X	X
Video review (video, audio, self, other)	X	X	X			X	X
Collaborative goal-setting	X	X	X				
Organizational strategies	X					X	X
Self-regulation (monitoring, reflecting) strategy instruction	X	X	X	X		X	X
Problem-solving strategy instruction	X	X					
Education/psychoeducation	X	X	X	X		X	X
Group process	X	X					

Note: GIST = Group Interactive Structured Treatment; IMPACT = Intervention for Metacognition and Social Participation; INSIGHT = Improving Natural Social Interaction: Group reHabilitation after Traumatic brain injury; VSM = Video Self-Monitoring; CommCope-I = Communication-specific Coping Intervention; DPT = Discourse Processing Treatment; NARNIA = Novel Approach to Real-life communication: Narrative Intervention in Aphasia.

participation and quality of interactions. In a follow-up study of INSIGHT delivered in a virtual format during the coronavirus pandemic, goal attainment scaling scores were again most sensitive to change and showed participants achieving personally relevant communication goals (Keegan et al., 2022).

Communication Partner Training

TBIconneCT. TBIconneCT is a communication partner training designed to provide people with TBI and someone close to them (e.g., parent, significant other, child) specific skills to support and encourage conversation and information exchange (Rietdijk et al., 2019). TBIconneCT is a streamlined version of the TBI Express program (Togher et al., 2013, Togher et al., 2016), so that many components are shared between the two. Recognizing that although group treatment is often preferable but rarely feasible (finding adequate numbers of clients for whom the training would be applicable, in addition to scheduling and reimbursement challenges), the key difference between the two is that TBI Express is a group treatment, whereas TBIconneCT is designed to provide the training to dyads (person with brain injury and a person close to them). Across 10 sessions, the clinician-led program provides education about TBI and its impact on communication along with training about supportive and unsupportive communication behaviors, such as effective listening, positive questioning, conversation roles, and how to facilitate communication as a shared act. Core strategies are built around collaboration and elaboration. In collaborative acts, conversation partners provide appropriate support

for changes after TBI. Partners may provide needed information rather than quizzing to support recall and memory (e.g., "We had a great time swimming at your aunt and uncle's last weekend. Do you want to see if we could go back to the lake this weekend?" rather than, "Remember what we did last weekend? Think back—you'll get it. It had to do with water."). Support may also be provided to organize the conversation for executive function needs (e.g., "You wanted to get some friends together next weekend? How about we figure out who you want to invite and then we can think about what you want to do."). Elaboration is about extending conversation through providing additional detail or noticing topics introduced by the person with TBI and exploring those together.

TBIconneCT has been shown to be equally effective when delivered in person or via telehealth (Rietdijk et al., 2020). Outcomes include fewer and less frequent conversation problems, better conversations (as rated by SLPs blinded to the intervention), and gains in specific communication skills (Rietdijk et al., 2019; Togher et al., 2013; Togher et al., 2016). Results relate to participants who completed at least 80% of TBIconneCT sessions, although clinicians are encouraged to consider which aspects may be most important or relevant to their particular client's needs.

Joint Video Self-Monitoring. Hoepner and colleagues (Hoepner & Olson, 2018; Hoepner et al., 2021) developed and tested a Joint Video Self-Monitoring intervention in which people with brain injury and their conversation partners used video self-monitoring (VSM) to review and learn from interactions happening in lived contexts. The person with brain injury and their partner record conversations between treatment sessions, then present these to the clinician during the session to be reviewed collaboratively. Some approaches to VSM use an errorless learning approach, focusing narrowly on successful interactions, then cataloging behaviors that led to that success. However, in the Joint VSM program, both successes and challenges were discussed, albeit with a focus on providing positive feedback (e.g., by encouraging that noticing challenges was a step toward avoiding them in the future). An inverted hierarchy of prompts from least to most was provided, moving from open-ended questions ("What did you think?") to open-ended questions about specific interactions, to asking the client to reflect on specific behaviors, and finally to directing the client to identification of specific behaviors. Motivational interviewing was used throughout to encourage metacognitive reflection. Results from two case studies (Hoepner & Olson, 2018; Hoepner et al., 2021) demonstrated improvement on personally relevant goal attainment scaling goals, awareness of communication problems in individuals with brain injury, and particular skills such as turn-taking and engagement. Overall, the approach was deemed feasible and appropriate for clinical use, holding promise for the development of self-regulated communication behaviors.

Individual and Discourse Treatments

The Communication-Specific Coping Intervention. Communication-Specific Coping Intervention (CommCope-I; Douglas et al., 2014; Douglas et al., 2019) is an intervention based on self-coaching principles (Ylvisaker, 2006), cognitive behavioral therapy, and context-sensitive social communication therapy. Productive strategies contributing to communicative success are identified, then shaped to increase their number and effectiveness, using these to replace less productive strategies. Clients are guided through three stages of the CommCope-I program: (a) development of self-awareness of coping strategy use, (b) practice with strategies in personally relevant contexts, and (c) self-assessment through video review. Ingredients used during these three stages include personally selected imagery, concrete cueing, repeated rehearsal, personally relevant scripts, communication partner reminder scripts, real-world practice, and self-evaluation. Results from studies examining outcomes following CommCope-I showed decreases in nonproductive strategy use for both comprehension and expression, similar increases for productive strategies as judged by close communication partners, and improvements to discourse as judged by trained raters blinded to the intervention. In addition, participants reported lower stress postintervention and qualitatively described feelings of accomplishment and independence as a result of completing the program.

Discourse Processing Treatment. A systematic review of narrative discourse interventions found few interventions, which were mostly of low quality due to small samples sizes (Steel et al., 2021). In addition, maintenance and generalization has proved challenging, perhaps due in part to limited personalization of the interventions. Even so, there is some emerging evidence toward procedures and approaches likely to result in improvement to narrative organization and quality of information exchange. For example, Kintz and colleagues (2018) based their Discourse Processing Treatment (DPT) on use of a visual story guide that included six sequentially arranged categories of information to include when describing sequentially arranged story cards (setting, problem, internal response, action/plan, results, and resolution). Following education about use of the story guide, the intervention moved through five steps, with the visual story guide present through the first four steps. First, the clinician presented the story cards and asked comprehension questions to ensure the person understood the story being presented. Cueing was provided in a least to most hierarchy. Second, the person with brain injury told the story, with a prompt to provide a story with a "beginning, middle, and end" (Kintz et al., 2018, p. 54). This story was recorded, then reviewed in Step 3 using the story guide. In Step 4, missing features were identified, with support provided by the clinician as necessary to ensure all categories were represented. In Step 5, the story guide was removed, and the person with brain injury retold the story independently. Results showed improvements on untrained stories in completeness and informativeness, as well as short-term improvements in coherence.

Novel Approach to Real-Life Communication: Narrative Intervention in Aphasia. In a trial of the Novel Approach to Real-Life Communication: Narrative Intervention in Aphasia (NARNIA; Whitworth et al., 2015), as applied to four participants with mixed acquired brain injury, a similar story framework was provided to organize and encourage communication effectiveness (Whitworth et al., 2020). Task types varied from personal events, procedures, exposition, and narrative retells (i.e., the Cinderella story). Video review and prompting was employed, with prompts being reduced over the course of the 6-week treatment period. Mind maps were used to organize narratives, and main events were identified along with specific verbs and nouns that would fit with each event. Although changes to the macrostructural organization of narratives were not observed, participants did increase quantity and efficiency of output. Importantly, cognitive profiles appeared to play an important role in response to treatment, and should be considered in future, larger studies, as well as clinically when tailoring the intervention and supports to an individual.

Brian's Treatment Plan

Brian's overall goal was to return to work. Goal attainment scaling (Table 3–17) and motivational interviewing techniques were used to collaboratively establish meaningful, achievable goals. This was accomplished through discussion of his experiences to date ("Tell me more about what happened when you tried to return to work. Why do you think that was a problem? Is there anything you could you do differently to perform your job more successfully? Given these issues, what do you think you could reasonably accomplish by the end of

Table 3–17. Sample Goal Attainment Scaling With Brian

Value Number	Meaning	Example
+2	Much more than expected level of outcome	I will meet five customers per week, using strategies
+1	Somewhat more than expected level of outcome	I will meet four customers per week, using strategies
0	Expected level of outcome	I will meet three customers per week, using strategies
−1	Somewhat less than expected level of outcome	I will meet two customers per week, using strategies
−2	Much less than expected level of outcome	I will meet two customers per month, using strategies

Note: Brian reported meeting with two to three customers per day prior to his accident.

therapy?"). Following these discussions, it was determined that scheduling and attending appointments would be the primary aim of treatment, and targets of treatment would include improving organization, planning, time management, and flexibility.

A variety of organizational strategies were used to address the problems Brian was experiencing with meeting customers. A task analysis of the activity was completed collaboratively. Brian brainstormed to write out all steps related to meeting with a client (sequential order was not necessary at this point), which helped him become aware of the complexity of the task. Brian was then prompted to reorganize all the steps into categories (preparation, scheduling the appointment, and traveling to the appointment), and cueing was provided as needed to add details. Templates, checklists, and a script were created over the next several sessions to provide structure and

reduce the load on working memory (Table 3–18).

In the early stage of treatment, templates were used to review Brian's customers' purchasing records and enter information from technical manuals for the products into templates. Consistent use of the templates was trained using elements of GMT (e.g., Levine et al., 2011) to help Brian stay on task and monitor his performance (What am I doing? Why am I doing it? Did I compare and contrast the most important features of the product?). Prediction was used to help with time management (How long will it take me to complete these forms? How long did it take?). After practicing completing the templates during sessions, Brian continued the activity for homework.

To facilitate scheduling, a script was generated and practiced using systematic instruction techniques (e.g., Ownsworth et al., 2017; Sohlberg & Turkstra, 2023). Immediate, corrective feedback

Table 3–18. Sample Template and Checklist for Brian

PLANNING		Notes
Review the customer's records	1. When did we last meet?	1.
	2. What did he buy?	2.
	3. Is there a newer model? (check catalogues)	3.
	a. How is it different?*	3a.
	b. Other models?*	3b.
	4. What else was he interested in?	4.
	5. Is there any other product that would be helpful for the customer? Why?	5.
	*Complete equipment template with information for customer's current product and one recommended product	

SCHEDULING	Notes
Gather props: Calendar, relevant cheat sheets 1. Hi Mr. _____ 2. It's been a while. We haven't had a chance to talk since _____ 3. How is the _____ working? 4. Is it meeting your needs? 5. Are there other jobs or tasks you need some help with? 6. I'd like to come see you again and show you some new products. 7. What day works for you? *Check calendar* *If there is nothing on your calendar, ask:* 8. What time? *If you already have something scheduled, state:* 9. I'm sorry, I already have an appointment that day. What other day are you available? *Write down customer's name and time of appointment in your calendar.* 10. Great! I look forward to meeting with you on _____.	

Table 3–18. *continued*

TRAVEL	
Two days before appointment	*Check off when completed*
1. Find address on Google Maps	1.
2. Note time it takes to get there	2.
3. Add 30 minutes	3.
4. Calculate total time you need to get there	4.
5. Calculate the time you need to leave	5.
6. Write time you need to leave and time of appointment in calendar	6.
7. Gather relevant cheat sheets and brochures	7.
Day before appointment	*Check off when completed*
1. Find address on Google Maps	1.
2. Print out route—read through 3 times	2.
3. Check appointment time and time you need to leave	3.
4. Review relevant cheat sheets and brochures	4.
Morning of appointment	*Check off when completed*
1. Check Google Maps—any change in time to get there? (accident, rush hour)	1.
2. Adjust time for travel, if necessary, remembering to add 30 minutes	2.
3. Review cheat sheets	3.
4. Put cheat sheets and print-out of route in car	4.

was provided if a step was missed (e.g., did not write the appointment in his calendar), and the script was started again from the beginning. As Brian became accustomed to using the script successfully, constraints or problems were spontaneously introduced to encourage problem solving and flexibility. A similar procedure was used for training use of the travel template.

Once the templates were trained, Brian began scheduling appointments using the goal-plan-do-review strategy to monitor and evaluate his performance (e.g., Feeney & Ylvisaker, 2003) (e.g., Goal—schedule appointment; Plan—complete templates; Do—meet with customer; Review—Was the meeting successful? Why or why not? What was easy or challenging?).

During the following sessions, successes and challenges of Brian's meetings with customers were reviewed. An emphasis was placed on identifying problems and potential solutions using elements of the STEP program (Cantor et al., 2014) (What was the problem? Why do you think it happened? What could you have done differently?). The templates and scripts were adjusted as needed to foster success.

Brian was seen for treatment twice a week (45-minute sessions) for 10 weeks to develop and practice the script and use of the templates, then once a week for 8 more weeks, during which time he attempted to schedule appointments with customers. By the 18th week, he had successful meetings with three customers per week for 3 consecutive weeks and met his goal (goal attainment scaling score of 0 = expected level of outcome) and he was discharged from therapy.

Carmi's Treatment Plan

Carmi's overarching goal was to return to school, and thus treatment began with collaborative goal setting to build the treatment plan toward that larger purpose. This began with motivational interviewing during the second assessment session but continued into the first treatment session as well (see Table 3–5 for examples of questions from the assessment and Table 3–13 for example change statements evoked during treatment). Carmi was focused on three areas: developing organizational strategies to manage tasks, improving her communication so that she could participate in class discussions or complete writing assignments, and identifying a new major.

Because of Carmi's needs and the complexity of returning to school, an interdisciplinary approach was necessary, so a referral was made to her local vocational rehabilitation services office to assist with her third goal area—identifying a new major. This office can provide vocational assessments for Carmi to explore other majors and also coordinate with her disability services office when she returns to school. In addition, Carmi continued to see a team of behavioral health professionals to address her posttraumatic stress from her injury. The remaining two goals around organizational strategies to manage tasks and organization of spoken discourse were then scaled using Goal Attainment Scaling (Table 3–19). Although writing was also a goal, Carmi decided to focus on speaking first. Carmi attended two 50-minute sessions each week—one in person and one delivered via telehealth—for 12 weeks.

During discussion with Carmi, she described using several organizational systems and planners but had not found one that worked for her. In reviewing some options together with the clinician, it became clear that she had a sense of what was needed and that no single planner had all of those features. She had also mentioned several times that she enjoyed designing flyers and social media postings in her volunteer work, so that it became clear that having Carmi design her own planner would allow her to perform a task analysis of what was needed, evaluate its effectiveness, and then redesign the planner as she used it. This process of design and redesign was framed in the language

Table 3–19. Sample Goal Attainment Scaling With Carmi

Value Number	Meaning	Assignments	Communication
+2	Much more than expected level of outcome	Using my planner and GPDR, I will manage my assignments independently and ask for help when I need it.	I will explain what I am learning, providing 100% of the most relevant information, using strategies.
+1	Somewhat more than expected level of outcome	Using my planner and GPDR, I will manage my assignments but have someone review them with me once a week.	I will explain what I am learning, providing 80% of the most relevant information, using strategies.
0	Expected level of outcome	Using my planner and GPDR, I will manage my assignments with help three times a week.	I will explain what I am learning, providing 60% of the most relevant information, using strategies.
−1	Somewhat less than expected level of outcome	Using my planner and GPDR, I will manage my assignments with help every day.	I will explain what I am learning, providing 40% of the most relevant information, using strategies.
−2	Much less than expected level of outcome	Using my planner and GPDR, I will have side-by-side help managing my assignments with help every day.	I will explain what I am learning, providing less than 40% of the most relevant information, using strategies.

of self-regulation, training it is a concrete example of monitoring how well things were going by practicing scheduling during the session, then making adjustments as need be, then checking again to see if performance improved. Initially, the clinician supported identification of needs through a task analysis, and having Carmi have control over the layout of the planner fostered much deeper connection to components of it that supported her organization and task completion. Once the planner was in a "beta" version, Carmi began testing it at home with a free online course, and a new goal was scaled to establish the habit of using the planner consistently (Figure 3–6).

As a related target, Carmi also began using a goal-plan-do-review form to plan and track her academic activities while taking the online course. In

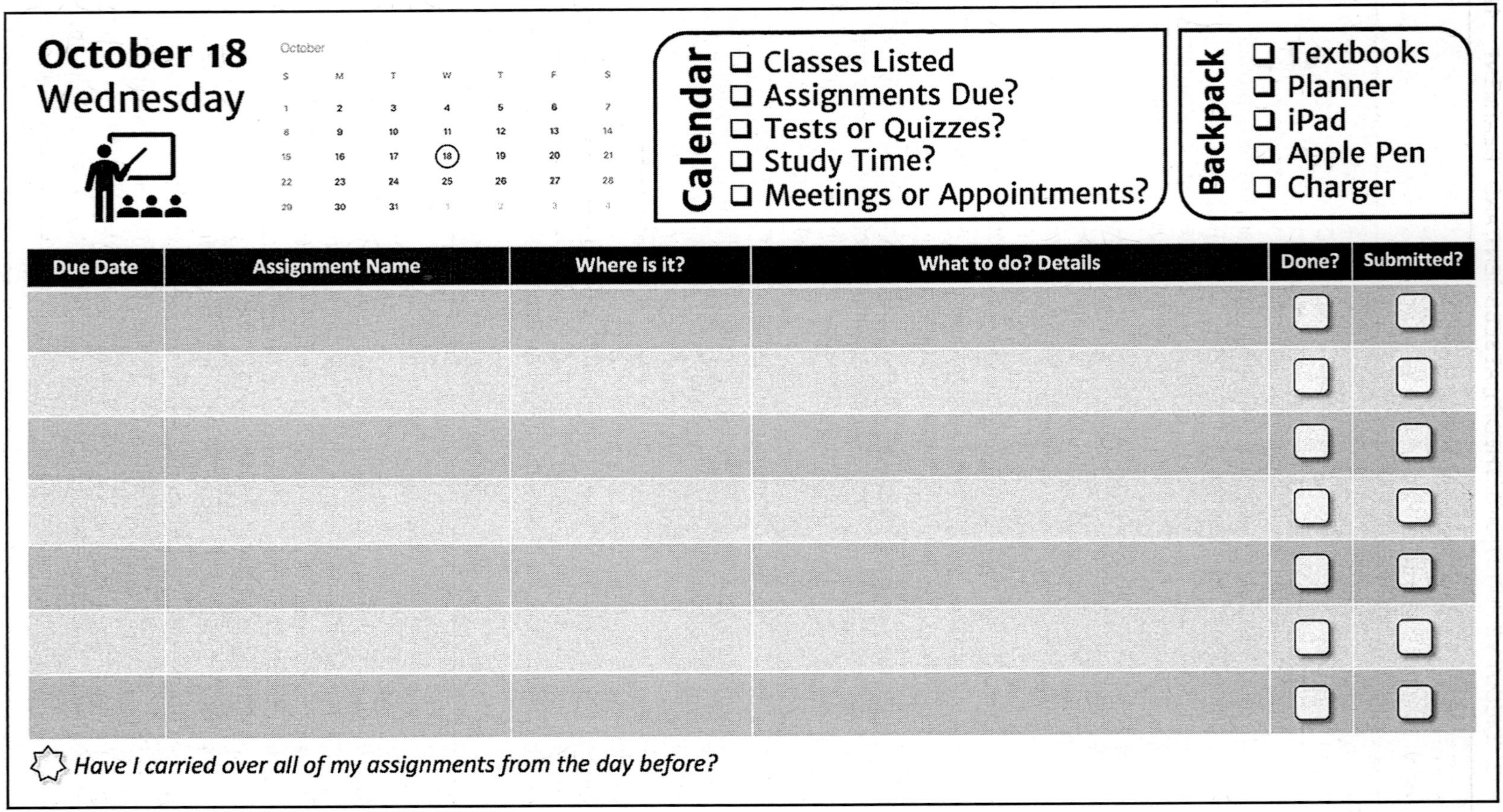

October 18
Wednesday

October

S	M	T	W	T	F	S
1	2	3	4	5	6	7
8	9	10	11	12	13	14
15	16	17	(18)	19	20	21
22	23	24	25	26	27	28
29	30	31	1	2	3	4

Calendar
- ☐ Classes Listed
- ☐ Assignments Due?
- ☐ Tests or Quizzes?
- ☐ Study Time?
- ☐ Meetings or Appointments?

Backpack
- ☐ Textbooks
- ☐ Planner
- ☐ iPad
- ☐ Apple Pen
- ☐ Charger

Due Date	Assignment Name	Where is it?	What to do? Details	Done?	Submitted?
				☐	☐
				☐	☐
				☐	☐
				☐	☐
				☐	☐
				☐	☐
				☐	☐

☆ *Have I carried over all of my assignments from the day before?*

Figure 3–6. Carmi's co-designed assignment page.

particular, because of Carmi's inefficiency at completing tasks, she was instructed to predict the time it would take to complete her assignments, then monitor how long it took to complete tasks. As described by Kennedy and Krause (2011), Carmi became better calibrated at predicting how long it would take her to complete tasks, thus allowing her to more accurately plan time for studying, reading, writing, and emailing in her daily schedule. She also then began working in regular breaks to allow herself "brain breaks" rather than trying to complete everything in one sitting.

For her communication, Carmi and her clinician developed a visual guide to support a discourse intervention approach. Carmi particularly struggled to explain her schoolwork and worried about the impacts this would have in the classroom during discussions. Because Carmi was much more successful when she paced herself and paused to give herself time to plan, they developed a guide based on the acronym STOP: (1) Slow down, (2) Think it through, (3) Organize it, and (4) Proceed and pause if needed. Carmi practiced summarizing content from her online course and also explaining how to use the online portal for the class. Each session, a brief strategy guide for Step 3, "Organize it" was trained, including chronological ordering, relating by importance, then compare and contrast, and finally problem and solution. Carmi created cue cards for each of these strategies as well, then would select the card that best fit the demands of the given task, which were drawn from her textbook prompts at the end of each chapter. After being given the task, she would slow down, pausing

to give herself time to think and plan rather than starting to speak. Next, she would think through which organizational strategy might be the best fit, and then in Step 3, she would implement the selected organizational approach. Finally, once she began speaking, she would pause if needed to either review the organizational strategy or confirm that her listener was following her message.

By week 12, Carmi had exceeded her assignment goal, achieving a level of +1 and had met her communication goal (Level 0). Working with her vocational rehabilitation counselor, she had also decided to take some courses in graphic design to determine if that might be a good fit for a new major. She enrolled in two courses at a local community college and agreed to reevaluate at the end of that semester to determine her readiness to return to her university. She would also meet with her physician at that time to determine if referral for a new episode of care with her SLP would be appropriate to support transition to a more demanding setting.

Summary

Executive dysfunction is a common consequence of brain injury and other neurologic disease processes. Comprehensive assessment and careful attention to the design and implementation of treatment can result in positive outcomes and improved participation in meaningful activities. Goal attainment scaling should be employed to develop personally relevant goals as well as build insight into the self and the therapeutic process. Motivational interviewing aids in identification of needs (including barriers and facilitators), development of the therapeutic relationship, and change in representations during treatment. The RTSS is useful in mapping targets/goals to acquisition of skills and habits or change in mental representations and selecting appropriate ingredients based on proposed mechanisms of action. Structured protocols exist to guide treatment approaches, although common ingredients across treatment emphasize the need for person-centered goals, metacognitive strategy instruction, and self-reflection and monitoring activities that foster the development of insight and awareness. In addition, group treatments and virtual reality should be considered where available, feasible, and appropriate for client goals.

References

Academy of Neurologic Communication Disorders and Sciences (ANCDS) Traumatic Brain Injury Writing Committee, Byom, L., O'Neil-Pirozzi, T. M., Lemoncello, R., MacDonald, S., Meulenbroek, P., . . . Sohlberg, M. M. (2020). Social communication following adult traumatic brain injury: A scoping review of theoretical models. *American Journal of Speech-Language Pathology, 29*(3), 1735–1748.

Agarwal, S., Highton-Williamson, E., Caga, J., Matamala, J. M., Dharmadasa, T., Howells, J., . . . Kiernan, M. C. (2018). Primary lateral sclerosis and the amyotrophic lateral sclerosis-frontotemporal dementia spectrum. *Journal of Neurology, 265*(8), 1819–1828. https://doi.org/10.1007/s00415-018-8917-5

Aitken, S., Chase, S., McClue, M., & Ratcliff, G. (1993). An American adaptation of the Multiple Errands Test: Assessment of executive abilities in everyday life. *Archives of Neurology, 8,* 212.

Alashram, A. R., Annino, G., Padua, E., Romagnoli, C., & Mercuri, N. B. (2019). Cognitive rehabilitation post traumatic brain injury: A systematic review for emerging use of virtual reality technology. *Journal of Clinical Neuroscience, 66,* 209–219. https://doi.org/10.1016/j.jocn.2019.04.026

American Speech-Language-Hearing Association. (2004). *Preferred practice patterns for the profession of speech-language pathology* [Preferred practice patterns]. http://www.asha.org/policy

Avila, J. F., Verney, S. P., Kauzor, K., Flowers, A., Mehradfar, M., & Razani, J. (2019). Normative data for Farsi-speaking Iranians in the United States on measures of executive functioning. *Applied Neuropsychology: Adult, 26*(3), 229–235. https://doi.org/10.1080/23279095.2017.1392963

Avramović, P., Kenny, B., Power, E., McDonald, S., Tate, R., Hunt, L., . . . Togher, L. (2017). Exploring the relationship between cognition and functional verbal reasoning in adults with severe traumatic brain injury at six months post injury. *Brain Injury, 31*(4), 502–516. https://doi.org/10.1080/02699052.2017.1280854

Baggetta, P., & Alexander, P. A. (2016). Conceptualization and operationalization of executive function. *Mind, Brain, and Education, 10*(1), 10–33. https://doi.org/10.1111/mbe.12100

Barker, M., Young, B., & Robinson, G. (2017). Cohesive and coherent connected speech deficits in mild stroke. *Brain and Language, 168,* 23–36. https://doi.org/10.1016/j.bandl.2017.01.004

Barnes, D. E., & Yaffe, K. (2011). The projected effect of risk factor reduction on Alzheimer's disease prevalence. *The Lancet Neurology, 10*(9), 819–828. https://doi.org/10.1016/S1474-4422(11)70072-2

Basilakos, A., Hula, W. D., Johnson, L. P., Kiran, S., Walker, G. M., & Fridriksson, J.

(2021). Defining the neurobiological mechanisms of action in aphasia therapies: Applying the RTSS framework to research and practice in aphasia. *Archives of Physical Medicine and Rehabilitation, 103*(3), 581–589. https://doi.org/10.1016/j.apmr.2021.10.017

Bedard, M., Steffener, J., & Taler, V. (2020). Long-term cognitive impairment following single mild traumatic brain injury with loss of consciousness: Findings from the Canadian Longitudinal Study on aging. *Journal of Clinical and Experimental Neuropsychology, 42*(4), 344–351. https://doi.org/10.1080/13803395.2020.1714552

Belanger, H., Spiegel, E., & Vanderploeg, R. (2010). Neuropsychological performance following a history of multiple self-reported concussions: A meta-analysis. *Journal of the International Neuropsychological Society, 16*(2), 262–267.

Benton, A. L., Hamsher, K., Rey, G. J., & Sivan, A. B. (1994). *Multilingual Aphasia Examination* (3rd ed.). Psychological Corporation.

Bertens, D., Kessels, R. P., Fiorenzato, E., Boelen, D. H., & Fasotti, L. (2015). Do old errors always lead to new truths? A randomized controlled trial of errorless Goal Management Training in brain-injured patients. *Journal of the International Neuropsychological Society, 21*(8), 639–649. https://doi.org/10.1017/S1355617715000764

Bertens, D., Kessels, R. P. C., Boelen, D. H. E., & Fasotti, L. (2016). Transfer effects of errorless Goal Management Training on cognitive function and quality of life in brain-injured persons. *NeuroRehabilitation, 38*(1), 79–84. https://doi.org/10.3233/NRE-151298

Bettcher, B. M., Mungas, D., Patel, N., Elofson, J., Dutt, S., Wynn, M., . . . Kramer, J. H. (2016). Neuroanatomical substrates of executive functions: Beyond prefrontal structures. *Neuropsychologia, 85*, 100–109. https://doi.org/10.1016/j.neuropsychologia.2016.03.001

Bhat, A., & Biswas, A. (2022). Cognitive profile of large-vessel vascular dementia—An observational study from a tertiary care center in Kolkata. *Journal of Neurosciences in Rural Practice, 13*(3), 411–416. https://doi.org/10.1055/s-0042-1744467

Blake, M. L. (2021). Communication deficits associated with right hemisphere brain damage. In J. Damico, N. Muller, & M. Ball (Eds.), *The handbook of language and speech disorders* (2nd ed., pp. 571–589). Wiley Blackwell.

Bogart, E., Togher, L., Power, E., & Docking, K. (2012). Casual conversations between individuals with traumatic brain injury and their friends. *Brain Injury, 26*(3), 221–233. https://doi.org/10.3109/02699052.2011.648711

Bogdanova, Y., Yee, M. K., Ho, V. T., & Cicerone, K. D. (2016). Computerized cognitive rehabilitation of attention and executive function in acquired brain injury: A systematic review. *The Journal of Head Trauma Rehabilitation, 31*(6), 419–433. https://doi.org/10.1097/HTR.0000000000000203

Borkowska, A. R., Daniluk, B., & Adamczyk, K. (2021). Significance of the diagnosis of executive functions in patients with relapsing-remitting multiple sclerosis. *International Journal of Environmental Research and Public Health, 18*(19), 10527. https://doi.org/10.3390/ijerph181910527

Boyd, T. M., Sautter, S., Bailey, M. B., Echols, K. D., & Douglas, J. W. (1987, Feb.). *Reliability and validity of a measure of everyday problem solving*. Paper presented at the annual meeting of the International Neuropsychological Society, Washington, DC.

Braden, C., Hawley, L., Newman, J., Morey, C., Gerber, D., & Harrison-Felix, C. (2010). Social communication skills group treatment: A feasibility study for persons with traumatic brain injury and comorbid conditions. *Brain Injury, 24*(11), 1298–1310.

Braswell, D., Hartey, A., Hoornbeek, S., Johansen, A., Johnson, L., Schultz, J., & Sohlberg, M. (1992). *The Profile of Executive Control System*. Northern Rehabilitation Services.

Brookshire, B. L., Chapman, S. B., Song, J., & Levin, H. S. (2000). Cognitive and linguistic correlates of children's discourse after closed head injury: A three-year follow-up. *Journal of the International Neuropsychological Society*, 6(7), 741–751. https://doi.org/10.1017/s1355617700677019

Brown, J., & Hux, K. (2017). Ecologically valid assessment of prospective memory for task planning and execution by adults with acquired brain injury. *American Journal of Speech-Language Pathology*, 26(3), 819–831. https://doi.org/10.1044/2017_AJSLP-16-0092

Brunner, M., Hemsley, B., Togher, L., & Palmer, S. (2017). Technology and its role in rehabilitation for people with cognitive-communication disability following a traumatic brain injury (TBI). *Brain Injury*, 31(8), 1028–1043. https://doi.org/10.1080/02699052.2017.1292429

Bryan, K. L., & Hale, J. B. (2001). Differential effects of left and right cerebral vascular accidents on language competency. *Journal of the International Neuropsychological Society*, 7, 655–664.

Byom, L., & Turkstra, L. (2017). Cognitive task demands and discourse performance after traumatic brain injury. *International Journal of Language and Communication Disorders*, 52(4), 501–513.

Caeyenberghs, K., Leemans, A., Leunissen, I., Gooijers, J., Michiels, K., Sunnaert, S., & Swinnen, S. (2014). Altered structural networks and executive deficits in traumatic brain injury patients. *Brain Structure and Function*, 219, 193–209.

Cannizzaro, M., & Coelho, C. (2013). Analysis of narrative discourse structure as an ecologically relevant measure of executive function in adults. *Journal of Psycholinguistic Research*, 42, 527–549. https://doi.org/10.1007/s10936-012-9231-5

Cantor, J., Ashman, T., Dams-O'Connor, K., Dijkers, M., Gordon, W., Spielman, L., . . . Oswald, J. (2014). Evaluation of the Short-Term Executive Plus intervention for executive dysfunction after traumatic brain injury: A randomized controlled trial with minimization. *Archives of Physical Medicine and Rehabilitation*, 95(1), 1–9. https://doi.org/10.1016/j.apmr.2013.08.005

Casarin, F. S., Pagliarin, K. C., Altmann, R. F., Parente, M. A. D. M. P., Ferré, P., Côté, H., . . . Fonseca, R. P. (2020). Montreal Communication Evaluation Brief Battery–MEC B: Reliability and validity. *CoDAS*, 32(1), 1–7.

Channon, S., & Watts, M. (2003). Pragmatic language interpretation after closed head injury: Relationship to executive functioning. *Cognitive Neuropsychiatry*, 8, 243–260.

Charters, E., Gillett, L., & Simpson, G. K. (2015). Efficacy of electronic portable assistive devices for people with acquired brain injury: A systematic review. *Neuropsychological Rehabilitation*, 25(1), 82–121. https://doi.org/10.1080/09602011.2014.942672

Chu, Y., Brown, P., Harniss, M., Kautz, H., & Johnson, K. (2014). Cognitive support technologies for people with TBI: Current usage and challenges experienced. *Disability and Rehabilitation: Assistive Technology*, 9(4), 279–285. https://doi.org/10.3109/17483107.2013.823631

Churilov, I., Brock, K., Churilov, J. M., Sutton, E., Murphy, D., MacIsaac, R. J., & Ekinci, E. I. (2020). Goal attainment scaling outcomes in general inpatient rehabilitation: Association with functional independence and perceived goal importance and difficulty. *Journal of Rehabilitation Medicine*, 52(4), jrm00054. https://doi.org/10.2340/16501977-2675

Cicerone, K. D., Goldin, Y., Ganci, K., Rosenbaum, A., Wethe, J. V., Langenbahn, D. M., . . . Harley, J. P. (2019). Evidence-based cognitive rehabilitation: Systematic review of the literature from 2009 through 2014. *Archives of Physical Medicine and Rehabilitation*, *100*(8), 1515–1533. https://doi.org/10.1016/j.apmr.2019.02.011

Cicerone, K. D., Langenbahn, D. M., Braden, C., Malec, J. F., Kalmar, K., Fraas, M., . . . Ashman, T. (2011). Evidence-based cognitive rehabilitation: Updated review of the literature from 2003 through 2008. *Archives of Physical Medicine and Rehabilitation*, *92*(4), 519–530. https://doi.org/10.1016/j.apmr.2010.11.015

Coelho, C. (1995). Impairments of discourse abilities and executive functions in traumatically brain-injured adults. *Brain Injury*, *9*(5), 471–477.

Coelho, C. (2002). Story narratives of adults with closed head injury and non-brain injured adults: Influence of socioeconomic status, elicitation task, and executive functioning. *Journal of Speech, Language, and Hearing Research*, *45*, 1232–1248.

Coelho, C. (2007). Management of discourse deficits following traumatic brain injury: Progress, caveats, and needs. *Seminars in Speech Language*, *28*(2), 122–128. https://doi.org/10.1055/s-2007-970570

Coelho, C., Grela, B., Corso, M., Gamble, A., & Feinn, R. (2005). Microlinguistic deficits in the narrative discourse of adults with traumatic brain injury. *Brain Injury*, *19*(13), 1139–1145. https://doi.org/10.1080/02699050500110678

Coelho, C., Lê, K., Mozeiko, J., Hamilton, M., Tyler, E., Krueger, F., & Grafman, J. (2013). Characterizing discourse deficits following penetrating head injury: A preliminary model. *American Journal of Speech-Language Pathology*, *22*(2), S438–S448. https://doi.org/10.1044/1058-0360(2013/12-0076)

Cohen, M., Ylvisaker, M., Hamilton, J., Kemp, L., & Claiman, B. (2010). Errorless learning of functional life skills in an individual with three aetiologies of severe memory and executive function impairment. *Neuropsychological Rehabilitation*, *20*(3), 355–376.

Collins, A., & Koechlin, E. (2012). Reasoning, learning, and creativity: Frontal lobe function and human decision-making. *PLoS Biology*, *10*(3), e1001293. https://doi.org/10.1371/journal.pbio.1001293

Constantinidou, F., Thomas, R. D., & Robinson, L. (2008). Benefits of categorization training in patients with traumatic brain injury during post-acute rehabilitation: Additional evidence from a randomized controlled trial. *The Journal of Head Trauma Rehabilitation*, *23*(5), 312–328. https://doi.org/10.1097/01.HTR.0000336844.99079.2c

Cook, L. G., Caulkins, N. N., & Chapman, S. B. (2020). A strategic memory advanced reasoning training approach for enhancing higher order cognitive functioning following sports- and recreation-related mild traumatic brain injury in youth using telepractice. *Perspectives of the ASHA Special Interest Groups*, *5*(1), 67–80. https://doi.org/10.1044/2019_PERSP-19-00106

Copley, A., Smith, K., Savill, K., & Finch, E. (2015). Does metacognitive strategy instruction improve impaired receptive cognitive-communication skills following acquired brain injury? *Brain Injury*, *29*(11), 1309–1316. https://doi.org/10.3109/02699052.2015.1043343

Cornis-Pop, M., Mashima, P. A., Roth, C. R., MacLennan, D. L., Picon, L. M., Hammond, C. S., . . . Frank, E. M. (2012). Cognitive-communication rehabilitation for combat-related mild traumatic brain injury. *The Journal of Rehabilitation Research and Development*, *49*(7), xi. https://doi.org/10.1682/jrrd.2012.03.0048

Cristofori, I., Zhong, W., Chau, A., Solomon, J., Krueger, F., & Graftman, J. (2015). White and gray matter contributions to executive function recovery after traumatic brain injury. *Neurology*, *84*(14) 1394–1401. https://doi.org/10.1212/WNL.0000000000001446

Cuberos-Urbano, G., Caracuel, A., Valls-Serrano, C., García-Mochón, L., Gracey, F., & Verdejo-García, A. (2018). A pilot investigation of the potential for incorporating lifelog technology into executive function rehabilitation for enhanced transfer of self-regulation skills to everyday life. *Neuropsychological Rehabilitation*, *28*(4), 589–601. https://doi.org/10.1080/09602011.2016.1187630

Dahlberg, C., Hawley, L., Morey, C., Newman, J., Cusick, C. P., & Harrison-Felix, C. (2006). Social communication skills in persons with post-acute traumatic brain injury: Three perspectives. *Brain Injury*, *20*(4), 425–435. https://doi.org/10.1080/02699050600664574

Dassanayake, T. L., Hewawasam, C., Bamiwatta, A., & Ariyasinghe, D. I. (2021). Regression-based, demographically adjusted norms for Victoria Stroop Test, Digit Span, and Verbal Fluency for Sri Lankan adults. *The Clinical Neuropsychologist*, *35*(Suppl. 1), S32–S49. https://doi.org/10.1080/13854046.2021.1973109

Davis, G. A., & Coelho, C. (2004). Referential cohesion and logical coherence of narration after closed head injury. *Brain and Language*, *89*, 508–523.

Delis, D. C., Kaplan, E., & Kramer, J. H. (2001). *Delis-Kaplan Executive Function System examiner's manual*. Psychological Corporation.

De Luca, R., Maggio, M. G., Maresca, G., Latella, D., Cannavò, A., Sciarrone, F., . . . Calabrò, R. S. (2019). Improving cognitive function after traumatic brain injury: A clinical trial on the potential use of the semi-immersive virtual reality. *Behavioural Neurology*, *2019*,1–7. https://doi.org/10.1155/2019/9268179

Diamond A. (2013). Executive functions. *Annual Review of Psychology*, *64*, 135–168. https://doi.org/10.1146/annurev-psych-113011-143750

Dirette, D., & Plaisier, B. (2007). The development of self-awareness of deficits from 1 week to 1 year after traumatic brain injury: Preliminary findings. *Brain Injury*, *21*(11), 1131–1136. https://doi.org/10.1080/02699050701687326

Douglas, J. M., Bracy, C. A., & Snow, P. C. (2007). Measuring perceived communicative ability after traumatic brain injury: Reliability and validity of the La Trobe Communication Questionnaire. *The Journal of Head Trauma Rehabilitation*, *22*(1), 31–38. https://doi.org/10.1097/00001199-200701000-00004

Douglas, J. M., Knox, L., De Maio, C., & Bridge, H. (2014). Improving communication-specific coping after traumatic brain injury: Evaluation of a new treatment using single-case experimental design. *Brain Impairment*, *15*(3), 190–201.

Douglas, J. M., Knox, L., De Maio, C., Bridge, H., Drummond, M., & Whiteoak, J. (2019). Effectiveness of Communication-specific Coping Intervention for adults with traumatic brain injury: Preliminary results. *Neuropsychological Rehabilitation*, *29*(1), 73–91. https://doi.org/10.1080/09602011.2016.1259114

Douglas, J. M., O'Flaherty, C., & Snow, P. (2000). Measuring perception of communicative ability: The development and evaluation of the La Trobe Communication Questionnaire. *Aphasiology*, *14*(3), 251–268.

Ehlhardt, L., Sohlberg, M., Kennedy, M., Coelho, C., Ylvisaker, M., Turkstra, L., & Yorkston, K. (2008). Evidence-based practice guidelines for instructing individuals with neurogenic memory impairments: What have we learned in the past 20 years? *Neuropsychological Rehabilitation*, *18*(3), 300–342. https://doi.org/10.1080/09602010701733190

Ehlhardt, L. A., Sohlberg, M. M., Glang, A., & Albin, R. (2005). TEACH-M: A pilot study evaluating an instructional sequence for persons with impaired memory and executive functions. *Brain injury*, *19*(8), 569–583. https://doi.org/10.1080/00269 9050400013550

Elbogen, E. B., Dennis, P. A., Van Voorhees, E. E., Blakey, S. M., Johnson, J. L., Johnson, S. C., . . . Beiger, A. (2019). Cognitive rehabilitation with mobile technology and social support for veterans with TBI and PTSD: A randomized clinical trial. *Journal of Head Trauma Rehabilitation*, 34(1), 1–10. https://doi.org/10.1097/HTR.0000000000000435

Emek-Savaş, D. D., Yerlikaya, D., Yener, G. G., & Oktem Tanor, O. (2019). Validity, reliability and normative data of The Stroop Test Capa version. *Turkish Journal of Psychiatry, 1*(1), 9–21. https://doi.org/10.5080/u23549

Emmanouel, A., Kontrafouri, E., Nikolaos, P., Kessels, R. P. C., & Fasotti, L. (2018). Incorporation of a working memory strategy in GMT to facilitate serial-order behaviour in brain-injured patients. *Neuropsychological Rehabilitation, 28*(7), 1–27. https://doi.org/10.1080/09602011.2018.1517369

Engel, L., Chui, A., Goverover, Y., & Dawson, D. R. (2019). Optimising activity and participation outcomes for people with self-awareness impairments related to acquired brain injury: An interventions systematic review. *Neuropsychological Rehabilitation, 29*(2), 163–198. https://doi.org/10.1080/09602011.2017.1292923

Eslinger, P. J., Moore, P., Anderson, C., & Grossman, M. (2011). Social cognition, executive functioning, and neuroimaging correlates of empathic deficits in frontotemporal dementia. *The Journal of Neuropsychiatry Clinical Neurosciences, 23*(1), 74–82. https://doi.org/10.1176/appi.neuropsych.23.1.74

Faustino, B., Oliveira, J., & Lopes, P. (2022). Normative scores of the Wisconsin Card Sorting Test in a sample of the adult Portuguese population. *Applied Neuropsychology: Adult, 29*(4), 767–777.

Feeney, T. J., & Ylvisaker, M. (2003). Context-sensitive behavioral supports for young children with TBI: Short-term effects and long-term outcome. *The Journal of Head Trauma Rehabilitation, 18*(1), 33–51.

Feeney, T. J., & Ylvisaker, M. (2006). Context-sensitive cognitive-behavioural supports for young children with TBI:

A replication study. *Brain Injury, 20*(6), 629–645. https://doi.org/10.1080/02699050600744194

Fernández López, R., & Antolí, A. (2020). Computer-based cognitive interventions in acquired brain injury: A systematic review and meta-analysis of randomized controlled trials. *PLoS One, 15*(7), e0235510. https://doi.org/10.1371/journal.pone.0235510

Finch, E., Copley, A., Cornwell, P., & Kelly, C. (2016). Systematic review of behavioral interventions targeting social communication difficulties after traumatic brain injury. *Archives of Physical Medicine and Rehabilitation, 97*, 1352–1365. https://doi.org/10.1016/j.apmr.2015.11.005

Finch, E., Copley, A., McLisky, M., Cornwell, P. L., Fleming, J. M., & Doig, E. (2018). Can Goal Attainment Scaling (GAS) accurately identify changes in social communication impairments following TBI? *Speech, Language and Hearing, 22*(3), 183–194. https://doi.org/10.1080/2050571x.2019.1611220

Finch, E., Cornwell, P., Copley, A., Doig, E., & Fleming, J. (2017). Remediation of social communication impairments following traumatic brain injury using metacognitive strategy intervention: A pilot study. *Brain Injury, 31*(13–14), 1830–1839.

Fischer, S., Trexler, L. E., & Gauggel, S. (2004). Awareness of activity limitations and prediction of performance in patients with brain injuries and orthopedic disorders. *Journal of the International Neuropsychological Society, 10*(2), 190–199. https://doi.org/10.1017/s1355617704102051

Flavell, J. H. (1979). Metacognition and cognitive monitoring: A new area of cognitive–developmental inquiry. *American Psychologist, 34*(10), 906–911. https://doi.org/10.1037/0003-066x.34.10.906

Francis, H. M., Osborne-Crowley, K., & McDonald, S. (2017). Validity and reliability of a questionnaire to assess social skills in traumatic brain injury: A preliminary study. *Brain Injury, 31*(3), 336–343. https://doi.org/10.1080/02699052.2016.1250954

Frankel, T., Penn, C., & Ormond-Brown, D. (2007). Executive dysfunction as an explanatory basis for conversation symptoms of aphasia: A pilot study. *Aphasiology, 21*(6–8), 814–828. https://doi.org/10.1080/02687030701192448

Fridriksson, J., Nettles, C., Davis, M., Morrow, L., & Montgomery, A. (2006). Functional communication and executive function in aphasia. *Clinical Linguistics & Phonetics, 20*(6), 401–410. https://doi.org/10.1080/02699200500075781

Friedman, N., & Robbins, T. (2022). The role of prefrontal cortex in cognitive control and executive function. *Neuropsychopharmacology, 47*(1), 72–89. https://doi.org/10.1038/s41386-021-01132-0

Frith, M., Togher, L., Ferguson, A., Levick, W., & Docking, K. (2014). Assessment practices of speech-language pathologists for cognitive communication disorders following traumatic brain injury in adults: An international survey. *Brain Injury, 28*(13–14), 1657–1666. https://doi.org/10.3109/02699052.2014.947619

Gadd, C., & Phipps, W. D. (2012). A Preliminary standardisation of the Wisconsin Card Sorting Test for Setswana-speaking university students. *South African Journal of Psychology, 42*(3), 389–398. https://doi.org/10.1177/008124631204200311

García-Escobar, G., Pérez-Enríquez, C., Arrondo-Elizarán, C., Pereira-Cuitiño, B., Grau-Guinea, L., Florido-Santiago, M., . . . Sánchez-Benavides, G. (2021). Estudios normativos españoles (Proyecto NEURONORMA Plus): Normas para las pruebas Delis Kaplan-Design Fluency Test (DK-DFT), Color Trails Tests (CTT) y Dual Task (DT). *Neurología*, S0213485321001134. https://doi.org/10.1016/j.nrl.2021.05.013

Gates, N. J., Vernooij, R. W., Di Nisio, M., Karim, S., March, E., Martinez, G., & Rutjes, A. W. (2019). Computerised cognitive training for preventing dementia in people with mild cognitive impairment. *Cochrane Database of Systematic Reviews, 3*(3), CD012279 https://doi.org/10.1002/14651858.CD012279.pub2

Gaubert, F., & Chainay, H. (2021). Decision-making competence in patients with Alzheimer's disease: A review of the literature. *Neuropsychology Review, 31*(2), 267–287. https://doi.org/10.1007/s11065-020-09472-2

Ghasemian-Shirvan, E., Shirazi, S. M., Aminikhoo, M., Zareaan, M., & Ekhtiari, H. (2018). Preliminary normative data of Persian Phonemic and Semantic Verbal Fluency Test. *Iranian Journal of Psychiatry, 13*(4), 288.

Godefroy, O., Bakchine, S., Verny, M., Delabrousse-Mayoux, J. P., Roussel, M., Pere, J. J., & REFLEX study group (2016). Characteristics of Alzheimer's disease patients with severe executive disorders. *Journal of Alzheimer's Disease, 51*(3), 815–825. https://doi.org/10.3233/JAD-150971

Gollwitzer, P. M. (1999). Implementation Intentions: Strong effects of simple plans. *American Psychologist, 54*(7), 493–503. https://doi.org/10.1037/0003-066X.54.7.493

Gollwitzer, P. M. (2014). Weakness of the will: Is a quick fix possible? *Motivation and Emotion, 38*(3), 305–322. https://doi.org/10.1007/s11031-014-9416-3

Goverover, Y., Johnson, M., Toglia, J., & Deluca, J. (2007). Treatment to improve self-awareness in persons with acquired brain injury. *Brain Injury, 21*(9), 913–923. https://doi.org/10.1080/02699050701553205

Grant, D. A., & Berg, E. A. (1948). A behavioral analysis of reinforcement and ease of shifting to new responses in a Weigel-type card-sorting problem. *Journal of Experimental Psychology, 38*, 404–411.

Grant, M., & Ponsford, J. (2014). Goal Attainment Scaling in brain injury rehabilitation: Strengths, limitations, and recommendations for future applications. *Neuropsychological Rehabilitation, 24*(5), 661–677. https://doi.org/10.1080/09602011.2014.901228

Hagen, C. (1997). *Ranchos Los Amigos Levels of Cognitive Functioning–Revised*. Ranchos Los Amigos Hospital.

Hagen, C., Malkamus, D., & Durham, P. (1972). *Levels of Cognitive Functioning*. Ranchos Los Amigos Hospital.

Halliday, M. (1994). *An introduction to functional grammar* (2nd ed.). Edward Arnold.

Hamilton, J., Sohlberg, M. M., & Turkstra, L. (2022). Opening the black box of cognitive rehabilitation: Integrating the ICF, RTSS, and PIE. *International Journal of Language & Communication Disorders*. Advance online publication. https://doi.org/10.1111/1460-6984.12774

Harrison-Felix, C., Newman, J. K., Hawley, L., Morey, C., Ketchum, J. M., Walker, W. C., . . . Howe, L. (2018). Social competence treatment after traumatic brain injury: A multicenter, randomized controlled trial of interactive group treatment versus noninteractive treatment. *Archives of Physical Medicine and Rehabilitation, 99*(11), 2131–2142.

Hart, T., Ketchum, J. M., O'Neil-Pirozzi, T. M., Novack, T. A., Johnson-Greene, D., & Dams-O'Connor, K. (2019). Neurocognitive status and return to work after moderate to severe traumatic brain injury. *Rehabilitation Psychology, 64*(4), 435–444. https://doi.org/10.1037/rep0000290.supp

Hart, T., Dijkers, M. P., Whyte, J., Turkstra, L. S., Zanca, J. M., Packel, A., . . . Chen, C. (2019). A theory-driven system for the specification of rehabilitation treatments. *Archives of Physical Medicine and Rehabilitation, 100*(1), 172–180.

Hart, T., & Evans, J. (2006). Self-regulation and goal theories in brain injury rehabilitation. *Journal of Head Trauma Rehabilitation, 21*(2), 142–155. http://pubmed.gov/16569988

Hartman-Maeir, A., Soroker, N., Ring, H., & Katz, N. (2002). Awareness of deficits in stroke rehabilitation. *Journal of Rehabilitative Medicine, 34*(4), 158–164.

Hawley, L. A., & Newman, J. K. (2010). Group interactive structured treatment (GIST): A social competence intervention for individuals with brain injury. *Brain Injury, 24*(11), 1292–1297. https://doi.org/10.3109/02699052.2010.506866

Heinz-Martin S., Oberauer, K., Wittmann, W., Wilhelm, O., & Schulze, R. (2002). Working-memory capacity explains reasoning ability—and a little bit more. *Intelligence, 30*, 261–288. https://doi.org/10.1016/S0160-2896(01)00100-3

Helm-Estabrooks, N. (2001). *Cognitive-Linguistic Quick Test*. Psychological Corporation.

Helm-Estabrooks, N. (2002). Cognition and aphasia: A discussion and a study. *Journal of Communication Disorders, 35*, 171–186.

Helm-Estabrooks, N. (2017). *Cognitive-Linguistic Quick Test–Plus*. Psychological Corporation.

Hill, E., Claessen, M., Whitworth, A., Boyes, M., & Ward, R. (2018). Discourse and cognition in speakers with acquired brain injury (ABI): A systematic review. *International Journal of Language & Communication Disorders, 53*(4), 689–717. https://doi.org/10.1111/1460-6984.12394

Hoepner, J. K., & Olson, S. E. (2018). Joint video self-modeling as a conversational intervention for an individual with traumatic brain injury and his everyday partner: A pilot investigation. *Clinical Archives of Communication Disorders, 3*(1), 22–41.

Hoepner, J. K., Sievert, A., & Guenther, K. (2021). Joint video self-modeling for persons with traumatic brain injury and their partners: A case series. *American Journal of Speech-Language Pathology, 30*(2S), 863–882.

Hunkin, N. M., Squires, E. J., Aldrich, F. K., & Parkin, A. J. (1998). Errorless learning and the acquisition of word processing skills. *Neuropsychological Rehabilitation, 8,* 433–449.

Indorewalla, K. K., Osher, J., Lanca, M., Kartik, R., Vaidya, N., & Moncata, S. (2022). A normative study of the Color Trails Test in the adult Indian population. *Applied Neuropsychology: Adult, 29*(5), 899–906. https://doi.org/10.1080/23279095.2020.1819279

Jang, J., Lee, J., & Yoo, D. (2015). Effects of spaced retrieval training with errorless learning in the rehabilitation of patients with dementia. *Journal of Physical Therapy Science, 27*(9), 2735–2738.

Jeffay, E., Ponsford, J., Harnett, A., Janzen, S., Patsakos, E., Douglas, J., . . . Green, R. (2023). INCOG 2.0 Guidelines for cognitive rehabilitation following traumatic brain injury, Part III: Executive functions. *Journal of Head Trauma Rehabilitation, 38*(1), 52–64. https://doi.org/10.1097/htr.0000000000000834

Joanette, Y., Ska, B., Cote, H., Ferre, P., LaPointe, L., Coppens, P., & Small, S. L. (2015). *Montreal Protocol for the Evaluation of Communication (MEC).* ASSBI Resources.

Johnen, A., Landmeyer, N. C., Bürkner, P. C., Wiendl, H., Meuth, S. G., & Holling, H. (2017). Distinct cognitive impairments in different disease courses of multiple sclerosis—A systematic review and meta-analysis. *Neuroscience and Biobehavioral Reviews, 83,* 568–578. https://doi.org/10.1016/j.neubiorev.2017.09.005

Joint Committee on Interprofessional Relations Between the American Speech-Language-Hearing Association and Division 40 (Clinical Neuropsychology) of the American Psychological Association. (2007). *Structure and function of an interdisciplinary team for persons with acquired brain injury.* http://www.asha.org/policy

Kagan, A., Simmons-Mackie, N., Rowland, A., Huijbregts, M., Shumway, E., McEwen, S., . . . Sharp, S. (2007) Counting what counts: A framework for capturing real-life outcomes of aphasia intervention. *Aphasiology, 21,* 39–66.

Kagan, A., Winckel, J., Black, S., Duchan, J. F., Simmons-Mackie, N., & Square, P. (2004). A set of observational measures for rating support and participation in conversation between adults with aphasia and their conversation partners. *Topics in Stroke Rehabilitation, 11*(1), 67–83.

Kasper, E., Schuster, C., Machts, J., Bittner, D., Vielhaber, S., Benecke, R., . . . Prudlo, J. (2015). Dysexecutive functioning in ALS patients and its clinical implications. *Amyotrophic Lateral Sclerosis & Frontotemporal Degeneration, 16*(3–4), 160–171. https://doi.org/10.3109/21678421.2015.1026267

Keegan, L. C., Murdock, M., Suger, C., & Togher, L. (2020). Improving natural social interaction: Group rehabilitation after traumatic brain injury. *Neuropsychological Rehabilitation, 30*(8), 1497–1522. https://doi.org/10.1080/09602011.2019.1591464

Keegan, L. C., Reilley, K., Stover, M., & Togher, L. (2022). Virtual INSIGHT: Improving natural social interaction: Group reHabilitation after traumatic brain injury. *International Journal of Language & Communication Disorders.* Advance online publication. https://doi.org/10.1111/1460-6984.12790

Keil, K., & Kaszniak, A. W. (2002). Examining executive function in individuals with brain injury: A review. *Aphasiology, 16*(3), 305–335.

Kennedy, M. R. (2010). *Self-regulation & executive functions after TBI: Evidence-based assessment and intervention approaches in cognitive rehabilitation.* Midwest Adult Communication Disorders Group.

Kennedy, M. R., & Coelho, C. (2005). Self-regulation after traumatic brain injury: A framework for intervention of memory and problem solving. *Seminars in Speech and Language, 26*(4), 242–255.

Kennedy, M. R., Coelho, C., Turkstra, L., Ylvisaker, M., Sohlberg, M. M., Yorkston, K., . . . Kan, P.F. (2008). Intervention for executive functions after traumatic brain injury: A systematic review, meta-analysis and clinical recommendations. *Neuropsychological Rehabilitation, 18*, 257–299.

Kennedy, M. R. T., & Krause, M. O. (2011). Self-regulated learning in a dynamic coaching model for supporting college students with traumatic brain injury. *Journal of Head Trauma Rehabilitation, 26*(3), 212–223. https://doi.org/10.1097/htr.0b013e318218dd0e

Kessels, R., & Hensken, L. (2009). Effects of errorless skill learning in people with mild-to-moderate or severe dementia: A randomized controlled pilot study. *NeuroRehabilitation, 25*(4), 307–312. https://doi.org/10.3233/NRE-2009-0529

Kim, H., Au, R., Thomas, R. J., Yun, C-H., Lee, S. K., Han, C., & Shin, C. (2017). Cognitive performance norms from the Korean Genome and Epidemiology Study (KoGES). *International Psychogeriatrics, 29*(11), 1909–1924. https://doi.org/10.1017/S1041610217000990

Kinnunen, K. M., Greenwood, R., Powell, J. H., Leech, R., Hawkins, P. C., Bonnelle, V., . . . Sharp, D. J. (2011). White matter damage and cognitive impairment after traumatic brain injury. *Brain, 134*(2), 449–463. https://doi.org/10.1093/brain/awq347

Kintz, S., Hibbs, V., Henderson, A., Andrews, M., & Wright, H. H. (2018). Discourse-based treatment in mild traumatic brain injury. *Journal of Communication Disorders, 76*, 47–59. https://doi.org/10.1016/j.jcomdis.2018.08.001

Kiselica, A. M., & Benge, J. F. (2021). Quantitative and qualitative features of executive dysfunction in frontotemporal and Alzheimer's dementia. *Applied Neuropsychology Adult, 28*(4), 449–463. https://doi.org/10.1080/23279095.2019.1652175

Kleim, J. A., & Jones, T. A. (2008). Principles of experience-dependent neural plasticity: Implications for rehabilitation after brain damage. *Journal of Speech, Language, and Hearing Research, 51*(1), S225–S239. https://doi.org/10.1044/1092-4388(2008/018)

Kohli, A., & Kaur, M. (2006). Wisconsin Card Sorting Test: Normative data and experience. *Indian Journal of Psychiatry, 48*(3), 181. https://doi.org/10.4103/0019-5545.31582

Krpan, K. M., Stuss, D. T., & Anderson, N. D. (2011). Coping behaviour following traumatic brain injury: What makes a planner plan and an avoider avoid? *Brain Injury, 25*(10), 989–996. https://doi.org/10.3109/02699052.2011.597045

Kudlicka, A., Clare, L., & Hindle, J. V. (2011). Executive functions in Parkinson's disease: Systematic review and meta-analysis. *Movement Disorders, 26*, 2305–2315.

Lê, K., Coelho, C., Mozieko, J., Krueger, F., & Grafman, J. (2014), Does brain volume loss predict cognitive and narrative discourse performance following traumatic brain injury? *American Journal of Speech Language Pathology, 23*, S271–S284.

Lehman-Blake, M., Duffy, J. R., Myers, P. S., & Tompkins, C. A. (2002). Prevalence and patterns of right hemisphere cognitive/communicative deficits: Retrospective data from an inpatient rehabilitation unit. *Aphasiology, 16*, 537–547.

Levine, B., Schweizer, T., O'Connor, C., Turner, G., Gillingham, S., Stuss, D., . . . Robertson, I. (2011). Rehabilitation of executive functioning in patients with frontal lobe brain damage with Goal Management Training. *Frontiers in Human Neuroscience, 5*(9), 1–9.

Lezak, M., Howieson, D., Bigler, E., & Tranel, D. (2012). *Neuropsychological assessment* (5th ed.). Oxford University Press.

Linscott, R., Knight, R., & Godfrey, H. (1996). The Profile of Functional Impairment in Communication (PFIC): A measure of communication impairment for clinical use. *Brain Injury, 10*(6), 397–412.

Linscott, R., Knight, R., & Godfrey, H. (2003). *Profile of Pragmatic Impairment in Communication (PPIC)*. University of Otago.

Ma, J., Zhang, Y., & Guo, Q. (2015). Comparison of vascular cognitive impairment —No dementia by multiple classification methods. *The International Journal of Neuroscience, 125*(11), 823–830. https://doi.org/10.3109/00207454.2014.972504

MacDonald, S. (2005). *Functional Assessment of Verbal Reasoning and Executive Strategies.* CCD Publishing.

MacDonald, S. (2017). Introducing the model of cognitive-communication competence: A model to guide evidence-based communication interventions after brain injury. *Brain Injury, 31*(13–14), 1760–1780. https://doi.org/10.1080/02699052.2017.1379613

MacDonald, S., & Johnson, C. (2005). Assessment of subtle cognitive-communication deficits following acquired brain injury: A normative study of the Functional Assessment of Verbal Reasoning and Executive Strategies (FAVRES). *Brain Injury, 19*(2), 895–902. https://doi.org/10.1080/02699050400004294

MacPherson, S. E., Wagner, G. P., Murphy, P., Bozzali, M., Cipolotti, L., & Shallice, T. (2014). Bringing the Cognitive Estimation Task into the 21st century: Normative data on two new parallel forms. *PLoS ONE, 9*(3), e92554. https://doi.org/10.1371/journal.pone.0092554

Manchester, D., Priestley, N., & Jackson, H. (2004). The assessment of executive functions: Coming out of the office. *Brain Injury, 18*(11), 1067–1081.

Manly, T., Hawkins, K., Evans, J., Woldt, K., & Robertson, I. (2002). Rehabilitation of executive function: Facilitation of effective goal management on complex tasks using periodic auditory tests. *Neuropsychologia, 40,* 271–281.

Marcotte, K., McSween, M.-P., Pouliot, M., Martineau, S., Pauzé, A.-M., Wiseman-Hakes, C., & MacDonald, S. (2017). Normative study of the Functional Assessment of Verbal Reasoning and Executive Strategies (FAVRES) Test in the French-Canadian population. *Journal of Speech, Language, and Hearing Research, 60*(8), 2217–2227. https://doi.org/10.1044/2017_JSLHR-L-17-0012

Marini, A., Zettin, M., & Galetto, V. (2014). Cognitive correlates of narrative impairment in moderate traumatic brain injury. *Neuropsychologia, 64,* 282–288.

Marquine, M. J., Yassai-Gonzalez, D., Perez-Tejada, A., Umlauf, A., Kamalyan, L., Morlett Paredes, A., . . . Heaton, R. K. (2021). Demographically adjusted normative data for the Wisconsin Card Sorting Test-64 item: Results from the neuropsychological norms for the U.S.–Mexico border region in Spanish (NP-NUMBRS) project. *The Clinical Neuropsychologist, 35*(2), 339–355. https://doi.org/10.1080/13854046.2019.1703042

Marsh, N., Ludbrook, M., & Gaffaney, L. (2016). Cognitive functioning following traumatic brain injury: A five-year follow-up. *NeuroRehabilitation, 38*(1), 71–78. https://doi.org/10.3233/NRE-151297

Marshall, R. C., Karow, C. M., Morelli, C. A., Iden, K. K., Dixon, J., & Cranfill, T. B. (2004). Effects of interactive strategy modeling training on problem-solving by persons with traumatic brain injury. *Aphasiology, 18*(8), 659–673.

Martin, A., Dzafic, I., Ramdave, S., & Meinzer, M. (2017). Causal evidence for task-specific involvement of the dorsomedial prefrontal cortex in human social cognition. *Social Cognitive and Affective Neuroscience, 12*(8), 1209–1218. https://doi.org/10.1093/scan/nsx063

McCue, M., Pramuka, M., Chase, S., & Fabry, P. (1995). Functional assessment procedures for individuals with severe cognitive disabilities. *American Rehabilitation, 20*(3), 17–27.

McDonald, S., Gowland, A., Randall, R., Fisher, A., Osborn Crowley, K., & Honan, B. (2014). Cognitive factors underpinning poor expressive communication skills after traumatic brain injury: Theory of mind or executive function? *Neuropsychology, 28,* 801–811.

McDonald, S., Togher, L., & Code, C. (2013). *Social and communication disorders follow-*

ing traumatic brain injury (2nd ed.). Psychology Press.

McEwen, S., Polatajko, H., Baum, C., Rios, J., Cirone, D., Doherty, M., & Wolf, T. (2015). Combined cognitive-strategy and task-specific training improve transfer to untrained activities in subacute stroke: An exploratory randomized controlled trial. *Neurorehabilitation and Neural Repair, 29*(6), 526–536. https://doi.org/10.1177/1545968314558602

McInnes, K., Friesen, C. L., MacKenzie, D. E., Westwood, D. A., & Boe, S. G. (2017). Mild Traumatic Brain Injury (mTBI) and chronic cognitive impairment: A scoping review. *PLoS ONE, 12*(4), e0174847. https://doi.org/10.1371/journal.pone.0174847

Medley, A., & Powell, T. (2010). Motivational interviewing to promote self-awareness and engagement in rehabilitation following acquired brain injury: A conceptual review. *Neuropsychological Rehabilitation, 20*(4), 481–508. https://doi.org/10.1080/09602010903529610

Meulenbroek, P., Ness, B., Lemoncello, R., Byom, L., MacDonald, S., O'Neil-Pirozzi, T. M., & Moore Sohlberg, M. (2019). Social communication following traumatic brain injury part 2: Identifying effective treatment ingredients. *International Journal of Speech-Language Pathology, 21*(2), 128–142. https://doi.org/10.1080/17549507.2019.1583281

Meulenbroek, P., & Turkstra, L. (2016). Job stability in skilled work and communication ability after moderate-severe traumatic brain injury. *Disability and Rehabilitation, 38*(5), 452–461. https://doi.org/10.3109/09638288.2015.1044621

Miller, W. R., & Rollnick, S. (2012). *Motivational interviewing: Helping people change.* Guilford.

Minga, J., Sheppard, S. M., Johnson, M., Hewetson, R., Cornwell, P., & Blake, M. L. (2022). Apragmatism: The renewal of a label for communication disorders associated with right hemisphere brain damage. *International Journal of Language & Communication Disorders.* Advance online publication. https://doi.org/10.1111/1460-6984.12807

Miranda, A. R., Franchetto Sierra, J., Martínez Roulet, A., Rivadero, L., Serra, S. V., & Soria, E. A. (2020). Age, education and gender effects on Wisconsin card sorting test: Standardization, reliability and validity in healthy Argentinian adults. *Aging, Neuropsychology, and Cognition, 27*(6), 807–825. https://doi.org/10.1080/13825585.2019.1693491

Miyake, A., & Friedman, N. P. (2012). The nature and organization of individual differences in executive functions: Four general conclusions. *Current Directions in Psychological Science, 21*(1), 8–14. https://doi.org/10.1177/0963721411429458

Mohammadnia, S., Bigdeli, I., Mashhadi, A., Ghanaei Chamanabad, A., & Roth, R. M. (2022). Behavior Rating Inventory of Executive Function–Adult version (BRIEF-A) in Iranian university students: Factor structure and relationship to depressive symptom severity. *Applied Neuropsychology: Adult, 29*(4), 786–792. https://doi.org/10.1080/23279095.2020.1810689

Morrison, M., Giles, G., Ryan, J., Baum, C., Dromerick, A., Polatajko, H., & Edwards, D. (2013). Multiple Errands Test–Revised (MET-R): A performance-based measure of executive function in people with mild cerebrovascular accident. *American Journal of Occupational Therapy, 13*(4), 460–468.

Mosher, F. A., & Hornsby, J. R. (1966). On asking questions. In J. S. Bruner, R. Oliver, & J. R. Greenfield (Eds.), *Studies in cognitive growth* (pp. 86–102). Wiley.

Mozeiko, J., Le, K., Coelho, C., Krueger, F., & Grafman, J. (2011). The relationship of story grammar and executive function following TBI. *Aphasiology, 25*(6–7), 826–835.

Mueller, J., & Dollaghan, C. (2013). A systematic review of assessments for identifying executive function impairment in adults with acquired brain injury. *Journal of Speech, Language, and Hearing Research, 56,* 1051–1064.

Murray L. L. (2012). Attention and other cognitive deficits in aphasia: Presence and relation to language and communication measures. *American Journal of Speech-Language Pathology, 21*(2), S51–S64. https://doi.org/10.1044/1058-0360 (2012/11-0067)

National Institute of Neurological Disorders and Stroke (NINDS). (2019, August). *Motor neuron disease fact sheet* (NIH Pub. No. 19-NS-5371). https://www.ninds.nih.gov/motor-neuron-diseases-factsheet

Ng, A. S., Rademakers, R., & Miller, B. L. (2015). Frontotemporal dementia: A bridge between dementia and neuromuscular disease. *Annals of the New York Academy of Sciences, 1338*(1), 71–93. https://doi.org/10.1111/nyas.12638

Nicholas, M., & Connor, L. (2017). People with aphasia using AAC: Are executive functions important? *Aphasiology, 31*(7), 819–836. https://doi.org/10.1080/02687038.2016.1258539

Norman, M. A., Moore, D. J., Taylor, M., Franklin, D., Cysique, L., Ake, C., . . . the HNRC Group. (2011). Demographically corrected norms for African Americans and Caucasians on the Hopkins Verbal Learning Test–Revised, Brief Visuospatial Memory Test–Revised, Stroop Color and Word Test, and Wisconsin Card Sorting Test 64-Card Version. *Journal of Clinical and Experimental Neuropsychology, 33*(7), 793–804. https://doi.org/10.1080/13803395.2011.559157

Norman, D. A., & Shallice, T. (1986). Attention to action: Willed and automatic control of behaviour. In R. J. Davidson., G. E. Schwartz, & D. E. Shapiro (Eds.), *Consciousness and self-regulation* (pp. 1–14). Plenum Press.

Nousia, A., Martzoukou, M., Tsouris, Z., Siokas, V., Aloizou, A.-M., Liampas, I., . . . Dardiotis, E. (2020). The beneficial effects of computer-based cognitive training in Parkinson's disease: A systematic review. *Archives of Clinical Neuropsychology, 35*(4), 434–447. https://doi.org/10.1093/arclin/acz080

Novakovic-Agopian, T., Chen, A., Rome, S., Abrams, G., Castelli, H., Rossi, A., . . . D'Esposito, M. (2011). Rehabilitation of executive functioning with training in attention regulation applied to individually defined goals: A pilot study bridging theory, assessment, and treatment. *Journal of Head Trauma Rehabilitation, 26,* 325–338.

Novakovic-Agopian, T., Kornblith, E., Abrams, G., Burciaga-Rosales, J., Loya, F., D'Esposito, M., & Chen, A. (2018). Training in goal-oriented attention self-regulation improves executive functioning in veterans with chronic traumatic brain injury. *Journal of Neurotrauma, 35,* 2784–2795. https://doi.org/10.1089/neu.2017.5529

O'Brien, K. H., Wallace, T., Kemp, A. M., & Pei, Y. (2022). Cognitive-communication complaints and referrals for speech-language pathology services following concussion. *American Journal of Speech-Language Pathology, 31*(2), 790–807. https://doi.org/10.1044/2021_AJSLP-21-00254

O'Keeffe, F., Dockree, P., Moloney, P., Carton, S., & Robertson, I. H. (2007). Awareness of deficits in traumatic brain injury: A multidimensional approach to assessing metacognitive knowledge and online-awareness. *Journal of the International Neuropsychological Society, 13*(1), 38–49. https://doi.org/10.1017/s1355617707070075

Oliveira, J., Gamito, P., Souto, T., Conde, R., Ferreira, M., Corotnean, T., . . . Neto, T. (2021). Virtual reality-based cognitive stimulation on people with mild to moderate dementia due to Alzheimer's disease: A pilot randomized controlled trial. *International Journal of Environmental Research and Public Health, 18*(10), 5290.

Orfei, M. D., Caltagirone, C., & Spalletta, G. (2009). The evaluation of anosognosia in stroke patients. *Cerebrovascular Diseases*, 27(3), 280–289.

Otermans, P. C. J., Parton, A., & Szameitat, A. J. (2022). The working memory costs of a central attentional bottleneck in multitasking. *Psychological Research*, 86(6), 1774–1791. https://doi.org/10.1007/s00426-021-01615-1

Ownsworth, T., Fleming, J., Tate, R., Beadle, E., Griffin, J., Kendall, M., . . . Shum, D. (2017). Do people with severe traumatic brain injury benefit from making errors? A randomized controlled trial of error-based and errorless learning. *Neurorehabilitation and Neural Repair*, 31(12), 1072–1082. https://doi.org/10.1177/1545968317740635

Pagulayan, K., Temkin, N., Machamer, J., & Dikmen, S. (2007). The measurement and magnitude of awareness difficulties after traumatic brain injury: A longitudinal study. *Journal of the International Neuropsychological Society*, 13(4), 561–570. https://doi.org/10.1017/S1355617707070713

Pearce, B., Cartwright, J., Cocks, N., & Whitworth, A. (2016). Inhibitory control and traumatic brain injury: The association between executive control processes and social communication deficits. *Brain Injury*, 30(13–14), 1708–1717. https://doi.org/10.1080/02699052.2016.1202450

Pender, N., Pinto-Grau, M., & Hardiman, O. (2020). Cognitive and behavioral impairment in amyotrophic lateral sclerosis. *Current Opinion in Neurology*, 33(5), 649–654. https://doi.org/10.1097/WCO.0000000000000862

Pettemeridou, E., Kennedy, M. R. T., & Constantinidou, F. (2020). Executive functions, self-awareness and quality of life in chronic moderate-to-severe TBI. *Neuro-Rehabilitation*, 46(1), 109–118. https://doi.org/10.3233/NRE-192963

Powell, J. M., Machamer, J. E., Temkin, N. R., & Dikmen, S. S. (2001). Self-report of extent of recovery and barriers to recovery after traumatic brain injury: A longitudinal study. *Archives of Physical Medicine and Rehabilitation*, 82(8), 1025–1030.

Powell, L., Glang, A., Ettel, D., Todis, B., Sohlberg, M., & Albin, R. (2012). Systematic instruction for individuals with acquired brain injury: Results of a randomized controlled trial. *Neuropsychological Rehabilitation*, 22(1), 85–112. https://doi.org/10.1080/09602011.2011.640466

Powell, L., Glang, A., Pinkelman, S., Albin, R., Harwick, R., Ettel, D., & Wild, M. (2015). Systematic instruction of assistive technology for cognition (ATC) in an employment setting following acquired brain injury: A single case, experimental study. *NeuroRehabilitation*, 37, 437–447. https://doi.org/10.3233/NRE-151272

Powell, L. E., Harwick, R., Glang, A., Todis, B., Ettel, D., Saraceno, C., . . . Albin, R. (2013). *TATE: Training Assistive Technology in the Environment Toolkit*. https://cbirt.org/research/completed-projects/tate-training-assistive-technology-environment-toolkit

Prescott, S., Fleming, J., & Doig, E. (2015). Goal setting approaches and principles used in rehabilitation for people with acquired brain injury: A systematic scoping review. *Brain Injury*, 29(13–14), 1515–1529. https://doi.org/10.3109/02699052.2015.1075152

Purdy, M. (2002). Executive functioning in aphasia. *Aphasiology*, 16 (4–6), 549–557. https://doi.org/10.1080/02687030240004000176

Purdy, M., Belanger, S., & Liles, B. (1993). Right brain damaged subjects' ability to use context in inferencing. In P. Lemme (Ed.), *Clinical aphasiology* (p. 21). Pro-Ed.

Purdy, M., & Koch, A. (2006). Prediction of strategy usage by adults with aphasia. *Aphasiology*, 20(2–4), 337–348. https://doi.org/10.1080/02687030500475085

Radomski, M., Giles, G., Finkelstein, M., Owens, J., Showers, M., & Zola, J. (2018).

Implementation intentions for self-selected occupational therapy goals: Two case reports. *The American Journal of Occupational Therapy, 72*(3), 7203345030p1–7203345030p6. https://doi.org/10.5014/ajot.2018.023135

Radomski, M., Giles, G. M., Owens, J., Showers, M., Rabusch, S., Kreiger, R., . . . Kath, K. (2022). Can service members with mild traumatic brain injury learn to develop implementation intentions for self-identified goals? *Disability and Rehabilitation, 44*(12), 2640–2647. https://doi.org/10.1080/09638288.2020.1841309

Radomski, M., Owens, J., Showers, M., Giles, G., Zola, J., & Kreiger, R. (2017). Limited feasibility evaluation of combining Implementation Intentions with Metacognitive Strategy Instruction. *Archives of Physical Medicine and Rehabilitation, 98*, e79. https://doi.org/10.1016/j.apmr.2017.08.248

Ramanan, S., Bertoux, M., Flanagan, E., Irish, M., Piguet, O., Hodges, J., & Hornberger, M. (2017). Longitudinal executive function and episodic memory profiles in behavioral-variant frontotemporal dementia and Alzheimer's disease. *Journal of the International Neuropsychological Society, 23*(1), 34–43. https://doi.org/10.1017/S1355617716000837

Rammal, S., Abi Chahine, J., Rammal, M., Fares, Y., & Abou Abbas, L. (2019). Modified Wisconsin Card Sorting Test (M-WCST): Normative data for the Lebanese adult population. *Developmental Neuropsychology, 44*(5), 397–408. https://doi.org/10.1080/87565641.2019.1652828

Rascovsky, K., Hodges, J. R., Knopman, D., Mendez, M. F., Kramer, J. H., Neuhaus, J., . . . Miller, B. L. (2011). Sensitivity of revised diagnostic criteria for the behavioural variant of frontotemporal dementia. *Brain, 134*(9), 2456–2477. https://doi.org/10.1093/brain/awr179

Raspelli, S., Pallavicini, F., Carelli, L., Morganti, F., Poletti, B., Corra, B., & Silani, V. (2011). Validation of a neuro virtual reality-based based version of the Multiple Errands Test for the assessment of executive functions. *Studies in Health Technology and Informatics, 167*(1), 92–97. https://doi.org/10.3233/978-1-60750-766-6-92

Ratiulon, P., Talos, F., Haker, S., Lieberman, D., & Everett, P. (2004). The tale of Phineas Gage, digitally remastered. *Journal of Neurotrauma, 21*(5), 637–643. https://doi.org/10.1089/089771504774129964

Ravizza, S. M., Goudreau, J., Delgado, M. R., & Ruiz, S. (2012). Executive function abilities in Parkinson's disease: Contributions of the fronto-striatal pathways to action and feedback processing. *Cognitive, Affective, & Behavioral Neuroscience, 12*(1), 193–206.

Raymer, A., Roitsch, J., Redman, R., Michalek, A., & Johnson, R. (2018). Critical appraisal of systematic reviews of executive function treatments in TBI. *Brain Injury, 32*(12–14), 1601–1611. https://doi.org/10.1080/02699052.2018.1522671

Richardson, C., McKay, A., & Ponsford, J. (2015). Factors influencing self-awareness following traumatic brain injury. *Journal of Head Trauma Rehabilitation, 30*(2), E43–E54. https://doi.org/10.1097/HTR.0000000000000048

Riedeman, S., & Turkstra, L. (2018). Knowledge, confidence, and practice patterns of speech-language pathologists working with adults with traumatic brain injury. *American Journal of Speech-Language Pathology, 27*(1), 181–191. https://doi.org/10.1044/2017_AJSLP-17-0011

Rietdijk, R., Power, E., Attard, M., & Togher, L. (2020). Acceptability of telehealth-delivered rehabilitation: Experiences and perspectives of people with traumatic brain injury and their careers. *Journal of Telemedicine and Telecare, 28*(2), 122–134. https://doi.org/10.1177/1357633x20923824

Rietdijk, R., Power, E., Brunner, M., & Togher, L. (2019). A single case experimental design study on improving social communication skills after traumatic brain injury using communication partner telehealth training. *Brain Injury*, 33(1), 1–11. https://doi.org/10.1080/02699052.2018.1531313

Robertson, I. H., & Garavan, H. (2000). Vigilant attention. In M. Gazzaniga (Ed.), *The new cognitive neurosciences* (2nd ed., pp. 563–578). MIT Press.

Robertson, K., & Schmitter-Edgecombe, M. (2015). Self-awareness and traumatic brain injury outcome. *Brain Injury*, 29(7–8), 848–858.

Román, G. C. (2003). Vascular dementia: Distinguishing characteristics, treatment, and prevention. *Journal of the American Geriatrics Society*, 51(5s2), S296–S304. https://doi.org/10.3109/02699052.2015.1005135

Roth, R., Isquith, P., & Gioia, G. (2005). *Behavior Rating Inventory of Executive Function–Adult Version (BRIEF-A)*. Psychological Assessment Resources.

Rousseaux, M., Verigneaux, C., & Kozlowski, O. (2010). An analysis of communication in conversation after severe traumatic brain injury. *European Journal of Neurology*, 17, 922–929.

Royall, D. R., Lauterbach, E. C., Cummings, J. L., Reeve, A., Rummans, T. A., Kaufer, D. I., . . . Coffey, C. E. (2002). Executive control function: A review of its promise and challenges for clinical research. A report from the Committee on Research of the American Neuropsychiatric Association. *The Journal of Neuropsychiatry and Clinical Neurosciences*, 14(4), 377–405.

Ruan, Q., Xiao, F., Gong, K., Zhang, W., Zhang, M., Ruan, J., . . . Yu, Z. (2020). Demographically corrected normative z scores on the Neuropsychological Test Battery in cognitively normal older Chinese adults. *Dementia and Geriatric Cognitive Disorders*, 49(4), 375–383. https://doi.org/10.1159/000505618

Rundek, T., Tolea, M., Ariko, T., Fagerli, E. A., & Camargo, C. J. (2022). Vascular cognitive impairment (VCI). *Neurotherapeutics, 19*(1), 68–88. https://doi.org/10.1007/s13311-021-01170-y

Schneck, M. (2008). Vascular dementia. *Top Stroke Rehabilitation*, 15(1), 22–26.

Schneider, W., & Chein, J. (2003). Controlled and automatic processing: Behavior, theory, and biological mechanisms. *Cognitive Science* 27(3), 525–559. https://doi.org/10.1207/s15516709cog2703_8

Schraw, G., & Moshman, D. (1995). Metacognitive theories. *Educational Psychology Review*, 7(4), 351–371. https://doi.org/10.1007/BF02212307

Shallice, T., & Burgess, P. (1991). Deficits in strategy application following frontal lobe damage in man. *Brain*, 114, 727–741.

Shan, I.-K., Chen, Y.-S., Lee, Y.-C., & Su, T.-P. (2008). Adult normative data of the Wisconsin Card Sorting Test in Taiwan. *Journal of the Chinese Medical Association*, 71(10), 517–522. https://doi.org/10.1016/S1726-4901(08)70160-6

Shao, K., Wang, W., Guo, S. Z., Dong, F. M., Yang, Y. M., Zhao, Z. M., . . . Wang, J. H. (2020). Assessing executive function following the early stage of mild ischemic stroke with three brief screening tests. *Journal of Stroke and Cerebrovascular Diseases*, 29(8), 104960.

Simblett, S. K., Ring, H., & Bateman, A. (2017). The Dysexecutive Questionnaire Revised (DEX-R): An extended measure of everyday dysexecutive problems after acquired brain injury. *Neuropsychological Rehabilitation*, 27(8), 1124–1141. https://doi.org/10.1080/09602011.2015.1121880

Simic, T., Rochon, E., Greco, E., & Martino, R. (2019). Baseline executive control ability and its relationship to language therapy improvements in post-stroke aphasia: A systematic review. *Neuropsychological Rehabilitation*, 29(3), 395–439. https://doi.org/10.1080/09602011.2017.1307768

Simon, D. K., Tanner, C. M., & Brundin, P. (2020). Parkinson disease epidemiology, pathology, genetics, and pathophysiology. *Clinics in Geriatric Medicine*, 36(1),

1–12. https://doi.org/10.1016/j.cger.2019.08.002

Smolker, H. R., Depue, B. E., Reineberg, A. E., Orr, J. M., & Banich, M. T. (2015). Individual differences in regional prefrontal gray matter morphometry and fractional anisotropy are associated with different constructs of executive function. *Brain Structure and Function, 220*, 1291–1306.

Sohlberg, M., Hamilton, J., & Turkstra, L. S. (2023). *Transforming cognitive rehabilitation: Effective instructional methods.* Guilford.

Sohlberg, M., Johnson, L., Paule, L., Raskin, S., & Mateer, C. (2001). *Attention Process Training (APT-II) manual.* Lash and Associates.

Sohlberg, M. M., Ehlhardt, L., & Kennedy, M. (2005). Instructional techniques in cognitive rehabilitation: A preliminary report. *Seminars in Speech and Language, 26*, 268–279.

Sohlberg, M. M., MacDonald, S., Byom, L., Iwashita, H., Lemoncello, R., Meulenbroek, P., . . . O'Neil-Pirozzi, T. M. (2019). Social communication following traumatic brain injury part one: State-of-the-art review of assessment tools. *International Journal of Speech-Language Pathology, 21*(2), 115–127. https://doi.org/10.1080/17549507.2019.1583280

Sohlberg, M. M., & Mateer, C. A. (2001). *Cognitive rehabilitation: An integrative neuropsychological approach.* Guilford.

Sohlberg, M. M., & Turkstra, L. (2011). *Optimizing cognitive rehabilitation: Effective instructional methods.* Guilford.

Spikman, J. M., Boelen, D. H., Lamberts, K. F., Brouwer, W. H., & Fasotti, L. (2010). Effects of a multifaceted treatment program for executive dysfunction after acquired brain injury on indications of executive functioning in daily life. *Journal of the International Neuropsychological Society, 16*(1), 118–129. https://doi.org/10.1017/S1355617709991020

Spitz, G., Ponsford, J. L., Rudzki, D., & Maller, J. J. (2012). Association between cognitive performance and functional outcome following traumatic brain injury: A longitudinal multilevel examination. *Neuropsychology, 26*(5), 604–612. https://doi.org/10.1037/a0029239

Stamenova, V., & Levine, B. (2019). Effectiveness of goal management training® in improving executive functions: A meta-analysis. *Neuropsychological Rehabilitation, 29*(10), 1569–1599. https://doi.org/10.1080/09602011.2018.1438294

Steel, J., Elbourn, E., & Togher, L. (2021). Narrative discourse intervention after traumatic brain injury. *Topics in Language Disorders, 41*(1), 47–72. https://doi.org/10.1097/tld.0000000000000241

Steel, J., Ferguson, A., Spencer, E., & Togher, K. (2017). Social communication assessment during post-traumatic amnesia and the post-acute period after traumatic brain injury. *Brain Injury, 31*(10), 1320–1330. https://doi.org/10.1080/02699052.2017.1332385

Steel, J., & Togher, L. (2018). Social communication assessment after TBI: A narrative review of innovations in pragmatic and discourse assessment methods. *Brain Injury, 33*(2), 48–61. https://doi.org/10.1080/02699052.2018.1531304

Steward, K. A., & Kretzmer, T. (2022). Anosognosia in moderate-to-severe traumatic brain injury: A review of prevalence, clinical correlates, and diversity considerations. *The Clinical Neuropsychologist, 36*(8), 2021–2040.

Strobach, T., Salminen, T., Karbach, J., & Schubert, T. (2014). Practice-related optimization and transfer of executive functions: A general review and a specific realization of their mechanisms in dual tasks. *Psychological Research, 78*(6), 836–851. https://doi.org/10.1007/s00426-014-0563-7

Struchen, M. A., Pappadis, M. R., Mazzei, D. K., Clark, A. N., Davis, L. C., & Sander, A. M. (2008). Perceptions of communication abilities for persons with traumatic brain injury: Validity of the La Trobe

Communication Questionnaire. *Brain Injury*, 22(12), 940–951. https://doi.org/10.1080/02699050802425410

Stubbs, E., Togher, L., Kenny, B., Fromm, D., Forbes, M., MacWhinney, B., . . . Power, E. (2018). Procedural discourse performance in adults with severe traumatic brain injury at 3 and 6 months post injury. *Brain Injury*, 32(2), 167–181. https://doi.org/10.1080/02699052.2017.1291989

Stuss, D. T. (2011). Functions of the frontal lobes: Relation to executive functions. *Journal of the International Neuropsychological Society*, 17(5), 759–765. https://doi.org/10.1017/s1355617711000695

Stuss, D. T., & Levine, B. (2005). Adult clinical neuropsychology: Lessons from studies of the frontal lobes. *Annual Review of Psychology*, 53(1), 401–433. https://doi.org/10.1146/annurev.psych.53.100901.135220

Tate, R., Kennedy, M., Ponsford, J., Douglas, J., Velikonja, D., Bayley, M., & Stergiou-Kita, M. (2014). INCOG recommendations for management of cognition following traumatic brain injury, Part III: Executive function and self-awareness. *Journal of Head Trauma Rehabilitation*, 29(4), 338–352. https://doi.org/10.1097/HTR.0000000000000068

Tavakoli, M., Barekatain, M., & Emsaki, G. (2015). An Iranian normative sample of the Color Trails Test. *Psychology & Neuroscience*, 8(1), 75–81. https://doi.org/10.1037/h0100351

Togher, L., Douglas, J., Turkstra, L. S., Welch-West, P., Janzen, S., Harnett, A., . . . Wiseman-Hakes, C. (2023). INCOG 2.0 Guidelines for cognitive rehabilitation following traumatic brain injury, Part IV: Cognitive-communication and social cognition disorders. *Journal of Head Trauma Rehabilitation*, 38(1), 65–82. https://doi.org/10.1097/htr.0000000000000835

Togher, L., McDonald, S., Tate, R., Power, E., & Rietdijk, R. (2013). Training communication partners of people with severe traumatic brain injury improves everyday conversations: A multicenter single blind clinical trial. *Journal of Rehabilitation Medicine*, 45, 637–645. https://doi.org/10.23 40/16501977

Togher, L., McDonald, S., Tate, R., Rietdijk, R., & Power, E. (2016). The effectiveness of social communication partner training for adults with severe chronic TBI and their families using a measure of perceived communication ability. *NeuroRehabilitation*, 38(3), 243–255.

Togher, L., Power, E., Tate, R., McDonald, S., & Rietdijk, R. (2010). Measuring the social interactions of people with traumatic brain injury and their communication partners: The adapted Kagan scales. *Aphasiology*, 24(6–8), 914–927. https://doi.org/10.1080/02687030903422478

Togher, L., Wiseman-Hakes, C., Douglas, J., Stergiou-Kita, M., Ponsford, J., Teasell, R., . . . Turkstra, L. (2014). INCOG recommendations for management of cognition following traumatic brain injury, Part IV: Cognitive communication. *Journal of Head Trauma Rehabilitation*, 29(4), 353–368. https://doi.org/10.1097/HTR.0000000000000071

Toglia, J., & Kirk, U. (2000). Understanding awareness deficits following brain injury. *NeuroRehabilitation*, 15, 57–70. https://doi.org/10.3233/NRE-2000-15104

Tompkins, C. A., Bloise, C. G. R., Timko, M. L., & Baumgaertner, A. (1994). Working memory and inference revision in brain-damaged and normally aging adults. *Journal of Speech and Hearing Research*, 37, 96–912.

Tornas, S., Lovstad, M., Solbakk, A., Evans, J., Endestad, T., Hol, P., . . . Stubberud, J. (2016). Rehabilitation of executive functions in patients with chronic acquired brain injury with goal management training, external cueing, and emotional regulation: A randomized controlled trial. *Journal of the International Neuropsychological Society*, 22, 436–452. https://doi.org/10.1017/S1355617715001344

Tornås, S., Løvstad, M., Solbakk, A.-K., Schanke, A.-K., & Stubberud, J. (2019). Use it or lose It? A 5-year follow-up study of Goal Management Training in patients with acquired brain injury. *Journal of the International Neuropsychological Society*, 25(10), 1082–1087. https://doi.org/10.1017/S1355617719000626

Tornås, S., Stubberud, J., Solbakk, A.-K., Evans, J., Schanke, A.-K., & Løvstad, M. (2019). Moderators, mediators and non-specific predictors of outcome after cognitive rehabilitation of executive functions in a randomised controlled trial. *Neuropsychological Rehabilitation*, 29(6), 844–865. https://doi.org/10.1080/09602011.2017.1338587

Trahan, E., Pepin, M., & Hopps, S. (2006). Impaired awareness of deficits and treatment adherence among people with traumatic brain injury or spinal cord injury. *Journal of Head Trauma Rehabilitation*, 21, 226–235. https://doi.org/10.1097/00001199-200605000-00003

Trenova, A. G., Slavov, G. S., Manova, M. G., Aksentieva, J. B., Miteva, L. D., & Stanilova, S. A. (2016). Cognitive impairment in multiple sclerosis. *Folia Medica*, 58(3), 157–163. https://doi.org/10.1515/folmed-2016-0029

Turkstra, L., & Flora, T. L. (2002). Compensating for executive function impairments after TBI: A single case study of functional intervention. *Journal of Communication Disorders*, 35, 467–482.

Turkstra, L. S., Norman, R., Whyte, J., Dijkers, M. P., & Hart, T. (2016). Knowing what we're doing: Why specification of treatment methods is critical for evidence-based practice in speech-language pathology. *American Journal of Speech-Language Pathology*, 25(2), 164–168. https://doi.org/10.1044/2015_ajslp-15-0060

Vanderah, T. W., Gould, D. J., & Nolte, J. (2021). *Nolte's The human brain: An introduction to its functional anatomy* (8th ed.). Elsevier.

Van Stan, J. H., Whyte, J., Duffy, J. R., Barkmeier-Kraemer, J. M., Doyle, P. B., Gherson, S., . . . Tolejano, C. J. (2021). Rehabilitation Treatment Specification System: Methodology to identify and describe unique targets and ingredients. *Archives of Physical Medicine and Rehabilitation*, 102(3), 521–531. https://doi.org/10.1016/j.apmr.2020.09.383

Vas, A., Chapman, S., Aslan, S., Spence, J., Keebler, M., Rodriguez-Larrain, G., . . . Krawczyk, D. (2016). Reasoning training in veteran and civilian traumatic brain injury with persistent mild impairment. *Neuropsychological Rehabilitation*, 26(4), 502–531. https://doi.org/10.1080/09602011.2015.1044013

Vas, A., Chapman, S., Cook, L., Elliott, A., & Keebler, M. (2011). Higher-order reasoning training years after traumatic brain injury in adults. *Journal of Head Trauma Rehabilitation*, 26(3), 224–239. https://doi.org/10.1097/HTR.0b013e318218dd3d

Vataja, R., Pohjasvaara, T., Mantyla, R., Ylikoski, R., Leppavuori, A., Leskela, M., . . . Erkinjuntti, T. (2003). MRI correlates of executive dysfunction in patients with ischaemic stroke. *European Journal of Neurology*, 10(6), 625–631.

Waid-Ebbs, J., Wen, P.-S., & Perlstein, W. (2022). Enhancing Goal Management Training with attention drill training. *Archives of Physical Medicine & Rehabilitation*, 103(3), e43. https://doi.org/10.1016/j.apmr.2022.01.119

Wallace, E. R., Segerstrom, S. C., van Horne, C. G., Schmitt, F. A., & Koehl, L. M. (2022). Meta-analysis of cognition in Parkinson's disease mild cognitive impairment and dementia progression. *Neuropsychology Review*, 32(1), 149–160. https://doi.org/10.1007/s11065-021-09502-7

Wallace, T. D., McCauley, K. L., Hodge, A. T., Moran, T. P., Porter, S. T., Whaley, M. C., & Gore, R. K. (2022). Use of person-centered goals to direct interdisciplinary care for military service members and veterans with chronic mTBI and co-occurring psychological conditions. *Frontiers in Neurology*, 13, 1015591. https://doi.org/10.3389/fneur.2022.1015591

Wallace, T. D., & Morris, J. T. (2020, September). SwapMyMood: User-centered design and development of a mobile app to support executive function. In K. Missenberger, R. Manduchi, M. Covarrubias Rodriguez, & P. Penaz (Eds), *International Conference on Computers Helping People with Special Needs* (pp. 259–265). Springer.

Weber, E., Spirou, A., Chiaravalloti, N., & Lengenfelder, J. (2018). Impact of frontal neurobehavioral symptoms on employment in individuals with TBI. *Rehabilitation Psychology, 63*(3), 383–391. https://doi.org/10.1037/rep0000208

Whitworth, A., Leitao, S., Cartwright, J., Webster, J., Hankey, G. J., Zach, J., . . . Wolz, V. (2015). NARNIA: A new twist to an old tale. A pilot RCT to evaluate a multilevel approach to improving discourse in aphasia. *Aphasiology, 29*(11), 1345–1382.

Whitworth, A., Ng, N., Timms, L., & Power, E. (2020, January). Exploring the viability of NARNIA with cognitive–communication difficulties: A pilot study. *Seminars in Speech and Language, 41*(1), 83–98.

Wilson, B. A., Alderman, N., Burgess, P. W., Emslie, H., & Evans, J. J. (1996). *Behavioural assessment of the dysexecutive syndrome*. Thames Valley Test Company.

World Health Organization. (2001). *International classification of functioning, disability, and health (ICF)*.

World Health Organization. (2022). *Dementia*. https://www.who.int/news-room/fact-sheets/detail/dementia

Yassai-Gonzalez, D., Marquine, M. J., Perez-Tejada, A., Umlauf, A., Kamalyan, L., Morlett Paredes, A., . . . Heaton, R. K. (2019). Normative data for Wisconsin Card Sorting Test-64 item in a Spanish speaking adult population living in the US/Mexico border region. *Archives of Clinical Neuropsychology, 34*(7), 1281. https://doi.org/10.1093/arclin/acz029.48

Yeo, Y. X., Pestell, C. F., Bucks, R. S., Allanson, F., & Weinborn, M. (2021). Metacognitive knowledge and functional outcomes in adults with acquired brain injury: A meta-analysis. *Neuropsychological Rehabilitation, 31*(3), 453–478. https://doi.org/10.1080/09602011.2019.1704421

Ylvisaker, M. (2006). Self-coaching: A context-sensitive, person-centred approach to social communication after traumatic brain injury. *Brain Impairment, 7*(3), 246–258. https://doi.org/10.1375/brim.7.3.246

Ylvisaker, M., & Feeney, T. J. (1998). *Collaborative brain injury intervention*. Singular Publishing.

Youse, K., Gathof, M., Fields, R., Lobianco, T., Bush, H., & Noffsinger, J. (2011). Conversational discourse analysis procedures: A comparison of two paradigms. *Aphasiology, 25*(1), 106–118. https://doi.org/10.1080/02687031003714467

Zimmermann, N., Cardoso, C. de O., Trentini, C. M., Grassi-Oliveira, R., & Fonseca, R. P. (2015). Brazilian preliminary norms and investigation of age and education effects on the Modified Wisconsin Card Sorting Test, Stroop Color and Word test and Digit Span test in adults. *Dementia & Neuropsychologia, 9*(2), 120–127. https://doi.org/10.1590/1980-5764 2015DN92000006

Zimmermann, N., Gindri, G., deOliveira, C., & Fonseca, R. (2011). Pragmatic and executive functions in traumatic brain injury and right brain damage: An exploratory comparative study. *Dementia & Neuropsychologia, 5*(4), 337–345.

4

Cognitive Communication Deficits Associated With Right Hemisphere Damage

Petrea L. Cornwell, Ronelle Hewetson,
and Margaret Lehman Blake

Chapter Learning Objectives

After reading this chapter you will be able to:

1. Describe the cognitive and communicative changes that are associated with right hemisphere damage.
2. Explain the impact that cognitive communication deficits associated with right hemisphere damage have on an individual's life.
3. Select appropriate assessments to comprehensively assess the cognitive communication deficits arising secondary to right hemisphere damage.
4. Identify, describe, and apply evidence-based approaches to intervention for cognitive communication disorder associated with right hemisphere damage.

History

The right hemisphere patient appears peculiarly unconcerned about the impact of his message, insensitive to his situation or to the environment . . . inevitably his interaction with others will change. (Myers, 1978, p. 50)

Throughout the mid- to late 20th century, deficits associated with damage to the right hemisphere were observed and reported. Visuoperceptual deficits and symptoms of visuospatial neglect were reported in the 1940s (see Heilman et al., 1985); difficulties with comprehending or expressing emotion were described in the 1950s. In the 1960s and 1970s, reports of communication problems associated with right hemisphere damage (RHD) were published. The deficits reported included changes in processing abstract, emotional, and metaphorical information following damage to the right hemisphere (Critchley, 1991; Eisenson, 1962). Gardner and his colleagues (1973, 1978) published reports of communication deficits in individuals with RHD. Their awareness of these problems grew out of aphasia research, in which they included adults with RHD as a brain-damaged control group, to evaluate whether aphasic deficits were due to brain damage in general or to the left hemisphere specifically. When they examined the results for the RHD "control" group, they found that although these individuals did not exhibit typical aphasic language impairments, they also did not perform like a control group of individuals without brain damage. Deficits were observed in a variety of areas, including appreciating humor, understanding inferred versus dominant meanings, and appreciating metaphorical and other nonliteral meanings (Wapner et al., 1981). Around the same time, Myers (1979) was reporting similar deficits and discussing the role of the speech-language pathologist (SLP) in assessment and treatment of these clients.

A seminal article by Wapner and colleagues (1981) and a book about cognitive communication processes associated with the right hemisphere (Perecman, 1983) stimulated work in the 1980s. Many studies were conducted to explore the types of deficits exhibited by adults with RHD and to describe RHD profiles. Characteristics noted included a lack of specific, relevant information in narratives (Cimino et al., 1991; Joanette et al., 1986); difficulties understanding or relating emotional concepts in stories (Bloom et al., 1990; Borod et al., 1985); overpersonalization

of responses (Wapner et al., 1981); poor organization of story retellings (Myers, 1979; Wapner et al., 1981); inclusion of tangential or off-topic comments in their responses (Wapner et al., 1981); difficulties interpreting humor and responding appropriately to humor (Brownell et al., 1983; Gardner et al., 1978); reduced abilities in determining morals or themes of stories (Benowitz et al., 1990; Delis et al., 1983; Mackisack et al., 1987; Moya et al., 1986; Rehak et al., 1992); and impairments in understanding nonliteral or connotative meanings (Brownell et al., 1984; Gardner & Denes, 1973; Myers & Linebaugh, 1981; Van Lancker & Kempler, 1987). One conclusion drawn from the patterns observed was that RHD communication deficits affected the comprehension and use of complex linguistic material (Wapner et al., 1981). In the 1990s, theories were proposed to explain the underlying deficits. Myers (1990) suggested an **inference failure** was the basis for many deficits associated with RHD. This label was not meant to indicate a complete failure of inferencing processes but rather inefficient or incomplete inferencing (just as aphasia literally means "without language" but in practice means difficulties with language). The inference failure account was based on observations and reports of difficulties with inferring meanings in both verbal and visual modalities. It suggested that inferencing processes impacted both early and late stages of cognitive processing and that inferencing was a central deficit in adults with RHD. The hypothesis was never directly tested and has not been revisited in its original form.

Other accounts followed, several of which were designed to explain inferencing difficulties. One suggests the problems are caused by an inability to generate inferences (Beeman, 1998). Another account proposes that initial inference generation is intact but that the problem lies in the inhibition, or suppression, of meanings that are less likely or that become inappropriate for a given context (Tompkins et al., 2004; Tompkins et al., 2001a, 2001b). Other accounts implicate Theory of Mind (ToM), or one's ability to understand that other people have ideas, beliefs, and views that differ from one's own (Balaban et al., 2016; Griffin et al., 2006; Happe et al., 1999; Martin & McDonald, 2003); the complexity of processing required for interpreting discourse and pragmatics (Monetta & Joanette, 2003; Monetta et al., 2006); and the interruption of executive function networks based in the frontal lobes (Martin & McDonald, 2003). These theories are discussed in more detail later as they relate to discourse and pragmatic deficits in adults with RHD. They also are used as suggested foundations for developing theoretically based treatments in the absence of evidence for efficacy of treatment in these areas.

During the 21st century, there has been a growth in the use of functional neuroimaging techniques to explore the role of the right hemisphere in cognitive and communication skills. While this statement may suggest that neural correlates of cognitive and communication functions are unitary, current research in the field of neuroscience is demonstrating that while there are key domain-specific networks (e.g., attention networks), these are also interdependent on other brain regions or networks (Keerativittayayut et al., 2018; Menon & D'Esposito, 2022; Nebel et al., 2005).

There is no commonly used label for communication deficits associated with RHD. Some labels that routinely appear in both research and clinical diagnoses include cognitive communication deficits, cognitive-linguistic deficits, or nonaphasic language deficits. The label "right hemisphere syndrome" also has been used. A syndrome generally has specific signs and symptoms associated with it and given that with RHD there is a wide variety of deficits and no readily apparent pattern of those deficits (Blake et al., 2002; Ferré et al., 2012), the term right hemisphere (RH) syndrome is perhaps a misnomer. Two other labels previously suggested highlighted the centrality of pragmatic deficits to the communication problems associated with RHD. The labels were **pragmatic aphasia** (Joanette & Ansaldo, 1999) and **apragmatism** (Myers, 2001), with the latter being revisited recently by a group of international researchers working collaboratively. This group has again proposed apragmatism as a diagnostic label that encompasses the communication-specific impairments that occur following RHD (Minga et al., 2023). Apragmatism has been defined as "a disorder of conveying and/or comprehending meaning or intent through linguistic, paralinguistic and/or extralinguistic modes of context-dependent communication" (Minga et al., 2023, p. 11). Its description acknowledges that perceptual and cognitive deficits may co-occur and impact communication abilities, as well as the importance of context to communication. Neither apragmatism nor pragmatic aphasia were adopted for general clinical use when proposed over 20 years ago; however, due to the recency of a renewed proposal to use apragmatism as a label, the term cognitive communication disorder (CCD) will be used in this chapter to refer to existing knowledge of the cognitive and communication changes that occur following RHD.

Characteristics and Clinical Profiles

Heterogeneity in the clinical presentation of CCD after RHD has been noted repeatedly within the literature (Blake & Hoepner, 2021; Ferré et al., 2012). Figure 4–1 provides an overview of the broad areas of cognition and communication associated with CCD after RHD and how other impairments and communication context influence the presenting characteristics. Unlike its left hemisphere damage (LHD) counterpart, aphasia, where typologies have been described and accepted into clinical practice, there has been no adoption of clinical profiles of CCD after RHD into practice. This is despite research-

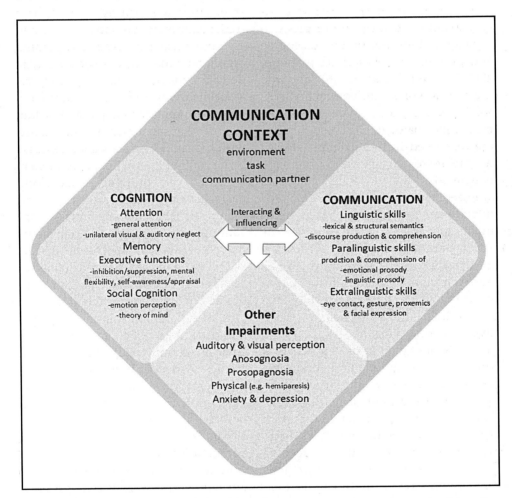

Figure 4–1. Overview of the cognitive and communication deficits and factors that interact or influence the clinical presentation of cognitive communication disorder after RHD.

ers having identified different profiles of impaired discourse production based on quantity and quality of production (Blake et al., 2002; Hillis Trupe & Hillis, 1985; Joanette et al., 1986) and proposing clinical profiles differing in terms of presence of impairment across semantics, prosody, discourse, and pragmatics (Ferré et al., 2012; Ferré & Joanette, 2016). The components of apragmatism—linguistic, paralinguistic, and extralinguistic—may facilitate such clinical profiles moving forward. The interaction between these clinical profiles and cognition remains unclear, although multiple hypotheses or theories such as the coarse coding (Beeman, 1998), suppression deficit (Tompkins et al., 2001a), and social cognitive deficit (Brownell & Martino, 1998) have been explored. Martin and McDonald (2003) concluded that no one of these hypotheses or theories could fully explain the clinical presentations of CCD seen in people with RHD.

Cognitive deficits associated with RHD include attention, memory, executive function, and social cognition. Attentional deficits include general deficits in the ability to focus attention, sustain attention over time, and alternate or divide attention between different tasks or stimuli. One specific type of attentional disorder strongly associated with RHD is unilateral neglect (UN), in which an individual has difficulty attending to stimuli presented on the side contralateral to the site of lesion. Evidence to support the presence of memory impairment after RHD damage is mixed and dependent on modality (visual or verbal) and nature of task (recognition vs. recall). Deficits in executive function impact organization, sequencing, problem solving, reason-

ing, judgment, and self-awareness. The social cognitive theory suggests that changes in communication after RHD arise due to deficits in social cognitive abilities, with emotion perception and ToM being the most discussed areas of difficulty. Patterns of co-occurrence of cognitive deficits have not been extensively studied, so conclusions are tentative, but deficits in learning/memory and attention may co-occur, as may executive functions (organizing, sequencing) and slowed processing.

Communication deficits associated with RHD can involve motor speech production (i.e., dysarthria) as well as linguistic, extralinguistic, and paralinguistic characteristics associated with CCD. Focusing on CCD, the communication deficits seen involve difficulty comprehending or conveying meaning using linguistic, paralinguistic, and extralinguistic skills (Minga et al., 2023). Linguistic deficits include challenges in interpreting or selecting contextually appropriate words, syntactic structures, or topics particularly at the level of discourse. This can lead to inefficient or ineffective conversational interactions. At the paralinguistic level, disruptions in the interpretation and/or production of prosodic contours to express meaning and emotion can occur. This is referred to as aprosodia. The ineffective or inappropriate use, or comprehension of body language and position, facial expression, gestures, or eye contact, represent extralinguistic deficits that may be observed after RHD but must be considered within the context of sociocultural norms and the nature of the communication exchange. Co-occurrence or patterns of communication deficits after RHD is still an area of emerging research. Ferré and Joanette (2016) have identified four clinical profiles characterized by (a) primarily prosodic impairments; (b) deficits during conversational discourse; (c) emotional prosody, narrative discourse, and semantic impairments that are generally mild to moderate in severity; and (d) severe deficits across multiple areas, including semantics, prosody, narrative discourse, and conversation. The occurrence of aprosodia with deficits in pragmatics or social interactions has also been highlighted as a common feature of CCD after RHD (Blake et al., 2002).

Causes and Prevalence

Many neurological conditions can cause RHD, including cerebrovascular accident (stroke), traumatic brain injury, brain tumors, and complications of their treatment. Beyond direct injury, the function of the right hemisphere can be altered by a variety of disorders and diseases of the nervous system, including seizure disorders, neurodegenerative diseases, and the effects of drugs and other toxins. The prevalence of RHD has most extensively been researched following cerebrovascular accidents. Right and left hemisphere strokes occur with comparable frequency when identified through neurological imaging; 48.1% right-sided, 51.9% left-sided (Portegies et al., 2015). When initial diagnosis of stroke relies on behavioral observation alone, a higher incidence of left-sided strokes is reported, suggesting that left-sided strokes are recognized more easily or perceived as more severe and conversely that right-sided strokes may have been missed (Portegies et al.,

2015). A lack of sensitivity of clinical tools to detect acute right hemisphere stroke and poor recognition and/or awareness of symptoms by patients and their family members have been implicated as the cause of perceived higher frequency of left-sided stroke (Blake 2016; Portegies et al., 2015). A laterality bias in the National Institutes of Health Stroke Scale (NIHSS; Lyden et al., 1999), a global clinical stroke tool, that awards greater points for impaired functions associated with the left hemisphere and does not include items such as aprosodia that are highly predictive of RHD further impacts accurate clinically derived frequency data (Dara et al., 2014; McCluskey et al., 2016; Woo et al., 1999).

Considering the frequency of diagnosed cognitive communication disorders, studies have suggested that 66% of first-onset right hemisphere strokes across both acute and rehabilitation settings were diagnosed with CCD (Hewetson et al., 2017), which increases to over 80% of adults with RHD within inpatient rehabilitation settings (Côté et al., 2007). The population of adults with RHD is extremely heterogeneous in terms of presentation. Cognitive deficits, including attention, unilateral neglect, memory, and executive function, are reportedly diagnosed more often than communication deficits (e.g., aprosodia, impaired spoken discourse) (Blake et al., 2002; Ramsey & Blake, 2020); however, it is unclear whether this pattern truly reflects the incidence of various deficits or if it is a by-product of assessment practices.

Spoken discourse and aprosodia emerged as the most frequent communication impairments from an examination of 112 individuals with RHD using the Protocole Montréal d'Evaluation de la Communication (Protocole MEC; Joanette et al., 2004). When spoken communication impairments are present, their frequency varies across the patterns of hyporesponsive (slow responses, unelaborated speech) and hyperresponsive (verbose, tangential), representing 48% and 51% prevalence out of 123 cases, respectively (Blake et al., 2002). This variation in quantity of content was recently replicated by Berube and colleagues (2022) where 19% of their participants with RHD presented with verbosity as determined by calculating syllables per content unit. During conversational discourse, a quarter of individuals with RHD may present with off-topic content and up to 50% with turn-taking quantity impairments (Kennedy, 2000; Prutting & Kittchner, 1987). Aprosodia incidence data vary from 24% (Blake et al., 2002) to 70% (Ferré & Joanette, 2016; Sheppard et al., 2020) depending on the time after stroke onset, with a higher incidence recorded during the acute phase. Fewer studies have reported the prevalence of linguistic and pragmatic impairments, noted to be present in 26% and 16.3% of 123 individuals with RHD, respectively (Blake et al., 2002).

Impact of Cognitive Communication Deficits

Impairments in communication and cognition can have substantial effects on social, emotional, and vocational outcomes. Many personal and clinical variables influence long-term outcomes following an acquired brain injury. Personal variables such as older age and relationship status (living alone) are highly significant predictors of functional outcomes after both stroke and TBI (e.g., Baumann et al., 2012). Clinical variables such as the severity of physical impairment, presence of cognitive deficits, anosognosia, and unilateral neglect have been linked to the length of stay in acute and subacute settings as well as poststroke functional status upon discharge and the likelihood of being discharged to an independent living setting (e.g., Appelros, 2007; D'Alisa et al., 2005; Gillen et al., 2005; Vossel et al., 2013; Wee & Hopman, 2005).

The presence of impaired communication following RHD has similarly been shown to be a significant clinical variable that is predictive of poststroke outcomes (Hewetson et al., 2018). Individuals with RHD who were diagnosed acutely with a CCD were more likely than those without CCD to experience changes in social participation that affected several areas: occupational activities, interpersonal relationships (notably a loss of friends), and independent living skills (Hewetson et al., 2018). CCD following RHD can have similar devastating effects on life participation as found in individuals with aphasia following a left hemisphere stroke. A group of people with RHD with diagnosed communication and social cognition impairments noted spousal relationship change and a reduction in the size and frequency of contact with their social networks (Hewetson et al., 2021). Deficits associated with RHD can also impact caregivers (Davidson & Wallace, 2022). Hillis and Tippett (2014) found that caregivers were concerned about eight poststroke changes related to communication and interpersonal interactions (reading, writing, memory, mood, prosody, empathy, personality/

behavior, and cognition). Change in an RHD stroke survivor's level of empathy was the most important change reported by caregivers and was rated as more important than hemiparesis or cognitive deficits (Hillis & Tippett, 2014).

Cognition

Attention

All forms of attention, including focused, sustained, alternating, and divided attention (as discussed in Chapter 1), may be affected by RHD. These types of attention can be described as general attention deficits; however, the person with RHD may also present with neglect, which is a spatial attention deficit. Attention deficits may co-occur or be selectively impaired. Furthermore, general attention appears to modulate or influence spatial attention deficits as represented in a range of models of general attentional control (refer to Zebhauser et al., 2019, for an overview). The occurrence of attention deficits after stroke, irrespective of lesion location, ranges from 46% to 92% (Barker-Collo et al., 2010). Numerous lateralization studies have considered left versus right hemispheric involvement across types of attention. The right hemisphere has a particular role in attention processes of alertness and vigilance while both hemispheres play a role in more complex types of attention, with more severe impairment in divided attention documented in those with RHD (Spaccavento et al., 2019).

Deficits in attention may negatively affect communication. A person with impaired attention due to RHD may find it difficult to maintain focus on conversations or reading material. The result of impaired attention is that information contained in a passage or spoken discourse may be missed by the person with RHD. This, in turn, may impact auditory and reading comprehension. If the information was not critical, then it is possible to refocus on the conversation and still get the gist of it. On the other hand, if critical information is omitted, then understanding will be incomplete at best or incorrect. Alternating and divided attention, in part, because they are more complex forms of attention, are frequently affected by RHD. A study by Leonard and Baum (2005) demonstrated the impact of attention on language-based activities in a group of people with RHD. Sentence stimuli were presented in three conditions: (a) isolation, (b) within a focused attention condition, and (c) in a divided attention task that included a competing auditory stimulus. It was particularly in the divided attention task where participants with RHD were less effective in using semantic context, thus supporting the need to consider processing demands inherent in different communication-based activities where attention has been impaired. Clinicians should consider that impaired attention may also influence assessment findings when planning treatment. For example, individuals with RHD may have difficulty focusing on assessment or treatment tasks, especially when there are distractors present. They also may have difficulty sustaining attention for several minutes at a time.

Neglect

Neglect (also known as spatial neglect or unilateral neglect) is multifactorial both in cause and presentation, with constituent deficits often co-occurring. Sometimes neglect is described as the person ignoring information from one hemispace. This term should be used cautiously, as the word ignore suggests that the person is aware of the stimulus and chooses not to attend to it. In contrast, neglect is not a conscious ignoring of information but a decreased ability to process that information. In fact, many people with neglect are not aware of their symptoms. It is, however, also known that unconscious processing of neglected information can occur (e.g., Vuilleumier et al., 2002; Vuilleumier et al., 2001). Individuals with visuospatial neglect demonstrate processing of color and shape, and even identity and meaning without conscious awareness of seeing the stimuli. This phenomenon can be used in treatment, as will be discussed later in this chapter.

Neglect may occur after damage to either cerebral hemisphere; however, it is more severe, more persistent, and more prevalent after right hemisphere stroke (33% to 82%), likely due to the neural network critical to spatial attention being predominantly located in the right side of the brain (Bowen et al., 1999; Esposito et al., 2021). Neglect arises both from specific lesions and due to intrahemispheric disconnection that impacts attention control broadly. The large prevalence range reported for neglect may be due to timing of assessment (acute vs. chronic), grouping data for all RHD participants without considering localization of brain lesions, or the variable sensitivity of tests for neglect. The latter is discussed in the section on assessment.

There are different ways to classify types of neglect, which can broadly be grouped as motor or sensory neglect.

Motor neglect can be observed during movements as a reduction, impersistence, or absence of spontaneous use of a limb opposite to the site of brain lesion, which occurs in the absence of hemiplegia (Sampanis & Riddoch, 2013). For example, an individual may not use their left arm to propel their wheelchair or for tasks that require both hands (e.g., unscrewing a lid), even if there is only mild weakness present. If sensory neglect is present, then the person may not be aware of, process, or be able to respond to sensory stimuli in the absence of impaired sensory pathways or lesions that might impact sensory processing. Sensory neglect is of relevance to communication as it may impact what is seen and heard and will be the focus of the following section.

Sensory neglect has been shown to impact rehabilitation outcomes, the ability to perform activities of daily life, and reading, and it is associated with greater family reported burden and stress (see Esposito et al., 2021, for an overview). Individuals with sensory neglect show reduced attention and fail to respond to stimuli (visual, auditory, tactile) presented on the side contralateral to the cerebral lesion (e.g., individuals do not process information from the left side of space after a lesion to the right hemisphere) (Rode et al., 2017). Ways of further conceptualizing sensory neglect is as personal, peripersonal, and extrapersonal space deficits or as allocentric (object-centered) neglect and egocentric (viewer-centered) neglect (see Table 4–1 and Figure 4–2 for descriptions and clinical examples) (Chatterjee, 1994; Zebhauser et al., 2019). More than 50% of people with RHD have both egocentric and allocentric neglect (Yue et al., 2012); however, dissociations also occur, which

Table 4–1. Example of How Neglect May Present Across Neglect Subtypes

Neglect Subtypes	Description	Examples of Clinical Presentation
Personal neglect (internal or body space)	Lack of exploration or use of contralesional limbs or head and/or impaired reactions to tactile stimuli Linked to damage to Brodmann area 40 in the right parietal lobe	May appear to • have a hemiplegia, or • avert posture and gaze toward the ipsilesional space. The person may fail to brush their hair on the left or shave only one side of their face or may fail to move their body to allow for appropriate eye contact with people on their left. Reactions to tactile stimuli may be impaired (e.g., not reacting to a hand caught in a wheel of a wheelchair).
Peripersonal neglect (within the person's reaching space)	Not attending to visual information that is within arm's reach Linked to lesions of the superior temporal gyrus, inferior frontal gyrus, and/or frontoparietal attentional networks	The person may only eat food on the right half of their plate, may not be able to locate items positioned within arm's reach on their left, or may omit the words (or parts of words) that are on the left side of a page during a reading task.
Extrapersonal neglect (far space or beyond the person's reaching space)	Inability to attend to sensory information on the left, beyond an arm's reach Similar lesion locations implicated in extrapersonal neglect as peripersonal neglect	Inability to notice when someone is speaking to them from the left side of a room or inability to point to an object located on the left. They may therefore not be able to "find" a window or TV or other object in the room. They are also at risk of bumping into items on the left when walking.
Allocentric neglect (object centered or stimulus centered)	Spatial inattention is specific to the contralesional side of an object irrespective of where the object is in relation to their view.	When asked to copy an image or produce a drawing of an object, the individual draws only the right side of the object regardless of where the line drawing or object is placed in their visual field.
Egocentric neglect (viewer centered or body centered)	Spatial inattention is specific to the contralesional area in relation to their midline or from their perspective.	Copying or describing only right-sided items of a picture, resulting in an incomplete representation of the visual scene or a descriptive discourse in which key elements of a picture are omitted

Source: Information compiled from Bartolomeo et al. (2007); Chatterjee et al. (1994); Zebhauser et al. (2019).

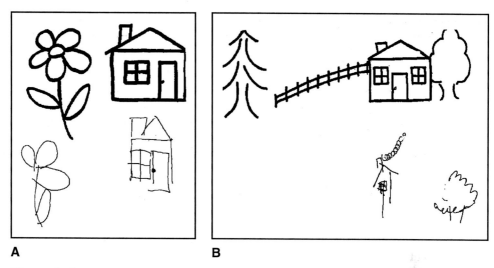

Figure 4–2. A. Viewer-centered neglect: The patient omitted the leftmost features of the drawing on the left side of the page. **B.** Object- and viewer-centered neglect: The patient omitted the left-sided detail of the two items he drew, as well as all items to the left of midline on the page.

means that a person might present with only personal but not peripersonal neglect and vice versa (Hillis, 2006).

The regions associated with neglect form a network of attention structures that likely contributes to a lack of clearly defined neuroanatomical origins of types of neglect (Corbetta & Shulman, 2011; Kenzie et al., 2015). Broadly, lesions in the temporoparietal junction and occipital lobe have been associated with allocentric neglect while more anterior lesion locations and the inferior parietal cortex are associated with egocentric neglect (e.g., see Hillis et al., 2005). Subcortical structures may also be involved, including the thalamus and the basal ganglia (Arene & Hillis, 2007; Karnath et al., 2004; Thiebaut de Schotten et al., 2014; Yue et al., 2012).

Visuospatial neglect symptoms (or unilateral visual neglect: UVN) are the most easily recognized in clinical contexts. UVN is not an all-or-none phenomenon: Some individuals can shift their attention to stimuli in the left visual space when cued to do so, some demonstrate delayed response times to left-sided stimuli, and others can attend to items in the left hemispace only when there are no competing stimuli on the right side (Anderson et al., 2000). There might also be a difficulty disengaging visual attention from a stimulus to shift attention to another one, resulting in a fixed gaze, which may seem pragmatically inappropriate (Sieroff et al., 2007).

UVN can affect discourse, reading, and writing. Berube and colleagues documented the impact of UVN on a descriptive discourse task using the Modern Cookie Theft picture where participants with RHD omitted important content units that were represented on the left side of the picture (Berube et al., 2022). The terms neglect dyslexia and neglect dysgraphia have been used to describe the deficits in reading and writing associated with UVN. An individual with neglect dyslexia may have difficulty reading the beginnings (leftmost characters) of words or sentences (Reinhart et al., 2013; Ronchi et al., 2016; Vallar et al., 2010). Thus, the word baseball may be read as ball or hiking as king. Sometimes there can be replacement of letters on the left side, resulting in snake being read as lake. This is thought to be due to the brain adding in letters to create a meaningful word given the nonword created by letters on the right side (-ake).

Neglect dysgraphia can have one or more of the following characteristics: writing that begins near the midline of a page as opposed to the left margin (for individuals who read languages written left to right), letter perseverations, perseverations of lines (e.g., crossing a T multiple times), and inappropriate gaps between letters in words (Cubelli et al., 2000; Ellis, 1998).

A person with **auditory neglect** may exhibit impairments in processing sounds that originate from the left side (Eramudugolla et al., 2007; Pavani et al., 2004; Zimmer et al., 2003). Auditory neglect can be difficult to identify because of the bilateral (although unequal) representation of sounds in the auditory cortex and from the transmission of sound through space such that sounds that originate on the left side are detected and processed by both ears (just softer and slightly later in time for the contralateral ear). Auditory neglect may manifest as a difficulty in localizing sounds, particularly those that originate from the left side of space (Brozzoli et al., 2006). Errors attributed to auditory neglect tend to correlate with the severity of visual neglect, suggesting a deficit of multimodal spatial processing (Pavani et al., 2002).

Another sensory neglect phenomenon is **extinction**, where an individual with RHD may accurately localize visual or tactile input when each side of the body is touched independently or objects are shown in each visual field separately but may not report sensation or the presence of visual stimuli on the left when the stimuli are presented bilaterally at the same time (Chechlacz et al., 2014; de Haan et al., 2012).

Executive Function

One theory to account for, in part, RHD communication deficits is that they arise because of executive dysfunction. Executive function (EF) deficits caused by stroke are well documented (Adamit et al., 2015; Levine et al., 2015; Middleton et al., 2014; Park et al., 2015). Unfortunately, the unique contribution made by discreet lesion locations cannot always be extrapolated as many studies report data for right and left hemisphere stroke together. Although EF deficits are not universally present in those with RHD, a significant association between poor inferential reasoning, which requires executive function, and greater difficulty with pragmatic interpretation has been noted (Martin & McDonald, 2006). As described in a previous chapter, many definitions of EF exist, and the components vary. This section will focus on inhibition, mental flexibility (generative or creative thinking), and self-awareness.

Champagne-Lavau and Joanette (2009) found that people with RHD may exhibit different patterns of EF impairment (either a lack of flexibility or a lack of inhibition) and that these impairments co-occur with different patterns of impairments evident on tasks that evaluate nonliteral interpretation. A deficit in inhibition may result in an interpretation of information based on the most salient or most likely content, which in turn suppresses multiple meanings. Similarly, it is postulated that a lack of mental flexibility may prevent activation of multiple or nonliteral interpretations. Impaired mental flexibility and/or inhibition may therefore impact communication ability.

Reduced verbal fluency (letter fluency and category fluency) reflects poor cognitive control related to mental flexibility and set shifting or the ability to move back and forward between different tasks (Mitrushina et al., 2005). People with RHD perform worse than neurologically normal controls on letter fluency tasks (divergent naming) where they must generate as many words as possible that start with a particular letter within a given time (Diggs & Basili, 1987; Hamilton et al., 2017).

Self-awareness can be conceptualized as metacognitive knowledge or self-knowledge, which includes stored knowledge and beliefs about task characteristics and understanding personal strengths and limitations (intellectual awareness), as well as and online awareness of performance, which includes self-appraisal and self-monitoring during a task or situation (emergent awareness) and anticipating future difficulties (anticipatory awareness) (Crosson et al., 1989; Toglia & Goverover, 2022). In people with RHD, metacognitive or general knowledge and online awareness are independent, and there is some evidence that distinct neuroanatomical systems underpin

these types of awareness deficit (Hoerold et al., 2013; Toglia & Chen, 2020). In a group of 44 individuals with RHD, online awareness varied across tasks, was related to the severity of cognitive deficits, and improved through experience with familiar and challenging tasks (Chen & Toglia, 2019).

Many of the conclusions drawn about EF deficits in adults with RHD are extrapolated from these individuals' deficits in visuoperception and complex communication tasks, including discourse and pragmatics. Although it makes sense logically that deficits in inferring communication-based meaning and problem-solving communication breakdowns may be due to more general executive function deficits in reasoning and problem solving, it needs to be explored further.

Memory

Research on verbal memory impairments in RHD are sparse and findings are mixed. A review of studies published between 1966 and 2003 found that 50% of studies on verbal memory impairments reported worse performance by individuals with RHD than control participants most notable on verbal recall (rather than verbal recognition) tasks (Gillespie et al., 2006). The inconsistency of presence of memory impairments should be interpreted in light of the assessment task that was used as the nature of the task is an important factor. The influence of task demands was demonstrated by Titone and colleagues (2001), who found that individuals with RHD obtained comparable results to controls (i.e., successfully recalled more main ideas than minor details of spoken passages) only when passages had highly predictable contexts and were spoken at normal speech rates. In comparison to verbal memory, more consistent evidence is available for visual memory. Individuals with RHD score lower than neurologically typical controls on tests of nonverbal or visual memory (Ferber et al., 2020; Kessels et al., 2002).

Impaired memory has the potential to negatively impact spoken discourse comprehension and reading comprehension. Further research is required to better understand the conditions under which people with RHD exhibit memory impairments, if difficulties are related to task complexity, and if such impairments are related to sites of lesion affecting the right hemisphere.

Social Cognition

One of the theories that has been proposed to explain the nature of communication deficits that arise following RHD is that these individuals have deficits in social cognition (Brownell & Martino, 1998). Social cognition encompasses cognitive processes for social perception, or the ability to interpret social cues; social understanding, which involves the appreciation of other's emotions, beliefs, and intentions; and social decision-making or responses to inferred meaning about others' intentions and emotions (Cassel et al., 2019; McDonald et al., 2013).

Deficits in social cognition are most evident at the interactional level of communication and are therefore often described as being part of, or contributing to, social communication abilities.

Social communication is a term that refers to the abilities that allow people to achieve social goals (Academy of Neurologic Communication Disorders and Sciences Traumatic Brain Injury [ANCDS TBI] Writing Committee, 2020), described as a "many-layered complex behavior composed of social and cognitive-communication skills" (Meulenbroek et al., 2019, p. 129). The underlying tenet of social communication is that communication should be interpreted at the levels of content and relationships, that individuals seek to reach common understanding, that sociocultural rules of communication are important but not sufficient to understand how meaning is created, and that communication is mediated by more than one system, be that verbal or nonverbal (Habermas et al., 1984; Paterno, 2020; Sigman, 1998). Pragmatic language is one of the skills required to be effective in social communication, as are cognitive skills (e.g., EF and ToM) and sociocultural knowledge (refer to ANCDS TBI Writing Committee, 2020, for a summary of social communication models).

Theory of Mind (ToM) is a social cognitive skill that refers to one's ability to understand that another person has ideas, beliefs, feelings, and emotions that differ from one's own (Aboulafia-Brakha et al., 2011; Balaban et al., 2016; Happe et al., 1999; Winner et al., 1998). Deficits affecting ToM can cause problems with interpretation of sarcasm or irony, recognizing social faux pas, and some aspects of language production, including the use of pronouns and explicit references that depend on consideration of what a listener knows to avoid ambiguity (Balaban et al., 2016).

ToM is thought to be controlled by a "mentalizing network" of regions in both right and left hemispheres that control understanding others' ideas and beliefs (cognitive ToM), as well as understanding others' feelings and emotions (affective ToM) (Hillis & Tippett, 2014; Shamay-Tsoory et al., 2003). A functional interdependence and overlap in brain networks involved in EF and ToM are noted. Performance on ToM tasks correlates strongly with aspects of EF in the presence of diffuse brain injury while a dissociation has also been reported when considering localized lesions (Aboulafia-Brakha et al., 2011; Rowe et al., 2001; Shamay-Tsoory et al., 2003). The exact relationship between difficulties in interpreting others' thoughts and feelings and impaired cognition, including EF, continues to be evaluated. The right hemisphere has a crucial role in supporting ToM ability even when controlling for the presence of other cognitive and perceptual factors that might influence the ability to attribute mental states (Hamilton et al., 2017).

Social cognition also encompasses cognitive processes for social perception, or the ability to interpret social cues. Emotion expression through facial expressions is one example of a social cue. A difficulty both producing and interpreting facial emotions may occur after RHD (Abbott et al., 2014; Blonder et al., 2005), which is discussed in more detail in the extralinguistic section to follow. Impairments in affect recognition from facial expressions in those with RHD have been found to relate to social participation and relationship satisfaction (Borod et al., 2002; Hewetson et al., 2021; O'Connell et al., 2021). Social cognition is considered essential to successful interpersonal interaction (McDonald et al., 2013) and warrants

evaluation in people with RHD, alongside assessment of attention, EF, and linguistic and paralinguistic components of communication.

Communication difficulties post-RHD are most evident during complex communication tasks and likely due to an interplay between communication, neurocognitive (e.g., attention and EF), and social cognition impairments. The unique contribution, co-occurrence, and interplay between these three domains remain an ongoing area of inquiry.

Communication

The ability to communicate effectively and efficiently after RHD can be affected by damage to the motor system, leading to a diagnosis of dysarthria or, as is the focus of this chapter, by changes in cognitive and/or communication abilities inclusive of deficits in linguistic (word and syntax), paralinguistic (vocal communication), and extralinguistic (nonverbal communication) skills. While the overall clinical presentation of people with RHD might represent a cognitive communication disorder, the term apragmatism focuses specifically on the communication-specific components of the disorder (see Figure 4–1). That is, apragmatism is characterized by changes in a person's ability to comprehend and/or produce meaning within the context of communicative interactions due to deficits in one or multiple areas of pragmatic language (linguistic, paralinguistic, or extralinguistic) (Minga et al., 2023). The situational nature of the changes of communication is integral to our understanding of the disorders reminding us to consider that a person with RHD's communication may be influenced by the context in which it occurs. As shown in Figure 4–1, the way we communicate is influenced by the interactional goal, the conversational partner(s), the environment (e.g., familiar vs. unfamiliar, quiet vs. busy), and sociocultural considerations.

Linguistics

Linguistic impairments arising after RHD can broadly be characterized as occurring within the areas of semantics (lexical and structural) and discourse (e.g., storytelling and conversation), resulting in a reduced ability to comprehend or produce language to achieve the communication goal. While each area of apragmatism can be described in isolation, it is important to note that the components can be interdependent, whereby conveying or comprehending the meaning of a message relies on integration of linguistic, paralinguistic, and extralinguistic elements (Minga et al., 2023).

Comprehension

Historically, discussions of comprehension impairments at the linguistic level with RHD have been strongly associated with difficulty in interpreting nonliteral language. Deficits have been reported in comprehension of metaphors, similes, idioms, and indirect questions (e.g., Can you tell me the time?). Nonliteral phrases have both a literal meaning and the intended nonliteral meaning. In the example of the indirect question above, a literal interpretation of the question would require a yes/no answer (e.g., "Yes, I am able

to tell you the time"). However, the intended meaning typically is "Would you tell me what time it is?" Typically, the listener would use contextual information to determine the likely intended meaning to make an appropriate response. For example, an adult talking with a 5-year-old child who has been learning to tell the time might use the question to check on their progress of learning this skill (literal meaning), while when a stranger stops you on the sidewalk to ask the same question, the intended meaning is likely to be the nonliteral form.

Moving beyond linguistic comprehension of literal and nonliteral interpretations at the phrase or sentence level is the ability to make inferences within discourse. Discourse can broadly be defined as two or more connected sentences and relies on appropriate links (explicit or implicit) between sentences or ideas and integration of information across sentences (Van Dijk, 2011). An inference is made when information that is not explicitly stated is inferred from the context. There are different types of inferences, categorized by the type of information to be inferred and the amount of time and/or mental resources needed to make the inference. Local or "bridging" coherence is a linguistic mechanism that links adjacent sentences to make a coherent story. This includes the use of linking pronouns to their proper antecedents. For example, in the text, "Sandy held Francis's hand as they crossed the street. She and her son were going to the playground." Bridging inferences are needed to link "she" to "Sandy" and "son" to "Francis." These are considered bridging inferences because they are necessary to link (or bridge) the two sentences together. Bridging inferences are generated quickly by healthy young adults, older adults, and adults with RHD and reliant on limited cognitive resourcing (Graesser et al., 1994; Kiefer, 1993; McKoon & Ratcliff, 1992).

Another mechanism that can assist in comprehension of meaning across sentences is an elaborative inference whereby a conclusion can be reached through drawing on additional information provided or drawing on shared world knowledge. These inferences are not necessary for comprehension but can enhance one's interpretation and may speed up processing of future information (Garrod et al., 1990; Matsuki et al., 2011). In the example above, one would not need to infer that Francis is a child. However, this elaboration may be made based on other clues in the story (e.g., he was holding his mother's hand and they were going to a playground) and integration of this information with one's world knowledge: It would be unusual for a grown man to hold his mother's hand or go to a playground with his mother. Another type of elaborative inference is a predictive inference, in which the recipient of the message predicts what will happen next. One might predict that Francis will use the swing or slide at the playground. Again, these inferences are not necessary to comprehend the short discourse. But if the story continues, "Francis first ran to the slide. He climbed up the ladder and slid down, landing with a bump," the listener processes this information more quickly if it matched their prediction.

Generation of inferences requires use of contextual cues. There has been controversy in the literature regarding whether adults with RHD can use con-

text. Some work indicates that they are unable to use context to generate some types of inferences (Beeman, 1998; Hough, 1990; Rehak et al., 1992). Other work indicates that the use of context is relatively preserved (Blake & Lesniewicz, 2005; Blake et al., 2015; Brownell et al., 1986; Lehman-Blake & Tompkins, 2001; Leonard et al., 1997; Tompkins & Scott, 2013). The truth likely lies somewhere in between: It is not an all-or-none deficit, and further research is needed to determine the conditions under which difficulties are minimized. The long-standing description of difficulties with inferencing and nonliteral language has depicted adults with RHD as overly literal and incapable of appreciating nonliteral meanings or information that is not explicitly stated. Recent research, along with careful examination of older reports, indicates that this conclusion is not tenable. In fact, adults with RHD can make inferences. Myers (1999) provides examples of generation of inferences. One task was to describe Norman Rockwell's *Waiting Room* picture. The picture shows three men and a boy all looking in the same direction, consternation on some faces, and a bandage on one man's head. Responses included comments such as, "they're sitting in a pew at church," "they've returned home from war," and "they're watching a movie." All these responses involve inferences about what is portrayed in the picture. However, none of them integrate all available cues to arrive at the most **appropriate interpretation**: that they are in a doctor's waiting room.

The alibility to integrate multiple cues and to be able to revise an initial interpretation appears to be one source of the difficulties underlying nonliteral language and inferencing, not the generation of inferences per se. In a study by Blake and Lesniewicz (2005), both individuals with RHD and adults without brain damage were found to be able to generate predictive inferences when reading stories where the stimuli were highly predictable. Differences between the two groups, however, were noted in terms of certainty of inference and generation of additional outcomes. Adults without brain damage generated the anticipated outcome without additional solution, while in contrast, those with RHD identified multiple outcomes, including the target. A second component is the ability to revise initial interpretations based on new information. Research has demonstrated that adults with RHD can have difficulties when they must change an initial interpretation (Brownell et al., 1986; Tompkins et al., 1994). A classic example is, "Barbara grew tired of the history book. She had already spent 5 years writing it." After reading only the first sentence, most might conclude that Barbara was reading the book. The second sentence changes that interpretation, from reading to writing the book. Adults with RHD can revise an initial interpretation, but it takes longer for them to do than adults without brain damage (Tompkins et al., 1994). The cost of taking time to revise the interpretation may lead to more general comprehension problems. If this story occurred within a conversation, listeners may lose track of what is said next if they are slow to revise their initial interpretation. Alternatively, if they continue to process new incoming information and do not take the time to make the revision, they may continue to think that Barbara was reading the book, which again would cause general comprehension problems.

Adults with RHD have been reported to have difficulty appreciating humor (Cheang & Pell, 2006; Shammi & Stuss, 1999; Winner et al., 1998). Humor often relies on revising interpretations. Consider the joke, "When she was 65, my grandmother started walking two miles a day. Now she's 71 and we have no idea where she is." To appreciate the humor, listeners must revise their interpretation of "walking two miles a day" from someone returning home each day after a walk to someone walking away, two miles at a time, resulting in being thousands of miles away. Individuals with RHD again may have difficulty with this reinterpretation process, resulting in confusion and lack of appreciation of the humorous intent.

A brief review of models of comprehension is needed to help explain the difficulties described above. Several models propose a two-stage comprehension process (Gernsbacher, 1990; McKoon & Ratcliff, 1992). The first is an activation or construction phase, which is context free. Multiple meanings and ideas are generated. When one hears the word "spring," for example, a variety of meanings and features are generated. These might include a season, flowers blooming, a wire coil, a mattress, and a small creek. The second phase is an integration phase, in which meanings are integrated into a context. Irrelevant or less important meanings are pruned away, or suppressed, to focus the interpretation of the material. If the word appeared in the sentence, "He went fishing in the spring," one would quickly suppress the "coil" meaning of the word but may keep the "season" and the "water" meanings activated, waiting for more information to help resolve the ambiguity. If the sentence is followed by, "There were more fish there than in the polluted pond," then one would suppress the "season" meaning based on the contextual bias toward the "water" meaning. Within a two-stage comprehension framework, most evidence suggests that RHD comprehension deficits occur primarily at the integration stage. These individuals generally can generate meanings and inferences (even multiple meanings) but have difficulty with integrating information to select the most appropriate interpretation. Some research indicates that some deficits may occur in the construction phase, particularly in activating and sustaining activation of distantly related meanings (Beeman et al., 2000; Bouaffre & Faita-Ainseba, 2007; Tompkins et al., 2008).

Production

Discourse production refers to the content and organization of verbal output, whereas pragmatics refers to the use of language in communicative interactions. Linguistic breakdown at the level of discourse production is commonly associated with RHD with impairments observed across the areas of meaning, appropriateness of content for context, cohesion or organization, or efficiency of production. Unlike aphasia, which arises due to left hemisphere damage, linguistic skills at the phonological, morphological, and/or syntactic levels are relatively spared after RHD, but deficits in semantic abilities (lexical and structural) have been reported frequently (Davis et al., 1997; Ferré & Joanette, 2016). The centrality of semantics to the communication disorder associated with RHD was evident in early descriptions that individuals were ineffective or inefficient in conveying their message, typified by discourse

that was concrete or literal in meaning (Myers, 1979).

The theories of semantic processing such as the coarse coding (Beeman, 1998) and suppression deficit hypothesis (Tompkins et al., 2000) explored with reference to linguistic comprehension are likely to also influence how meaning is created during discourse production. Semantics as a branch of linguistics studies how meaning is created at the word level (lexical-semantics) and the sentence level (structural semantics). Deficits in lexical-semantics have been identified when comparing those with RHD to non-brain-damaged adults on both convergent and divergent naming tasks (Adamovich & Brookes, 1981; Diggs & Basili, 1987; Gainotti et al., 1983) with abstract meaning more difficult to generate (Eisenson, 1962). The only link between these findings and vocabulary use at the discourse level related to emotional content, with people with RHD less likely to include emotional content (Bloom et al., 1983). Meaning conveyed at the sentence level goes beyond the string of lexical items (words) connected to how the structural units (i.e., phrase, clauses) are arranged. Phrases and clauses are the message units within the sentence and while people with RHD do not experience difficulty in creating syntactically correct sentences, there is evidence of a reduced number of message units being produced (Diggs & Basili, 1987). This reduction is greater for discourse produced in response to abstract rather than concrete stimuli.

Discourse production after RHD has been more extensively studied above the level of semantics examining the areas of appropriateness, cohesion, and efficiency. Research to date has used a variety of tasks, including story retell, picture description, procedural discourse, personal narrative, and conversation. Each of these tasks represents a different communicative context and/or goal, which along with other influencing factors (see Figure 4–1) can result in different patterns of discourse production. The heterogeneity seen both across the RHD population and within an individual likely result from these interactions, and despite early work to identify discourse profiles, these have not been extensively used in research or clinical practice. Hillis Trupe and Hillis (1985) identified five patterns of discourse production based on the appropriateness of content and efficiency of production, while more recently, Blake and colleagues (2002) proposed two patterns also linked to the appropriateness and efficiency of production: hyperresponsive and hyporesponsive. Furthermore, three of the four clinical communication profiles identified by Ferré and Joanette (2016) include deficits in narrative and/or conversational discourse production.

Achieving a communication goal through appropriate discourse production is grounded in context and how the content conveying meaning is organized. Discourse tasks that have been used to evaluate communication impairment after RHD represent different genre structures with different communicative purposes that must be considered when determining the appropriateness of discourse production. Speaker knowledge of the tasks' goal allows us to structure or organize our verbal output and use interactional structures (e.g., providing or taking turns) to be considered appropriate for the context. In addition, appropriate discourse production requires us to include meaningful content relevant to the topic. Each of these features has been reported as areas of difficulty for people with RHD (Chantraine et al., 1998; Garcia et al., 2021).

Achieving a communication goal through appropriate discourse production is grounded in context and how the content is organized. A review of the literature is unable to provide definitive statements about the appropriateness of discourse produced by the RHD population, but descriptors such tangential, disorganized, and/or egocentric are often used to describe the discourse of some people with RHD (Brady et al., 2006; Chantraine et al., 1998; Kennedy, 2000; Marini et al., 2005). These characteristics refer to a problem with coherence, which refers to how a story fits together as a whole: whether all the pieces are relevant and appropriately tied together to achieve the communicative goal. The greater constraints around structure and topics to be included in procedural, descriptive, and narrative discourse have been proposed as an explanation as to the relative absence of literature identifying problems with coherence in these genres (Brady et al., 2005). Of importance, however, is when taking a closer look at how coherence is maintained, people with RHD use different strategies to non-brain-damaged adults. Examples include use of fewer utterances per topic or statements about the task or task performance (Brady et al., 2003; Kim et al., 2022). In a structured conversation task, Brady and colleagues (2003) also reported that adults with RHD did not clearly demarcate between main topics and subtopics, but rather each piece of information was given equal importance. This causes confusion to listeners, who have difficulty discerning the main points from the asides. Adults with RHD may have difficulty staying on topic, being whisked away by tangential thoughts and details that are elaborated upon. Poor coherence may contribute to confusion over the intent of the discourse. Listeners may walk away from a conversation with someone with RHD, wondering what the point was. Research has, however, again highlighted the heterogeneity of the RHD population, with coherence not an issue for all individuals during conversation. Studies have indicated that between 25% and 40% of people with RHD have difficulty with topic maintenance through inclusion of off-topic or misplaced content (Kennedy, 2000).

The content of discourse produced by adults with RHD may not always be appropriate even where topic maintenance is achieved. They may be egocentric in their discourse through overpersonalizing their verbal output (Chantraine et al., 1988; Kim et al., 2022; Mackenzie et al., 1999; Wapner et al., 1981). This may be expressed as a personal comment or antidote (Brady et al., 2003; Kim et al., 2022) or personally sensitive topics that are inappropriate to the context (Kim et al., 2022).

As mentioned previously, to understand the problems people with RHD experience at the level of discourse production, a range of tasks across different genres have been used. Each of these has conventions that underpin and determine what is appropriate or not to include. The inability to follow these conventions can lead to confusion for the recipient of the message. Societal conventions are particularly evident in how we structure a narrative or inter-

act with others in conversation, but for procedural and descriptive discourse, individual task instructions guide the speaker as to expectations rather than societal conventions (Marini et al., 2005). Narrative and conversational discourse each have three key structural elements. An effective narrative is usually structured by beginning with the setting, moving to the complicating event, and then providing a resolution. In studies of story generation, people with RHD appear able to set the scene for their story, but varying results have emerged indicating difficulties in including the complicating event (Joanette et al., 1986), the resolution, or both the complicating event and resolution (Sherratt & Penn, 1990). As with narrative discourse, people with RHD have been found to include the initiation (greeting) phase of a conversation, whereas topic maintenance and termination phases are different (Kennedy, 2000). In particular, non-brain-damaged adults spend more time in topic maintenance than termination of the conversation than those with RHD who, in contrast, produce equal amounts of content in these two phases. This may influence how a conversational partner feels about the success or naturalness of the interaction. Contributing to these changes in conversational abilities for people with RHD may be difficulty identifying and/or interpreting interactional structures or cues. These interactional structures or cues can be linguistic (e.g., use of affirmative words to seek elaboration), paralinguistic (e.g., raising intonation to signal a question and turn change), or extralinguistic (e.g., head nod to encourage sharing of additional information).

The structural elements presented to date focus on how discourse production conveys the general message or gist, but also important to supporting clarity of discourse is its cohesiveness. This is achieved when a speaker makes effective and accurate connections between sentences. A range of different referents can be used to achieve cohesion, including conjunctions (and, but), pronouns (she, they), and lexical items (the dog) (Stockbridge et al., 2021). Research has shown that discourse produced by those with RHD may not always be cohesive, such that individual sentences are not clearly tied together. They may use ambiguous pronouns (e.g., John and Alex went to the store because he needed some milk), leaving the communication partner confused about who did what. There are varying reports about the nature of the difficulties with cohesion found in people with RHD, which may depend on the method of discourse elicitation. One study found significantly more cohesive errors in people with RHD during a story retell task when compared to adults without brain damage, but not on a narrative discourse using picture stimuli (Davis et al., 1997). Another study has suggested that the number of cohesive ties used is like other adults, but there is overuse of lexical markers of cohesion (Stockbridge et al., 2021), which may result in the listener feeling like the speaker has provided exces-sive detail.

Earlier it was mentioned that the discourse profiles of people with RHD have been associated with not only the appropriateness of content but also the efficiency of production with broadly two patterns: hyperresponsive and hyporesponsive (Blake et al., 2002). Some adults may exhibit verbosity in which they talk more than is socially acceptable (Hillis Trupe & Hillis, 1985; Mackisack et al., 1987). Those with verbosity may talk a lot but not convey much information. Their productions can lack informativeness. For example, they may assume that the listener knows what they do and not provide adequate background information. Alternatively, they may give too much information, including information that is not appropriate for the situation. Others may have paucity of speech, in which they say very little (Mackenzie et al., 1997). Verbosity and paucity of spoken output appear to be diagnosed with similar frequency in people with RHD (Blake et al., 2002).

Paralinguistics

Prosodic contours are used in spoken output to express meaning and emotions beyond that which is conveyed by words and sentences themselves, and this manipulation falls within the field of paralinguistics. The term aprosodia is used to describe deficits in the comprehension and production of prosody and is associated with RHD (Ross, 1981). Speakers manipulate prosodic contours through varying their volume, pitch, rate, and rhythm of speech to alter the meaning of utterance for grammatical, pragmatic, and emotional purposes (Minga et al., 2023). Grammatical prosody aids in segmenting clauses and differentiating word and sentence types, such as questions and statements (Peppé, 2009), while pragmatic prosody draws attention to specific information through emphasis to focus the listener or contrast with previous information, or alternatively signal handing over the "turn" to the listener. Emotional, also known as affective prosody, is used by speakers to convey their attitude, mood, and emotions.

In the RHD research, grammatical and pragmatic subtypes are commonly grouped together under the label **linguistic prosody**. Some reports suggest that linguistic prosody is controlled primarily by the left hemisphere, although other work suggests it is controlled bilaterally, or primarily by the right hemisphere (Baum & Pell, 1999; Walker et al., 2002; Walker et al., 2004). A recent systematic review and meta-analysis of aprosodia after RHD concluded that the comprehension of linguistic prosody at the word and phrase level is unaffected, but the ability to interpret prosodic features that convey meaning in speech acts (e.g., intonation pattern that indicates a question is being asked) was impaired (Stockbridge et al., 2022). Clinically, therefore, we need to ensure that comprehension of linguistic prosody is included as part of our assessment plan.

Emotional or affective prosody involves the use of intonation patterns to portray our mood, attitudes, or emotion beyond simply the meaning of the words (e.g., "I hate it when I do that," spoken in an off-handed or joking manner vs. the same statement proclaimed with anger). The recent systematic review by Stockbridge and colleagues (2022) confirmed what has long been proposed, a link between the right hemisphere and the comprehension and production of emotional prosody (Baum & Pell, 1999; Ethofer et al., 2006; Kotz et al., 2013; Walker et al., 2002; Wildgruber et al., 2009; Witteman et al., 2011). This conclusion is not surprising given that the right frontal, temporal, and anterior insula cortices alongside

subcortical structures such as the amygdala, basal ganglia, and thalamus have been identified as key neural correlates of emotional processing for some time (Blake & Hoepner, 2021).

Receptive emotional aprosodia involves difficulty interpreting mood or emotion expressed through prosodic features such a pitch or volume. This can affect identification of emotion (e.g., anger vs. disgust vs. surprise) but also the differentiation of strength of emotion (Pell, 2006). Some adults with aprosodia have difficulty interpreting attitude or intent, such as determining whether someone is conveying confidence or politeness through prosody (Pell, 2007). Recent neuroimaging research used a stroke population with RHD to confirm the damage to the right hemisphere posterolateral (ventral) stream; in particular, the superior temporal gyrus is associated with emotional prosody comprehension deficits (Sheppard et al., 2020). Extending on this work, Sheppard et al. (2021) explored different stages in the processing of the acoustic signals associated with emotion, their neural correlates, and potential patient clusters. Results indicated three subgroups of people with receptive aprosodia after RHD. The first subgroup had the mildest receptive emotional aprosodia, presenting primarily with frontotemporal lesions and difficulty with matching prosodic features to emotions. A second cluster presented with more severe receptive emotional aprosodia than the first group and had the most trouble on the task, requiring them to acoustically discriminate between tones. The sites of lesion most seen in this group were primarily posterior or thalamic. The final group presented with the most severe receptive aprosodia for emotions and had predominantly subcortical lesions, with the caudate a key structure.

Expressive emotional aprosodia is characterized by difficulty producing prosodic contours to convey mood, attitudes, or emotion. Speech produced by an individual with expressive aprosodia may be perceived to sound monotone or flat, that is, with limited inflection. Confirmation that the comprehension and production of emotional prosody is impaired in people with RHD was achieved through the recent meta-analysis (Stockbridge et al., 2021). Drawing on the findings of 47 peer-reviewed publications, the review identified that people with RHD have trouble using prosodic contours to understand the emotional content of a speaker's message. Additionally, people with RHD are unable to accurately signal emotional or affective meaning through the manipulation of prosodic markers associated with emotions. The neural network associated with expressive emotional aprosodia is frequently associated with a frontal lesion in the inferior frontal lobe and dorsal white matter tracts (Blake & Hoepner, 2021; Durfee, Sheppard, Blake, et al., 2021). Dorsal white matter structures such as the corona radiata, internal capsule, and superior longitudinal fasciculus have been linked to expressive emotional aprosodia, as have regions such as the insula, anterior-inferior parietal lobe, and anterior temporal lobe. Key regions of the right hemisphere linked to receptive and expressive emotional aprosodia are highlighted in Figure 4–3. The dorsal and ventral streams in the RH associated with aprosodia mirror those of the dual-stream language processing networks (Durfee, Sheppard, Blake, et al., 2021). The dorsal stream

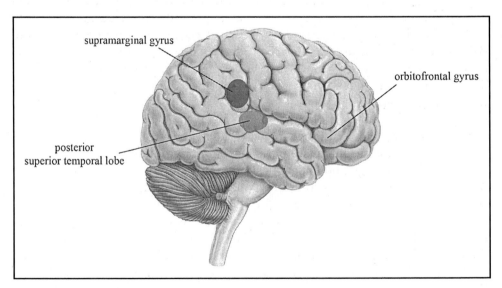

Figure 4–3. Right hemisphere regions involved in emotional prosody. From *Clinical Neuroscience for Communication Disorders: Neuroanatomy and Neurophysiology* (p. 250) by Lehman Blake, M., and Hoepner, J.K. Copyright © 2023 Plural Publishing, Inc. All rights reserved. Used with permission.

incorporates the orbitofrontal gyrus, supramarginal gyrus, and underlying white matter of the superior longitudinal fasciculus and is associated with expressive emotional aprosodia, while the ventral stream, which is linked to receptive emotional aprosodia, involves the posterior superior temporal lobe.

The impact and prevalence of aprosodia following RHD is unclear, with estimates of 20% to 80% (Blake et al., 2002; Dara et al., 2014). Communication partners of people with RHD rate prosodic deficits as being of equal significance to physical impairments such as left-sided hemiparesis (Hillis & Tippett, 2014). This finding is different from reports of functional outcomes following traumatic brain injury, where the ability to recognize emotion was not strongly correlated with outcomes (Milders et al., 2003; Osborne-Crowley & McDonald, 2016; Saxton et al., 2013).

Extralinguistics

As was highlighted in Figure 4–1, successful communication draws on three sets of skills; linguistic, paralinguistic, and extralinguistic and deficits in any or multiple sets of skills can lead to a diagnosis of apragmatism within the broader diagnosis of cognitive communication disorder for people with RHD. So far, details of linguistic and paralinguistic skills and deficits that arise after RHD have been explored, and now we consider what are extralinguistic skills and how are they impacted. The aspects of communication considered to be extralinguistic are nonverbal, including body language and proxemics, facial expression, eye contact, and gestures (Minga et al.,

2023). In people with RHD, again there is the potential for deficits to arise due to inefficient, ineffective, or inappropriate comprehension or use of nonverbal cues. Determination of what constitutes an impairment in extralinguistic skills varies based on the communication context, including the environment, communication partner(s), and sociocultural norms. These contextual factors should always be considered when evaluating whether an individual with RHD presents with extralinguistic deficits or not and in some cases may require seeking additional information from family and friends to understand preexisting skills and/or cultural norms.

People with RHD are frequently identified as presenting with nonverbal communication impairments that are persistent. In a longitudinal study of people with right hemisphere stroke, Mackenzie and colleagues (1997) found that nearly three quarters of participants were impaired in their use of facial expression and eye contact at 3 months poststroke with limited recovery at 12 months as two thirds had persistent impairments in use of facial expression and eye contact. Furthermore, people with RHD have been found to be less likely to convey emotion through facial expression, including smiling less than people with LHD (Blonder et al., 2005). This use of limited facial expression has also been shown to occur with limited use of emotional prosody; together, these can result in the person being described as presenting with a flat affect (Minga et al., 2023). Difficulty interpreting the facial emotions of others has been reported after RHD (Abbott et al., 2014; Kucharska-Pietura et al., 2004). People with RHD have been found to be less accurate in perceiving both positive and negative facial expressions (Gainotti, 2012). Although bilateral neural networks are involved in face perception (Nakamura et al., 2014), the right hemisphere may have a particular role in the processing of emotional information in faces.

Gestures as a form of communication are often used in conjunction with other extralinguistic, linguistic, and paralinguistic skills to enhance communication (Kelly et al., 1999). There is limited research about gesture interpretation and use in people with RHD, but there are a few studies that suggest that use of gestures may be impaired in some people with RHD (Cocks et al., 2007; Parola et al., 2016). There is some evidence that people with RHD may increase their use of inappropriate gestures during conversation such a grooming or scratching themselves (Cocks et al., 2007), while reduced gesture use was noted in relation to iconic gestures that supplement their message (Goksun et al., 2013) or when conveying emotional content (Cocks et al., 2007). Visual neglect or other visuoperceptual deficits may impact the interpretation or production of gestures, but poor performance cannot solely be accounted for based on the visuospatial skills present in most cases. Overall, it is important to acknowledge that impaired extralinguistic abilities after RHD like other aspects of apragmatism have the potential to negatively impact relationships. Studies have found an association between impaired ability to interpret facial emotions and other nonverbal cues on interpersonal relationships, particularly spousal and family relationships (Blonder et al., 2012; Hewetson et al., 2021).

Other Impairments

Individuals with right hemisphere damage have been shown to present with other impairments that may interact with or influence performance on cognitive and/or communication skills. Hemianopia, hemiplegia, and somatosensory deficits have all been noted as impairments present after RHD (Sterzi et al., 1993). Hemianopia is the term used to describe the loss of sight in one half of a person's visual field resulting from brain damage and is seen more commonly after RHD (18%) than LHD (7%). Somatosensory deficits are quite common after RHD, with approximately 40% experiencing a reduced ability to sense the body's position in space (proprioception) and 57% unable to feel pain (hemianesthesia). Hemiplegia or hemiparesis (paralysis or weakness on one side of the body) has been reported to occur in 95% of people with RHD. Cognitive impairments, including neglect and anosognosia (see following section for description), have been proposed as influencing or interacting with hemianopia, hemiplegia, and somatosensory deficits that influence rehabilitation outcome for those with RHD (Katz et al., 2000; Sterzi et al., 1993).

Anosognosia

Impaired self-awareness, seen in reduced appraisal, prediction, and regulation of performance during tasks and situations, fits within the scope of executive function, that is, mental processes that enable us to plan, appraise, and self-regulate. Individuals with impaired self-awareness may be aware of stroke-related impairments but may find it difficult to monitor for moments where impairments negatively impact a task or not be able to avoid the difficulty before it occurs (e.g., someone might have an intellectual understanding that they have aprosodia that impacts how they are perceived by others but may not be able to change their intonation patterns in the moment).

Anosognosia refers to a lack of awareness of some or all motor, sensory, perceptual, or cognitive impairments that occur following brain injury, as well as reduced insight as to the consequences of these impairments (Prigatano, 2010; Starkstein et al., 2010). Historically, anosognosia was a diagnostic term for unawareness of poststroke hemiplegia, which was extended to anosognosia for hemianopsia and more recently anosognosia for cognitive and language impairments and even unawareness of behavioral changes such as irritability and self-centeredness (Bisiach et al., 1986; Prigatano, 2010; Starkstein et al., 1996). A variety of theories have been proposed to explain the reduced awareness of deficits, including a relatively general deficit in cognition, an impairment in encoding new sensorimotor memories into long-term memory, and an interruption in a feed-forward process that sends sensory information forward to frontal motor systems for comparisons between anticipated actions and actual performance (for reviews, see Blake, 2018; Orfei et al., 2007).

Reduced awareness of deficits and their consequences is considered a hallmark of RHD, and evidence as to a RH bias in anosognosia is substantial (Morin, 2016). Estimates of prevalence range from 7% to 77% in individuals with unilateral strokes (Orfei et

al., 2007). The variability may be due to spontaneous recovery and the time point of evaluation or different sensitivities of assessment measures. Adults with RHD may have reduced awareness of cognitive, communication, and physical impairments and may not have a good awareness of the consequences of their deficits (e.g., accepting that they cannot drive because they have UN). When individuals with RHD report that they have deficits but do not seem to be overly bothered by them, then the term anosodiaphoria, meaning reduced concern about deficits, might be applied (Barrett et al., 2006; Orfei et al., 2007). Anosognosia also frequently co-occurs with neglect, noted in almost a quarter of 98 individuals with RH stroke (Dai et al., 2014).

The terms "denial" and "denial of deficits" frequently are used in relation to anosognosia following RHD, but these terms should be used with caution. Denial is considered a psychological issue, in which a patient is aware of a deficit on some level and fails to accept its existence either consciously or unconsciously. Differences in responses to feedback have been documented for individuals with psychological denial versus anosognosia or lack of awareness of deficits (Giacino & Cicerone, 1998; Prigatano, 2010). Individuals with denial may show resistance or anger to feedback about their deficits, while those with anosognosia are surprised or perplexed when shown their performance deficiencies.

Anosognosia has important consequences for interpretation of patient-reported questionnaires and for treatment. Overestimation of performance and function by individuals with RHD occurs often, 63% to 68% (McKay et al., 2011; Hewetson et al., 2018). Individuals who are not aware of their deficits or the consequences of those deficits are not as likely to actively participate in therapy and often have poorer outcomes (Jehkonen et al., 2001; Katz et al., 2000; Vossel et al., 2013).

Assessment

Assessment planning should be guided by a clear understanding of the full range of cognitive and communication changes that may occur following RHD and that heterogeneity of presenting impairments is expected. A second key consideration is that difficulties might be most evident within contexts that require integration of information or that are considered more complex in nature (e.g., a group conversation in a noisy environment vs. a one-on-one conversation with a SLP in a quiet clinic room). Not only should assessment include evaluation of cognition and communication, but standardized tools should also be supplemented with ecologically valid assessment tasks that replicate everyday communication. Observation of conversations with familiar and unfamiliar people, and observing the client in other settings, such as in a physical therapy gym, can provide valuable insights into how context influences communication. Lastly, we should analyze assessment findings considering an individual's age, educational attainment, linguistic and cultural background, and preinjury communication style.

Assessment of adults with RHD and diagnosis of cognitive and communication deficits can be challenging for several reasons. First, screening processes and tools used in acute care settings may not be able to detect mild cognitive communication disorders. While signs of a mild aphasia may be readily observed (e.g., word-retrieval difficulties), mild changes associated with RHD affecting discourse, pragmatics, prosody, executive function skills, and memory may not be evident from informal observation or brief screening assessments. Communication and cognition changes due to RHD may be underdiagnosed and those with mild impairments are at risk of premature discharge from hospital and restricted access to ongoing rehabilitation services (Hewetson et al., 2017). Second, there are few measures with strong psychometric properties (validity and reliability) that have been developed specifically for this population. Clinicians often use a variety of cognitive assessments that were developed primarily for adults with TBI given similarities in the types of cognitive impairments that might occur in RHD. There are also few comprehensive assessments that have been developed for or validated on diagnosing the communication deficits associated with RHD. Additionally, although profiles of communication impairments have been proposed, the exact pattern of co-occurrence of communication domains in addition to impairments in cognition requires further investigation. Sheppard and colleagues (2022) highlighted the need for research that might identify patterns of deficits in their systematic review of the co-occurrence of aprosodia and impairments in cognition. Thus, unlike with aphasia, subtypes of RHD are still being identified, which makes it difficult to extrapolate that if a client has difficulty with X, they will also have difficulty with Y, but Z will be preserved. Lastly, in the general population, there is a broad range of what is considered "normal" within the areas of cognition and communication affected by RHD; hence, it is difficult to set a solid cutoff to diagnose deficits.

To accurately diagnose an acquired communication impairment, especially apragmatism, the clinician should obtain information about preinjury communication style to ensure that what is being observed is not merely a communication difference, which could be related to personality or cultural preferences. For example, use of eye contact, the amount of personal sharing that is considered appropriate, and the use of direct versus indirect statements all can vary across cultures. Given the wide range of communicative behaviors seen in the general population, it is important to find out what behaviors are different from the client's preinjury state. Talking with family or close friends is thus essential for accurate diagnosis of pragmatic and other communication deficits. Speech-language pathologists, due to our in-depth knowledge of communication, may overdiagnose deficits when we see behaviors that appear inappropriate when family members report that the behaviors have not changed following the stroke (Baron et al., 1999). One study found that SLPs who were experienced in assessment and treatment of neurogenic communication disorders had distinct biases in judging discourse of healthy older adults versus discourse of individuals with RHD (Blake, 2006). Only a third of the clinicians accurately judged which samples belonged to healthy older adults versus those with RHD. This is a concerning finding as current speech-language pathology practice for this population often relies on clinician observation and use of informal assessment tasks, which may not be sensitive or lead to accurate diagnoses (Ramsey & Blake, 2020). Detecting receptive aprosodia, a sensitive indicator of RHD in the acute stroke setting (Dara et al., 2014), may be challenging for speech-language pathologists using observation alone.

Composite Assessment Tools

Several batteries have been designed specifically for RHD, each evaluating a different combination of communication and cognitive abilities. These include the Right Hemisphere Language Battery (RHLB; Bryan, 1994), the Mini Inventory of Right Brain Injury (MIRBI-R; Pimental & Kingsbury, 2000), the Burns Brief Inventory of Communication and Cognition (Burns Inventory; Burns, 1997), the Rehabilitation Institute of Chicago Evaluation Clinical Management of Right Hemisphere Dysfunction–Revised (RICE-3; Halper et al., 2010), and the Montreal Protocol for the Evaluation of Communication (MEC; Joanette et al., 2015).

Most of these batteries have subtests to measure attention; comprehension and/or use of abstract, metaphorical, or inferential language; discourse production and/or comprehension; pragmatics; and prosody or affect. Weaknesses in validity, reliability, and/or scope of many of these and other assessment tools have been identified in a review by Blake (2018). Many older tools were designed to measure symptoms reported in the literature and observed clinically but do not have a strong theoretical basis. Additionally, they may not be sensitive to mild deficits, and many of the subtests for pragmatics and other areas (e.g., prosody, discourse production) rely on subjective judgments. Currently available composite assessment tools for RHD allow description of presentation considering performance on individual subtests in comparison to normative data; however, they do not provide a clear criterion for diagnosis of apragmatism or establishing an overall severity. Some assessment tools designed for clients with TBI, described in other chapters in this book, may also be appropriate for adults with RHD. The reader is referred to reviews of formal (Turkstra et al., 2005) and nonstandardized (Coelho et al., 2005) assessment tools for an overview of possible assessment tools and tasks that may be valuable.

Assessment of Cognition

Attention

To understand the role that attention plays, either causative or contributory, to the communication impairment associated with RHD, it is also important to observe a client's performance during everyday communication tasks. Mark Ylvisaker's hypothesis testing approach to assessment is recommended when considering a client's performance during auditory attention tasks in varied settings, reading and responding to questions on texts that increase in length, and managing two tasks simultaneously such as writing down information provided during a phone conversation (see Coelho et al., 2005). Tests

of attention discussed in other chapters of this book may be appropriate for use with adults with RHD. When selecting a test of attention, it is helpful to consider if the test will support the identification of patterns of attention breakdown across sustained, selective, and divided attention. The Test of Everyday Attention (TEA; Robertson et al., 1994) is an example of a test that not only evaluates different aspects of attention but also uses everyday real-world materials, which increases the ecological validity.

Assessment of **Unilateral Visual Neglect** (UVN) generally involves one or more paper-and-pencil tasks, including line, letter, or shape cancellation tasks; line bisection; and copying and drawing tasks (e.g., clock drawing). The Behavioral Inattention Test (BIT; Wilson et al., 1987) is a standardized measure commonly used for assessing the presence and severity of neglect. In addition to conventional paper-and-pencil tasks (cancellation, line bisection, drawing, and copying tasks), there are subtests representing real-word activities such as reading a menu, dialing a phone number, and identifying items in a picture scene. It has become apparent that this and other standardized assessments are inadequate for several reasons. First, the tasks assess only peripersonal neglect in structured tasks. Arene and Hillis (2007) describe an individual who scored within normal limits on peripersonal neglect tasks but demonstrated difficulty with personal care tasks (personal neglect) and was unable to maneuver through a doorway without hitting the left side of the entrance (extrapersonal neglect). Second, the sensitivity of tasks varies considerably. Reports of sensitivity range from 19% to 100% for commonly used tasks and tests (Barrett et al., 2006). Lindell and colleagues (2007) administered 19 different neglect tests to a group of individuals with RHD. None of the tests, in isolation, identified more than 50% of people with neglect. The most sensitive tests were random shape cancellation, complex line bisection, and star cancellation, which together identified 88% of those with neglect. An additional three tasks (two-part picture, article reading, and finding objects in a pictured scene) had to be added to achieve 100% identification of peripersonal neglect. Representational drawing, such as drawing a clock or a person, was the least sensitive when used alone, identifying only 6% of cases.

Fewer assessment tools are available to diagnose auditory neglect, which has been referred to as the neglected neglect (Gokhale et al., 2013). Clinical bedside assessment of auditory neglect is challenging because of the binaural nature of auditory inputs in a free field context. Auditory neglect and auditory extinction can be detected using auditory tests such as sound localization tests and dichotic listening tasks, where different stimuli are presented through earphones simultaneously. Refer to Gokhale and colleagues (2013) for a summary of auditory tests that may support a diagnosis of auditory neglect. It is also worth noting that two types of auditory neglect, hemispatial inattention and spatial bias in auditory localization, have been proposed for people with RHD (Bellman et al., 2001).

Executive Function

There are no standardized tests of executive function specifically created for adults with RHD. However, the performance of a person with RHD on a general test of executive function can be compared to normative data, which provides valuable insights into executive function abilities. The Functional Assessment of Verbal Reasoning and Executive Strategies (FAVRES) is recommended as an ecologically valid assessment that incorporates real-world tasks such as planning an event, scheduling a workday, and building a case to solve a problem (MacDonald & Johnson, 2005). The FAVRES scores performance based on not just accuracy on a particular task but also the individual's rationale or reason that is provided for their responses and/or prioritization and the time required for completion. Although not designed as a comprehensive assessment of EF, the complexity and novel nature of the tasks elicit aspects of executive functioning (MacDonald & Johnson, 2005). A further example is the Controlled Oral Word Association Test (COWAT; Benton et al., 1983), which is also known as F-A-S or **verbal fluency** with orthographic constraint. COWAT requires executive function skills such as self-monitoring, inhibition, and cognitive flexibility (Golden et al., 2000). Words starting with a particular letter must be generated within a 1-minute period. Results can be analyzed against normative data based on age and educational level (see Tombaugh et al., 1999) and by considering the type of words generated and strategies used to do so. A variety of measures exist to explore **awareness of impairment** and **self-awareness**, including the Awareness Questionnaire (Sherer et al., 2003), the Patient Competency Rating Scale (Borgaro & Prigatano, 2003; Prigatano & Klonoff, 1998), and the Self Awareness of Deficit Interview (Fleming et al., 1996). Most were designed for adults with TBI but may be relevant and appropriate for individuals with RHD. Several include comparisons between responses from patients versus family or professionals (see also Blake, 2018; Orfei et al., 2007).

Memory

Several neuropsychological assessment tools that evaluate cognition include subtests on memory functioning. Frequently used screening tools include the Montreal Cognitive Assessment (MoCA; Nasreddine et al., 2005), Mini Mental State Exam (MMSE; Folstein et al., 1975), Addenbrooke's Cognitive Examination–Revised (ACE-R; Mioshi et al., 2006), and the Cognitive Linguistic Quick Test Plus (CLQT+; Helm-Estabrooks, 2001). When assessing memory, it is worth considering performance across different memory tasks. As examples, the Ross Information Processing Assessment-2 (RIPA-2; Ross-Swain, 1996), Rivermead Behavioural Memory Test–Third Edition (RBMT-3; Wilson et al., 2008), and the Repeated Battery for the Assessment of Neurospychological Status (RBANS; Randolph et al., 1998) consider immediate and delayed recall across verbal and visual memory tasks. In addition to standardized assessments, it is valuable to document the type of errors made on tasks of memory function, awareness of impaired memory, and the impact of memory impairments on communication, for example, the need for information and/or instructions to be repeated.

Social Cognition

The Awareness of Social Inference Test (TASIT; McDonald, Flanagan, & Rollins, 2003) evaluates a person's ability to integrate cues from facial expressions, prosody, gesture, and social contexts to interpret emotions, beliefs, and intentions (ToM). The TASIT consists of a series of video vignettes. A short form (screening version) of this assessment is also available (TASIT-S; Honan et al., 2016), which takes 20 to 30 minutes to administer. Performance of individuals with RHD has been reported in the literature using The Faux Pas Recognition Test (Stone et al., 1998), in which short stories need to be interpreted based on the presence or absence of a faux pas or social blunder, and false belief tasks (see Bomfim et al., 2021, for a review).

Assessment of Communication

Composite assessment tools, as described earlier in this chapter, that have been designed to assess cognitive and/or communication deficits after RHD provide a series of tasks that address primarily the linguistic and paralinguistic deficits characteristic of apragmatism. Evaluation of extralinguistic skills within these composite tools, however, is often restricted to questionnaires or checklists. The emergence of screening tools to identify those people with RHD at risk of cognitive and/or communication deficits may, in the future, allow SLPs to target their assessments to specific areas of concern. The following sections provide guidance on assessment tools and tasks that allow for targeted assessment of linguistic, paralinguistic, and/or extralinguistic skills. Diagnosis of a communication disorder can be specified by the areas affected, such as "apragmatism characterized by linguistic and paralinguistic deficits."

Linguistics

The assessment of linguistic abilities in adults with RHD can be divided into those that assess semantics (lexical or structural) or discourse (comprehension or production). Table 4–2 provides a summary of assessment tools or tasks that, while not designed to be exhaustive, provides options for assessing the linguistic domain of apragmatism.

The composite assessment tools previously outlined have a strong focus on assessing the lexical-semantics through semantic attributes of words, or comprehension of metaphors, and abstract or figurative language. Tasks focused on comprehension at the level of structural semantics is not routinely included in RHD assessment batteries, but subtests from assessment tools designed for diagnosing aphasia can be used if there are concerns about deficits at this level of linguistics (see Table 4–2). A strength of these tasks is the availability of normative data; however, they are not positioned within communicative context and so may not reflect performance beyond the assessment context. Two standardized assessments at the level of discourse comprehension, The Discourse Comprehension (DCT revised; Brookshire & Nicholas, 1997) and The Awareness of Social Inferences Test (TASIT; McDonald, Flanagan, & Rollins, 2003), allow for evaluation of inferred, implied, or abstract meaning. DCT is a measure of reading and auditory comprehension. Stories are 10 to 15 sentences long, and questions target details and main ideas that are either explicitly stated or must be inferred. TASIT consists of video vignettes where two or three actors interact in each scene, and the client

answers questions about the intent of statements conveyed. The two Social Inference subtests include interpretation of social exchanges, including sincere exchanges, white lies, and sarcasm. The test was designed for adults with TBI, and there are few data specific to RHD. It was constructed in Australia, so some individuals may have difficulty with the slight accents and some phrases that are not common in other dialects of English. Both the DCT and TASIT involve answering questions after the stimulus stories, thus creating memory demands that may affect performance.

Traditionally, the assessment of discourse production in people with RHD has been discussed alongside pragmatics due to overlap in the communication components. Assessment of pragmatics incorporates the linguistic, paralinguistic, and extralinguistic components of communication and how they contribute to the outcome of an interaction. As Penn (1999) suggested, when working with people with RHD, clinicians need to not only assess the individual components of communication but do so across different contexts and observe how the individual adapts to achieve communicative success. Divergent naming tasks are frequently included in composite assessment tools, or as part of assessing executive function, but the work by Diggs and Basili (1987) suggested that results from convergent and divergent naming tasks, particularly for more abstract items or tasks, provide value as part of a comprehensive assessment battery. They found that those that had more errors on convergent naming tasks and used fewer strategies to complete divergent naming activities were more likely to provide fewer meaning units carrying

Table 4–2. Overview of Assessment Tools and Tasks for the Evaluation of Linguistic Skills: Comprehension and Production

Areas Known to Be Impaired Post-RHD	Assessment Tools	Norms[a]
SEMANTICS		
Lexical Semantics		
Convergent Naming	Measure of Cognitive-Linguistic Abilities (MCLA; Ellmo, 1995) • Visual confrontation naming	Individuals without brain injury across age and educational bands
	Cognitive Linguistics Quick Test Plus (CLQT+; Helm-Estabrooks, 2017) • Confrontation naming	Norms for individuals without brain injury and aphasia across two age bands (18–69 and 70–89 years)
	Boston Naming Test (BNT; Kaplan et al., 2001)	Version dependent: norms are available for individuals without brain injury and following acquired brain injury
Divergent Naming	Montreal Protocol for the Evaluation of Communication (MEC; Joanette et al., 2015) • Free association, orthographic, semantic	Norms for individuals without brain injury, older adults, TBI RHD, TBI, norms for individuals without brain injury across age (18–90 years) and educational bands
	Measure of Cognitive-Linguistic Abilities (MCLA) • Orthographic, semantic, abstract	Individuals without brain injury across age and educational bands
	Cognitive Linguistics Quick Test Plus (CLQT+) • Generative naming	As above
Semantic attributes	Montreal Protocol for the Evaluation of Communication (MEC) • Semantic judgments	As above
Abstract or figurative language, metaphor	Montreal Protocol for the Evaluation of Communication (MEC) • Speech acts, metaphor interpretation	As above

234

Table 4–2. *continued*

Areas Known to Be Impaired Post-RHD	Assessment Tools	Norms[a]
Abstract or figurative language, metaphor *continued*	Measure of Cognitive-Linguistic Abilities (MCLA) • Verbal reasoning subtest	As above
	Communication Activities of Daily Living, Third Edition (CADL-3; Holland et al., 2018)	Norms for progressive and nonprogressive ABI
	Mini Inventory of Right Brain Injury (MIRBI-2; Pimental & Kingsbury, 2000)	RHD norms, control participants with no neurological injury and left hemisphere damage
	Rehabilitation Institute of Chicago Evaluation of Communication Problems in Right Hemisphere Dysfunction, Third Edition (RICE-3; Halper et al., 2010) • Metaphorical language	Individuals with RHD and no neurological injury
	Burns Brief Inventory of Communication and Cognition (Burns, 1997) • Inferences and metaphor	Right hemisphere inventory, left hemisphere inventory
Structural Semantics	Comprehensive Aphasia Test (CAT; Swinburn et al., 2023) • Sentence comprehension subtest	People with aphasia and individuals without brain injury
	Northwestern Assessment of Verbs and Sentences (NAVS; Thompson, 2011) • Sentence comprehension test	People with aphasia and primary progressive aphasia
DISCOURSE		
Comprehension	Montreal Protocol for the Evaluation of Communication (MEC) • Narrative discourse: comprehension questions	As above
	Discourse comprehension test (DCT; Brookshire & Nicholas, 1997) • Auditory comprehension • Reading comprehension	Stroke, TBI, individuals without brain injury

continues

Table 4–2. *continued*

Areas Known to Be Impaired Post-RHD	Assessment Tools	Norms[a]
Comprehension *continued*	Measure of Cognitive-Linguistic Abilities (MCLA)–paragraph (auditory) comprehension subtest • Functional and paragraph reading	As above
	Test of Awareness of Social Inference Test–Revised (TASIT; McDonald et al., 2003)[b] • Comprehension in social inferencing tests	Norms for adults and adolescents without brain injury and adults with TBI (21–64 years)
Production	Montreal Protocol for the Evaluation of Communication (MEC) • Story retell • Conversational discourse subtest	As above
	Measure of Cognitive-Linguistic Abilities (MCLA) • Spoken procedural, picture description, narrative, and conversation • Written narrative	As above
	Rehabilitation Institute of Chicago Evaluation of Communication Problems in Right Hemisphere Dysfunction, Third Edition (RICE-3)	As above
	RHDBank Protocol • Free speech, conversation, picture description, storytelling, procedural discourse, question asking	Norms under development
	LaTrobe Communication Questionnaire (LCQ; Douglas et al., 2007)	Norms for individuals without brain injury and adults with TBI

Table 4–2. *continued*

Areas Known to Be Impaired Post-RHD	Assessment Tools	Norms[a]
Production continued	Profile of Pragmatic Impairment in Communication (PPIC; Linscott & Knight, 2018)	n/a
	• Literal content	
	• General participation and quantity	
	• Subject matter	
	• Internal relation and external relation	
	• Clarity of expression	

[a]Details of normative data available are only provided for the first mention of an assessment tool. [b]TASIT Social Inferencing tests allow for assessment of linguistic, paralinguistic, and extralinguistic abilities in the same task.

informative content. As summarized in Table 4–2, the composite assessment tools for RHD included discourse production tasks, although not all include multiple discourse elicitation tasks, and only some include spoken and written discourse production. Recently, a group of researchers has initiated the RHDBank (https://rhd.talkbank.org) with a view to increase our understanding of discourse production in people with RHD (see Minga et al., 2021, for an overview). This has resulted in the development of a discourse assessment protocol across varying tasks inclusive of the required materials and resources and ultimately normative data to allow for comparison across individuals.

Paralinguistics

The assessment of aprosodia in people with RHD can be undertaken, as summarized in Table 4–3, through completing subtests within composite assessment tools such as the MEC (Joanette et al., 2015) or the RICE-3 (Halper et al., 2010), or more focused assessments such as the Florida Affect Battery (Bowers et al., 1991) or the Hillis Post-Stroke Prosody Battery (https://score.jhmi.edu/downloads.html; 2023). There is considerable variability in terms of the aprosodia type and type of task used across the assessment tools summarized in Table 4–3. The MEC includes evaluation of both receptive and expressive prosody tasks. Audio-recorded content is used to assess comprehension and repetition of linguistic and emotional meaning at the sentence level, while a final task examines the ability to convey emotional meaning at the sentence level in response to short text providing contextual information. The reliability of these tasks to correctly identify aprosodia is still unclear, but cut criteria are provided based on normative data.

Table 4–3. Overview of Assessment Tools and Tasks for Aprosodia

Assessment Tools	Areas Assessed	Norms
Montreal Protocol for the Evaluation of Communication (MEC)	Receptive aprosodia • Linguistic • Emotional Expressive aprosodia • Linguistic repetition • Emotional repetition • Emotion sentence production	RHD, TBI, norms for individuals without brain injury across age (18–90 years) and educational bands
Burns Brief Inventory of Communication and Cognition	Receptive aprosodia Spontaneous expressive aprosodia	Adults with stroke, TBI, Alzheimer's disease/dementia, small group adults without brain damage (18–80 years)
Measure of Cognitive-Linguistic Abilities (MCLA)	Spontaneous expressive aprosodia	Individuals without brain injury across age and educational bands
Mini Inventory of Right Brain Injury (MIRBI-2)	Expressive aprosodia • Expressing emotion	Adults without brain damage, adults with right or left hemisphere brain damage
Rehabilitation Institute of Chicago Evaluation of Communication Problems in Right Hemisphere Dysfunction, Third Edition (RICE-3)	Expressive aprosodia • Intonation in conversation	n/a
Hillis Post-Stroke Prosody Battery	Receptive aprosodia • Emotion recognition nonwords and real words • Acoustic feature recognition • Recognition of prosodic features Expressive aprosodia • Emotion production without cue • Emotion production with written cue • Emotion production with auditory cue	n/a

Table 4–3. *continued*

Assessment Tools	Areas Assessed	Norms
Florida Affect Battery	Receptive aprosodia • Linguistic discrimination • Emotional discrimination • Emotional comprehension	Adults without brain damage 17–85 years, adults with stroke and epilepsy
Test for Rating of Emotions in Speech	Receptive aprosodia • Emotion recognition • Emotion comprehension	Adults without brain damage
RHDBank Protocol	Expressive aprosodia • Spontaneous linguistic • Spontaneous emotional	
Test of Awareness of Social Inference Test (TASIT)	Receptive aprosodia	Norms for adults and adolescents without brain injury and adults with TBI (21–64 years)
Profile of Pragmatic Impairment in Communication (PPIC)	Expressive aprosodia • Aesthetics	n/a

Hillis's battery focuses on emotional prosody only, with task development based in neuroscience (Sheppard et al., 2021), whereby different regions of the brain are responsible for prosodic feature recognition, semantic knowledge, and the integration of the two for accurate comprehension of intended meaning. The expressive prosody tasks in this battery vary the level of cue (e.g., written vs. auditory) to determine the basis of the deficit. In many of the earlier assessment tools, expressive aprosodia was evaluated based on spontaneous verbal output during discourse tasks using rating scales. While there is strong ecological validity in using spontaneous speech, the choice of task to elicit the sample may influence the ability to evaluate a range of linguistic and emotional markers of prosody.

Extralinguistics

Standardized assessment of the extralinguistic aspects of communication is limited to pragmatic checklists or rating scales. There are several batteries available to assess affect in the form of emotion in facial expression, including the Florida Affect Battery (Bowers et al., 1991) and the New York Emotion Battery (Borod et al., 1992). The reliability and validity of these assessments are generally considered weak or unavailable, except for the Florida Affect Battery, which has reasonable psychometric properties.

Composite assessment tools such as the MEC and Measures of Cognitive-Linguistic Abilities (MCLA; Ellmo, 1995) contain rating scales or checklists that guide clinicians to evaluate extralinguistic abilities in areas such as facial expression, eye contact, gestures, and body distancing (proxemics). For example, the MCLA Discourse Rating Scale requires the clinician to rate communication across linguistic, paralinguistic, and extralinguistic domains on a 5-point scale. The ratings provided should be based on formal and informal interactions with the person with RHD across assessment sessions and reflect the percentage of time the individual was adequately or appropriately using the skills (e.g., score of 1 = 0%–25%, 5 = 85%–100%). Similarly, the Profile of Pragmatic Impairment in Communication (PPIC) includes items that span linguistic, paralinguistic, and extralinguistic aspects of communication (Linscott et al., 2003). Extralinguistic aspects of communication sit, alongside paralinguistic skills, within the "Aesthethics" subscale, where the clinician rates observations on a 4-point scale with the descriptors ranging from *not at all* to *nearly always/always*. Additionally, an overall impairment for the subscale can be made ranging from *normal* to *very severely impaired*. The procedure outlined in the MCLA highlights that if clinicians are using any of these checklists or rating scales to assess extralinguistic capabilities, scoring should be based on observation across multiple tasks, contexts, and assessment sessions. The value of confirming observations and ratings with someone who knew the person with RHD prior to injury should not be understated as we know that the environment and communication part-

ner influence the outcome of communicative interactions in this population.

Assessment of the Impact of a Cognitive Communication Disorder

The World Health Organization International Classification of Functioning, Disability and Health (WHO, 2001) prompts us to consider an individual beyond an impairment level by exploring the impact of CCD on their lives. A comprehensive assessment plan of an individual with RHD should include tasks and tools that provide insight into activity limitations and participation restrictions post brain injury. Impairments in cognition and communication can significantly influence the ability to resume and/or retain vocational and other community roles as well as interpersonal interactions and relationships. Several examples of relevant tools are provided here. The clinician is reminded to consider two things when selecting and interpreting findings. First, the nature and frequency of engagement in community activities and with members of a social network is highly individual. Assumptions about what constitutes a typical amount of activity or contact should not be clinician or tool based but rather informed by a change that has occurred for every individual who experiences RHD. Second, the presence of anosognosia and anosodiaphoria, as discussed earlier in this chapter, may result in poor awareness of the consequences of impairments. It is therefore important to supplement self-ratings of the impact of CCD with significant other (family member, friend) reports of how activities and social interactions have changed since the onset of RHD.

The domains of occupational activities and independent living skills may be explored using the Sydney Psychosocial Reintegration Scale (SPRS-2; Tate, 2012), the Stroke Specific Quality of Life Scale (SS-QOL; Williams et al., 1999), Quality of Life after Brain Injury (QOLIBRI; Von Steinbüchel et al., 2010), and the Craig Handicap Assessment and Reporting Technique (CHART/CHART-SF; Whiteneck et al., 1992). When exploring social network size, composition, frequency of contact with valued network members, and satisfaction with interpersonal relationships, it is recommended that self- and other-report questionnaires are supplemented with interviews to best understand factors that are influencing interpersonal relationships. The SPRS-2, Community Integration Questionnaire (CIQ; Willer et al., 1993, or CIQ-R: Callaway et al., 2016), Social Support Survey (SSS; Sherbourne & Stewart, 1991), and the Stroke Social Network Scale (SSNS; Northcott & Hilari, 2013) are examples of tools that consider social participation and relationship domains.

Treatment

An evidence-based practice model provides a framework for making clinical decisions regarding intervention. Clinicians should consider (a) current best evidence, (b) client and other stakeholder perspectives, (c) clinical knowledge and experience, and (d) client performance or data-informed treatment planning as proposed in the diamond or four-component construct of evidence-based practice (EBP) (Higginbotham & Satchidanand, 2019).

Clinical expertise in RHD, as with any neurogenic cognitive or communication disorder, begins with a solid knowledge of normal processes and the effects of brain injury on such processes. Knowledge about treatment procedures is also needed. The knowledge then must be coupled with clinical experiences to aid in the recognition and accurate diagnosis of the deficits and development of treatments. Opportunities for obtaining such knowledge are more challenging than for other neurogenic communication disorders. In contrast to the commendable body of literature on aphasia, TBI, and dementia, much less is published on the cognitive and communication changes associated with RHD. This disparity is evident in a review of trends in clinical practice research published in the American Speech-Language-Hearing Association's (ASHA) journals from 2008 to 2018, where CCD following RHD was the communication impairment with the fewest intervention-focused research papers and presentations (Roberts et al., 2020).

Consideration of a client's needs, preferences, and priorities is an important component of any treatment plan. These help a clinician to construct treatment goals with clients and to propose tasks and stimuli that are of interest to the client. The client should be actively involved in goal identification and goal setting as this helps to create ownership of treatment plans, which increases motivation and participation. This is especially important for individuals with anosognosia, who may not see the need for treatment.

In terms of current best evidence, there is a paucity of treatment efficacy research for disorders associated with RHD. The exception is UVN, for which there are many treatments, some with solid evidence of efficacy. There is a large body of research on cognitive deficits caused by TBI that can inform practice with RHD. Clinicians still must critically evaluate the use of such treatments and carefully measure outcomes to ensure that the treatments are creating meaningful change due to differences in the neurophysiology and neuropathology of TBI and stroke, as well as demographic differences in the populations (e.g., individuals with TBI are often young males while strokes tend to affect older adults) that could impact the effectiveness of treatment.

Treatment for Disorders of Cognition

Attention

Most treatments for **general attention deficits** have been designed for adults with attentional deficits caused by TBI (see Chapter 8). As discussed in that chapter, combinations of direct training and strategy training may be the most efficacious. As noted above, careful measurement of treatment outcomes is important because attentional deficits related to RHD may not respond to treatment in the same way as those caused by TBI. For example, results from a systematic review of randomized control trials indicated that participants with RHD had better outcomes following divided attention treatment than those with TBI (Virk et al., 2015). Another study (Sturm & Willmes, 1991)

reported that generalization from attention training to other cognitive and communication abilities was better for the group with TBI than participants with RHD. General attention or alertness treatments are designed to reduce the severity of neglect by targeting the general attentional system. Several treatments and programs have been developed, but the benefits generally are short-lived (DeGutis & Van Vleet, 2010; Robertson et al., 1995; Sturm et al., 2006; Thimm et al., 2006). Attention Process Training (e.g., APT; Sohlberg & Mateer, 2010) is an example of an attention treatment to improve selective attention, speed of information processing, and self-regulation through a series of exercises. The use of APT has been shown to result in related improvements in reading comprehension and rate (Sinot & Coelho, 2007). APT programs are seldom implemented in isolation. When direct attention training is combined with strategy instruction (i.e., metacognitive strategy instruction), significant improvements are possible, as reported for individuals with TBI (Butler et al., 2008; Cicerone, 2002).

Treatment for **neglect** has been studied more than any other deficit associated with RHD, and many reviews of neglect treatment have been published (Bowen et al., 2013; Cappa et al., 2005; Cicerone et al., 2011; Luauté et al., 2006; Pernet et al., 2013; Yang et al., 2013). Conclusions from the research indicate that there is substantial evidence to support the use of visual scanning and prism adaptation treatments in adults with USN, and there are several other treatments that have some empirical support, for example, mirror therapy, auditory spatial cueing while listening to preferred music, and virtual reality–

based treatments (Kaufman et al., 2022; Tavaszi et al., 2021). USN treatment studies of assessment and treatment consider predominantly ecocentric or viewercentred, peripersonal neglect. There are only a few studies of treatments for other forms of neglect (Barrett et al., 2006; Hillis, 2006). Few studies determine how the presence of one or more forms of neglect might impact response to treatment or if there is generalization from one form to another.

Treatments for neglect can be categorized as either top-down or bottom-up. Top-down attentional treatments improve individuals' performance via cognitive strategies (Azouvi et al., 2017; Dintén-Fernández et al., 2019). Visual scanning falls into this category. Bottom-up treatments, in contrast, are designed to increase attention to left-sided stimuli through manipulation of attentional systems or the stimuli themselves. Bottom-up treatments include general attention treatments, prism adaptation, external sensory stimulation, and treatments designed to expand the attentional window. Some treatments include both bottom-up and top-down features, such as visuomotor treatments (Barrett et al., 2006; Hillis, 2006; Saevarsson et al., 2011). Visual scanning training is recommended as a practice standard (Cicerone et al., 2011). Specific methods vary, but the essential component is repeated scanning for targets, which can be words, objects, or images, from left to right and back again. Scanning treatments often involve a hierarchy. Manipulation of the number, size, and visual complexity of the targets and the use of distractors can be used to alter difficulty. Remembering that USN is an attentional deficit will aid in developing a hierarchy of difficulty. Things that are likely to grab attention can be used to make the task easier. Examples of how to manipulate targets are provided in Table 4–4. Evidence from visual scanning treatment studies suggests that while improvements routinely occur on the tasks practiced in therapy, generalization to other tasks or situations does not always occur. Thus, it is important to match the therapy tasks to the goals. For example, if the patient's goal is to read books, then scanning treatment needs to involve text arranged in a hierarchy from words, sentences, and paragraphs.

Limb Activation Training (Bailey et al., 2002; Robertson et al., 2002) is a form of visuomotor treatment based on the idea that activation of right hemisphere motor regions associated with movement of the left limbs might enhance activation of right hemisphere attentional circuits. In this therapy, the patient is prompted to move their left arm or leg during scanning tasks. Movement of the left limbs requires right hemisphere activation; the pairing of such movement with visual scanning is thought to be more effective than the scanning alone. The Lighthouse Strategy takes the visuomotor training one step further by adding visualization of the beam of a lighthouse paired with the movement of the head from left to right and back again (Niemeier et al., 2001). Outcomes from visuomotor treatments differ across studies, but improvement has been reported on neglect measures, reading, motor function, and navigation in the environment (Luukkainen-Markkula et al., 2009; Priftis et al., 2013).

Externally driven bottom-up treatments include prism glasses and

Table 4–4. Sample Stimulus Manipulations for Treatment of Unilateral Visuospatial Neglect

Feature	Manipulation	Rationale
Size of target	Large → small	Greater visual demands in identifying smaller targets
Number of targets	Few → many	Greater attentional demands with more stimuli
Visual saliency of targets	Bright colors → subdued colors Blinking targets → solid targets	Greater visual demands in distinguishing targets that do not "pop out" from background
Emotional or personal saliency of targets	Emotionally stimulating targets (spiders, snakes, beautiful sunrise, pictures of patient or family members) → neutral targets (cow, tree, pictures of unknown people)	Meaningful or emotionally laded pictures/words may stimulate unconscious processing that grabs attention; neutral items will not
Presence of distractors	None → many	Greater attentional, visual, and cognitive demands in differentiating targets from distractors and inhibiting responses to distractors
Similarity of distractors	Visually distinct from targets → visually similar to targets	Greater attentional and visual demands in differentiating targets from distractors
Location of targets	Few on right side → many on right side	More items on right side will stimulate the "magnetic attraction" to the right side and hinder attentional shifts to left visual space

sensory stimulation. These must be conducted in collaboration with the appropriate colleagues (e.g., neurologists, neurophthalmologists) because they involve multiple sensory and neural systems. Prism glasses distort the visual images to one side. Initially, if the visual field is distorted to the right, the viewer will reach too far to the right to reach an object. Over time, the brain adapts to the distortion so that the reach is on target. When the glasses are removed, viewers experience a reversal of the perceptual distortion to the left side, with greater processing of items in the left side of space

(Barrett & Muzaffar, 2014; Fortis et al., 2010; Newport & Schenk, 2012; Rossetti et al., 1998; Rusconi & Carelli, 2012). Positive effects from prism glasses have been reported to last hours to days. Sensory stimulation techniques increase eye movement and attentional focus to the left side through, for example, neck vibration or optokinetic stimulation (watching vertical lines move leftward across a screen). Sensory stimulation techniques have resulted in at least transient reduction in severity of UN (Kerkhoff & Schenk, 2012; Reinhart et al., 2011; Ronchi et al., 2013), and added benefits have been reported for combinations of visual scanning and sensory stimulation techniques (Pitteri et al., 2013; Priftis et al., 2013).

The only published treatments for stimulus- or object-centered neglect are bottom-up treatments designed to draw attention leftward or expand the window of visual attention. The rationale for the latter is to expand the space of attentional focus so that for a small object, details on the left side of an object will fall within the window (Hillis et al., 1999). This was accomplished by interspersing different diameter circles. To perceive the larger diameter circles, the patient's attentional window had to expand. This resulted in the patient being able to identify features on the left side of a smaller diameter stimulus because that was well within the attentional window. The impact of object-centered neglect on word reading can be reduced by adding meaningless characters to the beginning of a word (Hillis, 2006). These characters become the leftmost region of a word and exist in the space that previously had been neglected. Other suggested treatments

that have not been studied empirically include manipulating stimuli to encourage leftward movement of attention, either explicitly or unconsciously (Myers, 1999; Tompkins, 1995). This can be done by having a client outline a paper with their finger before beginning a task, to establish the boundaries to be attended to. The use of stimuli that cross the midline also may shift attention leftward, particularly if the stimulus cannot be identified without processing details that appear on the left—for example, words presented at midline, for which no shorter word can be created by the letters on the left side of midline (e.g., "mountain" or "pencil"). Perceptual grouping and feature detection may impact the extent of USN on specific tasks (Brooks et al., 2005). Taking advantage of how human visual processing works can enable individuals with UVN to respond faster to stimuli on the left side of space: the presence of a connector joining left and right stimuli or when items are grouped by a peripheral border, such as a circle drawn around target stimuli. External cues such as red lines along the left margin or the examiner exhorting "look to the left" are commonly used in clinical practice to serve as anchors or reminders, or perhaps to capitalize on unconscious processing. For the latter, the presence of a bright or otherwise salient stimulus in the left margin may aid in an unconscious shift of attention toward the left. There is no evidence to support the use of external cues; often they are embedded into treatment programs but have not been independently assessed. There is extensive evidence from the TBI literature that external cues are not as effective as internal cues in the long term for a variety of reasons. First, performance gains usually are lost when the external cues are removed, and unless a client has someone to set the cues for them, they will obviously have no benefit. Second, in the cognitive disorder literature, there is a well-established disconnect between knowing and doing. While a patient may know that they need to look to the left and start at the left edge of a page, they may not be able to use those strategies in all situations.

Executive Function and Awareness

Currently, there are no efficacy data for treatment of EF deficits or anosognosia specifically resulting from RHD. Some studies include adults with cognitive deficits caused by either TBI or focal lesions, but most do not separate out results based on etiology or location of lesion, making it difficult to determine whether adults with RHD respond the same way as adults with TBI. In the absence of evidence specific to RHD, clinicians may use the questions provided below to evaluate treatments designed for adults with TBI described in previous chapters, to see if they might be appropriate for individual clients with RHD. Evidence for treatment of awareness deficits from the TBI literature suggests that feedback, experiential learning, and metacognitive strategies may be useful (Cheng & Man, 2006; Cicerone et al., 2011; Copley et al., 2020; Goverover et al., 2007). In group settings, verbal feedback can come not only from the clinician but also from other group members. For some clients, feedback from peers may be more powerful in creating awareness than feedback from

a clinician. Video feedback reduces the metacognitive demands of monitoring performance online. It may be difficult for some clients to catch errors when they are focused on completing a task. Giving them the opportunity to view a video after the fact allows them to focus on evaluating the performance. Another benefit is that clients can see for themselves when errors are made, which again may be more powerful in increasing awareness than hearing feedback from a clinician.

Social Cognition

As with EF and awareness, the reader is referred to evidence of social cognition treatments shown to be effective with individuals with TBI. Many studies report improvements following social cognition training (e.g., Bornhofen & McDonald, 2008; Neuman et al., 2015; Radice-Neuman et al., 2009). However, studies often target only a single aspect of social cognition and focus largely on behavior modification, and evidence for generalization of social cognition skills to everyday communication contexts is scarce. Facial affect training has been researched more extensively than ToM training (Vallat-Azouvi et al., 2019). Broadly, all treatment approaches use drill or repetition of exercises, with some also including a strategy approach. Some examples of treatments are Training of Affect Recognition (TAR; Wölwer et al., 1996), virtual reality to represent interpersonal interaction situations, mental state attribution tasks, Treatment for Social Cognition and Emotion Regulation (T-ScEmo; Westerhof-Evers et al., 2017), and Cognitive Pragmatic Treatment (Gabbatore et al., 2015).

Treatment for Disorders of Communication (Apragmatism)

Linguistics

Despite the number of assessments available to assess linguistic abilities at both the semantic and discourse levels, there have been limited studies exploring treatments addressing comprehension and production specifically for people with RHD. A small number of treatments have been developed to target specific areas of language comprehension affected by RHD. Contextual Constraint Treatment (Blake et al., 2015; Tompkins et al., 2012) was designed to implicitly stimulate and increase the efficiency of coarse coding and suppression mechanisms to improve narrative comprehension. Stimuli were developed with a hierarchy of contextual bias to capitalize on the preserved use of strong contextual cues to aid in comprehension. Results from a multiple-baseline design indicated gains not only in speed of responses to the individual items but, more importantly, to general comprehension. The treatment is not available for clinical use currently due to the complexity of individually programming the computerized administration. However, the takeaway is that broad language processes can be improved by increasing the efficiency of component processes (coarse coding and suppression). Offline, interactive treatments using the principles of contextual bias are described below.

A metaphor interpretation treatment was designed to improve comprehension of nonliteral meanings of novel phrases (Lundgren et al., 2011). The treatment involves generating meanings and features of words and linking overlapping meanings to create a nonliteral interpretation of a metaphor. For example, for the metaphor "a family is a cradle," features of the words "family" and "cradle" would be identified, and those that overlap would be connected to create a nonliteral meaning. Four of the five participants showed gains on the treatment task, but only one exhibited improvement on a standardized test of figurative language comprehension. No measures of generalization were reported, so it is unclear whether the gains affect general communication.

Spoken discourse interventions that have been designed and trialed in the RHD population are uncommon despite this often being considered a primary communicative challenge for the group. A recent systematic review by Lê and colleagues (2022) summarized the evidence for discourse and social communication interventions for people with TBI, with the latter focusing on interactions in a social context that draw on linguistic, paralinguistic, and extralinguistic abilities. Key components evident in interventions focused on discourse production were found to be the use of hierarchical training, metacognitive strategies, structured training prompts or scaffolding, and feedback protocols. Cannizzaro and Coehlo (2002) conducted one of the earliest studies to investigate interventions for narrative discourse production, and while they found an immediate impact on discourse ability, there was limited evidence of maintenance or generalization of learned skills. More recently, interventions have been designed to include tasks that simulate social contexts (Henderson et al., 2020; Whitworth et al., 2020) and functional practice of the learned skills (Whitworth et al., 2020) seeking to address issues of maintenance and generalization. Both studies again found immediate and 1-month post-treatment improvements in discourse outcomes, but effects beyond this period were mixed. Overall, the systematic review by Lê and colleagues (2022) indicated that discourse interventions were more effective for people with mild-to-moderate injury, while social communication interventions that addressed the multiple forms of communication were more effective for people with moderate-to-severe injury.

Paralinguistics

An emerging treatment for receptive aprosodia has been reported by Durfee, Sheppard, Meier, and colleagues (2021) based on a model of emotion prosody recognition described and refined by Wright et al. (2018) and Sheppard et al. (2020), respectively. There are three stages of processing required that begin with a perceptual stage, followed by integration of sensory and conceptual representations and then a cognitive evaluation based on semantic representations. The three-step training program by Durfee, Sheppard, Meier, and colleagues (2021) addresses Stage 1 (perceptual) and Stage 2 (conceptual) of the model of emotion prosody recognition, which are briefly described in Table 4–5. A study of 38 individuals with acute RHD has promising findings for the treatment of receptive aprosodia, with participants demonstrating significant improvements in their ability to recognize acoustic and prosodic features associated with emotion and matching the features with a named emotion. While these are extremely preliminary findings, how such gains

generalize to interpreting emotional prosody in everyday communication contexts is unclear, but this work is a positive step toward developing an effective treatment for receptive aprosodia.

Treatments for expressive aprosodia were first investigated by Leon and colleagues (2004). Two approaches to treatment were constructed based on theories of the underlying deficits causing aprosodia: (a) cognitive-linguistic and (b) motoric. The cognitive-linguistic treatment was based on the theory that expressive aprosodia results from an inability to access emotional linguistic structures and the prosodic patterns related to different emotions. The clinician provides the patient with information about prosodic characteristics that convey different emotions. A variety of cues, including the appropriate facial expression and a written description of the prosodic features, are provided, and the cues are gradually faded over a six step hierarchy (Table 4–6). A second treatment, the motoric imitative treatment, was based on the theory that aprosodia arises due to a motor speech deficit, whereby individuals are unable to program the speech mechanism to produce emotional prosodic patterns. The treatment focuses on the imitation of appropriate prosodic patterns, with cues faded over a six-step process (see Table 4–6).

As there was no clear support in the literature for one treatment (theory) over the other, all participants received both types of therapy, in random order. Results indicated that both treatments were efficacious. The one administered first was the most effective (regardless of type of treatment), and further gains were observed for most participants

Table 4–5. Emerging Receptive Aprosodia Treatment

Training Stage	Features of Task	Feedback/Training Schedule
Stage 1a: Acoustic Feature	• Pairs of pure-tone sequences presented • Pairs vary by one acoustic feature (rate, duration, volume, pitch) • Respond to multiple-choice presentation of acoustic features on computer screen • Person chooses which acoustic feature(s) differed between stimuli	• Visual and verbal feedback provided for both correct and incorrect responses • At end of trial set, client presented with pairs in error again with same feedback procedure • Up to three presentations of trial set allowed
Stage 1b: Prosodic Feature	• Presented with sentences conveying range of emotions • Presented with same acoustic features as in Stage 1a on a computer screen • Client required to identify two or three prosodic features from options	• Visual and verbal feedback provided for both correct and incorrect responses • Sentences only played once
Stage 2: ARACCE	• Emotion word presented in written format at the top of computer screen • Below this word same acoustic features as in Stage 1a/b are presented • Client asked to provide two or three prosodic features that convey the named emotion	• Visual and verbal feedback provided for both correct and incorrect responses

Note: Summary compiled from Durfee et al. (2021). ARACCE = Access to Abstract Representation of Acoustic Characteristics that Convey Emotion.

after the second therapy. Gains generalized within types of prosody trained. For example, after treatment, participants were able to produce a variety of "happy" sentences using appropriate "happy" prosody. Gains did not generalize to emotions not trained. Thus, participants were unable to produce appropriate fearful prosody after treatment, as fear was not trained during therapy. Four of the six participants available for follow-up demonstrated maintenance of gains 3 months after treatment ended.

Extralinguistics

Treatment for the extralinguistic aspects of communication is often incorporated into programs that address social

Table 4–6. Expressive Aprosodia Treatment Hierarchies

Cognitive-Linguistic Treatment for Emotional Aprosodia
Sample sentence:"You are insulting me"
1. Clinician provides a written description of tone of voice; client explains it back to the clinician.
2. Client matches name of emotion to description and matches picture of facial expression to description.
3. Client reads target sentence with appropriate prosody. Description, name, and face are available.
4. Client reads sentence with appropriate prosody. Name and face available.
5. Client reads sentence with appropriate prosody. Only face is available.
6. Client reads sentence with appropriate prosody. No cues are available.
Motoric-Imitative Treatment for Emotional Aprosodia
Sample sentence:"We just had a new baby"
1. Clinician reads sentence with appropriate prosody and facial expression. Client and clinician produce the sentence in unison.
2. Clinician reads sentence with appropriate prosody and facial expression. Client repeats the sentence.
3. Clinician reads sentence with appropriate prosody (covers face to remove visual cues). Client repeats the sentence.
4. Clinician reads sentence with neutral intonation. Client repeats the sentence with appropriate intonation.
5. Clinician asks a question to elicit the production of the target sentence. Client produces the sentence with appropriate prosody.
6. Client is asked to produce the sentence with appropriate prosody while imagining they are speaking to a family member.

Source: Adapted from Rosenbek et al. (2006).

communication and pragmatics, with most of these programs developed for other populations such as TBI and not people with RHD. Due to their focus on social communication, these programs will incorporate activities that address linguistic and paralinguistic skills within a range of communicative contexts such social, vocational, and interpersonal. The systematic review mentioned earlier by Lê and colleagues (2021) summarizes the evidence for social communication interventions for people with TBI that, due to their holistic approach to the treatment of cognitive communication disorder, have the potential to address para- and extralinguistic skills.

One specific extralinguistic skill where evidence-based treatments have been developed for the TBI population is emotion recognition, including facial expression. The Faces Intervention is an app-based treatment designed to address emotion recognition difficulties in people with TBI (Neumann et al., 2015). The focus is to train individuals to recognize emotions through facial expression through three constructs: (a) attending to relevant facial features and link these to specific emotions, (b) increasing awareness of own emotions through reflection and imitation to assist with identification in others, and (c) strengthening the conceptual and associative understanding of emotional responses. Study findings indicated that the Faces Intervention was the maintenance of this effect up to 6 months posttreatment.

Theoretically Based Treatments

There are theories of how the intact, healthy right hemisphere functions and how it contributes to language and communication (Beeman, 1998; Tompkins et al., 2013; Tompkins & Scott, 2013). These accounts suggest that the intact right hemisphere is important for discourse comprehension processes, including activating broad meanings of words (including abstract meanings, infrequent or less familiar meanings, and distantly related features), integrating ideas and information across sentences, generating inferences to determine main ideas, and integrating world knowledge with information being comprehended. Extrapolating to the RHD population, these accounts predict that damage to the RH will result in difficulties generating inferences and main ideas, as well as problems integrating across sentences. Although the predictions fit with general descriptions

of adults with RHD, the theories tend to overestimate the problems encountered in this population, for example, suggesting that all inferencing processes will be abolished. This is akin to predicting that because the left hemisphere is important for comprehending language, all left hemisphere strokes will severely impair comprehension. There is much evidence in the RHD literature suggesting that people with RHD do have some intact inferencing processes and that they can generate strongly suggested inferences. Thus, it is difficult to justify treatments based solely on the theories of intact RH functioning.

The suppression deficit hypothesis, described above, purports that adults with RHD have difficulty **suppressing** unwanted meanings to allow rapid selection of the most appropriate meaning for a given context. Treatments that emphasize the identification of contextual cues that guide the interpretation of meaning may be useful. Stories, cartoons, and statements in which a change or revision of an initial interpretation is needed can be used as stimuli. Puns and jokes can be a good source of material, such as the one presented earlier about Grandma walking two miles a day. Headlines are another source of stimuli, as they can sometimes have different meanings, such as, "Police chase snakes through downtown," in which the reader must determine if the police were chasing snakes or if their chase went through many downtown streets. Clients may be asked what their initial interpretation is, then given a new sentence that supports the alternate meaning (e.g., "Three boa constrictors escaped from an open cage in a downtown pet store"). The clients should be encouraged to identify clues in the context that indicates which meaning is correct.

Treatments that emphasize the use of context and contextual cues may facilitate processing in the integration phase of comprehension (see examples in Table 4–7). The clinician can discuss words or sentences that have alternative meanings and how those meanings can be informed by context. The English language is full of homographs and homophones that can be used (e.g., yard, pitcher). Context can be provided by presenting word pairs (e.g., yard-grass vs. yard-inch) or putting ambiguous words into sentences. Ambiguous sentences also can be used and then additional sentences added to provide a context with which to interpret the meaning.

If a client appears to have difficulty with nonliteral language (e.g., idioms or metaphors), it is important to determine if they have problems only when the idiom is presented in isolation or if the problem persists when it appears in context, also. Many idioms can be interpreted by surrounding context. For example, the expression "he's a tall drink of water" may not be familiar to some people. If this idiom is used in front of a classroom, some of the students will have no idea what it means. However, if spoken when standing in a bar, and a tall handsome man is standing on the other side of the room, the intended meaning may be more readily accessed. In increasingly multicultural societies, there are many individuals who may not be familiar with idioms of the dominant culture. If a client is unfamiliar with an idiom, a clinician can add context and guide the client in determining the meaning based on the context.

As noted earlier, contextual information is not restricted to language. Contextual cues are present in picture description stimuli, particularly those that are inferentially complex, such as Norman Rockwell paintings. Myers (1999) suggests guiding clients through picture descriptions, asking questions to draw attention to various facets. These may include determining relationships between characters in the picture (e.g., parents vs. children) or the roles of individuals (e.g., doctors, teachers). Various other features, such as facial expressions, signs, and postures, also can provide clues as to the full interpretation of a picture.

These techniques for identifying relevant contextual cues can also be used to address deficits of ToM or deficits based on the Social Inferencing account. Scenarios can be developed in which a client has to use information about relationships or what knowledge each person must use to determine the intent of a conversation or comment (Blake, 2007, 2018; Myers, 1999). For example, consider the following scenario: "Pasquale had a big surprise planned for Soraya. The previous day he had confirmed plans for a big screen TV to be delivered to their house while she was at work. When Soraya walked into the living room that evening, she exclaimed, 'I can't believe you did this without my knowing!'" Soraya's statement would be interpreted as expressing surprise at the gift. However, if the sentence, "Pasquale was upset when he realized that Soraya had been behind him as he confirmed the delivery time," was inserted into the scenario, then Soraya's exclamation would take on a new meaning, being teasing or sarcastic. Clients can read through such

Table 4–7. Examples of Stimuli for Contextually-Based Treatment

Homophones: Word Pairs
second–line vs. second–minute
fan–sports vs. fan–breeze
pitcher–water vs. pitcher–baseball
yard–grass vs. yard–distance
jam–toast vs. jam–cars

Homophones: Sentences
He was *second* in line. It took her a *second* to recognize him.
He took a *survey* of the land. He took a *survey* online.
The baseball *fan* cheered for his team. She wanted to buy a new ceiling *fan*.
He spilled the *pitcher* of water. The *pitcher* threw a curveball.
I sat in the *row* behind her. He did not know how to *row* the boat.
The dog ran through the neighbor's *yard*. He was tackled on the ten-*yard* line.

Ambiguous Sentences
The man stopped the robber with a bat. The man stopped the robber using his bat. OR The man stopped the robber who had a bat.
The woman was walking through the store with pillows. She walked with pillows in her hand through the store. OR She walked through the store which sells pillows.
The pitcher was full. The pitcher was full of water. OR The baseball pitcher just finished eating a whole pizza.

Common Idioms
You are dead meat.
That puts the icing on the cake.
He is working around the clock.
It's like finding a needle in a haystack.
She is about to open a can of worms.
My mother put her foot down about staying out late.
Have your cake and eat it too.

scenarios and discuss how new information (context) may change interpretations. Clients can be guided through determining which contextual cues are important and which are not.

Another account of RHD deficits is the executive function deficits model (Martin & McDonald, 2003), which proposes that many pragmatic deficits associated with RHD are a result of impairments in executive functioning. Martin and McDonald (2003) suggest that RHD causes damage to frontal lobes or the extensive executive function networks that are controlled primarily by the frontal lobes. They support their model with rough comparisons between cognitive deficits associated with frontal lobe damage and general RHD. It is not hard to find executive function explanations for RHD communication deficits. For example, difficulties with organizing and planning can result in problems telling a complete, coherent story; problem-solving deficits can result in difficulties fixing communication breakdowns when they occur. There have been no studies to examine whether benefits of treatment for general executive function deficits might generalize to communication. However, Ylvisaker and colleagues (2008) have reported that most successful cognitive treatments are focused and create benefits for circumscribed skills: Essentially, what you treat in therapy gets better, but there is not much generalization to other skills. Thus, it may not be prudent to expect improvements in communication from treatment of general executive function skills.

One final account of RHD deficits is the cognitive resources hypothesis (Monetta & Joanette, 2003; Monetta et al., 2006). According to this hypothesis, many deficits associated with RHD are due to complexity factors. Thus, problems arise not on simple, straightforward tasks but on those that are complex or require increased processing. The account is based on data indicating that performance by adults with RHD decreases as complexity level increases and that adults without brain damage can exhibit patterns of performance that are like adults with RHD when complexity increases. This latter result suggests that deficits associated with RHD are not qualitatively different from normal performance but quantitatively different. The authors emphasize that this hypothesis does not replace any of the others but should be considered in combination with others. SLPs generally are adept at modifying treatments to alter complexity. These can include manipulations such as the length of a stimulus passage, the number of cues and/or distractors present, the number of relevant versus irrelevant cues that must be considered, or the number of characters mentioned within a text.

Implementing Treatments Designed for Other Populations

When treatments designed specifically for a population of interest are not available, another option is to select treatments initially designed for other patient groups (Myers, 1999; Tompkins & Scott, 2013). This is a good first step, but careful consideration of the treatments and measurement of outcomes is needed. There are very few direct comparisons between TBI and RHD groups, and so while many of the deficits appear similar, it is not clear whether they may differ in terms of response to treatment.

Clinicians must carefully review the literature, examine the strength of the existing treatment studies, and then determine whether a specific treatment may be appropriate for any one client with RHD. The following six questions (Cicerone, 2005; based on Sackett et al., 2000) are used as a framework for guiding the selection of treatments for individuals with RHD.

1. *Is my client sufficiently similar, in most important ways, to those described in the treatment study?* The clinician must determine what personal and injury factors are important to consider when determining similarities and therefore suitability of the treatment. When considering treatments designed for other groups, the etiology of injury obviously differs in terms of location and extent of injury. For example, treatment studies designed for people with TBI generally have populations who have experienced diffuse damage (in addition to focal damage in some cases), but people with RHD have focal lesions. Another factor that may differ between these two populations is age. Young adults represent a significant proportion of groups studied in TBI treatment studies, while strokes occur in adults across a wider age range, including older adults. The course of both etiologies is stable or improving (i.e., neither is degenerative), highlighting that in both groups, the focus of treatment is on recovery rather than maintenance. Further, clients will move through acute and chronic stages of recovery. In acute stages, the potential for spontaneous recovery exists, and while we know that in chronic stages, recovery is still possible, clients may have had negative experiences due to their commu-

nication changes (e.g., a loss of friends due to pragmatic deficits), which influences engagement in treatment. During the chronic stage, individuals with TBI or RHD may actively seek out treatment with clear goals for participating in therapy. In contrast, those in acute stages may not have a clear understanding of their deficits or their implications and so may appear less engaged in treatment.

2. *Is the nature of my client's cognitive impairment similar to that targeted in the treatment research?* Deficits in attention, memory, executive function, and apragmatism have been reported to be similar across TBI and RHD groups. Caution in generalizing findings should ensue as similarities and differences between the groups have not been carefully evaluated to determine overlap features.

McDonald (Martin & McDonald, 2003, 2006; McDonald, 2000) has published several reviews of pragmatic disorders following brain injury. The reviews provide descriptions of pragmatic deficits based on the separate RHD and TBI literatures but do not directly compare the two groups on the same tasks. One conclusion drawn from the comparisons was that while adults with either RHD or TBI had problems interpreting nonliteral language (e.g., sarcasm), only difficulties due to RHD were linked to individuals' abilities to interpret emotional cues.

Prigatano (1996) directly compared adults with RHD to those with TBI in a study of awareness of deficits. Although both groups demonstrated better awareness of physical than social/emotional behaviors, participants with TBI were most likely to overestimate their abilities (as compared to relatives' ratings of the same behaviors). The self-ratings from the RHD group, in contrast to the other participants, did not correspond to their performance on a neurologic inventory. The few studies available suggest that while deficits in pragmatics and awareness may appear similar across TBI and RHD, the deficits are not necessarily equivalent. Future studies are needed to specifically compare deficits caused by diffuse TBI and focal RHD and determine to what extent the behavioral consequences of different types of etiologies can validly be equated.

3. *Are there coexisting physical and/ or cognitive impairments that are likely to influence the effectiveness of the treatment?* Likely problems associated with RHD include aprosodia, neglect, and anosognosia. Additional deficits in attention, executive function, or memory also may be present. Clinicians must judge the extent to which co-occurring deficits might impact the implementation of treatment or the potential gains. Self-awareness is especially important to consider. If individuals are not aware of their deficits, they may not be willing to participate in treatment or, if they do, may have trouble self-monitoring.

4. *Is it feasible to apply the intervention in this setting?* Feasibility concerns may include the amount of time available, the location/environment where treatment was conducted (e.g., inpatient, outpatient, academic research setting, intensive day program), and access to materials, including computers and software. For example, group-based treatments require consideration of appropriate facilities and resources that are available, as well as clients wishing to attend the groups.

5. *What are the expected benefits and potential costs of applying the interven-*

tion? Given that it is not clear how well treatments may generalize across populations, the benefits may be unknown. Clinicians must determine whether the potential for change is worth the cost of time and money for conducting the treatment. The situation is not too different from what is done in clinical practice currently, in which treatments with no established efficacy or effectiveness are used routinely due to the paucity of treatments for which evidence is available. Clinical expertise and experience with treatments should be considered in selection of treatments. Additionally, clinicians should consider whether potential treatments are consistent with existing theories of RHD deficits. If so, and if the treatment goals are commensurate with the client's values, then the potential benefits may outweigh the costs.

6. *Is the treatment consistent with the patient's own preferences, values, and expectations?* This question must be considered individually for each specific client. One consideration for clients with RHD is the presence of self-awareness deficits. As mentioned earlier, individuals who are not aware of their deficits or the consequences of those deficits may see no reason to participate in treatment. Cherney (2006) outlined four factors that should be considered in this type of situation and how much the clinician and/or family should work to provide treatment for a person who is not aware of their need for it: (a) **Medical indications** must be considered, including the diagnosis and prognosis (e.g., stable vs. progressive condition) and how this might influence progress and expectations. (b) The **client's preferences** must always be considered; however, the weight given to them may be dependent on

the client's level of understanding and decision-making ability. If the client with RHD is interested in improving social interactions, then discourse/pragmatic treatment may be appropriate. If not aware of their deficits and not interested in treatment, the need for treatment may be discussed with them if there is a risk of social isolation due to their communication skills. (c) **Quality of life** is a third component to consider. A client with cognitive communication inclusive of apragmatism may become increasingly isolated and lonely if family and friends are not comfortable interacting with them. The burden and subsequent change in quality of life of a caregiver should be considered. (d) **Contextual features** include economic and social circumstances. The clinician should consider the client's ability to access treatment based on services available to them due to location or cost. An individual trying to return to work may not be able to afford time during the week to attend treatments, while those living in a rural area or without transportation may not be able to reach a facility offering intervention. There are a range of other personal and environmental factors (e.g., religious, cultural, or personal beliefs) that influence a person's decisions to receive or opt out of treatment.

The series of questions can be used to select any treatment for any client. They are not restricted to selecting treatments originally designed for a different population. For example, a clinician may want to use the questions to determine if the motoric-imitative treatment for aprosodia is appropriate for a given client with RHD. It is important to remember that the quality of the

research behind any treatment must be evaluated first. If a treatment has little or no evidence of effectiveness and little or no theoretical basis, then it is probably inappropriate to use even if your client and situation match well with those in the treatment study.

Case Study—Patrick

Case Data

Patrick Johnson is a 55-year-old married father of two. Patrick is on the management committee of a community theater, where he has worked as a manager and actor for more than 20 years. He also enjoys working as a medical faculty simulated (standardized) patient at a nearby university. Prior to pursuing a career as an actor, Patrick obtained a bachelor's degree with a major in business. He describes himself as a social and physically active person. In his spare time, he enjoys social gatherings with friends and hiking with his wife, Theresa. Patrick sustained a middle cerebral artery stroke involving the right temporoparietal junction and caudate nucleus 3 months ago. During his hospital admission, changes in his communication and cognition were identified on screening assessments, and it was recommended that he continue with speech-language pathology rehabilitation on discharge from acute stroke care. Patrick resumed his vocational roles 2 months after his stroke. The transition back to work has not been smooth. Patrick reports that he is finding it difficult to retain details of his acting scripts and to use intonation to capture the characters that he must depict in simulation scenarios. Theresa noted that Patrick seems to miss details of conversations. There has been some marital tension as Theresa feels that Patrick is not able to interpret her emotions and that he is no longer the warm, charismatic person that he was before the stroke. Patrick has now commenced outpatient rehabilitation services. To guide goal identification and management planning, an assessment consisting of both standardized and informal tools and tasks, which gathers information from both Patrick and Theresa, will be completed.

Assessment Plan

Based on Patrick's stroke site of lesion and the case data already gathered, the following assessment tools and task have been selected. Patrick's age and years of education will be considered when evaluating his performance against normative data. Please note that the examples provided here were selected based on the current case data. It is very possible, and clinically appropriate, that additional areas of cognition (e.g., executive function) and/or communication may need to be explored as greater insight into Patrick's presenting difficulties and needs emerge.

1. To identify and describe impairments in attention and/or memory

Rationale: Patrick reports difficulty retaining details of scripts, while Theresa reports similar difficulties with attending to or recalling information conveyed during conversations. Both attention and memory impairments may account for Patrick's poststroke difficulty with recall. In additional to memory and general attention, unilateral visual neglect should also be evaluated as it is a frequent consequence of RHD, with allocentric neglect being associated with lesions in the temporoparietal junction.

Method: The following standardized assessments will be administered.

- RBANS to explore both verbal and visual memory ability
- TEA to consider different types of attention
- The Plan an Event subtest of the FAVRES to explore the impact of potential attention/memory impairments on completing real-world tasks of increased complexity and the time required to complete the task
- BIT to determine if unilateral neglect is present on both conventional tasks (e.g., letter cancellation) and ecologically valid tasks (e.g., article reading and address copying)

The above-listed standardized assessments should be supplemented by informal assessment tasks.

- Observe Patrick's ability to attend to and/or recall auditory and visual (written) information in the presence or absence of environmental distractions.
- Determine Patrick's ability to recall information of increasing length (i.e., to sustain his attention for increasing periods of time).

2. To identify and describe impairments in linguistic, paralinguistic,

and extralinguistic domains of communication

Rationale: Patrick's initial case data highlight particular difficulties in using prosodic features, interpreting emotional facial expressions, and possible linguistic comprehension difficulties (i.e., missing details during conversational discourse). These impairments are impacting his ability to complete vocational tasks and may be contributing to marital discord as reported by Theresa. A composite assessment of communication is appropriate as a starting point to more clearly identify impairments that are present across all three communication domains. Further assessment tools and tasks should be used to supplement the composite assessments where additional information is required to guide treatment planning.

Method: The following standardized/formal assessment tools will be administered.

- MEC to identify the presence/absence of impairments across linguistic (e.g., metaphor and speech act interpretation) and paralinguistic (e.g., receptive aprosodia) domains
- The Sentence Comprehension subtest from the Comprehensive Aphasia Test (Swinburn et al., 2023) to explore structural semantic comprehension
- DCR to explore variations in comprehension of stated or applied meanings in spoken and written narrative discourse
- TASIT-R to explore facial emotion recognition and social inferencing (ToM)

- LCQ to further explore significant-other observations of communication changes in real-world contexts. Patrick will also be asked to complete the LCQ. His responses will be compared to those of Theresa to explore Patrick's awareness of communication changes secondary to RHD.
- The Adapted Kagan Scales will be used to evaluate a recording of a conversation between Patrick and Theresa. This will allow exploration of Theresa's role in supporting communication exchanges.

The above-listed standardized assessments should be supplemented by informal observation of Patrick's awareness of communication changes and his ability to implement strategies and/or modify his answer/production based on feedback as the development of self-awareness may need to be a further treatment goal.

Assessment Findings

Patrick's assessment findings revealed impairments across both cognition and communication. The following is a diagnostic summary of results. Patrick presents with a cognitive communication disorder secondary to RHD characterized by impairments in sustained and divided attention, receptive and expressive emotional aprosodia, and neglect dyslexia. Mild difficulty in written and auditory discourse comprehension is present, which likely is due to neglect and impaired attention. Patrick's ability to complete valued vocational, social, and interpersonal roles and activities is negatively impacted by his CCD. Patrick is aware of the impairments and is motivated to engage in speech-language pathology treatment.

Treatment Goals and Suggested Approaches

The following treatment plan was informed by assessment findings and priorities as expressed by Patrick and Theresa. The goals represent a short-term plan (3 months), after which point the goals may be modified based on Patrick's progress and changes in his priorities and needs. During this time, Patrick will attend four 1-hourly sessions per week, of which three will be individual sessions and one will involve participation in a small group. Additional home-based practice activities will be provided to increase intensity of treatment and support maintenance and generalization.

> Long-term goal: For Patrick to maintain and participate successfully in work, social activities, and valued personal relationships

Treatment Area 1: Education and Communication Partner Training

Goal: Patrick and Theresa will develop their understanding of the cognitive and communication changes that occurred due to the right hemisphere stroke and strategies that will support their interpersonal communication.

Method:

- Individual session: Patrick and Theresa will attend a session

focused on information provision about CCD and strategies that will support communication. They will also be provided with print literature and suggested online resources (e.g., RightHemisphere.org) that can be shared with family members and friends about RHD.
- Future sessions: Ongoing discussion will occur to determine if information provision and treatment of aprosodia and attention resulted in improved communication between Patrick and Theresa. If difficulties persist, it may be suitable for them to complete a communication partner training program (e.g., TBI JOINT; Togher et al., 2016).

Treatment Area 2: Aprosodia

Goal: Patrick will correctly identify and produce prosodic features that are used to express emotions and intentions.

Method:

- Individual sessions: To improve interpretation of prosodic features, the Access to Abstract Representation of Acoustic Characteristics that Convey Emotion (ARACCE) treatment approach will be used. Expressive aprosodia will be treated using the Cognitive-Linguistic Treatment for Emotional Aprosodia.
- Group sessions: To support generalization of the ability to interpret and use prosodic features to express emotion, role-play activities will be used during small group sessions. Scenarios will be relevant to group members' work and/or leisure activities.

Treatment Area 3: Attention and Memory

Goal: Patrick will improve in his ability to attend to and retain text and/or spoken discourse that represent typical scripts used in his acting roles.

Method:

- Individual sessions: Implement the APT3 program during individual sessions and as part of home-based activities to improve sustained and selective attention. Reading comprehension strategies (e.g., identifying key words or main point and underlining them, or summarizing main points) will simultaneously be identified and practiced in line with a metacognitive strategy instruction approach.
- Group sessions: Patrick will actively evaluate his ability to utilize metacognitive strategies to support attention during group conversations to transfer/generalize attention strategy skills to a group conversation context.

Treatment Area 4: Neglect Dyslexia

Goal: Patrick will improve his reading comprehension and speed by reducing the impact of unilateral visual neglect.

Method: As Patrick presents with object-centered neglect, treatment will involve the inclusion of meaningless characters to the beginning of words in isolation and in phrases. Over time, this strategy will be reduced and replaced by metacognitive strategies in which Patrick develops self-monitoring and evaluation skills during reading tasks.

Speed of reading and reading comprehension will be developed using these strategies in text that increase in length.

References

Abbott, J. D., Wijerante, T., Hughes, A., Perre, D., & Lindell, A. K. (2014). The influence of left and right hemisphere brain damage on configural and featural processing of affective faces. *Laterality*, 19(4), 455–472. https://psycnet.apa.org/doi/10.1080/1357650X.2013.862256

Aboulafia-Brakha, T., Christe, B., Martory, M. D., & Annoni, J. M. (2011). Theory of mind tasks and executive functions: A systematic review of group studies in neurology. *Journal of Neuropsychology*, 5(1), 39–55. https://doi.org/10.1348/174866410x533660

Academy of Neurologic Communication Disorders Traumatic Brain Injury Writing Committee, Byom, L., O'Neil-Pirozzi, T. M., Lemoncello, R., MacDonald, S., Meulenbroek, P., . . . Sohlberg, M. M. (2020). Social communication following adult traumatic brain injury: A scoping review of theoretical models. *American Journal of Speech-Language Pathology*, 29(3), 1735–1748. https://doi.org/10.1044/2020_AJSLP-19-00020

Adamit, T., Maeir, A., Ben Assayag, E., Bornstein, N. M., Korczyn, A. D., & Katz, N. (2015). Impact of first-ever mild stroke on participation at 3 and 6 month post-event: The TABASCO study. *Disability and Rehabilitation*, 37(8), 667–673. https://doi.org/10.3109/09638288.2014.923523

Adamovich, B. L., & Brooks, R. L. (1981). A diagnostic protocol to assess the communication deficits of patients with right hemisphere damage. *Clinical Aphasiology: Proceedings of the Conference, 1981*, 244–253.

Anderson, B., Mennemeier, M., & Chatterjee, A. (2000). Variability not ability:

Another basis for performance decrements in neglect. *Neuropsychologia, 38*(6), 785–796. https://doi.org/10.1016/S00 28-3932(99)00137-2

Appelros, P. (2007). Prediction of length of stay for stroke patients. *Acta Neurologica Scandinavica, 116*(1), 15–19. https://doi .org/10. llll/j.1600-0404.2006.00756.x

Arene, N. U., & Hillis, A E. (2007). Rehabilitation of unilateral spatial neglect and neuroimaging. *Eura Medicophysiology, 43*(2), 255–269.

Azouvi, P., Jacquin-Courtois, S., & Luauté, J. (2017). Rehabilitation of unilateral neglect: Evidence-based medicine. *Annals of Physical and Rehabilitation Medicine, 60*(3), 191–197.

Bailey, M. J., Riddoch, M. J., & Crome, P. (2002). Treatment of visual neglect in elderly patients with stroke: A single-subject series using either a scanning and cueing strategy or a left-limb activation strategy. *Physical Therapy, 82*(8), 782–797.

Balaban, N., Friedmann, N., & Ziv, M. (2016). Theory of mind impairment after right hemisphere damage. *Aphasiology, 30*(12), 1–33. https://doi.org/10.1080/02 687038.2015.1137275

Barker-Collo, S. L., Feigin, V. L., Lawes, C. M., Parag, V., & Senior, H. (2010). Attention deficits after incident stroke in the acute period: Frequency across types of attention and relationships to patient characteristics and functional outcomes. *Topics in Stroke Rehabilitation, 17*(6), 463–476. https://doi.org/10.1310/tsr1706-463

Baron, C., Goldsmith, T., & Beatty, P. W. (1999). Family and clinician perceptions of pragmatic communication skills following right hemisphere stroke. *Topics in Stroke Rehabilitation, 5*(4), 55–64. https://doi .org/10.1310/78XM-RVMK-NNJ1-3NV9

Barrett, A. M., Buxbaum, L. J., Coslett, H. B., Edwards, E., Heilman, K. M., Hillis, A. E., . . . Robertson, I. H. (2006). Cognitive rehabilitation interventions for neglect and related disorders: Moving from bench to bedside in stroke patients. *Journal of Cognitive Neuroscience, 18*(7), 1223–1236. https://doi.org/10.1162/jocn .2006.18.7.1223

Barrett, A. M., & Muzaffar, T. (2014). Spatial cognitive rehabilitation and motor recovery after stroke. *Current Opinion in Neurology, 27*(6), 653–658. https://doi.org/ 10.1097/WCO.0000000000000148

Bartolomeo, P., Thiebaut de Schotten, M., & Doricchi, F. (2007). Left unilateral neglect as a disconnection syndrome. *Cerebral Cortex, 17*(11), 2479–2490. https://doi .org/10.1093/cercor/bhl181

Baum, S. R., & Pell, M. D. (1999). The neural bases of prosody: Insights from lesion studies and neuroimaging. *Aphasiology, 13*(8), 581–608. https://doi.org/ 10.1080/026870399401957

Baumann, M., Couffignal, S., Le Bihan, E., & Chau, N. (2012). Life satisfaction two-years after stroke onset: The effects of gender, sex occupational status, memory function and quality of life among stroke patients (NewsQol) and their family caregivers (WhoQol Bref) in Luxembourg. *BMC Neurology, 12*(1), 105. https://doi .org/10.1186/1471-2377-12-105

Beeman, M. J. (1998). Coarse semantic coding and discourse comprehension. In M. Beeman & C. Chiarello (Eds.), *Right hemisphere language comprehension: Perspectives from cognitive neuroscience* (pp. 255–284). Lawrence Erlbaum.

Beeman, M. J., Bowden, E. M., & Gembacher, M. A (2000). Right and left hemisphere cooperation for drawing predictive and coherence inferences during normal story comprehension. *Brain and Language, 71*(2), 310–336. https://doi .org/10.1006/brln.1999.2268

Bellmann, A., Meuli, R., & Clarke, S. (2001). Two types of auditory neglect. *Brain, 124*(4), 676–687. https://doi.org/10.1093/ brain/124.4.676

Benowitz, L. I., Moya, K. L., & Levine, D. N. (1990). Impaired verbal reasoning and constructional apraxia in subjects with right hemisphere damage. *Neuro-*

psychologia, 28(3), 231–241. https://doi .org/10.1016/0028-3932(90)90017-I

Benton, A. L., Hamsher, d. S. K., & Sivan, A. B. (1983). *Controlled Oral Word Association Test (COWAT)*. APA PsycTests. https:// doi.org/10.1037/t10132-000

Berube, S. K., Goldberg, E., Sheppard, S. M., Durfee, A. Z., Ubellacker, D., Walker, A., . . . Hillis, A. E. (2022). An analysis of right hemisphere stroke discourse in the Modern Cookie Theft picture. *American Journal of Speech-Language Pathology, 31*(5S), 2301–2312. https://doi.org/10.10 44/2022_ajslp-21-00294

Bisiach, E., Vallar, G., Perani, D., Papagno, C., & Berti, A. (1986). Unawareness of disease following lesions of the right hemisphere: Anosognosia for hemiplegia and anosognosia for hemianopia. *Neuropsychologia, 24*(4), 471–482. https:// doi.org/10.1016/0028-3932(86)90092-8

Blake, M. L. (2006). Clinical relevance of discourse characteristics after right hemisphere brain damage. *American Journal of Speech-Language Pathology, 15*(3), 256–267. https://doi.org/10.1044/1058-0360 (2006/024)

Blake, M. L. (2007). Perspectives on treatment for communication deficits associated with right hemisphere brain damage. *American Journal of Speech-Language Pathology, 16*(4), 331–342. https://doi .org/10.1044/1058-0360(2007/037)

Blake, M. L. (2016). Right hemisphere strokes. *Perspectives of the ASHA Special Interest Groups, 1*(2), 63–65. https://doi .org/10.1044/persp1.SIG2.63

Blake, M. L. (2018). *The right hemisphere and disorders of cognition and communication: Theory and clinical practice.* Plural Publishing.

Blake, M. L., Duffy, J. R., Myers, P. S., & Tompkins, C. A. (2002). Prevalence and patterns of right hemisphere cognitive/communicative deficits: Retrospective data from an inpatient rehabilitation unit. *Aphasiology, 16*(4–6), 537–547. https:// doi.org/10.1080/02687030244000194

Blake, M. L., & Hoepner, J. K. (2021). *Clinical neuroscience for communication disorders: Neuroanatomy and neurophysiology.* Plural Publishing.

Blake, M. L., & Lesniewicz, K. (2005). Contextual bias and predictive inferencing in adults with and without right hemisphere brain damage. *Aphasiology, 19*(3–5), 423–434. https://doi.org/10.1080/02 687030444000868

Blake, M. L., Tompkins, C. A., Scharp, V. L., Meigh, K. M., & Wambaugh, J. (2015). Contextual Constraint Treatment for coarse coding deficit in adults with right hemisphere brain damage: Generalisation to narrative discourse comprehension. *Neuropsychological Rehabilitation, 25*(1), 15–52. https://doi.org/10.1080/09 602011.2014.932290

Blonder, L. X., Heilman, K. M., Ketterson, T., Rosenbek, J. C., Raymer, A., Crosson, B., . . . Gonzalez-Rothi, L. (2005). Affective facial and lexical expression in aprosodic versus aphasic stroke patients. *Journal of the International Neuropsychological Society, 11*(6), 677–685. https://doi .org/10.1017/Sl355617705050794

Blonder, L. X., Pettigrew, L. C., & Kryscio, R. J. (2012). Emotion recognition and marital satisfaction in stroke. *Journal of Clinical and Experimental Neuropsychology, 34*(6), 634–642. https://doi.org/10.1080/ 13803395.2012.667069

Bloom, R. L., Borod, J. C., Obler, L. K., & Gerstman, L. J. (1983). Discourse following right and left brain damage. *Journal of Speech and Hearing Research, 36,* 1227–1235.

Bloom, R. L., Borod, J. C., Obler, L. K., & Koff, E. (1990). A preliminary characterization of lexical emotional expression in right and left brain-damaged patients. *International Journal of Neuroscience, 55*(2–4), 71–80. https://doi.org/ 10.3109/00207459008985952

Bomfim, A. J. D. L., Ferreira, B. L. C., Rodrigues, G. R., Pontes Neto, O. M., & Chagas, M. H. N. (2021). Lesion localization and performance on Theory of Mind tests in stroke survivors: A systematic review. *Archives of Clinical Psychiatry*, 47(5), 140–145. https://doi.org/10.1590/0101-60830000000250

Borgaro, S. R., & Prigatano, G. P. (2003). Modification of the Patient Competency Rating Scale for use on an acute neurorehabilitation unit: the PCRS-NR. *Brain Injury*, 17(10), 847–853. https://doi.org/10.1080/0269905031000089350

Bornhofen, C., & McDonald, S. (2008). Comparing strategies for treating emotion perception deficits in traumatic brain injury. *Journal of Head Trauma Rehabilitation*, 23(2), 103–115. https://doi.org/10.1097/01.HTR.0000314529.22777.43

Borod, J. C., Bloom, R. L., Brickman, A. M., Nakhutina, L., & Curko, E. A. (2002). Emotional processing deficits in individuals with unilateral brain damage. *Applied Neuropscyhology*, 9(1), 23–36. https://psycnet.apa.org/doi/10.1207/S15324826AN0901_4

Borod, J. C., Koff, E., Lorch, M. P., & Nicholas, M. (1985). Channels of emotional expression in patients with unilateral brain damage. *Archives of Neurology*, 42(4), 345–348. https://doi.org/10.1001/archneur.1985.04060040055011

Bouaffre, S., & Faita-Ainseba, F. (2007). Hemispheric differences in the time course of semantic priming processes: Evidence from event-related potentials (ERPs). *Brain and Cognition*, 63(2), 123–135. https://doi.org/10.1016/j.bandc.2006.10.006

Bowen, A., Hazelton, C., Pollock, A., & Lincoln, N. B. (2013). Cognitive rehabilitation for spatial neglect following stroke. *Cochrane Database of Systematic Reviews*, 2013(7), CD003586. https://doi.org/10.1002/14651858.cd003586.pub3

Bowen, A., McKenna, K., & Tallis, R. C. (1999). Reasons for variability in the reported rate of occurrence of unilateral spatial neglect after stroke. *Stroke*, 30(6), 1196–1202. https://doi.org/10.1161/01.str.30.6.1196

Bowers, D., Blonder, L., & Heilman, K. M. (1991). *The Florida Affect Battery*. Center for Neuropsychological Studies Cognitive Neuroscience Laboratory, University of Florida. http:/neurology.ufl.edu/files/2011/12/Florida-Affect-Battery-Manual.pdf

Brady, M., Armstrong, L., & Mackenzie, C. (2005). Further evidence on topic use following right hemisphere brain damage: Procedural and descriptive discourse. *Aphasiology*, 19(8), 731–747. https://doi.org/10.1080/02687030500141430

Brady, M., Armstrong, L., & Mackenzie, C. (2006). An examination over time of language and discourse production abilities following right hemisphere brain damage. *Journal of Neurolinguistics*, 19(4), 291–310. https://doi.org/10.1016/jneuroling.2005.12.001

Brady, M., Mackenzie, C., & Armstrong, L. (2003). Topic use following right hemisphere brain damage during three semi-structured conversational discourse samples. *Aphasiology*, 17(9), 881–904. https://doi.org/10.1080/02687030344000292

Brooks, J. L., Wong, Y., & Robertson, L. C. (2005). Crossing the midline: Reducing attentional deficits via interhemispheric interactions. *Neuropsychologia*, 43(4), 572–582. https://doi.org/10.1016/j.neuropsychologia.2004.07.009

Brookshire R. H., & Nicholas L. E. (1997). *Discourse Comprehension Test: Test manual (Revised)*. BRK.

Brownell, H., & Martino, G. (1998). Deficits in inference and social cognition: The effects of right hemisphere brain damage. In M. Beeman & C. Chiarello (Eds.), *Right hemisphere language comprehension: Perspectives from cognitive neuroscience* (pp. 309–328). Lawrence Erlbaum.

Brownell, H. H., Michel, D., Powelson, J., & Gardner, H. (1983). Surprise but not coherence: Sensitivity to verbal humor in right-hemisphere patients. *Brain and Language*, 18(1), 20–27. https://doi.org/10.1016/0093-934X(83)90002-0

Brownell, H. H., Potter, H. H., & Bihrle, A. M. (1986). Inference deficits in right brain damaged patients. *Brain and Language, 27*(2), 310–321. https://doi.org/10.1016/0093-934X(86)90022-2

Brownell, H. H., Potter, H. H., Mishelow, D., & Gardner, H. (1984). Sensitivity to lexical decision and connotation in brain damaged patients: A double dissociation? *Brain and Language, 22*, 253–265. https://doi.org/10.1016/0093-934x(84)90093-2

Brozzoli, C., Dematte, M. L., Pavani, F., Frassinetti, F., & Fame, A. (2006). Neglect and extinction: Within and between sensory modalities. *Restorative Neurology and Neuroscience, 24*(4–6), 217–232.

Bryan, K. (1994). *Right Hemisphere Language Battery-2*. John Wiley & Sons.

Burns, M. S. (1997). *Burns Brief Inventory of Communication and Cognition*. PsychCorp.

Butler, R. W., Copeland, D. R., Fairclough, D. L., Mulhern, R. K., Katz, E. R., Kazak, A. E., . . . Sahler, O. J. Z. (2008). A multicenter, randomized clinical trial of a cognitive remediation program for childhood survivors of a pediatric malignancy. *Journal of Consulting and Clinical Psychology, 76*(3), 367–378. https://doi.org/10.1037/0022-006x.76.3.367

Callaway, L., Winkler, D., Tippett, A., Herd, N., Migliorini, C., & Willer, B. (2016). The Community Integration Questionnaire-Revised: Australian normative data and measurement of electronic social networking. *Australian Occupational Therapy Journal, 63*(3), 143–153. https://doi.org/10.1111/1440-1630.12284

Cannizzaro, M. S., & Coehlo, C. A. (2002). Treatment of story grammar following traumatic brain injury: A pilot study. *Brain Injury, 16*(12), 1065–1073. https://doi.org/10.1080/02699050210155230

Cappa, S. F., Benke, T., Clarke, S., Rossi, B., Stemmer, B., & Heugten, C. M. (2005). EFNS guidelines on cognitive rehabilitation: Report of an EFNS task force. *European Journal of Neurology, 12*(9), 665–680. https://doi.org/10.1111/j.1468-1331.2005.01330.x

Casarin, F. S., Scherer, L. C., Ferré, P., Ska, B., de Mattos Parente, M. A. P., Joanette, Y., & Fonseca, R. P. (2013). Adaptação do protocole MEC de poche e da bateria MAC expandida: Bateria MAC breve. *Psico, 44*(2), 288–299.

Cassel, A., McDonald, S., Kelly, M., & Togher, L. (2019). Learning from the minds of others: A review of social cognition treatments and their relevance to traumatic brain injury. *Neuropsychological Rehabilitation, 29*(1), 22–55. https://doi.org/10.1080/09602011.2016.1257435

Champagne-Lavau, M., & Joanette, Y. (2009). Pragmatics, theory of mind and executive functions after a right-hemisphere lesion: Different patterns of deficits. *Journal of Neurolinguistics, 22*(5), 413–426. https://psycnet.apa.org/doi/10.1016/j.jneuroling.2009.02.002

Chantraine, Y., Joanette, Y., & Ska, B. (1998). Conversational abilities in patients with right hemisphere damage. *Journal of Neurolingusitics, 11*(1–2), 21–32. https://doi.org/10.1016/S0911-6044(98)00003-7

Chatterjee, A. (1994). Picturing unilateral spatial neglect: Viewer versus object centred reference frames. *Journal of Neurology, Neurosurgery, and Psychiatry, 57*(10), 1236–1240. https://doi.org/10.1136/jnnp.57.10.1236

Cheang, H. S., & Pell, M. D. (2006). A study of humour and communicative intention following right hemisphere stroke. *Clinical Linguistics & Phonetics, 20*(6), 447–462. https://doi.org/10.1080/02699200500135684

Chechlacz, M., Rotshtein, P., Demeyere, N., Bickerton, W. L., & Humphreys, G. W. (2014). The frequency and severity of extinction after stroke affecting different vascular territories. *Neuropsychologia, 54*(1), 11–17. https://doi.org/10.1016/j.neuropsychologia.2013.12.016

Chen, P., & Toglia, J. (2019). Online and offline awareness deficits: Anosognosia for spatial neglect. *Rehabilitation Psychology, 64*(1), 50–64. https://doi.org/10.1037/rep0000207

Cheng, S. K. W., & Man, D. W. K. (2006). Management of impaired self-awareness in persons with traumatic brain injury. *Brain Injury, 20*(6), 621–628. https://doi.org/10.1080/02699050600677196

Cherney, L. R. (2006). Ethical issues involving the right hemisphere stroke patient: To treat or not to treat? *Topics in Stroke Rehabilitation, 13*(4), 47–53. https://doi.org/10.1310/tsr1304-47

Cicerone, K. (2002). Remediation of "working attention" in mild traumatic brain injury. *Brain Injury, 16*(3), 185–195. https://doi.org/10.1080/02699050110103959

Cicerone, K. D. (2005). Methodological issues in evaluating the effectiveness of cognitive rehabilitation. In P. W. Halligan & D. T. Wade (Eds.), *Effectiveness of rehabilitation for cognitive deficits* (pp. 43–58). Oxford University Press.

Cicerone, K. D., Langenbahn, D. M., Braden, C., Malec, J. F., Kalmar, K., Fraas, M., . . . Ashman, T. (2011). Evidence-based cognitive rehabilitation: Updated review of the literature from 2003 through 2008. *Archives of Physical Medicine and Rehabilitation, 92*(4), 519–530. https://doi.org/10.1016/j.apmr.2010.11.015

Cimino, C. R., Verfaellie, M., Bowers, D., & Heilman, K. M. (1991). Autobiographical memory: Influence of right hemisphere damage in emotionality and specificity. *Brain and Cognition, 15*(1), 106–118. https://doi.org/10.1016/0278-2626(91)90019-5

Cocks, N., Hird, K., & Kirsner, K. (2007). The relationship between right hemisphere damage and gesture in spontaneous discourse. *Aphasiology, 21*(3–4), 299–319. https://doi.org/10.1080/02687030600911393

Coelho, C., Ylvisaker, M., & Turkstra, L. S. (2005, November). Nonstandardized assessment approaches for individuals with traumatic brain injuries. *Seminars in Speech and Language, 26*(4), 223–241. https://doi.org/10.1055/s-2005-922102

Copley, A., Smith, C., Finch, E., Fleming, J., & Cornwell, P. (2020). Does metacognitive strategy instruction improve impaired self-awareness in adults with cognitive-communication disorders following an acquired brain injury? *Speech, Language and Hearing, 25*(2), 1–13. https://doi.org/10.1080/2050571X.2020.1816403

Corbetta, M., & Shulman, G. L. (2011). Spatial neglect and attention networks. *Annual Review of Neuroscience, 34*, 569–599. https://doi.org/10.1146/annurev-neuro-061010-113731

Côté, H., Payer, M., Giroux, F., & Joanette, Y. (2007). Towards a description of clinical communication impairment profiles following right-hemisphere damage. *Aphasiology, 21*(6–8), 739–749. https://doi.org/10.1080/02687030701192331

Critchley, E. M. R. (1991). Speech and the right hemisphere. *Behavioural Neurology, 4*(3), 143–151. https://doi.org/10.3233/BEN-1991-4302

Crosson, B., Barco, P. P., Velozo, C. A., Bolesta, M. M., Cooper, P. V., Werts, D., & Brobeck, T. C. (1989). Awareness and compensation in post-acute head injury rehabilitation. *Journal of Head Trauma Rehabilitation, 4*(3), 46–54. https://doi.org/10.1097/00001199-198909000-00008

Cubelli, R., Guiducci, A., & Consolmagno, P. (2000). Afferent dysgraphia after right cerebral stroke: An autonomous syndrome? *Brain and Cognition, 44*(3), 629–644. https://doi.org/10.1006/brcg.2000.1239

Dai, C. Y., Liu, W. M., Chen, S. W., Yang, C. A., Tung, Y. C., Chou, L. W., & Lin, L. C. (2014). Anosognosia, neglect and quality of life of right hemisphere stroke survivors. *European Journal of Neurology, 21*(5), 797–801. https://doi.org/10.1111/ene.12413

D'Alisa, S., Baudo, S., Mauro, A., & Miscio, G. (2005). How does stroke restrict participation in long-term post-stroke survivors? *Acta Neurologica Scandinavia, 112*(3), 157–162. https://doi.org/10.1111/j.1600-0404.2005.00466.x

Dara, C., Bang, J., Gottesman, R. F., & Hillis, A. E. (2014). Right hemisphere dysfunction is better predicted by emotional prosody impairments as compared to neglect. *Journal of Neurology and Translational Neuroscience*, 2(1), 1037. https://www.ncbi.nlm.nih.gov/pmc/articles/PMC4059678/

Davidson, C. S., & Wallace, S. E. (2022). Information needs for carers following a family member's right hemisphere stroke. *Aphasiology*, 36(3), 291–316. https://doi.org/10.1080/02687038.2021.1873906

Davis, G. A., O'Neil-Pirozzi, T. M., & Coon, M. (1997). Referential cohesion and logical coherence of narration after right hemisphere stroke. *Brain and Language*, 56(2), 183–210. https://doi.org/10.1006/brln.1997.1741

DeGutis, J. M., & Van Vleet, T. M. (2010). Tonic and phasic alertness training: A novel behavioral therapy to improve spatial and non-spatial attention in patients with hemispatial neglect. *Frontiers in Human Neuroscience*, 4, 1–17. https://doi.org/10.3389/fnhum.2010.00060

de Haan, B., Karnath, H.-O., & Driver, J. (2012). Mechanisms and anatomy of unilateral extinction after brain injury. *Neuropsychologia*, 50(6), 1045–1053. https://doi.org/10.1016/j.neuropsychologia.2012.02.015

Delis, D. C., Wapner, W., Gardner, H., & Moses, J. A. J. (1983). The contribution of the right hemisphere to the organization of paragraphs. *Cortex*, 19(1), 43–50. https://doi.org/10.1016/s0010-9452(83)80049-5

Diggs, C. C., & Basili, A. G. (1987). Verbal expression of right cerebrovascular accident patients: Convergent and divergent language. *Brain and Language*, 30(1), 130–146. https://doi.org/10.1016/0093-934x(87)90033-2

Dintén-Fernández, A., Fernández-González, P., Koutsou, A., Alguacil-Diego, I. M., Laguarta-Val, S., & Molina-Rueda, F. (2018). Top-down and bottom-up approaches for the treatment of unilateral spatial neglect in stroke patients: A sys-

tematic review. *Rehabilitacion*, 53(2), 93–103.

Douglas, D., Bracy, C., & Snow, P. (2007). Measuring perceived communicative ability after traumatic brain injury: reliability and validity of the La Trobe Communication Questionnaire. *Journal of Head Trauma Rehabilitation*, 22(1), 31–38. https://doi.org/10.1097/00001199-200701000-00004

Durfee, A. Z., Sheppard, S. M., Blake, M. L., & Hillis, A. E. (2021). Lesion loci of impaired affective prosody: A systematic review of evidence from stroke. *Brain and Cognition*, 152, 105759. https://doi.org/10.1016/j.bandc.2021.105759

Durfee, A. Z., Sheppard, S. M., Meier, E. L., Bunker, L., Cui, E., Crainiceanu, C., & Hillis, A. E. (2021). Explicit training to improve affective prosody recognition in adults with acute right hemisphere stroke. *Brain Sciences*, 11(5), 667. https://doi.org/10.3390/brainsci11050667

Eisenson, J. (1962). Language and intellectual modifications associated with right cerebral damage. *Language and Speech*, 5(2), 49–53. https://doi.org/10.1177/002383096200500201

Ellis, A. W. (1998). Normal writing processes and peripheral acquired dysgraphias. *Language and Cognitive Processes*, 3(2), 99–127. https://doi.org/10.1080/01690968808402084

Ellmo, W. J. (1995). *Measure of Cognitive-Linguistic Abilities*. The Speech Bin.

Eramudugolla, R., Irvine, D. R. F., & Mattingley, J. B. (2007). Association between auditory and visual symptoms of unilateral spatial neglect. *Neuropsychologia*, 45, 2631–2637. https://doi.org/10.1016/j.neuropsychologia.2007.03.015

Esposito, E., Shekhtman, G., & Chen, P. (2021). Prevalence of spatial neglect post-stroke: A systematic review. *Annals of Physical and Rehabilitation Medicine*, 64(5), 101459. https://doi.org/10.1016/j.rehab.2020.10.010

Ethofer, T., Anders, S., Wiethoff, S., Erb, M., Herbert, C., Saur, R., . . . Wildgruber,

O. (2006). Effects of prosodic emotional intensity on activation of associative auditory cortex. *NeuroReport, 17*(3), 249–253. https://doi.org/10.1097/01.wnr.0000199466.32036.5d

Ferber, S., Ruppel, J., & Danckert, J. (2020). Visual working memory deficits following right brain damage. *Brain and Cognition, 142*, 105566. https://doi.org/10.1016/j.bandc.2020.105566

Ferré, P., & Basaglia-Pappas, S. (2015). *Protocole Montréal d'évaluation de la Communication de Poche (protocole MEC-P ET I-MEC Fr)*. Ortho Édition.

Ferré, P., Fonseca, R. P., Ska, B., & Joanette, Y. (2012). Communicative clusters after a right-hemisphere stroke: Are there universal clinical profiles? *Folia Phoniatrica et Logopaedica, 64*(4), 199–207. https://doi.org/10.1159/000340017

Ferré, P., & Joanette, Y. (2016). Communication abilities following right hemisphere damage: Prevalence, evaluation, and profiles. *Perspectives of the ASHA Special Interest Groups, 1*(2), 106–115. https://doi.org/10.1044/persp1.SIG2.106

Fleming, J. M., Strong, J., & Ashton, R. (1996). Self-awareness of deficits in adults with traumatic brain injury: How best to measure? *Brain Injury, 10*(1), 1–16. https://psycnet.apa.org/doi/10.1080/026990596124674

Folstein, M. F., Folstein, S. E., & McHugh, P. R. (1975). "Mini-mental state": A practical method for grading the cognitive state of patients for the clinician. *Journal of Psychiatric Research, 12*(3), 189–198. https://doi.org/10.1016/0022-3956(75)90026-6

Fortis, P., Maravita, A., Gallucci, M., Ronchi, R., Grassi, E., Senna, I., . . . Vallar, G. (2010). Rehabilitating patients with left spatial neglect by prism exposure during a visuomotor activity. *Neuropsychology, 24*(6), 681–697. https://doi.org/10.1037/a0019476

Gabbatore, I., Sacco, K., Angeleri, R., Zettin, M., Bara, B. G., & Bosco, F. M. (2015). Cognitive pragmatic treatment: A reha-bilitative program for traumatic brain injury individuals. *Journal of Head Trauma Rehabilitation, 30*(5), E14–E28. https://doi.org/10.1097/htr.0000000000000087

Gainotti, G. (2012). Unconscious processing of emotions and the right hemisphere. *Neuropsychologia, 50*(2), 205–218. https://doi.org/10.1016/j.neuropsychologia.2011.12.005

Gainotti, G., Caltagirone, C., & Miceli, G. (1983). Selective impairment of semantic-lexical discrimination in right-brain-damaged patients. *Brain and Language, 13*(2), 201–211. https://doi.org/10.1016/0093-934x(81)90090-0

Garcia, E. L., Ferré, P., & Joanette, Y. (2021). Right-hemisphere language disorders. In L. Cummings (Ed.) *Handbook of pragmatic language disorders: Complex and underserved populations* (pp. 313–334). Springer.

Gardner, H., & Denes, G. (1973). Connotative judgements by aphasic patients on a pictorial adaptation of the semantic differential. *Cortex, 9*(2), 183–196. https://doi.org/10.1016/s0010-9452(73)80027-9

Gardner, H., Silverman, J., Wapner, W., & Zurif, E. (1978). The appreciation of antonymic contrasts in aphasia. *Brain and Language, 6*(3), 301–317. https://doi.org/10.1016/0093-934x(78)90064-0

Garrod, S., Brien, E. J. O., Morris, R. K., & Rayner, K. (1990). Elaborative inferencing as an active or passive process. *Journal of Experimental Psychology: Learning, Memory, and Cognition, 16*(2), 250–257. https://psycnet.apa.org/doi/10.1037/0278-7393.16.2.250

Gernsbacher, M. A. (1990). *Language comprehension as structure building*. Psychology Press.

Giacino, J. T., & Cicerone, K. D. (1998). Varieties of deficit unawareness after brain injury. *Journal of Head Trauma Rehabilitation, 13*(5), 1–15. https://doi.org/10.1097/00001199-199810000-00003

Gillen, R., Tennen, H., & McKee, T. (2005). Unilateral spatial neglect: Relation to rehabilitation outcomes in patients with right hemisphere stroke. *Archives of Physical Medicine and Rehabilitation, 86*, 763–767. https://doi.org/10.1016/j.apmr.2004.10.029

Gillespie, D. C., Bowen, A., & Foster, J. K. (2006). Memory impairment following right hemisphere stroke: A comparative meta-analytic and narrative review. *The Clinical Neuropsychologist, 20*(1), 59–75. https://doi.org/10.1080/13854040500203308

Gokhale, S., Lahoti, S., & Caplan, L. R. (2013). The neglected neglect: Auditory neglect. *JAMA Neurology, 70*(8), 1065–1069. https://psycnet.apa.org/doi/10.1001/jamaneurol.2013.155

Goksun, T., Lehet, M., Malykhina, K., & Chatterjee, A. (2013). Naming and gesturing spatial relations: Evidence from focal brain-injured individuals. *Neuropsychologia, 51*(8), 1518–1527. https://doi.org/10.1016/j.neuropsychologia.2013.05.006

Golden, C. J., Espe-Pfeifer, P., & Wachsler-Felder, J. (2000). *Neuropsychological interpretation of objective psychological tests.* Kluwer Academic/Plenum.

Goverover, Y., Johnston, M. V, Toglia, J., & Deluca, J. (2007). Treatment to improve self-awareness in persons with acquired brain injury. *Brain Injury, 21*(9), 913–923. https://doi.org/10.1080/02699050701553205

Graesser, A. C., Singer, M., & Trabasso, T. (1994). Constructing inferences during narrative text comprehension. *Psychological Review, 101*(3), 371–395. https://psycnet.apa.org/doi/10.1037/0033-295X.101.3.371

Griffin, R., Friedman, O., Ween, J., Winner, E., Happe, F., & Brownell, H. H. (2006). Theory of mind and the right cerebral hemisphere: Refining the scope of impairment. *Laterality, 11*(3), 195–225. https://doi.org/10.1080/13576500500450552

Habermas, J., McCarthy, T., & McCarthy, T. (1984). *The theory of communicative action* (Vol. 1, p. 308). Beacon.

Halper, A. S., Cherney, L. R., & Burns, M. S. (2010). *The Rehabilitation Institute of Chicago Evaluation of Communication Problems in Right Hemisphere Dysfunction* (3rd ed.). Rehabilitation Institute of Chicago.

Hamilton, J., Radlak, B., Morris, P. G., & Phillips, L. H. (2017). Theory of mind and executive functioning following stroke. *Archives of Clinical Neuropsychology, 32*(5), 507–518. https://doi.org/10.1093/arclin/acx035

Happe, F., Brownell, H. H., & Winner, E. (1999). Acquired 'theory of mind' impairments following stroke. *Cognition, 70*(3), 211–240. https://doi.org/10.1016/s0010-0277(99)00005-0

Heilman, K. M., Watson, R. T., & Valenstein, E. (1985). Neglect and related disorders. In K. M. Heilman & E. Valenstein (Eds.), *Clinical neuropsychology* (2nd ed., pp. 243–293). Oxford University Press.

Helm-Estabrooks, N. (2017). *Cognitive linguistic Quick Test: CLQT.* Psychological Corporation.

Henderson, A., Roeschlein, M. A., & Wrigth, H. H. (2020). Improving discourse following traumatic brain injury: A tale of two treatments. *Seminars in Speech and Language, 41*(5), 365–382. https://doi.org/10.1055/s-0040-1712116

Hewetson, R., Cornwell, P., & Shum, D. (2017). Cognitive-communication disorder following right hemisphere stroke: Exploring rehabilitation access and outcomes. *Topics in Stroke Rehabilitation, 24*(5), 330–336. https://doi.org/10.1080/10749357.2017.1289622

Hewetson, R., Cornwell, P., & Shum, D. (2018). Social participation following right hemisphere stroke: Influence of a cognitive-communication disorder. *Aphasiology, 32*(2), 164–182. https://doi.org/10.1080/02687038.2017.1315045

Hewetson, R., Cornwell, P., & Shum, D. H. K. (2021). Relationship and social network change in people with impaired social cognition post right hemisphere stroke. *American Journal of Speech-Language*

Pathology, 30(S2), 962. https://doi.org/10.1044/2020_AJSLP-20-00047

Hewetson, R., Covich, R., Cornwell, P., Ferré, P., Love, A., Joanette, Y., & McDonald, S. (2023, May). *Pocket MEC: A cognitive-communication screening test supported by Australian norms.* Speech Pathology Australia Conference Abstract, Tasmania.

Higginbotham, J., & Satchidanand, A. (2019). *From triangle to diamond: Recognizing and using data to inform our evidence-based practice.* ASHA Journals. https://academy.pubs.asha.org/2019/04/from-triangle-to-diamond-recognizing-and-using-data-to-inform-our-evidence-based-practice/

Hillis, A. E. (2006). Rehabilitation of unilateral spatial neglect: New insights from magnetic resonance perfusion imaging. *Archives of Physical Medicine and Rehabilitation, 87*(12, Suppl.), 43–49. https://doi.org/10.1016/j.apmr.2006.08.331

Hillis, A. E. (2023). *Hillis Post-stroke Prosody Battery.* https://score.jhmi.edu/downloads.html

Hillis, A. E., Mordkoff, J. T., & Caramazza, A. (1999). Mechanisms of spatial attention revealed by hemispatial neglect. *Cortex, 35*(3),433–442. https://doi.org/10.1016/s0010-9452(08)70811-6

Hillis, A. E., Newhart, M., Heidler, J., Barker, P. B., Herskovits, E. H., & Degaonkar, M. (2005). Anatomy of spatial attention: Insights from perfusion imaging and hemispatial neglect in acute stroke. *Journal of Neuroscience, 25*(12), 3161–3167. https://doi.org/10.1523/jneurosci.4468-04.2005

Hillis, A. E., & Tippett, D. C. (2014). Stroke recovery: Surprising influences and residual consequences. *Advances in Medicine, 2014,* 378263. https://doi.org/10.1155/2014/378263

Hillis Trupe, E., & Hillis, A. (1985). Paucity vs. verbosity: Another analysis of right hemisphere communication deficits. *Clinical Aphasiology, 15,* 83–96. http://aphasiology.pitt.edu/id/eprint/841

Hoerold, D., Pender, N. P., & Robertson, I. H. (2013). Metacognitive and online error awareness deficits after prefrontal cortex lesions. *Neuropsychologia, 51*(3), 385–391. https://psycnet.apa.org/doi/10.1016/j.neuropsychologia.2012.11.019

Holland, A., Fromm, D., & Wozniak, L. (2018). *Communication Activities of Daily Living (3rd ed.).* Pro-Ed.

Honan, C. A., McDonald, S., Sufani, C., Hine, D. W., & Kumfor, F. (2016). The Awareness of Social Iinference test: Development of a shortened version for use in adults with acquired brain injury. *The Clinical Neuropsychologist, 30*(2), 243–264. https://psycnet.apa.org/doi/10.1080/13854046.2015.1136691

Hough, M. (1990). Narrative comprehension in adults with right and left hemisphere brain damage: Theme organisation. *Brain and Language, 38*(2), 253–277. https://doi.org/10.1016/0093-934X(90)90114-V

Jehkonen, M., Ahonen, J.-P., Dastidar, P., Koivisto, A.-M., Laippala, P., Vilkki, J., & Molnar, G. (2001). Predictors of discharge to home during the first year after right hemisphere stroke. *Acta Neurologica Scandinavica, 104*(3), 136–141. https://doi.org/10.1034/j.1600-0404.2001.00025.x

Joanette, Y., & Ansaldo, A. I. (1999). Clinical note: Acquired pragmatic impairments and aphasia. *Brain and Language, 68*(3), 529–534. https://doi.org/10.1006/brln.1999.2126

Joanette, Y., Goulet, P., Ska, B., & Nespoulous, J.-L. (1986). Informative content of narrative discourse in right-brain-damaged right-handers. *Brain and Language, 29*(1), 81–105. https://doi.org/10.1016/0093-934X(86)90035-0

Joanette, Y., Ska, B., & Côté, H. (2004). *Protocole Montréal d'Évaluation de la Communication.* Ortho Édition.

Joanette, Y., Ska, B., Côté, H., Ferré, P., LaPointe, L., Coppens, P., & Small, S. L. (2015). *The Montreal Protocol for the Evaluation of Communication (MEC).* Australasian Society for the Study of Brain Impairment.

Kaplan, E., Goodglass, H., & Weintraub, S. (2001). *Boston Naming Test* (2nd ed.). Pro-Ed.

Karnath, H-O., Fruhmann Berger, M., Kuker, W., & Rarden, C. (2004). The anatomy of spatial neglect based on voxelwise statistical analysis: A study of 140 patients. *Cerebral Cortex*, *14*(10), 1164–1172. https://doi.org/10.1093/cercor/bhh076

Katz, N., Hartman-Maeir, A., Ring, H., & Soroker, N. (2000). Relationships of cognitive performance and daily function of clients following right hemisphere stroke: Predictive and ecological validity of the LOTCA battery. *The Occupational Therapy Journal of Research*, *20*(1), 3–17. https://psycnet.apa.org/record/2000-13701-001

Kaufmann, B. C., Cazzoli, D., Bartolomeo, P., Frey, J., Pflugshaupt, T., Knobel, S. E. J., . . . Nyffeler, T. (2022). Auditory spatial cueing reduces neglect after right-hemispheric stroke: A proof of concept study. *Cortex*, *148*, 152–167. https://doi.org/10.1016/j.cortex.2021.12.009

Keerativittayayut, R., Aoki, R., Taghizadeh Sarabi, M., Jimura, K., & Nakahara, K. (2018). Large-scale network integration in the human brain tracks temporal fluctuations in memory encoding performance. *ELife*, *7*, e32696. https://doi.org/10.7554/eLife.32696

Kelly, S. D., Barr, D. J., Church, R. B.& Lynch, K. (1999). Offering a hand to pragmatic understanding: The role of speech and gesture in comprehension and memory. *Journal of Memory and Language*, *40*(4), 577–592. https://doi.org/10.1006/jmla.1999.2634

Kennedy, M. R. (2000). Topic scenes in conversations with adults with right-hemisphere brain damage. *American Journal of Speech-Language Pathology*, *9*(1), 72–86. https://doi.org/10.1044/1058-0360.0901.72

Kenzie, J. M., Girgulis, K. A., Semrau, J. A., Findlater, S. E., Desai, J. A., & Dukelow, S. P. (2015). Lesion sites associated with allocentric and egocentric visuospatial neglect in acute stroke. *Brain Connectivity*, *5*(7), 413–422. https://psycnet.apa.org/doi/10.1089/brain.2014.0316

Kerkhoff, G., & Schenk, T. (2012). Rehabilitation of neglect: An update. *Neuropsychologia*, *50*(6), 1072–1079. https://doi.org/10.1016/j.neuropsychologia.2012.01.024

Kessels, R. P., Kappelle, L. J., de Haan, E. H., & Postma, A. (2002). Lateralization of spatial-memory processes: Evidence on spatial span, maze learning, and memory for object locations. *Neuropsychologia*, *40*(8), 1465–1473. https://doi.org/10.1016/s0028-3932(01)00199-3

Kiefer, R. F. (1993). The role of predictive inferences in situation model construction. *Discourse Processes*, *16*(1–2), 99–124. https://doi.org/10.1080/01638539309544831

Kim, Y. J., Jeong, H. Y., Choi, H. C., Sohn, J. H., Kim, C., Lee, S. H., . . . Yoon, J. H. (2022). Effect of right hemispheric damage on structured spoken conversation. *PLoS ONE*, *17*(8), e0271727. https://doi.org/10.1371/journal.pone.0271727

Kotz, S. A., Kalberlah, C., Bahlmann, J., Friederici, A. D., & Haynes, J.-D. (2013). Predicting vocal emotion expressions from the human brain. *Human Brain Mapping*, *34*(8), 1971–1981. https://doi.org/10.1002/hbm.22041

Kucharska-Pietura, K., Nikolaou, V., Masiak, M., & Treasure, J. (2004). The recognition of emotion in the faces and voice of anorexia nervosa. *International Journal of Eating Disorders*, *35*(1), 42–47. https://doi.org/10.1002/eat.10219

Lê, L., Coehlo, C., & Fiszdon, J. (2022). Systematic review of discourse and social communication interventions in traumatic brain injury. *American Journal of Speech-Language Pathology*, *31*(2), 991–1022. https://doi.org/10.1044/2021_AJSLP-21-00088

Lehman-Blake, M. T., & Tompkins, C. A. (2001). Predictive inferencing in adults with right hemisphere brain damage. *Journal of Speech, Language, and Hearing Research, 44,* 639–654. https://doi.org/10.1044/1092-4388(2001/052)

Leon, S. A., Rosenbek, J. C., Crucian, G. P., Hieber, B., Holiway, B., Rodriguez, A. D., . . . Gonzalez-Rothi, L. (2004). Active treatments for aprosodia secondary to right hemisphere stroke. *Journal of Rehabilitation Research and Development, 41*(1), 93. https://doi.org/10.1682/JRRD.2003.12.0182

Leonard, C. L., & Baum, S. R. (2005). Research note: The ability of individuals with right-hemisphere damage to use context under conditions of focused and divided attention. *Journal of Neurolinguistics, 18*(6), 427–441. https://doi.org/10.1016/j.jneuroling.2005.03.001

Leonard, C. L., Waters, G. S., & Caplan, D. (1997). The use of contextual information related to general world knowledge by right brain-damaged individuals in pronoun resolution. *Brain and Language, 57*(57), 343–359. https://doi.org/10.1006/brln.1997.1744

Levine, D. A., Galecki, A. T., Langa, K. M., Unverzagt, F. W., Kabeto, M. U., Giordani, B., & Wadley, V. G. (2015). Trajectory of cognitive decline after incident stroke. *JAMA, 314*(1), 41–51. https://doi.org/10.1001/jama.2015.6968

Lindell, A. B., Jalas, M. J., Tenovuo, O., Brunila, T., Voeten, M. J. M., & Hamalainen, H. (2007). Clinical assessment of hemispatial neglect: Evaluation of different measures and dimensions. *The Clinical Neuropsychologist, 21*(3), 479–497. https://doi.org/10.1080/13854040600630061

Linscott, R., & Knight, R. (2018). *Profile of pragmatic impairment in communication.* Lulu Publishing.

Lo, R. S., Cheng, J. O., Wong, E. M., Tang, W. K., Wong, L. K., Woo, J., & Kwok, T. (2008). Handicap and its determinants of change in stroke survivors: One-year follow-up study. *Stroke, 39*(1), 148–153. https://doi.org/10.1161/strokeaha.107.491399

Luauté, J., Halligan, P., Rode, G., Rossetti, Y., & Boisson, D. (2006). Visuo-spatial neglect: A systematic review of current interventions and their effectiveness. *Neuroscience and Biobehavioral Reviews, 30*(7), 961–982. https://doi.org/10.1016/j.neubiorev.2006.03.001

Lundgren, K., Brownell, H. H., Cayer-Meade, C., Milione, J., & Kearns, K. (2011). Treating metaphor interpretation deficits subsequent to right hemisphere brain damage: Preliminary results. *Aphasiology, 5*(4), 456–474. https://doi.org/10.1080/02687038.2010.500809

Luukkainen-Markkula, R., Tarkka, I. M., Pitkanen, K., Sivenius, J., & Hamalainen, H. (2009). Rehabilitation of hemispatial neglect: A randomized study using either arm activation or visual scanning training. *Restorative Neurology and Neuroscience, 27*(6), 663–672. https://doi.org/10.3233/RNN-2009-0520

Lyden, P., Lu, M. Jackson, C., Marler, J., Kothari, R., Brott, T., & Zivin, J. (1999). Underlying structure of the National Institutes of Health Stroke Scale: Results of a factor analysis. *Stroke, 30*(11), 2347–2354. https://doi.org/10.1161/01.STR.30.11.2347

Macdonald, S., & Johnson, C. J. (2005). Assessment of subtle cognitive communication deficits following acquired brain injury: A normative study of the Functional Assessment of Verbal Reasoning and Executive Strategies (FAVRES). *Brain Injury, 19*(11), 895–902. https://doi.org/10.1080/02699050400004294

Mackenzie, C., Begg, T., Brady, M., & Lees, K. R. (1997). The effects on verbal communication skills of right hemisphere stroke in middle age. *Aphasiology, 11*(10), 929–945. https://doi.org/10.1080/02687039708249420

Mackenzie, C., Begg, T., Lees, K. R., & Brady, M. (1999). The communication effects of right brain damage on the very old and the not so old. *Journal of Neurolinguistics, 12*, 79–93. https://doi.org/10.1016/S0911-6044(99)00004-4

Mackisack, E. L., Myers, P. S., & Duffy, J. R. (1987). Verbosity and labelling behavior: The performance of right hemisphere and non-brain-damaged adults on an inferential picture description task. In R. H. Brookshire (Ed.) *Clinical aphasiology conference proceedings* (pp. 143–151). BRK Publishers.

Marini, A., Carlomagno, S., Caltagirone, C., & Nocentini, U. (2005). The role played by the right hemisphere in the organization of complex textual structures. *Brain and Language, 93*(1), 46–54. https://10.1016/j.bandl.2004.08.002

Martin, I., & McDonald, S. (2003). Weak coherence, no theory of mind, or executive dysfunction? Solving the puzzle of pragmatic language disorders. *Brain and Language, 85*(3), 451–466. https://doi.org/10.1016/S0093-934X(03)00070-1

Martin, I., & McDonald, S. (2006). That can't be right! What causes pragmatic language impairment following right hemisphere damage? *Brain Impairment, 7*(3), 202–211. https://doi.org/10.1375/brim.7.3.202

Matsuki, K., Chow, T., Hare, M., Elman, J. L., Scheepers, C., & McRae, K. (2011). Event-based plausibility immediately influences on-line language comprehension. *Journal of Experimental Psychology: Learning, Memory, and Cognition, 37*(4), 913–934. https://doi.org/10.1037/a0022964

McCluskey, G., Wade, C., McKee, J., McCarron, P., McVerry, F., & McCarron, M. O. (2016). Stroke laterality bias in the management of acute ischemic stroke. *Journal of Stroke and Cerebrovascular Diseases, 25*(11), 2701–2707. https://doi.org/10.1016/j.jstrokecerebrovasdis.2016.07.019

McDonald, S. (2000). Exploring the cognitive basis of right-hemisphere pragmatic language disorders. *Brain and Language,* 75(1), 82–107. https://doi.org/10.1006/brln.2000.2342

McDonald, S., Flanagan, S., & Rollins, J. (2003). *The Awareness of Social Inference Test (TASIT).* Australasian Society for the Study of Brain Impairment.

McDonald, S., Togher, L., & Code, C. (2013). *Social and communication disorders following traumatic brain injury.* Psychology Press.

McKay, C., Rapport, L. J., Coleman Bryer, R., & Casey, J. (2011). Self-evaluation of driving simulator performance after stroke. *Topics in Stroke Rehabilitation, 18*(5), 549–561. https://doi.org/10.1310/tsr1805-549

McKoon, G., & Ratcliff, R. (1992). Inference during reading. *Psychological Review, 99*(3), 440–466. https://psycnet.apa.org/doi/10.1037/0033-295X.99.3.440

Menon, V., & D'Esposito, M. (2022). The role of PFC networks in cognitive control and executive function. *Neurpsychopharmacology, 47*, 90–103. https://doi.org/10.1038/s41386-021-01153-w

Mesulam, M.-M. (2000). Attentional networks, confusional states and neglect syndromes. In M. M. Mesulam (Ed.). *Principles of behavioral and cognitive neurology* (2nd ed., pp. 174–256). Oxford University Press.

Meulenbroek, P., Ness, B., Lemoncello, R., Byom, L., MacDonald, S., O'Neil-Pirozzi, T. M., & Moore Sohlberg, M. (2019). Social communication following traumatic brain injury part 2: Identifying effective treatment ingredients. *International Journal of Speech-Language Pathology, 21*(2), 128–142. https://doi.org/10.1080/17549507.2019.1583281

Middleton, L. E., Lam, B., Fahrni, H., Black, S. E., McIlroy, W. E., Stuss, D. T., . . . Turner, G. R. (2014). Frequency of domain-specific cognitive impairment in sub-acute and chronic stroke. *NeuroRehabilitation, 34*(2), 305–312. https://doi.org/10.3233/nre-131030

Milders, M., Fuchs, S., & Crawford, J. R. (2003). Neuropsychological impairments and changes in emotional and social behaviour following severe traumatic brain injury. *Journal of Clinical and Experimental Neuropsychology, 25*(2), 157–172. https://doi.org/10.1076/jcen.25.2.157.13642

Minga, J., Johnson, M., Blake, M. L., Fromm, D., & McWhinney, B. (2021). Making sense of right hemisphere discourse using RHDBank. *Topics in Language Disorders, 4*(1), 99–122. https://doi.org/10.1097/tld.0000000000000244

Minga, J., Sheppard, S. M., Johnson, M., Hewetson, R., Cornwell, P., & Blake, M. L. (2023). Apragmatism: The renewal of a label for communication disorders associated with right hemisphere brain damage. *International Journal of Language & Communication Disorders, 58*(2), 651–666. https://doi.org/10.1111/1460-6984.12807

Mioshi, E., Dawson, K., Mitchell, J., Arnold, R., & Hodges, J. R. (2006). The Addenbrooke's Cognitive Examination Revised (ACE-R): A brief cognitive test battery for dementia screening. *International Journal of Geriatric Psychiatry, 21*(11), 1078–1085. https://doi.org/10.1002/gps.1610

Mitrushina, M., Boone, K. B., Razani, J., & D'Elia, L. F. (2005). *Handbook of normative data for neuropsychological assessment.* Oxford University Press.

Monetta, L., & Joanette, Y. (2003). Specificity of the right hemisphere's contribution to verbal communication: The cognitive resources hypothesis. *Journal of Medical Speech-Language Pathology, 11*(4), 203–211.

Monetta, L., Ouellet-Plamondon, C., & Joanette, Y. (2006). Simulating the pattern of right-hemisphere-damaged patients for the processing of the alternative metaphorical meanings of words: Evidence in favor of a cognitive resources hypothesis. *Brain and Language, 96*(2), 171–177. https://doi.org/10.1016/j.bandl.2004.10.014

Morin, A. (2016). The "self-awareness-anosognosia" paradox explained: How can one process be associated with activation of, and damage to, opposite sides of the brain. *Laterality: Asymmetries of Body, Brain and Cognition, 22*(1), 105–119. https://doi.org/10.1080/1357650X.2016.1173049

Moya, K. L., Benowitz, L. I., Levine, D. N., & Finklestein, S. (1986). Covariant defects in visuospatial abilities and recall of verbal narrative after right hemisphere stroke. *Cortex, 22*(3), 381–397. https://doi.org/10.1016/s0010-9452(86)80003-x

Myers, P. S. (1978). Analysis of right hemisphere communication deficits: Implications for speech pathology. *Aphasiology,* 1–7. http://aphasiology.pitt.edu/414/

Myers, P. S. (1979). Profiles of communication deficits in patients with right cerebral hemisphere damage: Implications for diagnosis and treatment. In R H. Brookshire (Ed.). *Clinical aphasiology conference proceedings* (pp. 38–46). BRK Publishers.

Myers, P. S. (1990). Inference failure: The underlying impairment in right-hemisphere communication disorders. In T. E. Prescott (Ed.), *Clinical aphasiology conference proceedings* (pp. 167–180). Pro-Ed.

Myers, P. S. (1999). *Right hemisphere damage: Disorders of communication and cognition.* Singular Publishing.

Myers, P. S. (2001). Toward a definition of RHD syndrome. *Aphasiology, 15*(10–11), 913–918. https://doi.org/10.1080/02687040143000285

Myers, P. S., & Linebaugh, C. W. (1981). Comprehension of idiomatic expressions by right-hemisphere-damaged adults. In R. Brookshire (Ed.), *Clinical aphasiology conference proceedings* (pp. 254–261). BRK Publishers.

Nakamura, A., Maess, B., Knösche, T. R., & Friederici, A. D. (2014). Different hemispheric roles in recognition of happy expressions. *PLoS ONE, 9*(2), e88628. https://doi.org/10.1371/journal.pone.0088628

Nasreddine, Z. S., Phillips, N. A., Bédirian, V., Charbonneau, S., Whitehead, V., Collin, I., . . . Chertkow, H. (2005). The

Montreal Cognitive Assessment, MoCA: A brief screening tool for mild cognitive impairment. *Journal of the American Geriatrics Society, 53*(4), 695–699. https://doi.org/10.1111/j.1532-5415.2005.53221.x

Nebel, K., Wiese, H., Stude, P., de Greiff, A., Diener, H., & Keidel, M. (2005). On the neural basis of focused and divided attention. *Cognitive Brain Research, 25,* 760–776. https://doi.org/10.1016/j.cogbrainres.2005.09.011

Neumann, D., Babbage, D. R., Zupan, B., & Willer, B. (2015). A randomized controlled trial of emotion recognition training after traumatic brain injury. *The Journal of Head Trauma Rehabilitation, 30*(3), E12–E23. https://doi.org/10.1097/htr.0000000000000054

Newport, R., & Schenk, T. (2012). Prisms and neglect: What have we learned? *Neuropsychologia, 50*(6), 1080–1091. https://doi.org/10.1016/j.neuropsychologia.2012.01.023

Niemeier, J. P., Cifu, D. X., & Kishore, R. (2001). The Lighthouse Strategy: Improving the functional status of patients with unilateral neglect after stroke and brain injury using a visual imagery intervention. *Topics in Stroke Rehabilitation, 8,* 10–18. https://doi.org/10.1310/7UKK-HJ0F-GDWF-HHM8

Northcott, S., & Hilari, K. (2013). Stroke Social Network Scale: Development and psychometric evaluation of a new patient-reported measure. *Clinical Rehabilitation, 27*(9), 823–833. https://doi.org/10.1177/0269215513479388

O'Connell, K., Marsh, A. A., Edwards, D. F., Dromerick, A. W., & Seydell-Greenwald, A. (2021). Emotion recognition impairments and social well-being following right-hemisphere stroke. *Neuropsychological Rehabilitation, 23*(7), 1–19. https://doi.org/10.1080/09602011.2021.1888756

Orfei, M. O., Robinson, R. G., Prigatano, G. P., Starkstein, S., Rusch, N., Bria, P., . . . Spalletta, G. (2007). Anosognosia for hemiplegia after stroke is a multifaceted phenomenon: A systematic review of the literature. *Brain, 130*(Pt. 12), 3075–3090. https://doi.org/10.1093/brain/awm106

Osborne-Crowley, K., & McDonald, S. (2016). Hyposmia, not emotion perception, is associated with psychosocial outcome after severe traumatic brain injury. *Neuropsychology, 37*(7), 820–829. https://doi.org/10.1037/neu0000293

Park, Y. H., Jang, J. W., Park, S. Y., Wang, M. J., Lim, J. S., Baek, M. J., . . . Kim, S. (2015). Executive function as a strong predictor of recovery from disability in patients with acute stroke: A preliminary study. *Journal of Stroke and Cerebrovascular Diseases, 24*(3), 554–561. https://doi.org/10.1016/j.jstrokecerebrovasdis.2014.09.033

Parola, A., Gabbatore, I., Bosco, F. M., Bara, B. G., Cossa, F. M., Gindri, P., & Sacco, K. (2016). Assessment of pragmatic impairment in right hemisphere damage. *Journal of Neurolinguistics, 39,* 10–25. https://doi.org/10.1016/j.jneuroling.2015.12.003

Paterno, D. (2020). Social communication theory revisited: The genesis of medium in communication. *Atlantic Journal of Communication, 28*(3), 153–164. https://doi.org/10.1080/15456870.2019.1616735

Pavani, F., Husain, M., Ladavas, E., & Driver, J. (2004). Auditory deficits in visuospatial neglect patients. *Cortex, 40,* 347–365. https://doi.org/10.1016/S0010-9452(08)70130-8

Pavani, F., Ladavas, E., & Driver, J. (2002). Selective deficit of auditory localisation in patients with visuospatial neglect. *Neuropsychologia, 40*(3), 291–301. https://doi.org/10.1016/s0028-3932(01)00091-4

Pell, M. D. (2006). Cerebral mechanisms for understanding emotional prosody in speech. *Brain and Language, 96*(2), 221–234. https://doi.org/10.1016/j.bandl.2005.04.007

Pell, M. D. (2007). Reduced sensitivity to prosodic attitudes in adults with focal right hemisphere brain damage. *Brain and Language, 101*(1), 64–79. https://doi.org/10.1016/j.bandl.2006.10.003

Penn, C. (1999). Pragmatic assessment and therapy for persons with brain damage: What have clinicians gleaned in two decades? *Brain and Language, 68*(3), 535–552. https://doi.org/10.1006/brln.1999.2127

Peppé, S. J. (2009). Why is prosody in speech-language pathology so difficult? *International Journal of Speech-Language Pathology, 11*(4), 258–271. https://doi.org/10.1080/17549500902906339

Perecman, E. (Ed.). (1983). *Cognitive processing in the right hemisphere.* Academic Press.

Pernet, L., Jughters, A., & Kerckhofs, E. (2013). The effectiveness of different treatment modalities for the rehabilitation of unilateral neglect in stroke patients: A systematic review. *NeuroRehabilitation, 33*(4), 611–620. https://doi.org/10.3233/NRE-130986

Pimental, P. A., & Kingsbury, N. A. (2000). *Mini Inventory of Right Brain Injury.* Pro-Ed.

Pitteri, M., Arcara, G., Passarini, L., Meneghello, F., & Priftis, K. (2013). Is two better than one? Limb activation treatment combined with contralesional arm vibration to ameliorate signs of left neglect. *Frontiers in Human Neuroscience, 7,* 1–10. https://doi.org/10.3389/fnhum.2013.00460

Portegies, M. L., Selwaness, M., Hofman, A., Koudstaal, P. J., Vernooij, M. W., & Ikram, M. A. (2015). Left-sided strokes are more often recognized than right-sided strokes: The Rotterdam study. *Stroke, 46*(1), 252–254. https://www.ahajournals.org/doi/10.1161/STROKEAHA.114.007385

Priftis, K., Passarini, L., Pilosio, C., Meneghello, F., & Pitteri, M. (2013). Visual scanning training, limb activation treatment, and prism adaptation for rehabilitating left neglect: Who is the winner? *Frontiers in Human Neuroscience, 7,* 1–12. https://doi.org/10.3389/fnhum.2013.00360

Prigatano, G. P. (1996). Behavioral limitations TBI patients tend to underestimate: A replication and extension to patients with lateralized cerebral dysfunction. *Clinical Neuropsychologist, 10*(2), 191–201. https://doi.org/10.1080/13854049608406680

Prigatano, G. P. (2010). *The study of anosognosia.* Oxford University Press.

Prigatano, G. P., & Klonoff, P. S. (1998). A clinician's rating scale for evaluating impaired self-awareness and denial of disability after brain injury. *The Clinical Neuropsychologist, 12*(1), 56–67. https://doi.org/10.1076/clin.12.1.56.1721

Prutting, C. A., & Kittchner, D. M. (1987). A clinical appraisal of the pragmatic aspects of language. *Journal of Speech and Hearing Disorders, 52*(2), 105–119. https://doi.org/10.1044/jshd.5202.105

Radice-Neumann, D., Zupan, B., Tomita, M., & Willer, B. (2009). Training emotional processing in persons with brain injury. *The Journal of Head Trauma Rehabilitation, 24*(5), 313–323. https://doi.org/10.1097/htr.0b013e3181b09160

Ramsey, A., & Blake, M. L. (2020). Speech-language pathology practices for adults with right hemisphere stroke: What are we missing? *American Journal of Speech-Language Pathology, 29*(2), 741–759. https://doi.org/10.1044/2020_ajslp-19-00082

Randolph, C., Tierney, M. C., Mohr, E., & Chase, T. N. (1998). The Repeatable Battery for the Assessment of Neuropsychological Status (RBANS): Preliminary clinical validity. *Journal of Clinical and Experimental Neuropsychology, 20*(3), 310–319. https://doi.org/10.1076/jcen.20.3.310.823

Rehak, A., Kaplan, J. A., Weylman, S. T., Kelly, B., Brownell, H. H., & Gardner, H. (1992). Story processing in right-hemisphere brain-damaged patients. *Brain and Language, 42*(3), 320–336. https://doi.org/10.1016/0093-934X(92)90104-M

Reinhart, S., Schaadt, A. K., Adams, M., Leonhardt, E., & Kerkhoff, G. (2013). The frequency and significance of the word length effect in neglect dyslexia. *Neuro-*

psychologia, 51(7), 1273–1278. https://doi
.org/10.1016/j.neuropsychologia.2013
.03.006

Reinhart, S., Schindler, I., & Kerkhood, G.
(2011). Optokinetic stimulation affects
word omissions but not stimulus-centered
reading errors in paragraph reading in
neglect dyslexia. *Neuropsychologia, 49*(9),
2728–2735. https://doi.org/10.1016/j
.neuropschologia.2011.05.022

Roberts, M. Y., Sone, B. J., Zanzinger, K. E.,
Bloem, M. E., Kulba, K., Schaff, A., . . .
Goldstein, H. (2020). Trends in clinical
practice research in ASHA journals: 2008–
2018. *American Journal of Speech-Language
Pathology, 29*(3), 1629–1639. https://doi
.org/10.1044/2020_ajslp-19-00011

Robertson, I. H., McMillan, T. M., MacLeod,
E., Edgeworth, J., & Brock, D. (2002).
Rehabilitation by limb activation training
reduces left-sided motor impairment in
unilateral neglect patients: A single-blind
randomised control trial. *Neuropsychological Rehabilitation, 12*(5), 439–454. https://
doi.org/10.1080/09602010244000228

Robertson, I. H., Tegner, R., Tham, K., Lo,
A., & Nimmo-Smith, I. (1995). Sustained
attention training for unilateral neglect:
Theoretical and rehabilitation implications. *Journal of Clinical and Experimental
Neuropsychology, 17*(3), 416–430. https://
doi.org/10.1080/01688639508405133

Robertson, I. H., Ward, T., Ridgeway, V., &
Nimmo-Smith, I. (1994). *The Test of Everyday Attention.* Pearson Assessment.

Rode, G., Pagliari, C., Huchon, L., Rossetti, Y.,
& Pisella, L. (2017). Semiology of neglect:
An update. *Annals of Physical and Rehabilitation Medicine, 60*(3), 177–185. https://
doi.org/10.1016/j.rehab.2016.03.003

Ronchi, R., Algeri, L., Chiapella, L., Gallucci, M., Spada, M. S., & Vallar, G. (2016).
Left neglect dyslexia: Perseveration and
reading error types. *Neuropsychologia,
89*, 453–464. https://doi.org/10.1016/j
.neuropsychologia.2016.07.023

Ronchi, R., Rode, G., Cotton, F., Farne, A.,
Rossetti, Y., & Jacquin-Courtis, S. (2013).

Remission of anosognosia for right hemiplegia and neglect after caloric vestibular stimulation. *Restorative Neurology and
Neuroscience, 31*(1), 19–24. https://doi
.org/10.3233/RNN-120236

Rosenbek, J. C., Crucian, G. P., Leon, S. A.,
Hieber, B., Rodriguez, A. D., Holiway,
B., . . . Gonzalez-Rothi, L. (2004). Novel
treatments for expressive aprosodia:
A phase I investigation of cognitive
linguistic and imitative interventions.
*Journal of the International Neuropsycho-
logical Society, 10*, 786–793. https://doi
.org/10.1017/S135561770410502X

Rosenbek, J. C., Rodrigeuz, A. D., Hieber,
B., Leon, S. A., Crucian, G. P., Ketterson,
T. U., . . . Gonzales-Rothi, L. J. (2006).
Effects of two treatment for aproso-
dia secondary to acquired brain injury.
*Journal of Rehabilitation and Development,
43*(3), 379–390. https://doi.org/10.1682/
jrrd.2005.01.0029

Ross, E. D. (1981). The aprosodias: Func-
tional-anatomic organization of the
affective components of language in the
right hemisphere. *Archives of Neurology,
38*, 561–569. https://doi.org./10.1001/
archneur.1981.00510090055006

Rossetti, Y., Rode, G., Pisella, L., Farné, A.,
Boisson, M. T., & Lyon, D. (1998). Prism
adaptation to a rightward optical deviation rehabilitates left hemispatial neglect.
Nature, 395, 8–11. https://doi.org/10.10
38/25988

Ross-Swain, D. (1996). *Ross Information Processing Assessment-Second edition (RIPA-2).*
Pro-Ed.

Rowe, A. D., Bullock, P. R., Polkey, C. E., &
Morris, R. G. (2001). Theory of mind
impairments and their relationship to
executive functioning following frontal
lobe excisions. *Brain, 124*(3), 600–616.
https://doi.org/10.1162/0898929033215
93063

Rusconi, M. L., & Carelli, L. (2012). Long-
term efficacy of prism adaptation on
spatial neglect: Preliminary results on
different spatial components. *Scientific*

World Journal, 2012, 618528. https://doi.org/10.1100/2012/618528

Sackett, D. L., Straus, E., Richardson, W. S., Rosenberg, W., & Haynes, R. B. (2000). *Evidence-based medicine: How to practice and teach EBM.* Churchill Livingstone.

Sampanis, D. S., & Riddoch, J. (2013). Motor neglect and future directions for research. *Frontiers in Human Neuroscience, 28*(7), 110. https://doi.org/10.3389/fnhum.2013.00110

Saevarsson, S., Halsband, U., & Kristjánsson, A. (2011). Designing rehabilitation programs for neglect: Could 2 be more than 1 + 1? *Applied Neuropsychology, 18*(2), 95–106. https://doi.org/10.1080/09084282.2010.547774

Saxton, M. E., Younan, S. S., & Lah, S. (2013). Social behaviour following severe traumatic brain injury: Contribution of emotion perception deficits. *NeuroRehabilitation, 33*(2), 263–271. https://doi.org/10.3233/NRE-130954

Shamay-Tsoory, S. G., Tomer, R., Berger, B. D., & Aharon-Peretz, J. (2003). Characterization of empathy deficits following prefrontal brain damage: The role of the right ventromedial prefrontal cortex. *Journal of Cognitive Neuroscience, 15*(3), 324–337. https://doi.org/10.1162/089892903321593063

Shammi, P., & Stuss, D. T. (1999). Humour appreciation: A role of the right frontal lobe. *Brain, 122*(4), 657–666. https://doi.org/10.1093/brain/122.4.657

Sheppard, S. M., Keator, L. M., Breining, B. L., Wright, A. E., Saxena, S., Tippett, D. C., & Hillis, A. E. (2020). Right hemisphere ventral stream for emotional prosody identification: Evidence from acute stroke. *Neurology, 94*(10), e1013–e1020. https://doi.org/10.1212/wnl.0000000000008870

Sheppard, S. M., Meier, E. L., Durfee, A. Z., Walker, A., Shea, J., & Hillis, A. E. (2021). Characterizing subtypes and neural correlates of receptive aprosodia in acute right hemisphere stroke. *Cortex, 141,* 36–54. https://doi.org/10.1016/j.cortex.2021.04.003

Sheppard, S. M., Stockbridge, M. D., Keator, L. M., Murray, L. L., Blake, M. L., Right Hemisphere Damage Working Group, & Evidence-Based Clinical Research Committee. (2022). The company prosodic deficits keep following right hemisphere stroke: A systematic review. *Journal of the International Neuropsychological Society, 28*(10), 1075–1090. https://doi.org/10.1017/s1355617721001302

Sherbourne, C. D., & Stewart, A. L. (1991). The MOS social support survey. *Social Science & Medicine, 32*(6), 705–714. https://doi.org/10.1016/0277-9536(91)90150-b

Sherer, M., Hart, T., & Nick, T. G. (2003). Measurement of impaired self-awareness after traumatic brain injury: A comparison of the Patient Competency Rating Scale and the Awareness Questionnaire. *Brain Injury, 17*(1), 25–37. https://doi.org/10.1080/0269905021000010113

Sherratt, S. M., & Penn, C. (1990). Discourse in right-hemisphere brain-damaged subject. *Aphasiology, 4*(6), 539–560. https://doi.org//10.1080/02687039008248506

Sieroff, E., Decaix, C., Chokron, S., & Bartolomeo, P. (2007). Impaired orienting of attention in left unilateral neglect: A componential analysis. *Neuropsychology, 21*(1), 94–113. https://doi.org/10.1037/0894-4105.21.1.94

Sigman, S. J. (1998). Relationships and communication: A social communication and strongly consequential View. In R. L. Conville & L. E. Rogers (Eds.), *The meaning of relationship in interpersonal communication* (pp. 47–68). Praeger.

Sinott, M., & Coelho, C. (2007). Attention training for reading in mild aphasia: A follow-up study. *Neurorehabilitation, 22*(4), 303–310. https://doi.org/10.1080/02699050110103959

Sohlberg, M. M., & Mateer, C. A. (2010). *APT-III: Attention process training: A direct attention training program for persons with acquired brain injury.* Lash & Associates Publishing/Training Incorporated.

Spaccavento, S., Marinelli, C. V., Nardulli, R., Macchitella, L., Bivona, U., Piccardi,

L., . . . Angelelli, P. (2019). Attention deficits in stroke patients: The role of lesion characteristics, time from stroke, and concomitant neuropsychological deficits. *Behavioural Neurology*, *2019*, 7835710. https://doi.org/10.1155/2019/7835710

Starkstein, S. E., Jorge, R. E., & Robinson, R. G. (2010). The frequency, clinical correlates, and mechanism of anosognosia after stroke. *The Canadian Journal of Psychiatry*, *55*(6), 355–361. https://doi.org/10.1177/070674371005500604

Starkstein, S. E., Sabe, L., Chemerinski, E., Jason, L., & Leiguarda, R. (1996). Two domains of anosognosia in Alzheimer's disease. *Journal of Neurology, Neurosurgery & Psychiatry*, *61*, 485–490. https://doi.org/10.1136/jnnp.61.5.485

Sterzi, R., Bottini, G., Celani, M.G., Righetti, E., Lamassa, M., Ricci, S., & Vallar, G. (1993). Hemianopia, hemianaesthesia, and hemiplegia after right and left hemisphere damage. A hemispheric difference. *Journal of Neurology, Neurosurgery, and Psychiatry*, *56*(3), 308–310. https://doi.org/10.1136/jnnp.56.3.308

Stockbridge, M. D., Fridriksson, J., Sen, S., Bonilha, L., & Hillis, A. E. (2021). Protocol for Escitalopram and Language Intervention for Subacute Aphasia (ELISA): A randomized, double blind, placebo-controlled trial. *PLoS ONE*, *16*(12), e0261474. https://doi.org/10.1371/journal.pone.0261474

Stockbridge, M. D., Sheppard, S. M., Keator, L. M., Murray, L. L., Blake, M. L., Right Hemisphere Disorders Working Group, & Evidence-Based Clinical Research Committee. (2022). Aprosodia subsequent to right hemisphere brain damage: A systematic review and meta-analysis. *Journal of the International Neuropsychological Society*, *28*(7), 709–735. https://doi.org/10.1017/s1355617721000825

Stone, V. E., Baron-Cohen, S., & Knight, R. T. (1998). Frontal lobe contributions to theory of mind. *Journal of Cognitive Neuroscience*, *10*, 640–656. https://doi.org/10.1162/089892998562942

Sturm, W., Thimm, M., Kust, J., Karbe, H., & Fink, G. R. (2006). Alertness-training in neglect: Behavioral and imaging results. *Restorative Neurology and Neuroscience*, *24*(4–6), 371–384.

Sturm, W., & Willmes, K. (1991). Efficacy of a reaction training on various attentional and cognitive functions in stroke patients. *Neuropsychological Rehabilitation*, *1*(4), 259–280. https://doi.org/10.1080/09602019108402258

Swinburn, K., Porter, G., & Howard, D. (2023). *Comprehensive Aphasia Test* (2nd ed.). Routledge.

Tate, R., Simpson, G., Lane-Brown, A., Soo, C., de Wolf, A., & Whiting, D. (2012). Sydney Psychosocial Reintegration Scale (SPRS-2): Meeting the challenge of measuring participation in neurological conditions. *Australian Psychologist*, *47*(1), 20–32. https://doi.org/10.1111/j.1742-9544.2011.00060.x

Tavaszi, I., Nagy, A. S., Szabo, G., & Fazekas, G. (2021). Neglect syndrome in post-stroke conditions: Assessment and treatment (scoping review). *International Journal of Rehabilitation Research*, *44*(1), 3–14. https://doi.org/10.1097/mrr.0000000000000438

Thiebaut de Schotten, M., Tomaiuolo, F., Aiello, M., Merola, S., Silvetti, M., Lecce, F., . . . Doricchi, F. (2014). Damage to white matter pathways in subacute and chronic spatial neglect: A group study and 2 single-case studies with complete virtual "in vivo" tractography dissection. *Cerebral Cortex*, *24*(3), 691–706. https://doi.org/10.1093/cercor/bhs351

Thimm, M., Fink, G. R., Kiist, J., Karbe, H., & Sturm, W. (2006). Impact of alertness training on spatial neglect: A behavioural and fMRI study. *Neuropsychologia*, *44*(7), 1230–1246. https://doi.org/10.1016/j.neuropsychologia.2005.09.008

Thompson, C. (2011). *Northwestern Assessment of Verbs and Sentences*. Northwestern University.

Titone, D., Wingfield, A., Caplan, D., Waters, G., & Prentice, K. (2001). Memory and encoding of spoken discourse following right hemisphere damage: Evidence from the auditory moving window (AMW) technique. *Brain and Language*, 77(1), 10–24. https://doi.org/10.1006/brln.2000.2419

Togher, L., McDonald, S., Tate, R., Rietdijk, R., & Power, E. (2016). The effectiveness of social communication partner training for adults with severe chronic TBI and their families using a measure of perceived communication ability. *Neurorehabilitation*, 38(3), 243–255. https://doi.org/10.3233/NRE-151316

Togher, L., Power, E., Tate, R., McDonald, S., & Rietdijk, R. (2010). Measuring the social interactions of people with traumatic brain injury and their communication partners: The adapted Kagan scales. *Aphasiology*, 24(6–8), 914–927. https://doi.org/10.1080/02687030903422478

Toglia, J., & Chen, P. (2020). Spatial exploration strategy training for spatial neglect: A pilot study. *Neuropsychological Rehabilitation*, 32(5), 792–813. https://doi.org/10.1080/09602011.2020.1790394

Toglia, J., & Goverover, Y. (2022). Revisiting the dynamic comprehensive model of self-awareness: A scoping review and thematic analysis of its impact 20 years later. *Neuropsychological Rehabilitation*, 32(8), 1676–1725. https://doi.org/10.1080/09602011.2022.2075017

Tombaugh, T. N., Kozak, J., & Rees, L. (1999). Normative data stratified by age and education for two measures of verbal fluency: FAS and animal naming. *Archives of Clinical Neuropsychology*, 14(2), 167–177. https://doi.org/10.1016/S0887-6177(97)00095-4

Tompkins, C. A. (1995). *Right hemisphere communication disorders: Theory and management.* Singular Publishing.

Tompkins, C. A., Baumgaertner, A., Lehman, M. T., & Fassbinder, W. (2000). Mechanisms of discourse comprehension impairment after right hemisphere brain damage: Suppression in lexical ambiguity resolution. *Journal of Speech, Language, and Hearing Research*, 43(1), 62–78. https://doi.org/10.1044/jslhr.4301.62

Tompkins, C. A., Bloise, C. G. R., Timko, M. L., & Baumgaertner, A. (1994). Working memory and inference revision in brain-damaged and normally aging adults. *Journal of Speech and Hearing Research*, 37(4), 896–912. https://doi.org/10.1044/jshr.3704.896

Tompkins, C. A., Fassbinder, W., Blake, M. L., Baumgaertner, A., & Jayaram, N. (2004). Inference generation during text comprehension by adults with right hemisphere brain damage: Activation failure versus multiple activation. *Journal of Speech, Language, and Hearing Research*, 47(6), 1308–1395. https://doi.org/10.1044/1092-4388(2004/103)

Tompkins, C. A., Lehman-Blake, M. T., Baumgaertner, A., & Fassbinder, W. (2001a). Divided attention impedes suppression by right-brain-damaged and non-brain damaged adults. *Brain and Language*, 79(1), 57–59.

Tompkins, C. A., Lehman-Blake, M. T., Baumgaertner, A., & Fassbinder, W. (2001b). Mechanisms of discourse comprehension after right hemisphere brain damage: Inferential ambiguity resolution. *Journal of Speech, Language, and Hearing Research*, 44, 400–415. https://doi.org/10.1044/jslhr.4301.62

Tompkins, C. A., Scharp, V. L., Meigh, K., Blake, M. L., & Wambaugh, J. (2012). Generalization of a novel, implicit treatment for coarse coding deficit in right hemisphere brain damage: A single subject experiment. *Aphasiology*, 26(5), 698–708. https://doi.org/10.1080/02687038.2012.676869

Tompkins, C. A., Scharp, V. L., Meigh, K. M., & Fassbinder, W. (2008). Coarse coding and discourse comprehension in adults with right hemisphere brain damage. *Aphasiology*, 22(2), 204–223. https://doi.org/10.1080/02687030601125019

Tompkins, C. A., & Scott, A.G. (2013). Treatment of right hemisphere disorders. In I. Papathanasiou, P. Coppens, & C. Potagas (Eds.), *Aphasia and related neurogenic communication disorders* (pp. 345–364). Jones & Bartlett.

Turkstra, L., Ylvisaker, M., Coelho, C., Kennedy, M., Sohlberg, M. M., Avery, J., & Yorkston, K. (2005). Practice guidelines for standardized assessment for persons with traumatic brain injury. *Journal of Medical Speech-Language Pathology, 13*(2), ix–xxxviii. https://link.gale.com/apps/doc/A133706263/AONE?u=anon~a63b7feb&sid=googleScholar&xid=ac60382e

Vallar, G., Burani, C., & Arduino, L. S. (2010). Neglect dyslexia: A review of the neuropsychological literature. *Experimental Brain Research, 206*(2), 219–235. https://doi.org/10.1007/s00221-010-2386-0

Vallat-Azouvi, C., Azouvi, P., Le-Bornec, G., & Brunet-Gouet, E. (2019). Treatment of social cognition impairments in patients with traumatic brain injury: A critical review. *Brain Injury, 33*(1), 87–93. https://doi.org/10.1080/02699052.2018.1531309

Van Dijk, T. (2011). *Discourse studies: A multidisciplinary introduction.* (2nd ed.). Sage.

Van Lancker, D. R., & Kempler, D. (1987). Comprehension of familiar phrases by left- but not by right-hemisphere damaged patients. *Brain and Language, 32*(2), 265–277. https://doi.org/10.1016/0093-934x(87)90128-3

Virk, S., Williams, T., Brunsdon, R., Suh, F., & Morrow, A. (2015). Cognitive remediation of attention deficits following acquired brain injury: A systematic review and meta-analysis. *NeuroRehabilitation, 36*(3), 367–377. https://doi.org/10.3233/NRE-151225

Von Steinbüchel, N., Wilson, L., Gibbons, H., Hawthorne, G., Höfer, S., Schmidt, S., . . . Truelle, J. L. (2010). Quality of Life after Brain Injury (QOLIBRI): Scale development and metric properties. *Journal of Neurotrauma, 27*(7), 1167–1185. https://doi.org/10.1089/neu.2009.1076

Vossel, S., Weiss, P. H., Eschenbeck, P., & Fink, G. R. (2013). Anosognosia, neglect, extinction and lesion site predict impairment of daily living after right-hemispheric stroke. *Cortex, 49*(7), 1782–1789. https://doi.org/10.1016/j.cortex.2012.12.011

Vuilleumier, P., Schwartz, S., Clarke, K., Husain, M., & Driver, J. (2002). Testing memory for unseen visual stimuli in patients with extinction and spatial neglect. *Journal of Cognitive Neuroscience, 14*(6), 875–886. https://doi.org/10.1162/089892902760191108

Vuilleumier, P., Schwartz, S., Husain, M., Clarke, K., & Driver, J. (2001). Implicit processing and learning of visual stimuli in parietal extinction and neglect. *Cortex, 37*(5), 741–744. https://doi.org/10.1016/S0010-9452(08)70629-4

Walker, J. P., Daigle, T., & Buzzard, M. (2002). Hemispheric specialisation in processing prosodic structures: Revisited. *Aphasiology, 16*(12), 1155–1172. https://doi.org/10.1080/02687030244000392

Walker, J. P., Pelletier, R., & Reif, L. (2004). The production of linguistic prosodic structures in subjects with right hemisphere damage. *Clinical Linguistics & Phonetics, 18*(2), 85–106. https://psycnet.apa.org/doi/10.1080/026992003100015 96179

Wapner, W., Hamby, S., & Gardner, H. (1981). The role of the right hemisphere in the apprehension of complex linguistic materials. *Brain and Language, 14*(1), 15–33. https://doi.org/10.1016/0093-934X(81)90061-4

Wee, J. Y. M., & Hopman, W. M. (2005). Stroke impairment predictors of discharge function, length of stay, and discharge destination in stroke rehabilitation. *American Journal of Physical Medicine and Rehabilitation, 84*(8), 604–612. https://doi.org/10.1097/01.phm.0000171005.08744.ab

Westerhof-Evers, H. J., Visser-Keizer, A. C., Fasotti, L., Schönherr, M. C., Vink, M., van der Naalt, J., & Spikman, J. M. (2017). Effectiveness of a treatment for impairments in social cognition and emotion regulation (T-ScEmo) after traumatic brain injury: A randomized controlled trial. *Journal of Head Trauma Rehabilitation, 32*(5), 296–307. https://doi.org/10.1097/htr.0000000000000332

Whiteneck, G. G., Charlifue, S. W., Gerhart, K. A., Overholser, J. D., & Richardson, G. N. (1992). Quantifying handicap: A new measure of long-term rehabilitation outcomes. *Archives of Physical Medicine and Rehabilitation, 7,* 519–526.

Whitworth, A., Ng, N., & Timms, L., & Power, E. (2020). Exploring the viability of NARNIA with cognitive-communication difficulties: A pilot study. *Seminars in Speech and Language, 41*(01), 83–97. https://doi.org/10.1055/s-0039-3400512

Wildgruber, D., Ethofer, T., Grandjean, D., & Kreifelts, B. (2009). A cerebral network model of speech prosody comprehension. *International Journal of Speech-Language Pathology, 11*(4), 277–281. https://doi.org/10.1080/17549500902943043

Willer, B., Rosenthal, M., Kreutzer, J. S., Gordon, W. A., & Rempel, R. (1993). Assessment of community integration following rehabilitation for traumatic brain injury. *The Journal of Head Trauma Rehabilitation, 8*(2), 75–87. https://psycnet.apa.org/doi/10.1097/00001199-199308020-00009

Williams, L. S., Weinberger, M., Harris, L.E., Clark, D. O., & Biller J. (1999). Development of a stroke-specific quality of life scale. *Stroke, 30*(7), 1362–1369. https://doi.org/10.1161/01.str.30.7.1362

Wilson, B. A., Cockburn, J., & Halligan, P. W. (1987). *Behavioural Inattention Test.* Pearson Assessment.

Wilson, B. A., Greenfield, E., & Clare, L. (2008). *The Rivermead Behavioural Memory Test–third Edition (RBMT-3).* Pearson Assessment.

Winner, E., Brownell, H. H., Happe, F., Blum, A., & Pincus, D. (1998). Distinguishing lies from jokes: Theory of Mind deficits and discourse interpretation in right hemisphere brain-damaged patients. *Brain and Language, 62*(62), 89–106. https://doi.org/10.1006/brln.1997.1889

Witteman, J., van Ijzendoorn, M. H., van de Velde, D., van Heuven, V. J. J. P., & Schiller, N. O. (2011). The nature of hemispheric specialization for linguistic and emotional prosodic perception: A meta-analysis of the lesion literature. *Neuropsychologia, 49*(13), 3722–3738. https://doi.org/10.1016/j.neuropsychologia.2011.09.028

Wölwer, W., Streit, M., Gaebel, W., & Polzer, U. (1996). Facial affect recognition in the course of schizophrenia. *European Archives of Psychiatry and Clinical Neuroscience, 246*(3), 165–170. https://doi.org/10.1007/bf02189118

Woo, D., Broderick, J. P., Kothari, R. U., Lu, M., Brott, T., Lyden, P. D., . . . Grotta, J. C. (1999). Does the National Institutes of Health Stroke Scale favor left hemisphere strokes? *Stroke, 30*(11), 2355–2359. https://doi.org/10.1161/01.str.30.11.2355

World Health Organization. (2001). *International classification of functioning, disability and health: ICF.* https://apps.who.int/iris/handle/10665/42407

Wright, A. E., Saxena, S., Sheppard, S. M., & Hillis, A. E. (2018). Selective impairments in components of affective prosody in neurologically impaired individuals. *Brain and Cognition, 124,* 29–36. https://doi.org/10.1016/j.bandc.2018.04.001

Yang, N. Y. H., Zhou, D., Chung, R. C. K., Li-Tsang, C. W. P., & Fong, K. N. K. (2013). Rehabilitation interventions for unilateral neglect after stroke: A systematic review from 1997–2012. *Frontiers in Human Neuroscience, 10*(7), 1–11. https://doi.org/10.3389/fnhum.2013.00187

Ylvisaker, M., Szekeres, S. F., & Feeney, T. J. (2008). Communication disorders associated with traumatic brain injury. In R. Chapey (Ed.), *Language intervention strategies in aphasia and related neurogenic communication disorders* (5th ed., p. 879). Lippincott Williams & Wilkins.

Yue, Y., Song, W., Huo, S., & Wang, M. (2012). Study on the occurrence and neural bases of hemispatial neglect with different reference frames. *Archives of Physical Medicine and Rehabilitation, 93*(1), 156–162. https://doi.org/10.1016/j.apmr.2011.07.192

Zebhauser, P. T., Vernet, M., Unterburger, E., & Brem, A. K. (2019). Visuospatial ne-glect—A theory-informed overview of current and emerging strategies and a systematic review on the therapeutic use of non-invasive brain stimulation. *Neuropsychology Review, 29*(4), 397–420. https://doi.org/10.1007/s11065-019-09417-4

Zimmer, U., Lewald, J., & Karnath, H. (2003). Disturbed sound lateralization in patients with spatial neglect. *Journal of Cognitive Neuroscience, 15*(5), 694–703. https://doi.org/10.1162/089892903322307410

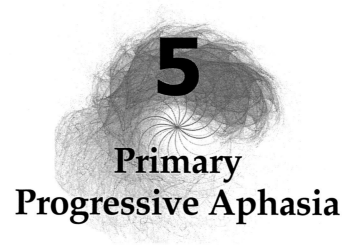

5

Primary Progressive Aphasia

Heather Dial and Maya Henry

Chapter Learning Objectives

After reading this chapter you will be able to:

1. Explain the diagnostic criteria for identifying primary progressive aphasia (PPA).
2. Explain the distinguishing characteristics and etiologies among the three PPA variants.
3. Identify appropriate assessment strategies and tests for each of the PPA variants.
4. Select appropriate treatment approaches to address the speech, language, and cognitive deficits associated with PPA.

Introduction

Primary progressive aphasia, or PPA, is a neurodegenerative disorder in which speech and language functions gradu-

ally deteriorate. This loss of function occurs in the presence of relatively spared general cognition, at least in the initial stages of the disease (Gorno-Tempini et al., 2011; Mesulam, 1982, 2001). Although the existence of this language-specific dementia was first documented in the late 1800s (Déjerine & Sérieux, 1897; Kertesz & Kalvach, 1996; Pick, 1892/1977), in-depth research into PPA symptoms, progression, and treatment is a relatively new endeavor. Since speech and language impairments are the primary deficits observed in this relatively rare form of dementia, speech-language pathologists (SLPs) serve an important role in the diagnosis and management of this disorder. SLPs who have worked with stroke-induced aphasia already have many of the skills and tools needed to work with individuals with PPA. However, to provide the best care for individuals with PPA, SLPs require a thorough understanding of the nature of the deficits observed in PPA, its typical patterns of progression, and potential treatment options.

Brief History

PPA was first described by Arnold Pick in 1892 (Kertesz & Kalvach, 1996; Pick, 1892/1977). Pick, a psychiatrist at a medical university in Prague, had seen several patients who presented with gradually worsening aphasia. Following the patients' deaths, he examined their brains, observing that atrophy was relatively circumscribed to areas of the brain that had recently been identified as related to language. This led him to refer to the disorder as a "focal" dementia. Nearly 100 years after the first documentation of this "focal," language-based dementia, Marsel Mesulam described a "slowly progressive aphasia without generalized dementia" (Mesulam, 1982). In this seminal work, Mesulam presented his clinical impressions regarding several individuals who had experienced gradually worsening language impairments. Most of the individuals presented with anomia, with two individuals also presenting with "nonfluent aphasias similar to the Broca type" (p. 597). He noted that these individuals were fairly young, with four of the cases in their late 40s to early 60s, suggesting an average age of onset that is younger than the more common Alzheimer's dementia. Mesulam noted that, as the disease progressed, many of the individuals developed additional deficits in language comprehension, repetition, and general cognitive processing.

Other researchers and clinicians began to document individuals who had anomia and a progressive loss of semantic knowledge (Hodges et al., 1992; Snowden et al., 1989; Warrington, 1975). Warrington (1975) described three individuals who had word-finding difficulties and loss of knowledge for everyday objects and common words, with relatively preserved visuospatial processing and episodic memory. Snowden and colleagues presented three similar cases and coined the diagnostic term "semantic dementia." A few years later, Hodges and colleagues presented five more cases of semantic dementia, noting that the likely underlying cause was frontotemporal lobar degeneration (FTLD; Hodges et al., 1992). Around the same time, Grossman et al. (1996) described a progressive language disorder characterized by a predominantly nonfluent profile, which was termed "progressive nonfluent aphasia." The link between semantic dementia, progressive aphasia, and FTLD was formalized by David Neary and colleagues, who outlined clinical criteria for syndromic diagnosis of frontotemporal dementia, semantic dementia, and progressive nonfluent aphasia (Neary et al., 1998). Shortly thereafter, Mesulam introduced clinical criteria for diagnosis of PPA (Mesulam, 2001). By the mid-2000s, three PPA phenotypes had been delineated: semantic variant (svPPA), nonfluent variant (nfvPPA), and a newly characterized logopenic variant (lvPPA; Gorno-Tempini et al., 2004), and formal diagnostic criteria for each subtype quickly followed (Bonner et al., 2010; Gorno-Tempini et al., 2011; Henry & Gorno-Tempini, 2010).

There is a history of inconsistent and evolving nomenclature associated with PPA, with terms including focal dementia, slowly progressive aphasia, fluent progressive aphasia, nonfluent progressive aphasia, and semantic dementia being used in the 1970s, 1980s, and 1990s for conditions that are now considered to be subtypes of PPA. Focal dementia and slowly progressive aphasia have been used to describe PPA generally, fluent progressive aphasia and semantic dementia likely refer to svPPA, and nonfluent progressive aphasia has, historically, encompassed both lvPPA and nfvPPA. When considering research from this period to aid in the development of appropriate treatment plans for individuals with PPA, care should be taken in interpreting diagnostic labels. Although the relevance of the various nosologic traditions may not be immediately obvious, it is important to be aware of the various naming conventions to gain a thorough understanding of the PPA literature.

Clinical Criteria for PPA Diagnosis

Formalized diagnostic criteria for PPA and its subtypes were formalized over the last two decades. Whereas Neary et al. (1998) presented the first diagnostic criteria for FTLD variants, which included semantic dementia and progressive nonfluent aphasia, Mesulam was the first to present diagnostic criteria for PPA proper (Mesulam, 2001). According to Mesulam (2001), to be conferred a diagnosis of PPA, an individual's language disturbance must have had a gradual onset and should be the initial and primary symptom for at least the first 2 years and must remain the most prominent impairment throughout disease progression. In the early stages of the disease, any disruptions in daily life should be related to language problems. PPA diagnosis is not appropriate if visuospatial processing impairments, episodic memory deficits, or behavioral disruptions are prominent in the initial stages of the disease or if deficits can be clearly

linked to stroke, brain tumor, traumatic brain injury, or psychiatric conditions. Once a diagnosis of PPA is made, diagnosis by clinical subtype, if possible, follows.

Gorno-Tempini et al. (2011) reiterated the diagnostic criteria for PPA that were originally enumerated by Mesulam (2001), with the only modification being that the language disturbance must be isolated in the "initial phases of the disease" (p. 1008) rather than the first 2 years. Additionally, they presented clinical criteria for diagnosing three PPA subtypes: the semantic variant (svPPA), the logopenic variant (lvPPA), and the nonfluent variant (nfvPPA; Table 5–1). In broad terms, lexical retrieval difficulties are the most prominent impairment in svPPA and lvPPA, due to a loss of core semantic knowledge in svPPA and phonological processing impairments in lvPPA. For example, an individual with relatively mild svPPA may mistakenly identify an octopus as a jellyfish, which is both semantically and visually similar, whereas an individual with relatively mild lvPPA may have difficulty assembling the constituent sounds and produce something like /ɑkpətʊs/. In nfvPPA, agrammatism and/or apraxia of speech are the first symptoms, leading to syntactically simple utterances and/or distorted speech (Gorno-Tempini et al., 2011; see Montembeault et al., 2018, for a review of clinical and anatomical correlates of each PPA subtype). The core linguistic deficits observed in each PPA variant are most distinct in the mild to moderate stages of the disorder. As the symptoms and underlying disease progress, the behavioral profile of each PPA subtype becomes less distinct (Cerami et al., 2017; Rogalski et al., 2011).

Table 5–1. Consensus Clinical Criteria for Diagnosis by PPA Subtype

PPA Subtype	Core Clinical Features	Supporting Features
Semantic Variant	**Both** of the following: 1. Picture naming deficit 2. Single-word comprehension deficit	At least **three** of the following: 1. Loss of object knowledge 2. Surface dyslexia/dysgraphia 3. Relatively preserved repetition 4. Intact grammar and motor speech
Logopenic Variant	**Both** of the following: 1. Difficulty with single-word retrieval in spontaneous speech and picture naming 2. Phrase and sentence repetition deficit	At least **three** of the following: 1. Phonemic paraphasias in spontaneous speech and picture naming 2. Relatively preserved comprehension of single words and intact object knowledge 3. Lack of motor speech impairments 4. Spared syntactic processing
Nonfluent Variant	At least **one** of the following: 1. Agrammatism 2. Apraxia of speech	At least **two** of the following: 1. Syntax comprehension deficit, particularly for complex syntax 2. Relatively preserved comprehension of single words 3. Relatively preserved object knowledge

Source: Criteria originally presented by Gorno-Tempini et al. (2011).

PPA Subtypes and Etiology

Semantic Variant

SvPPA is characterized by a loss of semantic knowledge. This manifests as a progressively worsening anomia and single-word comprehension impairment, the two core clinical features for svPPA diagnosis (Bonner et al., 2010; Gorno-Tempini et al., 2011; Hodges & Patterson, 2007; see Table 5–1). Although the primary cause of anomia is loss of semantic knowledge, anomia may also be related to a weakening of the link between a concept and its verbal label, such that the person knows what they are trying to say but cannot retrieve the word for it (Wilson et al., 2017). Individuals are likely to make semantic errors or errors of omission in language production when the incorrect verbal label is selected, but in some mild cases, they may be able to successfully cue themselves or their conversation partners via circumlocution.

In addition to the core linguistic impairments, at least three of the following supporting features must be present: loss of object knowledge, surface dyslexia/dysgraphia, spared repetition, and intact grammatical processing and motor speech. Individuals with svPPA may fail to recognize items and objects, especially those that are relatively uncommon. With progressive loss of object knowledge, they may begin to use objects inappropriately. Another potential consequence of loss of semantic knowledge is surface dyslexia and dysgraphia, in which individuals have selective difficulty reading and spelling irregular words (Coltheart et al., 2001), leading individuals with svPPA to produce regularization errors when reading or spelling irregular words. For example, the word *island* might be read as /ɪzlænd/. By contrast, reading and spelling of regular words and nonwords remains relatively intact. Phonological processing is typically unaffected, such that performance on repetition tasks is generally within normal limits, especially in the early stages of the disease. Grammatical processing impairments or motor speech deficits are not observed in svPPA, as regions in the brain that are devoted to these processes are generally spared.

As the disease progresses, language production becomes progressively empty, while remaining largely intelligible and grammatical. Additionally,

individuals may develop behavioral symptoms consistent with frontotemporal dementia such as compulsive behaviors, disinhibition, changes in personality, and altered eating preferences (Cerami et al., 2017; Macoir et al., 2017; Seeley et al., 2005). For example, Macoir and colleagues (2017) describe an individual with svPPA who, after visiting the clinic for 3 years, began insisting that all assessment materials be thoroughly disinfected immediately prior to use.

The deficits observed in svPPA are related to temporal lobe atrophy, with greatest atrophic changes in the anterior temporal lobe in the language dominant hemisphere (Gorno-Tempini et al., 2004; Figure 5–1). This is consistent with a proposed role for the anterior temporal lobes in semantic memory (Patterson et al., 2007; Simmons & Martin, 2009). With progression, the frontal, parietal, and medial temporal lobes will also be affected by the disease process (Cerami et al., 2017; Wisse et al., 2021). The underlying cause of neurodegeneration may vary across individuals, but the most likely pathological finding is FTLD-TDP, with one study observing that 83% of a sample of 29 svPPA cases had FTLD-TDP pathology at autopsy (Spinelli et al., 2017). Knowledge of the underlying disease process may ultimately inform decisions regarding pharmaceutical intervention. Unfortunately, there is currently no way to confirm FTLD-TDP pathology in vivo (Neumann et al., 2021) and no pharmacological intervention currently exists for treating the underlying disease (Suarez-Gonzalez et al., 2021). However, several clinical trials are currently underway, and medications may be prescribed to alleviate

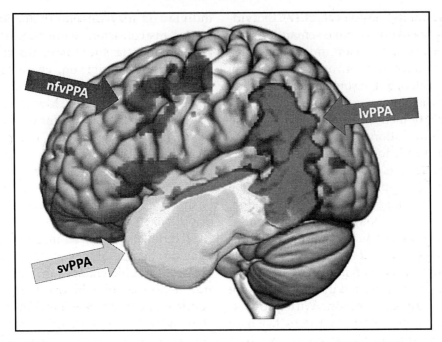

Figure 5–1. Left hemisphere cortical atrophy patterns in svPPA, lvPPA, and nfvPPA.

behavioral symptoms (e.g., selective serotonin reuptake inhibitors [SSRIs]; Young et al., 2018).

Logopenic Variant

LvPPA is the most recently identified PPA subtype and is characterized by a phonological processing impairment that results in anomia and deficits in repeating phrases and sentences, the two core clinical features for lvPPA diagnosis (see Table 5–1). Individuals with lvPPA struggle with confrontation naming, and spontaneous speech may contain frequent pauses due to lexical retrieval difficulties, contributing to a slow rate of production. In addition, these individuals have trouble repeating phrases and sentences and may rely upon semantic memory when performing repetition tasks, causing them

to produce semantically similar but not identical utterances (Gorno-Tempini et al., 2008; Henry & Gorno-Tempini, 2010; Leyton & Hodges, 2013).

At least three of the following supporting features must also be present for an lvPPA diagnosis: phonemic paraphasias in spontaneous speech and picture naming, intact single-word comprehension and object knowledge, intact motor speech, and spared syntactic processing. In spontaneous speech and picture naming, individuals with lvPPA may produce phonemic paraphasias via substitution, transposition, deletion, or addition of phonemes. For example, one individual with relatively mild lvPPA, when presented with a picture of a candelabra, remarked that "I've got parts of this rattling around in my head. It's like having two out of three syllables. It's a cal, a candeluh, candelagra." These errors suggest difficulty assembling and producing the phonemes necessary to successfully say "candelabra." However, the proximity to the correct phonological form suggests intact object knowledge for this low-frequency word. Indeed, most individuals with lvPPA, at least in the early stages of the disease process, have intact comprehension of single words and spared object knowledge. In this example, the errors produced were nondistorted sound errors of a phonological nature and not attributable to apraxia of speech. This provides evidence for the supporting clinical feature of intact motor speech. Finally, although individuals with lvPPA may appear to be agrammatic at times, this can be attributed to their lexical retrieval and phonological working memory deficits, and frank agrammatism is not typically noted.

As the disease progresses, individuals may develop jargon-like language, including semantic paraphasias and neologisms (Caffara et al., 2013). At this point, the message the individual is attempting to convey may be indecipherable. Comprehension deficits are also likely to occur in later stages of the disease (Caffara et al., 2013). Lastly, individuals may begin to have difficulty with verbal memory and to develop episodic memory impairment and other symptoms consistent with Alzheimer's dementia (Brambati et al., 2015; Cerami et al., 2017; Rohrer et al., 2013).

The deficits observed in lvPPA are attributed to temporo-parietal atrophy that is greater in the language-dominant hemisphere (Gorno-Tempini et al., 2004; see Figure 5–1), consistent with a role for this region in phonological processing and phonological working memory (Buchsbaum et al., 2001; Henry et al., 2016). The parietal lobe atrophy in lvPPA may also affect an individual's ability to perform simple arithmetic, and so these individuals may struggle with math calculations (Henry & Gorno-Tempini, 2010; Rohrer et al., 2010). Although the observed neurodegeneration may be related to different disease processes in different lvPPA cases, an atypical manifestation of Alzheimer's disease is the most likely cause, with recent research reporting that 100% of a sample of 11 lvPPA cases had Alzheimer's pathology at autopsy (Spinelli et al., 2017). Unlike svPPA, which is caused by FTLD, there are pharmaceutical interventions designed to manage Alzheimer's disease, such as cholinesterase inhibitors, although the efficacy of these drugs may vary across individuals (Kobayashi et al., 2016; Trinh et al., 2003). As with svPPA, drugs may also be prescribed to target symptoms associated with disease progression (e.g., antianxiety medication).

Nonfluent Variant

In nfvPPA, the core clinical features are agrammatism and apraxia of speech, with some individuals presenting with both features and some presenting with one or the other (Gorno-Tempini et al., 2011; Henry, Meese, et al., 2013). Individuals with agrammatism produce short, simple utterances and may omit function words, resulting in telegraphic output. Speech output of individuals with apraxia of speech is slow, effortful, and aprosodic, often with prominent distortions that affect intelligibility. Although dysarthria is not a diagnostic feature of nfvPPA, it may co-occur with apraxia of speech (Ogar et al.,

2007). In rare instances, progressive apraxia of speech may be observed in the absence of agrammatism. Although this falls under the umbrella of nfvPPA under the Gorno-Tempini et al. (2011) criteria, the diagnostic term "primary progressive apraxia of speech" has also been utilized (Duffy et al., 2021; Duffy & Josephs, 2012; Josephs et al., 2012).

To confirm nfvPPA diagnosis, at least two of the following supporting features must be present: comprehension deficit for syntactically complex utterances, intact single-word comprehension, and intact object knowledge. Individuals with nfvPPA may have difficulty understanding noncanonical utterances. For example, an individual with nfvPPA might interpret the passive voice sentence "The cat was chased by the dog" as if it were active voice, with the resulting interpretation that a cat was chasing a dog. It is unlikely that an individual with nfvPPA will have difficulty understanding single words, as comprehension deficits are related to a syntactic processing impairment. Finally, object knowledge is typically spared in nfvPPA.

As the disease progresses, language becomes increasingly agrammatic and speech increasingly unintelligible. In some cases, an individual may become completely mute early in the disease process in the presence of relatively spared general cognitive function (Gorno-Tempini et al., 2006). Depending on the underlying etiology, many individuals with nfvPPA will develop a generalized movement disorder such as corticobasal syndrome or progressive supranuclear palsy (Cerami et al., 2017). Therefore, regular swallowing evaluations are warranted to moni-

tor for signs of dysphagia (Langmore et al., 2007).

The deficits observed in nfvPPA are related to fronto-insular atrophy, with a greater degree of atrophy in the language-dominant hemisphere (Gorno-Tempini et al., 2004; see Figure 5–1). This area is critically involved in grammatical processing (Friederici, 2002; Friederici et al., 2003) and motor programming for speech (Dronkers, 1996). As with svPPA and lvPPA, the etiology of the neurodegenerative process may vary across individuals, but in nfvPPA, the most likely cause is FTLD-tau, in the form of Pick's disease, progressive supranuclear palsy, or corticobasal degeneration. Spinelli and colleagues recently reported that 88% of a sample of 25 nfvPPA cases had FTLD-tau pathology at autopsy (Spinelli et al., 2017). As with svPPA, there are no approved pharmaceutical options to target the underlying disease process, although medications may be prescribed to address symptoms, and clinical trials for drugs targeting tau are currently being conducted (Novak et al., 2019).

Mixed PPA

In some cases, an individual may present with clinical features that do not fit within one of the three PPA subtypes described above, leading to a classification of mixed PPA (Mesulam et al., 2009; Mesulam et al., 2012; Sajjadi et al., 2014). Sajjadi and colleagues argue that mixed PPA is most often observed in PPA with Alzheimer's pathology and that the inclusion criteria for lvPPA may be too narrow to capture the full range of observed deficits in this clinical syndrome (Sajjadi et al., 2014; see also Leyton et al., 2015). Alternatively, the underlying pathology may be a disease process known to target frontal and temporal regions, such as Pick's disease. For example, an individual with Pick's disease may present with lexical retrieval difficulties, single-word comprehension impairment, and apraxia of speech, thus meeting core criteria for both svPPA and nfvPPA (Spinelli et al., 2017). Still others have argued that the current clinical consensus criteria simply do not capture all possible PPA phenotypes (Harris et al., 2013). When designing clinical care plans and behavioral interventions for individuals with a mixed PPA presentation, it is important to consider each individual's profile of linguistic and motoric deficits as well as their unique functional needs.

Assessment and Diagnosis

Cognitive-linguistic assessment and diagnosis by PPA subtype are important components of clinical care (see Henry & Grasso, 2018, for a thorough discussion of PPA assessment). Knowledge of PPA subtype will help patients and families better understand the nature of the disease and its likely progression, will serve to inform potential treatment options, and may help in determining underlying etiology, which has implications for pharmaceutical interventions and clinical trials. In order to determine an accurate PPA diagnosis, it is important to obtain relevant case history and perform a comprehensive cognitive-linguistic evaluation. Following confirmation of a general PPA diagnosis,

clinicians should use assessments that evaluate relevant speech and language domains implicated in svPPA, lvPPA, and nfvPPA, as enumerated in current consensus criteria.

General PPA Diagnosis

As in any speech-language evaluation, a comprehensive case history is obtained to determine the pattern of onset and progression of speech-language symptoms and to discern areas of greatest functional communication impairment from the patient and family's perspective. Table 5–2 presents a series of questions that may be helpful in acquiring the most relevant information. For example, clinicians should ask questions regarding the individual's initial symptoms, how long they have been experiencing these symptoms, and whether they have noticed progression or worsening of deficits. Demographic information and medical history will be of value when attempting to rule out alternative causes for speech-language impairment. In some instances, especially in more advanced cases, the individual with PPA may have difficulty understanding and responding to questions. It is recommended that, whenever possible, the patient be accompanied by a family member or friend who may assist in answering questions.

Second, it is important to confirm a general PPA diagnosis. Speech and language can be evaluated using batteries developed for use in stroke-induced aphasia, such as the Western Aphasia Battery–Revised (WAB-R; Kertesz, 2007), the Boston Diagnostic Aphasia Exam (BDAE; Goodglass et al., 2001),

Table 5–2. Screening Questions to Obtain Relevant Case History and to Inform PPA Diagnosis and Treatment

To Acquire Information Regarding	Example Questions	Responses That Do Not Support PPA Diagnosis
Demographics and medical history	1. What was/is your occupation? 2. What is your highest level of education? If you completed college, what field of study?	
	3. Do you have a history of brain injury, stroke, heart disease, seizures, alcohol or drug abuse, depression, diabetes, brain tumor, etc.? 4. Do you speak more than one language? If so, what languages do you speak? In what settings do you use each language?	History of brain injury, stroke, heart disease, brain tumor, alcohol or drug abuse, psychiatric condition, etc. that are the likely cause of observed impairments
	5. Have you consulted with a neurologist regarding your communication difficulties? If so, what were the results of the consultation?	If an individual has not yet consulted with a neurologist, a neurological assessment should be recommended to rule out other causes of speech-language decline.
Symptoms and disease progression	1. What were the first symptoms you noticed that made you realize something was wrong? Do you ever have trouble with: a. finding or pronouncing words? b. calling things the wrong name? c. speaking in sentences? d. reading or writing? e. recognizing objects or words? f. remembering the names of people you know? g. recognizing people you know?	First signs and symptoms include episodic memory loss or general cognitive impairment. If the individual indicates they experience memory loss, query further to determine whether this refers specifically to words and names or whether this includes memory for events. Early changes in mobility and loss of motor control beyond the speech domain.

Table 5–2. *continued*

To Acquire Information Regarding	Example Questions	Responses That Do Not Support PPA Diagnosis
Symptoms and disease progression	2. When did you first notice these symptoms? 3. Have you noticed that your symptoms are getting worse? 4. What are your greatest communication challenges at present? 5. Do you also experience difficulty with remembering things such as conversations, events, or where you left objects? If so, when did you first notice these symptoms? 6. Have you ever gotten lost in a familiar place? 7. Do you also experience difficulty with gross motor skills such as walking or fine motor skills such as tying shoes? If so, when did you first notice these symptoms?	Symptoms do not show evidence of progression.
Premorbid language abilities	1. Before your current symptoms, began, how would you rate your ability to read? 2. Before your current symptoms began, how would you rate your ability to spell? 3. Do you have a history of developmental language impairment? Did you receive special help in school for speech or language?	Premorbid speech-language impairment is not exclusionary, but should be noted in order to inform interpretation of language assessments.

and the Comprehensive Aphasia Test (CAT; Swinburn et al., 2004). However, aphasia classification systems used in stroke-induced aphasia should not be applied in PPA. In addition to formal test batteries, engaging in conversation (i.e., getting a spontaneous speech sample) provides insight into an individual's overall speech and language function while serving to build rapport.

It is critical that clinicians also examine other domains, including general cognitive function, visuospatial processing and visual memory, episodic memory, motor skills, and emotional processing, to rule out alternative diagnoses. Cognitive screening tools such as the Mini-Mental State Exam (Folstein et al., 1975) or the Montreal Cognitive Assessment (Nasreddine et al., 2005) may be used to assess general cognitive function, although these are linguistically loaded, and so interpretation of performance should be carefully considered in the context of the language impairment. Visuospatial processing and visual memory should also be evaluated, which can be accomplished using a complex figure copy and recall task. If complex figure copy is performed without error, poor recall of the figure may indicate visual or episodic memory impairment. Episodic memory can be further evaluated via self- and caregiver-report. Poor performance on complex figure copy could be related to impaired motor control and is most likely to be observed in moderate-to-severe nfvPPA. Emotion processing can be evaluated via observation and using tests such as the Emotional Evaluation subtest of the Awareness of Social Inference Test (TASIT; McDonald et al., 2003; discussed in relation to PPA in Binney et al., 2016). Disrup-

tions in emotional processing are often observed in svPPA as the disease process begins to encroach upon the amygdala and right anterior temporal lobe (Binney et al., 2016; Cerami et al., 2017; Miller et al., 2012; Rosen et al., 2002). If emotion processing deficits are more pronounced than verbal semantic deficits, a diagnosis of behavioral variant or right temporal lobe variant of frontotemporal dementia should be considered (Neary et al., 1998; Rascovsky et al., 2007; Ulugut Erkoyun et al., 2020; Younes et al., 2022). Whereas nonlanguage cognitive impairments may be observed in PPA, speech and language impairments should constitute the most prominent deficits for confirmation of PPA diagnosis.

Diagnosis by PPA Subtype

After confirming a PPA diagnosis, clinicians can diagnose the PPA subtype via examination of patterns of performance on tasks designed to assess core and supporting clinical features for each variant. A good first step is to evaluate spontaneous speech (see Table 5–3 for sample responses to the "Cat Rescue" picture; Nicholas & Brookshire, 1993). Wilson and colleagues presented information on speech rate and error patterns on the WAB-R picnic description for individuals with svPPA, lvPPA, and nfvPPA, which can be helpful in considering diagnosis by PPA subtype (Wilson et al., 2010). In svPPA, connected speech was characterized as fluent with a large proportion of high-frequency nouns, pronouns, and verbs, reflecting lexical retrieval difficulties, and a normal speech rate. In nfvPPA, connected speech was characterized as nonfluent,

Table 5–3. Sample Transcriptions of the Cat Rescue Picture Description (Nicholas & Brookshire, 1993) for Each PPA Subtype

PPA Subtype	Sample Cat Rescue Description
Semantic Variant	"There's a little girl and she's . . . got her . . . dog . . . cat up on the roof or I mean up in the tree . . . and she has a little . . . not a bike . . . it has three . . . .um, you know, the round things for moving . . . and there's an animal on the tree or just trying to . . . um . . . yell, not yell, he's just barking at the tree and there's a guy up on the things that come out of the tree and, um, there's another little animal on the tree on the other side and he's happy and there's, um, men who stop the fires running over to get the guy off the . . . device for climbing . . . and they have a . . . fire truck in the back and they also have another device that is sitting in the back of the tree. And this thing over here, I don't recognize."
Logopenic Variant	"Ok we have, um . . . a big tree that is, uh . . . he's in trouble because he's up on top and he needs to get down out of there. So, we have a . . . um . . . depart the fire department is coming up with two of them and their great big, uh, thing that drives it, and the, um . . . away from him well the guy who's up on top he has a young daughter that is on the ground looking up at a cat that is up above where she can't get to it and the bicycle is still there. Then there is, um, something to go up some, um, things to, um, you can, it's not set up to be able to go up it because it's on the ground. A ladder! The dog is at the bot, the bottom of it, for the tree, and it's making noise for the man who is still up there, and there's a bird out on the right side."
Nonfluent Variant	"A girl . . . um . . . girl is . . . um . . . calling . . . um . . . up tree . . . cat . . . tree . . . dog there . . . it barks . . . .man in tree . . . sturk . . . uh . . . stuck . . . in . . . tree . . . there bird . . . in . . . on banch . . . barnch . . . branch. Ferman run . . . have ladder . . . fertruck back there . . . oh . . . um . . . and girl . . . um . . . has . . . tri . . . cyc . . . le."

agrammatic, and slow, with frequent speech sound distortions. Speech rate for lvPPA was intermediate between svPPA and nfvPPA, with fewer syntactic errors than nfvPPA and lexical retrieval difficulties that were less severe than svPPA. Phonemic paraphasias were present in some individuals with lvPPA.

It may be of value to examine patterns of performance on batteries such as the WAB-R, BDAE, or CAT. Note, however, that the subtests of these batteries may not be sensitive enough to detect deficits in milder cases, so additional assessments should be utilized if normal performance is observed when a deficit is suspected by the clinician. In the context of the aphasia battery, individuals with svPPA perform poorly on auditory comprehension subtests, reflecting single-word comprehension deficits. Individuals with lvPPA and nfvPPA typically perform relatively well on auditory comprehension subtests, reflecting intact single-word comprehension. On naming subtests, impairments will be observed in svPPA and lvPPA. Individuals with svPPA typically produce semantic errors and errors of omission and may not be aided by phonemic cues. Individuals with lvPPA may produce phonological errors and are more likely to benefit from phonemic cues than individuals with svPPA. Individuals with nfvPPA often produce sound distortions, although these errors may be difficult to differentiate from phonological errors and should be interpreted in the context of other speech features (e.g., rate and prosody) that may be confirmatory for motor speech impairment. On phrase and sentence repetition subtests, individuals with lvPPA will have pronounced difficulty, whereas individuals with svPPA should perform relatively well. Individuals with nfvPPA may struggle with repetition, although impaired performance is linked to motor speech or grammatical processing impairments.

Regarding assessment of motor speech, evaluations such as those developed by Wertz et al. (1984) and Duffy (2013) may be employed, which include such tasks as diadochokinesis, repetition of words and sentences of increasing length and complexity, and passage reading. Individuals with nfvPPA will have the most difficulty with these tasks due to apraxia of speech and, often, concomitant dysarthria. However, individuals with lvPPA may struggle with sentence repetition and diadochokinesis because of phonological working memory and sequencing deficits. Individuals with svPPA demonstrate relative sparing on tasks assessing motor programming and coordination for speech.

Regular, irregular, and nonword reading and spelling can be used to inform PPA subtype diagnosis (Brambati, et al., 2009; Gorno-Tempini et al., 2011). Surface dyslexia/dysgraphia may be observed in svPPA, with patients exhibiting selective impairment of irregular word reading and spelling. Individuals with lvPPA often have impaired nonword reading and spelling due to phonological processing impairment. Reading and spelling in nfvPPA may be affected by motor speech deficits or limb apraxia, respectively, but error patterns (e.g., distortions) are less influenced by word regularity or word/nonword status.

Semantic processing should be evaluated in the nonverbal domain to identify loss of object knowledge. The picture version of the Pyramids and Palm Trees task (PPT; Howard & Patterson, 1992), an object association task, may be used (see also the Cambridge Semantic Memory Test Battery, which includes the Camels and Cactus Test; Adlam et al., 2010). Individuals with svPPA will have greatest difficulty with the PPT, whereas those with lvPPA and nfvPPA typically perform this type of task relatively well, reflecting intact object knowledge.

Finally, expressive and receptive grammatical processing should be assessed. The Northwestern Anagram Test (NAT; Weintraub et al., 2009) and the Sentence Comprehension Test/ Make a Sentence Test (SECT/MAST; Billette et al., 2015) may be useful for this purpose. The NAT, which requires that written words be arranged to describe pictures, is useful in assessing syntax production without the need for overt speech (which may be affected by motor speech impairment). Of the three variants, individuals with nfvPPA have the most difficulty performing this type of task. Individuals with svPPA and lvPPA typically perform the NAT relatively well, reflecting a lack of frank agrammatism. The SECT requires a single-word response to demonstrate comprehension of auditorily or visually presented sentences with varying degrees of syntactic complexity, and the MAST requires individuals to produce sentences of varying syntactic complexity when provided with four nouns and a verb in a specific order. Impaired comprehension of syntactically complex utterances is a supporting feature in nfvPPA, reflecting a core deficit in grammatical processing. The NAT may be preferable to the MAST for use in individuals with motor speech disorders as it does not rely on overt speech production.

There are now several assessments designed specifically for use in PPA, which may eventually obviate the need to use batteries designed for stroke-induced aphasia (see Battista et al., 2017, for review). One of these is the Sydney Language Battery (SydBat), which consists of a simple series of tasks designed to aid diagnosis by PPA subtype. The SydBat includes confrontation naming, auditory word-picture matching (select target picture from among six semantically or visually similar distractors), semantic association (select one of four pictures that is most closely associated with a target picture), and single-word

repetition subtests (Savage, Foxe, et al., 2013). Another assessment is the Repeat and Point Test, which was created to aid differential diagnosis of semantic dementia (svPPA) and progressive nonfluent aphasia. The Repeat and Point Test involves, not surprisingly, repeating a word or pointing to a picture following auditory presentation of a single word (Hodges et al., 2008). This test was shown to reliably distinguish between semantic dementia and progressive nonfluent aphasia, although its utility in distinguishing between lvPPA and nfvPPA has not been addressed. Both the SydBat and the Repeat and Point Test are freely available online (see web content).

Finally, two scales have been designed to aid in tracking disease severity in PPA. Both the Progressive Aphasia Severity Scale (PASS; Sapolsky et al., 2014) and the Progressive Aphasia Language Scale (PALS; Leyton et al., 2011) were developed to assess severity and progression of impairments within specific speech and language domains, such as articulation, grammar, word retrieval, and word comprehension. The PASS and the PALS both rely on a clinician's subjective ratings via a Likert scale (5-point or 3-point scale, respectively). Sapolsky and colleagues (2014) recommend the use of the PASS in evaluating treatment efficacy and determining the appropriateness of speech and language interventions (e.g., when to shift the focus of treatment to the use of alternative and augmentative communication strategies). The PALS was also designed as a means to aid in PPA subtyping via a simple algorithm and was demonstrated to have 94% concordance with diagnosis provided by

PPA experts (Leyton et al., 2011). Both scales are freely available online (see web content).

Although not strictly necessary, structural neuroimaging (magnetic resonance imaging [MRI], computed tomography [CT]) may aid in the diagnostic process. Note, however, that in early/mild PPA cases, radiological reports may indicate that an MRI scan is within normal limits, with subtle brain atrophy attributed to the aging process. In conjunction with the medical team, clinicians involved in PPA diagnosis should review MRI scans for patterns of asymmetry or focal brain atrophy, which may have been previously undetected. Notable features include lateralization of neural changes to the language-dominant (typically left) hemisphere. Focal changes are typically observed in the anterior temporal lobe in svPPA, the left temporo-parietal junction in lvPPA, and fronto-insular regions in nfvPPA (see Figure 5–1).

Treatment

The evidence base supporting the utility of restitutive speech and language intervention in PPA has grown over the last two and a half decades. The majority of these studies utilized single-case, case series, or single-subject experimental designs and were intended to treat lexical retrieval deficits (Cadório et al., 2017; Carthery-Goulart et al., 2013; Cotelli et al., 2020; Volkmer, Rogalski, et al., 2020). In svPPA, researchers have most often implemented treatment protocols in which a picture is paired and rehearsed with the spoken and/or written word form. The goal of this form of treatment is to strengthen the link between the phonological and/or orthographic representations and the semantic representation, which is presumed to be activated via presentation of the picture. These studies report improved naming performance for trained items in svPPA patients, but generalization to untrained items or contexts is rarely observed (e.g., Graham et al., 1999; Graham et al., 2001; Heredia et al., 2009; Jokel et al., 2006; Jokel & Anderson, 2012; Mayberry et al., 2011a, 2011b; Meyer et al., 2017; Savage, Ballard, et al., 2013; Savage et al., 2015; Snowden & Neary, 2002). Fewer studies have examined treatment outcomes past the immediate post-treatment phase, although some studies have reported maintenance of treatment-induced gains up to 6 months post-treatment (Heredia et al., 2009; Jokel et al., 2006; Savage et al., 2015).

The item- and context-specific gains demonstrated in these studies indicate that vocabulary relearning in svPPA may depend on episodic memory and rote memorization to compensate for degraded semantic representations (e.g., Graham et al., 1999; Graham et al., 2001; Snowden & Neary, 2002). In a direct test of this hypothesis, Hoffman and colleagues (2015) manipulated factors related to episodic memory. In an initial experiment, items were presented in either a fixed or a random order during the treatment phase, with random presentation hypothesized to prevent context- and order-dependent learning. In a second experiment, items were presented with a single exemplar or with multiple exemplars, with the use of multiple exemplars designed to prevent rigid relearning of picture-word pairs and to promote generalization to novel exemplars (Hoffman et al., 2015). The researchers found that treatment outcomes were greatest in the random presentation and multiple exemplars conditions, lending support to an episodic basis for relearning in svPPA. Recently, the structural integrity of the hippocampus, which supports episodic memory, has also been linked to treatment outcomes in svPPA, lending additional support to the episodic memory hypothesis for relearning in svPPA (Dial et al., 2023). There is, however, evidence that residual semantic knowledge also plays an important role in treatment outcomes, with research suggesting that items lacking residual conceptual knowledge are unlikely to be relearned (Jokel et al., 2006; Jokel et al., 2010; Jokel et al., 2012; Jokel et al., 2016).

A growing number of studies have implemented cueing hierarchies that utilize semantic feature analysis and encourage the retrieval of autobiographical and episodic information in relation to each picture. Participants are also trained to use phonological and orthographic cues to support word retrieval. Pictures are then presented with spoken or written word forms if cueing is unsuccessful (Beales et al., 2016; Bier et al., 2009; Dial et al., 2019; Dial et al., 2023; Dressel et al., 2010; Evans et al., 2016; Henry et al., 2008; Henry, Rising, et al., 2013; Henry et al., 2019; Jokel & Anderson, 2012; Jokel et al., 2010; Macoir et al., 2015; Newhart et al., 2009). These studies report improved naming of trained items, generalization to untrained items (Beales et al., 2016; Henry et al., 2008; Henry, Rising, et al. 2013; Jokel & Anderson, 2012; Jokel et al., 2010), and maintenance of gains at 1 month (e.g.,

Macoir et al., 2015), 3 months (e.g., Jokel et al., 2010; Jokel et al., 2012), 4 months (e.g., Dressel et al., 2010; Henry et al., 2008; Henry, Rising, et al., 2013), or 12 months posttreatment (e.g., Henry et al., 2019). This type of approach has also proven beneficial in bilingual individuals with PPA (Grasso et al., 2021). Overall, the evidence supporting treatment in svPPA indicates that episodic memory and residual semantic knowledge are important factors and that a richer variety of cueing modalities may enhance direct treatment effects as well as generalization and maintenance of gains.

As in svPPA, most treatment studies in lvPPA have targeted lexical retrieval deficits (cf. Tsapkini et al., 2013, and Tsapkini et al., 2014, for treatment designed to improve spelling in lvPPA and nfvPPA). In general, treatment targeting lexical retrieval in lvPPA has utilized similar approaches as those implemented with svPPA, namely, the pairing of pictures with spoken and/or written word forms (Croot et al., 2015; Meyer et al., 2015; Meyer, Getz, et al., 2016; Meyer, Tippett, et al., 2016; Meyer et al., 2017). In these studies, significant treatment effects were observed on trained items, but no maintenance was observed and no generalization to untrained items or contexts (e.g., connected speech) was found. Researchers have also implemented cueing hierarchies utilizing semantic, autobiographical, episodic, phonological, and orthographic cues to treat anomia in lvPPA. In these studies, improved naming of trained items was observed, as was generalization to untrained items. Moreover, maintenance of gains was observed at 6 months (Beales et al., 2016; Newhart et al., 2009; Henry, Rising, et al., 2013) or 12 months post-treatment (Henry et al., 2019). Finally, one study implemented semantic elaboration training and generative naming in a brief but intensive protocol (Beeson et al., 2011). Treatment effects in naming were significant for trained sets, with generalization observed for untrained sets. Gains were maintained for trained items up to 6 months post-treatment. As in svPPA, it seems that a richer variety of cues may lead to greater and longer-lasting gains.

Finally, as with svPPA and lvPPA, most intervention research in nfvPPA has focused on lexical retrieval treatment. In several studies, lexical retrieval treatment was implemented such that a picture was paired and rehearsed with the spoken and/or written word form (Cotelli et al., 2014; Cotelli et al., 2016; Croot et al., 2015; Jokel et al., 2009; Meyer, Getz, et al., 2016; Meyer, Tippett, et al., 2016; Meyer et al., 2017). In these studies, significant treatment effects were observed on treated items but did not generalize to untreated items, with maintenance observed at 1 month post-treatmnet in some participants (Jokel et al., 2009; Meyer, Getz, et al., 2016; Meyer, Tippett, et al., 2016; Meyer et al., 2017). Studies using a richer variety of training techniques (semantic feature analysis: Marcotte & Ansaldo, 2010; multimodality treatment: Farrajota et al., 2012) also documented gains on trained items; however, these studies did not measure generalization or maintenance of treatment-induced gains.

Other studies have focused on core linguistic and motoric deficits associated with the nfvPPA syndrome, such as word retrieval and grammar (Hameister et al., 2016), verb and sentence production (Machado et al., 2014; Schneider et

al., 1996), and apraxia of speech (Henry, Meese, et al. 2013; Henry et al., 2018). Hameister et al. (2016) used a "go-fish" style card game wherein participants requested cards via description of the action on the card. They observed significant gains for trained items, generalization to untrained items, and maintenance up to 2 months post-treatment. Schneider et al. (1996) utilized a treatment that involved repeating gestures and sentences with verbs in the past, present, or future tense. Following treatment, improvement was noted on the use of trained gestures and verbs, with generalization to untrained noun and verb phrase combinations. The use of gestures and the production of future-tense verbs was maintained up to 3 months post-treatment. Finally, Henry and colleagues (2018) utilized a video-implemented script training technique to address speech production and fluency in nfvPPA. In this study, participants rehearsed production of personalized scripts by speaking in unison with a video model of a healthy speaker. Independent practice with the audiovisual model was complemented by sessions with a clinician targeting memorization and conversational usage of scripts. Significant gains were observed in production of correct, intelligible words for trained scripts, as was generalized improvement in intelligibility and maintenance of gains for trained topics up to 1 year post-treatment.

There is a modest body of evidence supporting the use of noninvasive neuromodulation, either in isolation or, more typically, as an adjuvant to restitutive interventions in PPA (for reviews, see Coemans et al., 2021; Cotelli et al., 2020; Nissim et al., 2020; Sheppard,

2022). The most common neuromodulatory approaches are transcranial direct current stimulation (tDCS) and transcranial magnetic stimulation (TMS). The precise mechanisms by which tDCS and TMS modify neural activity is beyond the scope of this chapter, but both seek to change the baseline excitability of neurons to improve treatment outcomes. Neuromodulation has been linked to improved outcomes (relative to behavioral intervention alone) for treatment targeting spoken naming (e.g., Cotelli et al., 2014) and written naming and spelling (e.g., Fenner et al., 2019; Tspakini et al., 2014), with some studies documenting enhanced generalization and maintenance of treatment effects. Differential effects of neuromodulation have been observed across studies where neural targets (i.e., stimulation montage), PPA subtypes, participant demographic factors, and treatment approaches vary, and there is some evidence of publication bias in favor of studies reporting positive effects of neuromodulation (Nissim et al., 2020). Neuromodulatory techniques have proven safe and feasible in persons with PPA, and outcomes to date are promising; however, additional research is needed before neuromodulatory techniques are adopted for use in standard clinical practice. In particular, studies should seek to clarify ideal site and dosage for stimulation across clinical phenotypes and when paired with different types of behavioral intervention in PPA.

Across PPA variants and treatment designs, restitutive behavioral intervention for speech and language deficits has shown great promise, with the potential for enhanced outcomes when paired with neuromodulation. In most studies, treatment-induced gains have been observed immediately post-treatment, with some studies also documenting generalization to untrained items and tasks and maintenance of gains up to 1 year post-treatment. However, given the progressive nature of PPA, it is important that SLPs proactively consider the changing needs of the individual with PPA as well as the psychosocial sequelae that accompany the loss of communicative capacity. With progression, individuals gradually lose their spoken language skills. As such, functional interventions, such as augmentative and alternative communication (AAC), are an important complement to restitutive treatment. Although there is limited work examining psychosocial (Schaffer & Henry, 2021) or functional communication interventions (Volkmer, Spector, et al., 2020), results to date are encouraging.

In contrast to stroke-induced aphasia, where there is usually improvement in speech and language functions followed by relative stability, in PPA, there is an inevitable loss of function over time. This takes an emotional toll on the both the individual with PPA and their family, as individuals must continually confront new losses and adapt to changing life roles. SLPs are well positioned to offer psychosocial support, as it is within their scope of practice to provide informational counseling on PPA and its likely progression as well as personal adjustment counseling focused on the emotional response to the disorder. Several studies have addressed the impact of counseling on the emotional well-being of individuals with PPA. Preliminary findings from the Communication Bridge web app study, which includes a wide variety of restitutive tasks in addition to informational and emotional counseling, indicate that engaging with Communication Bridge leads to improved communication confidence (Rogalski & Khayum, 2018). A group intervention with an informational counseling component has been shown to improve understanding of PPA for individuals with PPA and their care partners (Jokel et al., 2017). Similarly, positive outcomes were observed following a guided support group for care partners of individuals with PPA that included both informational and emotional counseling (Schaffer & Henry, 2021). Lastly, a single-case experimental study of an individual with nfvPPA noted improvements on both speech-language measures and measures of psychosocial functioning following an intervention that combined script training with cognitive-behavioral therapy (Schaffer et al., 2021).

Among functional communication interventions, AAC has been examined most frequently, with several studies confirming its utility in persons with PPA (Volkmer, Spector, et al., 2020). In an early study, Cress and King (1999) trained two individuals with PPA (unspecified subtype) to use low-tech AAC boards. Both individuals were reported to produce more comprehensible and complex messages following development of the AAC boards. One individual's family reported that he was using his communication boards regularly, that their use aided communication, and that he maintained his ability to use the boards after a year, despite a decline in general cognition. Pattee et al. (2006) trained an individual with PPA and apraxia of speech to use a text-to-speech device and American Sign Language. Following treatment, the individual produced more content for trained targets, but generalization was not observed, and maintenance was not assessed. Of note, the participant stated a preference for the Sign Language approach and decided to discontinue use of the text-to-speech device. Mooney and colleagues (2018) trained participants with svPPA, lvPPA, and nfvPPA to use a beta version of an AAC application called CoChat (Mooney et al., 2018). With CoChat, participants take photos and share them with close friends and family, who then comment on the photos. The comments are analyzed using a natural language processor, which creates a list of the 10 most salient words and concepts and places the written words in an array around the photo (visual scene display). In this study, participants used the visual scene display to aid in story retell, leading to increased production of target words relative to a picture-only condition in most participants immediately post-treatment. Maintenance was assessed for only one of the participants, who showed maintenance of treatment-induced gains at 9 months post-treatment. AAC has also been incorporated into phased intervention approaches that target multiple communication skills longitudinally, with both restitutive and compensatory treatment components (Mahendra & Tadokoro, 2020; Murray, 1998). Murray (1998) presented a phased treatment approach for an individual with nonfluent primary progressive aphasia (consistent with Neary et al., 1998, criteria). Following an initial phase of restitutive intervention, the individual was trained to use drawing to communicate intended messages, leading to improved performance on a trained drawing task. In another phase of treatment, communication boards were developed, with symbols that were subsequently transferred to an electronic AAC device programmed with corresponding written and spoken statements. The individual used the device successfully both within and outside of therapy sessions, adding new symbols to the device, as needed. Several months later, she and her spouse reported that she had spontaneously started drawing to communicate messages and continued to use the AAC device. Despite limited evidence, findings from these studies are promising and warrant further research, including use of AAC in the context of group therapy for PPA, as recent evidence suggests that group therapy sessions targeting AAC may be beneficial (Mooney et al., 2018). In addition to AAC, conversation partner training can be used to improve communication within the home by shifting some of the burden away from the individual with PPA. "Better Conversations" is one example of an evidence-based approach to conversation partner training in stroke-induced aphasia (Beeke et al., 2013) that has been adapted for use in PPA. Clinical trial results are pending, and online tutorials are being developed to aid in administration (Volkmer et al., 2021).

It is important to consider compensatory approaches such as AAC relatively early in the disease course, as increased success may be observed if the individual begins to use compensatory strategies and devices before deficits in general cognitive function emerge. This generally fits within a phased approach to intervention, where treatment initially focuses on restoring lost functions and strength-

ening residual functions, and gradually shifts to more functional, compensatory approaches (Mahendra & Tadokoro, 2020; Murray, 1998). Together, the person with PPA, their care partner, and the SLP can develop an individually tailored course of treatment to best suit the individual.

Conclusion

PPA is a relatively rare neurodegenerative disorder that predominantly affects speech and language. In PPA, general cognitive and motoric abilities are spared in the initial stages of the disease process, although additional impairments emerge over time. There are three widely recognized PPA subtypes: the semantic variant, characterized by a loss of core semantic knowledge; the logopenic variant, characterized by phonological processing deficits; and the nonfluent variant, characterized by agrammatism and/or apraxia of speech. The underlying disease etiology varies across the three subtypes. In this chapter, we presented information regarding clinical criteria for PPA diagnosis, approaches to assessment in PPA, and evidence-based treatment approaches that have proven beneficial in this population. It is imperative that researchers continue to investigate the nature and progression of deficits in PPA and focus efforts on the development of novel approaches to intervention as well as optimization of existing treatment approaches for this population. Given their unique set of skills, speech-language pathologists will play a critical role in these endeavors.

Case Study

The following case serves to illustrate the principles of assessment, diagnosis, and intervention in PPA that were described in this chapter.

Ms. Smith is a 55-year-old lawyer who has been having increasing difficulty finding words. She first noticed the problem in high-stress situations, such as when arguing a case in court, but was generally able to compensate by substituting a different word for words she could not find. At first, she thought that she was just tired and stressed, so she tried getting more rest. However, the problem continued to worsen. Recently, her word-finding problems have been affecting her ability to communicate in a significant way and are negatively impacting her work performance. She sometimes uses the wrong word in conversation. She was particularly worried when she was preparing for a big case and did not recognize an important piece of evidence. She asked her partner what the object was, and after being told that it was a checkbook, she said that she "felt foolish and laughed it off." Her family began to notice that she was having more and more trouble, and at her daughter's suggestion, she visited a neurologist.

At the neurologist, she reports that there is something wrong with her memory. Given her relatively young age, the neurologist thinks this is stress related or that she may be anxious or depressed. In order to be thorough, an MRI scan is acquired and a comprehensive neurological and cognitive-linguistic exam are performed. The neurologist notes that she is well groomed and behaves in a socially appropriate matter. Lab tests confirm that she is generally healthy, although a radiologist notes atrophy in the temporal lobes bilaterally. She performs well on measures of visual memory, visuospatial processing, and motor speech but makes semantic errors on a confrontation naming task. She is mildly impaired on a nonverbal measure of semantic processing (an object association test) and the Mini Mental State Exam. With this formal testing, it becomes clear that she does not have an episodic memory problem but instead is experiencing lexical retrieval difficulties and a mild loss of semantic knowledge. The neurologist diagnoses her with svPPA and she is referred to a speech-language pathologist (SLP) for further evaluation and treatment. The neurologist asks her to schedule follow-up appointments every 6 months.

The SLP meets with Ms. Smith and her daughter. The clinician first engages in casual conversation with Ms. Smith to get a general idea of her current language abilities and to better understand the nature of the communication challenges from her perspective. Given the recent neuropsychological testing, she does not conduct a full language assessment but does conduct a dynamic assessment of naming, evaluating Ms. Smith's potential for generating residual semantic, phonological, and orthographic information in the event of naming difficulty and her potential to self-cue for word retrieval. The SLP also takes the opportunity to offer some counseling regarding the PPA diagnosis and answers questions the two women have regarding the nature and progression of svPPA. She also discusses potential treatment options with Ms. Smith and her daughter, and together they identify goals for treatment. In the first phase, they will work on word-finding via semantic and phonological self-cueing strategies, as Ms. Smith has demonstrated the ability to retrieve residual semantic and phonological information during word-retrieval difficulty. Subsequently, they begin to work on developing a simple alternative communication system (a picture book with functional items grouped by category and paired with written words). Even though Ms. Smith doesn't feel as though she needs the book at this point, she understands that it will be easier to use in the future if she begins working with it now and learning to use it as a conversational support. The SLP, Ms. Smith, and her daughter all agree that Ms. Smith can benefit from practicing word-finding strategies and using her communication book at home with her family's support so that she can get the most out of treatment. Additionally, the SLP engages in structured communication partner training with Ms. Smith's daughter, emphasizing ways to maximize and support communication for her mother such as using high-frequency vocabulary, giving plenty of time to speak, and using and modeling multimodality communication strategies (e.g., writing, drawing, and gesturing). After this round of treatment, Ms. Smith will have follow-up appointments every 6 months with her neurologist and SLP to monitor symptom progression and to discern whether new goals for treatment should be developed and an additional "dose" of treatment undertaken.

References

Adlam, A. L. R., Patterson, K., Bozeat, S., & Hodges, J. R. (2010). The Cambridge Semantic Memory Test Battery: Detection of semantic deficits in semantic dementia and Alzheimer's disease. *Neurocase*, *16*(3), 193–207.

Battista, P., Miozzo, A., Piccininni, M., Catricalà, E., Capozzo, R., Tortelli, R., . . . Logroscino, G. (2017). Primary progressive aphasia: A review of neuropsychological tests for the assessment of speech and language disorders. *Aphasiology*, *31*(12), 1359–1378.

Beales, A., Cartwright, J., Whitworth, A., & Panegyres, P. K. (2016). Exploring generalisation processes following lexical retrieval intervention in primary progressive aphasia. *International Journal of Speech-Language Pathology*, *18*(3), 299–314.

Beeke, S., Sirman, N., Beckley, F., Maxim, J., Edwards, S., Swinburn, K., & Best, W. (2013). *Better conversations with aphasia: An e-learning resource.* https://extend.ucl.ac.uk/

Beeson, P. M., King, R. M., Bonakdarpour, B., Henry, M. L., Cho, H., & Rapcsak, S. Z. (2011). Positive effects of language treatment for the logopenic variant of primary progressive aphasia. *Journal of Molecular Neuroscience*, *45*(3), 724–736.

Bier, N., Macoir, J., Gagnon, L., Van der Linden, M., Louveaux, S., & Desrosiers, J. (2009). Known, lost, and recovered: Efficacy of formal-semantic therapy and spaced retrieval method in a case of semantic dementia. *Aphasiology*, *23*(2), 210–235.

Billette, O. V., Sajjadi, S. A., Patterson, K., & Nestor, P. J. (2015). SECT and MAST: New tests to assess grammatical abilities in primary progressive aphasia. *Aphasiology*, *29*(10), 1135–1151.

Binney, R. J., Henry, M. L., Babiak, M., Pressman, P. S., Santos-Santos, M. A., Narvid, J., . . . Binney, R. J. (2016). Reading words and other people: a comparison of exception word, familiar face and affect processing in the left and right temporal variants of primary progressive aphasia. *Cortex*, *82*, 147–163.

Bonner, M. F., Ash, S., & Grossman, M. (2010). The new classification of primary progressive aphasia into semantic, logopenic, or nonfluent/agrammatic variants. *Current Neurology and Neuroscience Reports, 10*(6), 484–490.

Brambati, S. M., Amici, S., Racine, C. A., Neuhaus, J., Miller, Z., Ogar, J., . . . Gorno-Tempini, M. L. (2015). Longitudinal gray matter contraction in three variants of primary progressive aphasia: A tenser-based morphometry study. *NeuroImage: Clinical, 8*, 345–355.

Brambati, S. M., Ogar, J., Neuhaus, J., Miller, B. L., & Gorno-Tempini, M. L. (2009). Reading disorders in primary progressive aphasia: A behavioral and neuroimaging study. *Neuropsychologia, 47*(8–9), 1893–1900.

Buchsbaum, B. R., Hickok, G., & Humphries, C. (2001). Role of left posterior superior temporal gyrus in phonological processing for speech perception and production. *Cognitive Science, 25*(5), 663–678.

Cadório, I., Lousada, M., Martins, P., & Figueiredo, D. (2017). Generalization and maintenance of treatment gains in primary progressive aphasia (PPA): A systematic review. *International Journal of Language & Communication Disorders, 52*(5), 543–560.

Caffarra, P., Gardini, S., Cappa, S., Dieci, F., Concari, L., Barocco, F., . . . Prati, G. D. R. (2013). Degenerative jargon aphasia: Unusual progression of logopenic/phonological progressive aphasia? *Behavioural Neurology, 26*, 89–93.

Carthery-Goulart, M. T., Silveira, A. D. C. D., Machado, T. H., Mansur, L. L., Parente, M. A. D. M. P., Senaha, M. L. H., . . . Nitrini, R. (2013). Nonpharmacological interventions for cognitive impairments following primary progressive aphasia: A systematic review of the literature. *Dementia & Neuropsychologia, 7*, 122–131.

Cerami, C., Dodich, A., Greco, L., Iannaccone, S., Magnani, G., Marcone, A., . . . Perani, D. (2017). The role of single-subject brain metabolic patterns in the early differential diagnosis of primary progressive aphasias and in prediction of progression to dementia. *Journal of Alzheimer's Disease, 55*, 183–197.

Coemans, S., Struys, E., Vandenborre, D., Wilssens, I., Engelborghs, S., Paquier, P., . . . Keulen, S. (2021). A systematic review of transcranial direct current stimulation in primary progressive aphasia: Methodological considerations. *Frontiers in Aging Neuroscience, 13*, 710818.

Coltheart, M., Rastle, K., Perry, C., Langdon, R., & Ziegler, J. (2001). DRC: A dual route cascaded model of visual word recognition and reading aloud. *Psychological Review, 108*(1), 204.

Cotelli, M., Manenti, R., Ferrari, C., Gobbi, E., Macis, A., & Cappa, S. F. (2020). Effectiveness of language training and non-invasive brain stimulation on oral and written naming performance in primary progressive aphasia: A meta-analysis and systematic review. *Neuroscience & Biobehavioral Reviews, 108*, 498–525.

Cotelli, M., Manenti, R., Paternicò, D., Cosseddu, M., Brambilla, M., Petesi, M., . . . Borroni, B. (2016). Grey matter density predicts the improvement of naming abilities after tDCS intervention in agrammatic variant of primary progressive aphasia. *Brain Topography, 29*(5), 738–751.

Cotelli, M., Manenti, R., Petesi, M., Brambilla, M., Cosseddu, M., Zanetti, O., . . . Borroni, B. (2014). Treatment of primary progressive aphasias by transcranial direct current stimulation combined with language training. *Journal of Alzheimer's Disease, 39*(4), 799–808.

Cress, C. J., & King, J. M. (1999). AAC strategies for people with primary progressive aphasia without dementia: Two case studies. *Augmentative and Alternative Communication, 15*(4), 248–259.

Croot, K., Taylor, C., Abel, S., Jones, K., Krein, L., Hameister, I., . . . Nickels, L. (2015). Measuring gains in connected speech following treatment for word retrieval: A study with two participants with primary progressive aphasia. *Aphasiology*, *29*(11), 1265–1288.

Déjerine, J. J., & Sérieux, P. (1897). Un cas de surdité verbale pure, terminée par aphasie sensorielle, suivi d'autopsie. *Comptes Rendues des Séances de la Société de Biologie (Paris)*, *49*, 1074–1077.

Dial, H., Europa, E., Grasso, S. M., Mandelli, M. L., Schaffer, K. M., Hubbard, H. I., . . . Henry, M. L. (2023). Baseline structural imaging correlates of treatment outcomes in semantic variant primary progressive aphasia. *Cortex*, *158*, 158–175.

Dial, H., Hinshelwood, H., Grasso, S., Hubbard, H., Gorno-Tempini, M. L., & Henry, M. (2019). Investigating the utility of teletherapy in individuals with primary progressive aphasia. *Clinical Interventions in Aging*, *14*, 1–19.

Dressel, K., Huber, W., Frings, L., Kümmerer, D., Saur, D., Mader, I., . . . Abel, S. (2010). Model-oriented naming therapy in semantic dementia: A single-case fMRI study. *Aphasiology*, *24*(12), 1537–1558.

Dronkers, N. (1996). A new brain region for coordinating speech articulation. *Nature*, *384*, 159–161.

Duffy, J. R. (2013). *Motor speech disorders: Substrates, differential diagnosis, and management.* Elsevier Health Sciences.

Duffy, J. R., & Josephs, K. A. (2012). The diagnosis and understanding of apraxia of speech: Why including neurodegenerative etiologies may be important. *Journal of Speech, Language, and Hearing Research*, *55*(5), S1518–S1522.

Duffy, J. R., Utianski, R. L., & Josephs, K. A. (2021). Primary progressive apraxia of speech: From recognition to diagnosis and care. *Aphasiology*, *35*(4), 560–591.

Evans, W. S., Quimby, M., Dickey, M. W., & Dickerson, B. C. (2016). Relearning and retaining personally-relevant words using computer-based flashcard software in primary progressive aphasia. *Frontiers in Human Neuroscience*, *10*, 1–8.

Farrajota, L., Maruta, C., Maroco, J., Martins, I. P., Guerreiro, M., & De Mendonca, A.

(2012). Speech therapy in primary progressive aphasia: a pilot study. *Dementia and Geriatric Cognitive Disorders Extra*, *2*(1), 321–331.

Fenner, A. S., Webster, K. T., Ficek, B. N., Frangakis, C. E., & Tsapkini, K. (2019). Written verb naming improves after tDCS over the left IFG in primary progressive aphasia. *Frontiers in Psychology*, *10*, 1396.

Folstein, M. F., Folstein, S. E., & McHugh, P. R. (1975). "Mini-mental state": A practical method for grading the cognitive state of patients for the clinician. *Journal of Psychiatric Research*, *12*(3), 189–198.

Friederici, A. D. (2002). Towards a neural basis of auditory sentence processing. *Trends in Cognitive Sciences*, *6*(2), 78–84.

Friederici, A. D., Ruschemeyer, S.-A., Hahne, A., & Fiebach, C. J. (2003). The role of left inferior frontal and superior temporal cortex in sentence comprehension: Localizing syntactic and semantic processes. *Cerebral Cortex*, *13*, 170–177.

Goodglass, H., Kaplan, E., & Barresi, B. (2001). *The Boston Diagnostic Aphasia Examination (BDAE-3).* Lippincott Williams & Wilkins.

Gorno-Tempini, M. L., Brambati, S. M., Ginex, V., Ogar, J., Dronkers, N. F., Marcone, A., . . . Miller, B. L. (2008). The logopenic/phonological variant of primary progressive aphasia. *Neurology*, *71*(16), 1227–1234.

Gorno-Tempini, M. L., Dronkers, N. F., Rankin, K. P., Ogar, J. M., Phengrasamy, L., Rosen, H. J., . . . Miller, B. L. (2004). Cognition and anatomy in three variants of primary progressive aphasia. *Annals of Neurology*, *55*(3), 335–346.

Gorno-Tempini, M. L., Hillis, A. E., Weintraub, S., Kertesz, A., Mendez, M., Cappa, S. F., . . . Grossman, M. (2011). Classification of primary progressive aphasia and its variants. *Neurology*, *76*(11), 1006–1014.

Gorno-Tempini, M. L., Ogar, J. M., Brambati, S. M., Wang, P., Jeong, J. H., Rankin, K. P., . . . Miller, B. L. (2006). Anatomical correlates of early mutism in progressive nonfluent aphasia. *Neurology, 67,* 1849–1851.

Graham, K. S., Patterson, K., Pratt, K. H., & Hodges, J. R. (1999). Relearning and subsequent forgetting of semantic category exemplars in a case of semantic dementia. *Neuropsychology, 13*(3), 359.

Graham, K. S., Patterson, K., Pratt, K. H., & Hodges, J. R. (2001). Can repeated exposure to "forgotten" vocabulary help alleviate word-finding difficulties in semantic dementia? An illustrative case study. *Neuropsychological Rehabilitation, 11*(3–4), 429–454.

Grasso, S. M., Peña, E. D., Kazemi, N., Mirzapour, H., Neupane, R., Bonakdarpour, B., . . . Henry, M. L. (2021). Treatment for anomia in bilingual speakers with progressive aphasia. *Brain Sciences, 11*(11), 1371.

Grossman, M., Mickanin, J., Onishi, K., Hughes, E., D'Esposito, M., Ding, X. S., . . . Reivich, M. (1996). Progressive nonfluent aphasia: Language, cognitive, and PET measures contrasted with probable Alzheimer's disease. *Journal of Cognitive Neuroscience, 8*(2), 135–154.

Hameister, I., Nickels, L., Abel, S., & Croot, K. (2016). "Do you have mowing the lawn?"—Improvements in word retrieval and grammar following constraint-induced language therapy in primary progressive aphasia. *Aphasiology, 31*(13), 1–24.

Harris, J. M., Gall, C., Thompson, J. C., Richardson, A. M. T., Neary, D., du Plessis, D., . . . Jones, M. (2013). Classification and pathology of primary progressive aphasia. *Neurology, 81*(21), 1832–1839.

Henry, M., Beeson, P., & Rapcsak, S. (2008). Treatment for lexical retrieval in progressive aphasia. *Aphasiology, 22*(7–8), 826–838.

Henry, M., & Gorno-Tempini, M. L. (2010). The logopenic variant of primary progressive aphasia. *Current Opinion in Neurology, 23*(6), 633–637.

Henry, M., & Grasso, S. (2018). Assessment of individuals with primary progressive aphasia. *Seminars in Speech and Language, 39*(3), 231–241.

Henry, M. L., Hubbard, H. I., Grasso, S. M., Dial, H. R., Beeson, P. M., Miller, B. L., & Gorno-Tempini, M. L. (2019). Treatment for word retrieval in semantic and logopenic variants of primary progressive aphasia: Immediate and long-term outcomes. *Journal of Speech, Language, and Hearing Research, 62*(8), 2723–2749.

Henry, M. L., Hubbard, H. I., Grasso, S. M., Mandelli, M. L., Wilson, S. M., Sathishkumar, M. T., . . . Gorno-Tempini, M. L. (2018). Retraining speech production and fluency in non-fluent/agrammatic primary progressive aphasia. *Brain, 141*(6), 1799–1814.

Henry, M. L., Meese, M. V, Truong, S., Babiak, M. C., Miller, B. L., & Gorno-Tempini, M. L. (2013). Treatment for apraxia of speech in nonfluent variant primary progressive aphasia. *Behavioural Neurology, 26*(1–2), 77–88.

Henry, M. L., Rising, K., DeMarco, A. T., Miller, B. L., Gorno-Tempini, M. L., & Beeson, P. M. (2013). Examining the value of lexical retrieval treatment in primary progressive aphasia: Two positive cases. *Brain and Language, 127*(2), 145–156.

Henry, M. L., Wilson, S. M., Babiak, M. C., Mandelli, M. L., Beeson, P. M., Miller, Z. A., & Gorno-Tempini, M. L. (2016). Phonological processing in primary progressive aphasia. *Journal of Cognitive Neuroscience, 28*(2), 210–222.

Heredia, C. G., Sage, K., Lambon Ralph, M. A., & Berthier, M. L. (2009). Relearning and retention of verbal labels in a case of semantic dementia. *Aphasiology, 23*(2), 192–209.

Hodges, J. R., Martinos, M., Woollams, A. M., Patterson, K., & Adlam, A. R. (2008). Repeat and point: Differentiating semantic dementia from progressive non-fluent aphasia. *Cortex, 44,* 1265–1270.

Hodges, J. R., & Patterson, K. (2007). Semantic dementia: A unique clinicopathological syndrome. *Lancet Neurology*, *6*(11), 1004–1014.

Hodges, J. R., Patterson, K., Oxbury, S., & Funnell, E. (1992). Semantic dementia: Progressive fluent aphasia with temporal lobe atrophy. *Brain*, *115*(6), 1783–1806.

Hoffman, P., Clarke, N., Jones, R.W., & Noonan, K. A. (2015). Vocabulary relearning in semantic dementia: Positive and negative consequences of increasing variability in the learning experience. *Neuropsychologia*, *76*, 240–253.

Howard, D., & Patterson, K. (1992). *The Pyramids and Palm Trees Test: A test of semantic access from words and pictures*. Thames Valley Test Company.

Jokel, R., & Anderson, N. D. (2012). Quest for the best: Effects of errorless and active encoding on word re-learning in semantic dementia. *Neuropsychological Rehabilitation*, *22*(2), 187–214.

Jokel, R., Cupit, J., Rochon, E., & Leonard, C. (2009). Relearning lost vocabulary in nonfluent progressive aphasia with MossTalk words. *Aphasiology*, *23*(2), 175–191.

Jokel, R., Kielar, A., Anderson, N. D., Black, S. E., Rochon, E., Graham, S., . . . Tang-Wai, D. F. (2016). Behavioural and neuroimaging changes after naming therapy for semantic variant primary progressive aphasia. *Neuropsychologia*, *89*, 191–216.

Jokel, R., & Meltzer, J. (2017). Group intervention for individuals with primary progressive aphasia and their spouses: Who comes first? *Journal of Communication Disorders*, *66*, 51–64.

Jokel, R., Rochon, E., & Anderson, N. D. (2010). Errorless learning of computer-generated words in a patient with semantic dementia. *Neuropsychological Rehabilitation*, *20*(1), 16–41.

Jokel, R., Rochon, E., & Leonard, C. (2006). Treating anomia in semantic dementia: Improvement, maintenance, or both? *Neuropsychological Rehabilitation*, *16*(3), 241–256.

Josephs, K. A., Duffy, J. R., Strand, E. A., Machulda, M. M., Senjem, M. L., Master, A. V., . . . Whitwell, J. L. (2012). Characterizing a neurodegenerative syndrome: Primary progressive apraxia of speech. *Brain*, *135*(5), 1522–1536.

Kertesz, A. (2007). *Western Aphasia Battery–Revised*. The Psychological Corporation.

Kertesz, A., & Kalvach, P. (1996). Arnold Pick and German neuropsychiatry in Prague. *Archives of Neurology*, *53*(9), 935–938.

Kobayashi, H., Ohnishi, T., Nakagawa, R., & Yoshizawa, K. (2016). The comparative efficacy and safety of cholinesterase inhibitors in patients with mild-to-moderate Alzheimer's disease: A Bayesian network meta-analysis. *International Journal of Geriatric Psychiatry*, *31*(8), 892–904.

Langmore, S. E., Olney, R. K., Lomen-Hoerth, C., & Miller, B. L. (2007). Dysphagia in patients with frontotemporal lobar dementia. *Archives of Neurology*, *64*(1), 58–62.

Leyton, C. E., & Hodges, J. R. (2013). Towards a clearer definition of logopenic progressive aphasia. *Current Neurology and Neuroscience Reports*, *13*(11), 396.

Leyton, C. E., Hodges, J. R., McLean, C. A., Kril, J. J., Piguet, O., & Ballard, K. J. (2015). Is the logopenic-variant of primary progressive aphasia a unitary disorder? *Cortex*, *67*, 122–133.

Leyton, C. E., Villemagne, V. L., Savage, S., Pike, K. E., Ballard, K. J., Piguet, O., . . . Hodges, J. R. (2011). Subtypes of progressive aphasia: Application of the international consensus criteria and validation using β-amyloid imaging. *Brain*, *134*, 3030–3043.

Machado, T. H., Campanha, A. C., Caramelli, P., & Carthery-Goulart, M. T. (2014). Brief intervention for agrammatism in primary progressive nonfluent A case report. [Intervençã breve para agramatismo em afasia progressiva primária não fluente: relato de caso]. *Dementia e Neuropsychologia*, *8*(3), 291–296.

Macoir, J., Lavoie, M., Laforce, R., Brambati, S. M., & Wilson, M. A. (2017). Dysexecutive symptoms in primary progressive aphasia: Beyond diagnostic criteria. *Journal of Geriatric Psychiatry and Neurology, 30*(3), 151–161.

Macoir, J., Leroy, M., Routhier, S., Auclair-Ouellet, N., Houde, M., & Laforce, R. (2015). Improving verb anomia in the semantic variant of primary progressive aphasia: The effectiveness of a semantic-phonological cueing treatment. *Neurocase, 21*(4), 448–456.

Mahendra, N., & Tadokoro, A. (2020). Nonfluent primary progressive aphasia: Implications of palliative care principles for informing service delivery. *Topics in Language Disorders, 40*(3), E7–E24.

Marcotte, K., & Ansaldo, A.I. (2010). The neural correlates of semantic feature analysis in chronic aphasia: Discordant patterns according to etiology. *Seminars in Speech and Language, 31*, 52–63.

Mayberry, E., Sage, K., Ehsan, S., & Lambon Ralph, M. (2011a). An emergent effect of phonemic cueing following relearning in semantic dementia. *Aphasiology, 25*(9), 1069–1077.

Mayberry, E., Sage, K., Ehsan, S., & Lambon Ralph, M. (2011b). Relearning in semantic dementia reflects contributions from both medial temporal lobe episodic and degraded neocortical semantic systems: Evidence in support of the complementary learning systems theory. *Neuropsychologia, 49*, 3591–3598.

McDonald, S., Flanagan, S., Rollins, J., & Kinch, J. (2003). TASIT: A new clinical tool for assessing social perception after traumatic brain injury. *The Journal of Head Trauma Rehabilitation, 18*(3), 219–238.

Mesulam, M. M. (1982). Slowly progressive aphasia without generalized dementia. *Annals of Neurology, 11*(6), 592–598.

Mesulam, M. M. (2001). Primary progressive aphasia. *Annals of Neurology, 49*(4), 425–432.

Mesulam, M., Wieneke, C., Rogalski, E., Cobia, D., Thompson, C., & Weintraub, S. (2009). Quantitative template for subtyping primary progressive aphasia. *Archives of Neurology, 66*(12), 1545–1551.

Mesulam, M., Wieneke, C., Thompson, C., Rogalski, E., & Weintraub, S. (2012). Quantitative classification of primary progressive aphasia at early and mild impairment stages. *Brain, 135*(5), 1537–1553.

Meyer, A. M., Faria, A. V., Tippett, D. C., Hillis, A. E., & Friedman, R. B. (2017). The relationship between baseline volume in temporal areas and post-treatment naming accuracy in primary progressive aphasia. *Aphasiology, 31*, 1059–1077.

Meyer, A. M., Getz, H. R., Brennan, D. M., Hu, T. M., & Friedman, R. B. (2016). Telerehabilitation of anomia in primary progressive aphasia. *Aphasiology, 30*(4), 483–507.

Meyer, A. M., Snider, S. F., Eckmann, C. B., & Friedman, R. B. (2015). Prophylactic treatments for anomia in the logopenic variant of primary progressive aphasia: Cross-language transfer. *Aphasiology, 29*(9), 1062–1081.

Meyer, A. M., Tippett, D. C., & Friedman, R. B. (2016). Prophylaxis and remediation of anomia in the semantic and logopenic variants of primary progressive aphasia. *Neuropsychological Rehabilitation, 28*(3), 352–368.

Miller, L. A., Hsieh, S., Lah, S., Savage, S., Hodges, J. R., & Piguet, O. (2012). One size does not fit all: Face emotion processing impairments in semantic dementia, behavioural-variant frontotemporal dementia and Alzheimer's disease are mediated by distinct cognitive deficits. *Behavioural Neurology, 25*(1), 53–60.

Montembeault, M., Brambati, S. M., Gorno-Tempini, M. L., & Migliaccio, R. (2018). Clinical, anatomical, and pathological features in the three variants of primary progressive aphasia: A review. *Frontiers in Neurology, 9*, 692.

Mooney, A., Beale, N., & Fried-Oken, M. (2018). Group communication treatment for individuals with PPA and their partners. *Seminars in Speech and Language, 39*, 257–269.

Mooney, A., Bedrick, S., Noethe, G., Spaulding, S., & Fried-Oken, M. (2018). Mobile technology to support lexical retrieval during activity retell in primary progressive aphasia, *Aphasiology*, 32(6), 666–692.

Murray, L. L. (1998). Longitudinal treatment of primary progressive aphasia: A case study. *Aphasiology*, 12, 651–672.

Nasreddine, Z. S., Phillips, N. A., Bédirian, V., Charbonneau, S., Whitehead, V., Collin, I., . . . Chertkow, H. (2005). The Montreal Cognitive Assessment, MoCA: A brief screening tool for mild cognitive impairment. *Journal of the American Geriatrics Society*, 53(4), 695–699.

Neary, D., Snowden, J. S., Gustafson, L., Passant, U., Stuss, D., Black, S., . . . Benson, D. F. (1998). Frontotemporal lobar degeneration: A consensus on clinical diagnostic criteria. *Neurology*, 51(6), 1546–1554.

Neumann, M., Lee, E. B., & Mackenzie, I. R. (2021). Frontotemporal lobar degeneration TDP-43-immunoreactive pathological subtypes: Clinical and mechanistic significance. *Advances in Experimental Medicine and Biology*, 1281, 201–217. https://doi.org/10.1007/978-3-030-51140-1_13

Newhart, M., Davis, C., Kannan, V., Heidler-Gary, J., Cloutman, L., & Hillis, A. E. (2009). Therapy for naming deficits in two variants of primary progressive aphasia. *Aphasiology*, 23(7–8), 823–834.

Nicholas, L. E., & Brookshire, R. H. (1993). A system for quantifying the informativeness and efficiency of the connected speech of adults with aphasia. *Journal of Speech, Language, and Hearing Research*, 36(2), 338–350.

Nissim, N. R., Moberg, P. J., & Hamilton, R. H. (2020). Efficacy of noninvasive brain stimulation (tDCS or TMS) paired with language therapy in the treatment of primary progressive aphasia: An exploratory meta-analysis. *Brain Sciences*, 10(9), 597.

Novak, P., Zilka, N., Zilkova, M., Kovacech, B., Skrabana, R., Ondrus, M., . . .

Novak, M. (2019). AADvac1, an active immunotherapy for Alzheimer's disease and non-Alzheimer tauopathies: An overview of preclinical and clinical development. *The Journal of Prevention of Alzheimer's Disease*, 6, 63–69.

Ogar, J. M., Dronkers, N. F., Brambati, S. M., Miller, B. L., & Gorno-Tempini, M. L. (2007). Progressive nonfluent aphasia and its characteristic motor speech deficits. *Alzheimer Disease and Associated Disorders*, 21(4), S23–S30.

Pattee, C., Von Berg, S., & Ghezzi, P. (2006). Effects of alternative communication on the communicative effectiveness of an individual with a progressive language disorder. *International Journal of Rehabilitation Research*, 29(2), 151–153.

Patterson, K., Nestor, P. J., & Rogers, T. T. (2007). Where do you know what you know? The representation of semantic knowledge in the human brain. *Nature Reviews Neuroscience*, 8(12), 976–987.

Pick, A. (1892). Uber die Beziehungen der senilen Hirnatrophie zur Aphasie. *Prager Medizinische Wochenschrift*, 17, 165–167.

Pick, A. (1977). On the relation between aphasia and senile atrophy of the brain. In D. Rottenberg & F. Hochberg (Eds.), *Neurological classics in modern translation* (pp. 35–40). Hafner Press.

Rascovsky, K., Hodges, J. R., Kipps, C. M., Johnson, J. K., Seeley, W. W., Mendez, M. F., . . . Miller, B. M. (2007). Diagnostic criteria for the behavioral variant of frontotemporal dementia (bvFTD): Current limitations and future directions. *Alzheimer Disease & Associated Disorders*, 21(4), S14–S18.

Rogalski, E., Cobia, D., Harrison, T. M., Wieneke, C., Weintraub, S., & Mesulam, M.-M. (2011). Progression of language decline and cortical atrophy in subtypes of primary progressive aphasia. *Neurology*, 76(21), 1804–1810.

Rogalski, E. J., & Khayum, B. (2018). A life participation approach to primary progressive aphasia intervention. *Seminars in Speech and Language*, 39(3), 284–296.

Rohrer, J. D., Caso, F., Mahoney, C., Henry, M., Rosen, H. J., Rabinovici, G., . . . Gorno-Tempini, M. L. (2013). Patterns of longitudinal brain atrophy in the logopenic variant of primary progressive aphasia. *Brain and Language, 127*, 121–126.

Rohrer, J. D., Ridgway, G. R., Crutch, S. J., Hailstone, J., Goll, J. C., Clarkson, M. J., . . . Warrington, E. K. (2010). Progressive logopenic/phonological aphasia: Erosion of the language network. *Neuroimage, 49*(1), 984–993.

Rosen, H. J., Gorno-Tempini, M. L., Goldman, W. P., Perry, R. J., Schuff, N., Weiner, M., . . . Miller, B. L. (2002). Patterns of brain atrophy in frontotemporal dementia and semantic dementia. *Neurology, 58*, 198–208.

Sajjadi, S. A., Patterson, K., & Nestor, P. J. (2014). Logopenic, mixed, or Alzheimer-related aphasia? *Neurology, 82*(13), 1127–1131.

Sapolsky, D., Domoto-Reilly, K., & Dickerson, B. C. (2014). Use of the Progressive Aphasia Severity Scale (PASS) in monitoring speech and language status in PPA. *Aphasiology, 28*(8–9), 993–1003.

Savage, S. A., Ballard, K. J., Piguet, O., & Hodges, J. R. (2013). Bringing words back to mind—Improving word production in semantic dementia. *Cortex, 49*(7), 1823–1832.

Savage, S. A., Foxe, D., & Piguet, O. (2013). Distinguishing subtypes in primary progressive aphasia: Application of the Sydney Language Battery. *Dementia and Geriatric Cognitive Disorders, 35*, 208–218.

Savage, S. A., Piguet, O., & Hodges, J. R. (2015). Cognitive intervention in semantic dementia: Maintaining words over time. *Alzheimer Disease and Associated Disorders, 29*(1), 55–62.

Schaffer, K. M., Evans, W. S., Dutcher, C. D., Philburn, C., & Henry, M. L. (2021). Embedding aphasia-modified cognitive behavioral therapy in script training for primary progressive aphasia: A single-case pilot study. *American Journal of Speech-Language Pathology, 30*(5), 2053–2068.

Schaffer, K. M., & Henry, M. L. (2021). Counseling and care partner training in primary progressive aphasia. *Perspectives of the ASHA Special Interest Groups, 6*(5), 1015–1025.

Schneider, S. L., Thompson, C. K., & Luring, B. (1996). Effects of verbal plus gestural matrix training on sentence production in a patient with primary progressive aphasia. *Aphasiology, 10*(3), 297–317.

Seeley, W. W., Bauer, A. M., Miller, B. L., Gorno-Tempini, M. L., Kramer, J. H., Weiner, M., & Rosen, H. J. (2005). The natural history of temporal variant frontotemporal dementia. *Neurology, 64*(8), 1384–1390.

Sheppard, S. (2022). Noninvasive brain stimulation to augment language therapy for primary progressive aphasia. *Handbook of Clinical Neurology, 185*, 251–260.

Simmons, W. K., & Martin, A. (2009). The anterior temporal lobes and the functional architecture of semantic memory. *Journal of the International Neuropsychological Society, 15*, 645–649.

Snowden, J. S., Goulding, P. J., & Neary, D. (1989). Semantic dementia: A form of circumscribed cerebral atrophy. *Behavioural Neurology, 2*, 167–182.

Snowden, J. S., & Neary, D. (2002). Relearning of verbal labels in semantic dementia. *Neuropsychologia, 40*(10), 1715–1728.

Spinelli, E. G., Mandelli, M. L., Miller, Z. A., Santos-Santos, M. A., Wilson, S. M., Agosta, F., . . . Gorno-Tempini, M. L. (2017). Typical and atypical pathology in primary progressive aphasia variants. *Annals of Neurology, 81*(3), 430–443.

Suarez-Gonzalez, A., Savage, S. A., Bier, N., Henry, M. L., Jokel, R., Nickels, L., & Taylor-Rubin, C. (2021). Semantic variant primary progressive aphasia: Practical recommendations for treatment from 20 years of behavioral research. *Brain Sciences, 11*(12), 1552.

Swinburn, K., Porter, G., & Howard, D. (2004). *Comprehensive Aphasia Test*. Psychology Press.

Trinh, N. H., Hoblyn, J., Mohanty, S., & Yaffe, K. (2003). Efficacy of cholinesterase inhibitors in the treatment of neuropsychiatric symptoms and functional impairment in Alzheimer disease: A meta-analysis. *JAMA, 289*(2), 210–216.

Tsapkini, K., Frangakis, C., Gomez, Y., Davis, C., & Hillis, A. E. (2014). Augmentation of spelling therapy with transcranial direct current stimulation in primary progressive aphasia: Preliminary results and challenges. *Aphasiology, 28*(8–9), 1112–1130.

Tsapkini, K., & Hillis, A. E. (2013). Spelling intervention in post-stroke aphasia and primary progressive aphasia. *Behavioural Neurology, 26*, 55–66.

Ulugut Erkoyun, H., Groot, C., Heilbron, R., Nelissen, A., van Rossum, J., Jutten, R., . . . Pijnenburg, Y. (2020). A clinical-radiological framework of the right temporal variant of frontotemporal dementia. *Brain, 143*(9), 2831–2843.

Volkmer, A., Rogalski, E., Henry, M., Taylor-Rubin, C., Ruggero, L., Khayum, R., . . . Rohrer, J. D. (2020). Speech and language therapy approaches to managing primary progressive aphasia. *Practical Neurology, 20*(2), 154–161.

Volkmer, A., Spector, A., Meitanis, V., Warren, J. D., & Beeke, S. (2020). Effects of functional communication interventions for people with primary progressive aphasia and their caregivers: A systematic review. *Aging & Mental Health, 24*(9), 1381–1393.

Volkmer, A., Spector, A., Swinburn, K., Warren, J. D., & Beeke, S. (2021). Using the Medical Research Council framework and public involvement in the development of a communication partner training intervention for people with primary progressive aphasia (PPA): Better Conversations with PPA. *BMC Geriatrics, 21*, 1–17.

Warrington, E. K. (1975). The selective impairment of semantic memory. *The Quarterly Journal of Experimental Psychology, 27*(4), 635–657.

Weintraub, S., Mesulam, M. M., Wieneke, C., Rademaker, A., Rogalski, E. J., & Thompson, C. K. (2009). The Northwestern Anagram Test: Measuring sentence production in primary progressive aphasia. *American Journal of Alzheimer's Disease & Other Dementias, 24*(5), 408–416.

Wertz, R. T., LaPointe, L. L., & Rosenbek, J. C. (1984). *Apraxia of speech in adults: The disorder and its management*. Grune and Stratton.

Wilson, S. M., Dehollain, C., Ferrieux, S., Christensen, L. E. H., & Teichmann, M. (2017). Lexical access in semantic variant PPA: Evidence for a post-semantic contribution to naming deficits. *Neuropsychologia, 106*, 90–99.

Wilson, S. M., Henry, M. L., Besbris, M., Ogar, J. M., Dronkers, N. F., Jarrold, W., . . . Gorno-Tempini, M. L. (2010). Connected speech production in three variants of primary progressive aphasia. *Brain, 133*, 2069–2088.

Wisse, L. E., Ungrady, M. B., Ittyerah, R., Lim, S. A., Yushkevich, P. A., Wolk, D. A., . . . Grossman, M. (2021). Cross-sectional and longitudinal medial temporal lobe subregional atrophy patters in semantic variant primary progressive aphasia. *Neurobiology of Aging, 98*, 231–241.

Younes, K., Borghesani, V., Montembeault, M., Spina, S., Mandelli, M. L., Welch, A. E., . . . Gorno-Tempini, M. L. (2022). Right temporal degeneration and socioemotional semantics: Semantic behavioural variant frontotemporal dementia. *Brain, 145*(11), 4080–4096.

Young, J. J., Lavakumar, M., Tampi, D., Balachandran, S., & Tampi, R. R. (2018). Frontotemporal dementia: Latest evidence and clinical implications. *Therapeutic Advances in Psychopharmacology, 8*(1), 33–48.

6

Dementia: Concepts and Contemporary Practice

Nidhi Mahendra and Eduardo Europa

Chapter Learning Objectives

After reading this chapter you will be able to:

1. Compare and contrast mild cognitive impairment and dementia.
2. Summarize the decline of cognitive communication in persons with Alzheimer's disease.
3. Describe salient characteristics of common types of dementia, other than Alzheimer's disease.
4. Discuss the role of speech-language pathologists in serving persons with dementia or mild cognitive impairment.
5. Select appropriate screening and assessment measures for persons with dementia or mild cognitive impairment.
6. Identify evidence-based principles for managing cognitive-communicative impairments in persons with dementia.

Introduction

Population aging is considered one of the most pivotal social transformations of the 21st century. In 2018, for the first time in recorded history, globally, persons over the age of 65 years outnumbered children under the age of 5 years (United Nations, 2019). In the United States, the 2020 census revealed that in the past decade, the number of Americans aged 65 years or older grew by 34.2% or 13,787,044 people (United States Census Bureau, 2020). Global aging has significant implications for health care practitioners, including speech-language pathologists (SLPs) and audiologists, who serve increasing numbers of older adults on their caseloads. There is an urgent need for better understanding of biopsychosocial changes that accompany typical and pathological aging, as well as for ensuring that extensions in human life span go alongside improvements in health and quality of life.

One consequence of global demographic changes and accelerated aging is the increasing likelihood of dementia and of mild cognitive impairment or MCI—a state of cognitive function between that seen in normal aging and dementia (Petersen, 2016). Indeed, the World Health Organization (WHO, 2017) has recognized dementia as a public health priority and reported that more than 55 million people worldwide have dementia, with more than 60% living in low-income and middle-income countries (WHO, 2022). Dementia deserves the greatest attention because of its significant global incidence and prevalence, its progressive nature, the social and economic implications of care, and its tremendous impact on individuals and families.

Historically, there has always been a strong focus on basic and applied research to better understand dementia and its distinct types, characteristic cellular-molecular pathology and neuropathology, clinical symptomatology, progression, and pharmacological treatments. In the past 30 years, there has been much research aimed at enhancing early identification, timely diagnosis, nonpharmacological interventions, optimizing cognition and well-being in affected persons, palliative care, and caregiver-focused training and interventions. It is imperative that SLPs have expert knowledge of evidence-based practices and culturally responsive practices for optimally serving persons with dementia. Further, SLPs have an important role in leading research efforts and community education about modifiable risk factors and lifelong practices and activities that build cognitive reserve and stave off late-life cognitive decline. Speech-language pathologists have unique knowledge and skills to serve persons with dementia and MCI given their strong foundation in understanding typical and atypical changes in communication, cognition, swallowing, health status, and quality of life. Also, SLPs work with persons with dementia in varied clinical settings, including acute care, skilled nursing facilities, community-based centers (e.g., senior centers), and home-based health care. The following sections introduce the impact of dementia on racially and ethnically diverse populations and present a definition of dementia, MCI, and the latest diagnostic criteria.

Impact of Dementia on Racially and Ethnically Diverse Populations

Much research on health disparities reveals that the burden of neurological disorders and neurodegenerative conditions like dementia is not uniformly distributed across all persons, communities, and cultural groups. There is growing understanding that differential distribution of social determinants of health and many structural and systemic factors (e.g., unequal access to health care, prevalence of risk factors) underlie these differences. As the racial and ethnic composition of the U.S. population changes rapidly and global aging occurs at an unprecedented rate, there is a strong interest in studying the incidence and impact of dementia across persons of different races and ethnicities.

Recent reports reveal that age-adjusted dementia incidence rates are highest among Black and Hispanic adults, being significantly higher than non-Hispanic White adults (Alzheimer's Association, 2022; Kornblith et al., 2022; Mehta & Yeo, 2016). Dementia incidence and impact has been understudied in some groups like Native American and Alaska Native populations as well as among Asian Americans (Mayeda et al., 2016). These insufficient data on and limited outreach to Asian American communities are significant given the heterogeneity of this racial group and its status as the fastest-growing group in the United States (Lee et al., 2022). Beyond incidence, persons of color with dementia are more likely to experience discrimination in health settings at higher rates than White Americans (Alzheimer's Association, 2022) with resulting delays in early identification, diagnosis, and referrals to specialists. Persons of color with dementia are also more likely to experience disproportionately higher incidence of mental health issues (e.g., anxiety, depression) than their White counterparts (Novak et al., 2020).

Mild Cognitive Impairment, Dementia, and the *DSM-5* Criteria

Mild Cognitive Impairment (MCI)

Research on cognitive and physiologic biomarkers for the early detection of dementia led to the identification of mild cognitive impairment or MCI as a prodromal state for dementia. Persons with MCI demonstrate subtle yet measurable cognitive impairment with minimal impairment of instrumental activities of daily living or ADLs (Petersen, 2016). In 2001, the American Academy of Neurology (AAN; Ganguli et al., 2001) identified three criteria for a diagnosis of MCI: (a) self-report of memory problems, with corroboration from a family member or caregiver; (b) measurable memory impairment on standardized testing, outside the range expected for age- and education-matched healthy older adults; and (c) no impairments in reasoning, general thinking skills, or ability to perform ADLs. Thus, a diagnosis of MCI is made on the basis of mild, detectable changes in a person's cognitive functioning that are noticed by the affected person and confirmed by family members or significant others.

Based on a recent practice guideline update (Petersen et al., 2018), MCI can present as the earliest cognitive manifestation of Alzheimer's disease (AD) or another neurodegenerative disease or may result from other neurologic, systemic, or psychiatric disorders. In 2011, the Alzheimer's Association and the National Institute on Aging (McKhann et al., 2011) revised long-standing criteria for diagnosing dementia due to AD. With this revision, MCI was elevated in its importance because in some persons, MCI may represent an early stage of AD, particularly when specific biomarkers exist (e.g., neuronal atrophy, presence of beta-amyloid protein in the brain) and indicate a high probability of conversion to AD (Albert et al., 2011; Jack et al., 2010; Petersen & Negash, 2008). Currently, MCI is classified into two types (Mariani et al., 2007; Petersen, 2004, 2016)—**amnestic** MCI that initially affects memory only and **nonamnestic** MCI in which cognitive functions such as language, visuospatial function, or executive function are initially affected (Huey et al., 2013). Both amnestic and nonamnestic MCI may affect a single cognitive domain or multiple domains.

Figure 6–1 illustrates that in cases where MCI leads to dementia, a disease process may begin and progress in its pathogenesis for considerable time before any observable clinical symptoms appear (Amieva et al., 2005; Petersen & Negash, 2008). Identifying MCI is important because of the greater likelihood of possible progression to dementia (Jack et al., 2010; Mitchell & Shiri-Feshki, 2009), especially in an MCI profile dominated by memory impairment. Timely identification of MCI allows affected persons to initiate beneficial cognitive or lifestyle interventions (Alves et al., 2013; Petersen et al., 2018) and to monitor symptom progression over time. Discussed next are the latest criteria for dementia and

MCI from the fifth edition of the *Diagnostic and Statistical Manual of Mental Disorders* (*DSM-5*; American Psychiatric Association [APA], 2013; *DSM-5-TR*; APA, 2022).

Dementia

Dementia is a syndrome comprising a cluster of symptoms that can have many different causes. Dementia is characterized by acquired, persistent impairment of multiple cognitive domains that significantly alters communication, social interaction, occupational function, and the ability to perform instrumental ADLs (Grabowski & Damasio, 2004). Further, these pervasive cognitive impairments must exist in the absence of delirium (an acute confusional state) and any other neurologic or psychiatric disorder. In most dementia types, the most commonly affected

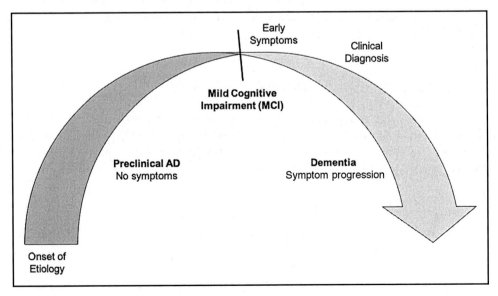

Figure 6–1. Relationship between preclinical AD, mild cognitive impairment (MCI), and dementia.

neuropsychological domain is memory, with related impairments in attention, executive function, language and communication, visuospatial function, and reduced ability to complete basic and instrumental ADLs (Figure 6–2).

Diagnostic and Statistical Manual of Mental Disorders (DSM-5) Criteria

The 2013 *DSM-5* criteria (APA, 2013) reframed dementia by placing it under two diagnostic categories of **Mild Neurocognitive Disorders** and **Major Neurocognitive Disorders** (NCDs). According to Ganguli and colleagues (2011), for a person to meet *DSM-5* diagnostic criteria for Major NCD, there must be evidence of significant cognitive decline (e.g., in memory, language/communication, or executive function) and this observed, quantifiable cognitive decline must be severe enough to disrupt independent completion of ADLs. To meet the *DSM-5* criteria for Mild NCD, persons must demonstrate evidence of slight cognitive decline that does not interfere with the ability to independently complete ADLs. Typically, a person with a Mild NCD can perform tasks requiring money management, taking medications, and remembering daily events or appointments, yet may report that these tasks are becoming more difficult. One clear advantage of the *DSM-5* criteria for Major NCD is that physicians are required to be specific about the cause of dementia—whether it is AD, frontotemporal lobar degeneration, vascular disease, Lewy body disease, Parkinson's disease, or multiple etiologies.

A recent Neurocognitive Disorders Supplement (*DSM-5-TR*; APA, 2022) updated its guidelines so that Mild NCD and Major NCD both may be attributed to a specific underlying disease process, to multiple coexisting etiologies, to other medical conditions, and to unknown etiology. This newer coding update also allows for recording whether Mild NCD or Major NCD is accompanied by any behavioral disturbance.

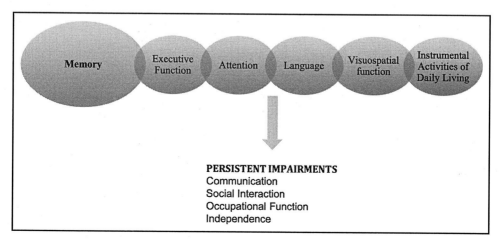

Figure 6–2. Affected domains of functioning in dementia.

Types of Dementia

Dementia may be caused by over 50 known conditions, and many types of dementia involve progressive and degenerative changes in neurons, neuronal networks, and entire cortical regions responsible for cognitive functions. However, in some cases, dementia-like symptoms may occur in the absence of degenerative brain disease, and the symptoms subside or reduce considerably when these reversible causes are treated. Some common causes of reversible dementia-like symptoms include depression, delirium, thyroid problems, Lyme disease, side effects of medications, untreated sleep apnea, specific vitamin deficiencies, and alcoholism (Alzheimer's Association, 2022).

Dementia is the progressive deterioration in cognitive and communicative functioning with decreased capacity for independent living. Each type of dementia is characterized by a particular presenting pattern and trajectory of symptoms as a result of brain disease (or neuropathology) that causes progressive degeneration of neurons, cortical regions, and entire brain networks. Although definitive diagnosis of brain disease can only be established postmortem, a dementia diagnosis can help rule out less likely brain diseases or to pinpoint the most probable underlying brain disease(s).[1] Neurologists diagnose types of dementia based on the current pattern and history of symptoms, progression, and other clinical information derived from brain scans, biological specimens (e.g., blood and cerebrospinal fluid), and behavioral observations. Speech-language pathologists play a critical role in the evaluation of speech, language, cognitive communication, and swallowing abilities, as well as the treatment and management of these impairments in people with dementia. In the next sections, we discuss specific patterns of symptom onset and progression, signature areas of neuropathology, and responses to cognitive communication interventions across dementia types.

Alzheimer's Disease (AD)

Alzheimer's disease (AD) is thought to result from a convergence of factors rather than a single cause and is the single most common cause of dementia, accounting for an estimated 60% to 80% of all dementia cases, currently affecting approximately 6.5 million Americans (Alzheimer's Association, 2022). In the United States, AD affects more women than men, affecting nearly 4 million women. The most significant nonmodifiable risk factors for developing AD are older age, positive family history (especially in a first-degree relative), and elevated genetic risk in the form of carrier status for the e4 allele of the apolipoprotein E (APOE) gene, which governs the production of a protein involved in cholesterol transport in the blood (Liu et al., 2013). Modifiable risk factors are those factors that can be managed to significantly reduce

---

[1]Some people use the name of the brain disease and the dementia syndrome interchangeably (e.g., "Alzheimer's disease" referring to the dementia syndrome and the neuropathology), while others make a distinction between the two (e.g., "Alzheimer's disease" is the underlying neuropathology of an "Alzheimer's dementia" syndrome).

the risk of cognitive decline and dementia. These include consuming a heart-healthy diet, maintaining regular physical activity, staying mentally and socially active, controlling cardiovascular disease risk factors, avoiding smoking, and preventing traumatic brain injury (TBI; Baumgart et al., 2015; WHO, 2019).

The earliest-appearing, hallmark symptoms of AD involve impairments of episodic memory (Bayles, 1991; Mahendra et al., 2018; Mahendra et al., 2011; Salmon & Bondi, 2009), working memory (Baddeley et al., 2001), and executive function (Kirova et al., 2015). The signature neuropathology of AD begins in the medial temporal lobe in the hippocampus and the entorhinal and perirhinal cortices—regions crucial to episodic memory. Further, from the early stages, prominent neuropathological abnormalities are detected in the posterior cortical regions of the brain, including the precuneus, posterior cingulate, retrosplenial, and lateral posterior parietal cortices (Buckner et al., 2005).

Episodic memory is the ability to consciously recall moments and unique personal experiences (Bayles et al., 2018; Baddeley, 2002; Squire & Zola-Morgan, 1991; Tulving, 1983), which allows us to perform everyday tasks like recalling a phone message or remembering recent conversations, names, and events (Dickerson & Eichenbaum, 2010). People with AD often present with significant impairments of attention (Foldi et al., 2002) and executive function in early stages of the disease (Collette et al., 2001; Kirova et al., 2015; Martyr & Clare, 2012). These executive function impairments adversely influence planning, goal setting, decision-making, self-monitoring, inhibition of interfering stimuli, and cognitive flex-ibility—all components of simple and complex daily activities. Thus, executive impairments precede impairments of praxis or the ability to carry out skilled motor procedures like driving (Martyr & Clare, 2012), dressing, and self-feeding (Baudic et al., 2006). Collectively, these impairments of attention, working memory, episodic memory, and executive function adversely affect linguistic communication—this is discussed later in this chapter.

Vascular Dementia (VaD)

Vascular dementia (VaD) results in impaired cognitive functions and ADL performance that is directly related to ischemic or hemorrhagic cerebrovascular disease, that is, circulatory disturbances that damage brain areas vital for memory and cognitive functions (Bir et al., 2021; Román, 2005). By itself, VaD accounts for between 5% and 10% of dementia cases; however, it occurs more commonly in combination with AD (Kapasi et al., 2017; Schneider et al., 2007). Conditions that increase the risk of developing VaD include large and small vessel disease, hypertension, hyperlipidemia, diabetes mellitus, and a history of smoking (Elzaguirre et al., 2017).

For a diagnosis of VaD or vascular NCD, there must be objective evidence of cardiac and/or other systemic vascular conditions and of cerebrovascular disease, etiologically tied to the onset of dementia symptoms. Focal neurological signs and symptoms (e.g., slow gait, poor balance) or neuroimaging evidence of ischemic, hemorrhagic, lacunar, or white matter lesions must be present while ensuring that VaD symptoms do not occur exclusively during delirium (Bir et al., 2021; Randolph,

1997). Symptoms of VaD tend to be more variable in presentation than AD and may be associated with sudden or chronic onset from accumulating ischemic brain changes over time. Unlike the early appearing memory impairments in AD, the initial symptoms in VaD are impaired decision-making, planning, and organizing.

In reviewing the literature on differences between AD and VaD across cognitive domains, Mahendra and Engineer (2009) summarized that persons with VaD perform better than those with AD on episodic memory, semantic memory, and category fluency tasks. Also, persons with VaD perform worse than those with AD on letter fluency, attention, executive function, and visuospatial tasks. Finally, consistent differences do not emerge between persons with VaD and AD on tasks assessing processing speed, language, digit span, and constructional ability. For a case study on the longitudinal effects of VaD on cognitive-communicative function, readers are directed to Mahendra and Engineer (2009).

Dementia With Lewy Bodies (DLB)

This dementia gets its name from Lewy bodies that are found in the cerebral cortex of affected persons. Lewy bodies are abnormal clumps of alpha-synuclein, a neuronal protein also implicated in the neuropathology of Parkinson's disease (PD). In PD, Lewy bodies are found in the substantia nigra and are responsible for the rapid degeneration of dopaminergic neurons. Thus, dementia with Lewy bodies (DLB) and PD share the distinctive pathological hallmark of Lewy bodies. Persons with DLB frequently have overlapping cognitive symptoms with those of AD yet are much more likely to present with early symptoms of sleep disturbance, visuospatial impairment and well-formed visual hallucinations (Ballard et al., 2013), fluctuating attention (Schneider et al., 2012), and motor impairment similar to PD (Hanson & Lippa, 2009). Other characteristics of DLB include executive dysfunction, cognitive inflexibility, and reduced speech rate and fluency (Ash et al., 2012). Notably, these symptoms occur in the absence of episodic memory impairments like those seen in AD (McKeith et al., 2016).

Frontotemporal Dementia (FTD)

Frontotemporal dementia (FTD) results from frontotemporal lobar degeneration (FTLD). This pattern of neuropathology is characterized by progressive, marked atrophy of the frontal and temporal brain regions with spongiform changes in the cortex and abnormal tau protein inclusions (Cairns et al., 2007; Sieben et al., 2012). Nearly 60% of persons with FTD are between 45 and 60 years of age (National Institute on Aging, 2022). This brain disease is associated with a heterogeneous group of rare neurodegenerative syndromes[2] that can result

---

[2]People refer to this group of syndromes as FTD, FTLD, frontotemporal disorders, or FTD- or FTLD-spectrum disorders. Similar to AD, some people use the name of the brain disease and the dementia syndrome interchangeably (e.g., "FTLD" referring to the dementia syndrome and the neuropathology), while others make a distinction between the two (e.g., "FTLD" is the underlying neuropathology of "FTD").

in significant impairments of communication and/or movement (National Institute on Aging, 2012). Unlike AD, which primarily affects memory, early symptoms of FTD generally develop in one of three domains—personality and behavior, speech and language, and movement and motor skills. Figure 6–3 illustrates the three main types of FTD.

The behavioral variant of FTD (bvFTD) accounts for about half of all FTD cases and is characterized by marked changes in personality, behavior, and social pragmatics. Speech and language impairments are usually less prominent in bvFTD but may include difficulties in naming, word comprehension, semantic knowledge, reading irregular words, and accurate recognition and expression of prosody (see Geraudie et al., 2021, for a review).

It is crucial for SLPs to note that isolated speech and language impairments are often the earliest-appearing symptoms of the FTD language syndromes: the semantic variant of primary progressive aphasia, characterized by fluent speech and rapid loss of semantic knowledge, and the non-fluent/agrammatic variant of primary progressive aphasia, characterized by effortful speech and/or grammatical impairments (Gorno-Tempini et al., 2004; Gorno-Tempini et al., 2011). There are three primary progressive aphasias, the third being the logopenic variant of primary progressive aphasia, which is more linked to AD pathology than to FTLD (Deramecourt et al., 2010; Europa et al., 2020; Josephs et al., 2008; Mahendra, 2012; Mesulam et al., 2008; Rohrer et al., 2012; Spinelli et al., 2017). Readers are referred to Chapter 5 in this text for a detailed discussion of PPA.

FTD motor syndromes include corticobasal syndrome, motor neuron disease, multiple system atrophy, and

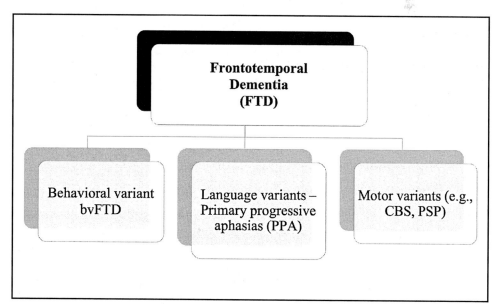

Figure 6–3. Types of frontotemporal dementia (FTD).

progressive supranuclear palsy syndrome. Some of the earliest-appearing symptoms in FTD motor syndromes may include motor speech problems. Expertise from SLPs may be helpful in motor speech diagnosis, treatment, and management.

HIV-Associated Neurocognitive Disorders (HAND)

Persons living with human immunodeficiency virus or HIV may develop a combination of cognitive, motor, and possible mood problems that are collectively referred to as HIV-associated Neurocognitive Disorders or HAND, previously known as the AIDS Dementia Complex (Antinori et al., 2007). It is estimated that roughly between 30% and 50% of persons living with HIV may present with HAND, and most present with mild forms (Heaton et al., 2010). Kopstein and Mohlman (2022) described that HAND symptoms may present as (a) asymptomatic neurocognitive impairment, characterized by mildly impaired neuropsychological test performance with ability to independently complete ADLs; (b) mild NCD, characterized by mild impact on ADLs; or (c) HIV-Associated Dementia (HAD), the most severe form of HAND, characterized by inability to complete ADLs. Persons affected with HAND in any form present with deficits in attention, concentration, and memory with slowed movements, low motivation, depression, and irritability. Notably, HAND does not have a typical course or definitely progresses to dementia. Indeed, HAND is not considered a progressive disorder due to the success and widespread availability of highly active antiretroviral treatments for HIV (Antinori et al., 2007).

Mixed Dementia

This section concludes with brief discussion about mixed pathologies as a common cause of dementia when an affected person shows the effects of brain changes resulting from more than one cause of dementia. Converging evidence from longitudinal studies, autopsy studies, brain imaging, and histopathologic investigations suggests that mixed dementia is quite common and may account for 50% or more of adults with dementia (Kapasi et al., 2017; Schneider et al., 2007) and that mixed dementia is most common in adults aged 85 years or older (Alzheimer's Association, 2022). Table 6–1 illustrates select parameters, based on published literature, that can be useful in differentially diagnosing AD from VaD, DLB, and FTD.

Impact of Dementia on Cognition and Communication

The syndrome of dementia impacts multiple cognitive domains severely. This impact on multiple cognitive domains adversely influences communication, social interactions, occupational function, and ADLs. Given that AD accounts for the majority of dementia cases, we discuss its broad impact on cognition and communication here. In AD, the earlier mentioned deficits in episodic memory, attention, working memory, and executive function

Table 6–1. Differential Diagnosis of Types of Dementia

	AD	VaD	DLB	FTD
Age of Onset	Mostly past age 65 years. Early onset AD is rarer	Mostly past age 65 years. Age of onset is variable	Most often past age 65 years	Most often between 45 and 64 years of age
Known Risk Factors	Genetic risk (APOE-e4 allele), older age, family history of AD in first-degree relative, cardiovascular risk factors, diabetes, hypertension, prior TBI, smoking	Cardiovascular disease, prior stroke/infarct, diabetes, hypertension, hyperlipidemia, smoking	Genetic risk, family history of PD, history of depression or anxiety, history of stroke	Genetic risk, family history of dementia, diabetes, prior TBI, autoimmune disease
Neuroimaging Findings	Classic medial temporal lobe damage to the hippocampus and surrounding cortex	Multiple ischemic lesions, silent strokes, lacunar infarcts, white matter lesions	Nigrostriatal degeneration, occipital area hypoperfusion affecting primary visual cortex and visual association areas, altered white matter integrity, spared medial temporal lobe	Focal atrophy of frontal and temporal brain regions, spongiform changes to cortex, tau protein inclusions
Earliest Symptoms	Episodic memory, working memory, executive function	Impaired judgment or impaired planning/decision-making	Sleep disturbance, visual or other sensory hallucination, confusion, motor impairment	Noticeable changes in behavior (bvFTD) or in speech and language (PPA)
Language	Early impairment in generative naming, discourse. Phonology, syntax, reading mechanics, and fluency are relatively spared	Impaired word retrieval and performance on semantic memory tasks, disorganized discourse	Impaired naming and severely impaired conceptual knowledge, reduced speech rate and fluency	Dramatic impairment of language and communication in PPA, worsens rapidly

negatively influence language processing and communicative function. Two aspects of linguistic communication affected earliest are naming ability and discourse performance. Confrontation naming and generative naming, or the ability to generate names of exemplars of a category, are significantly impaired in persons with AD when compared to age-matched healthy older adults (Arkin & Mahendra, 2001; Clark et al., 2009; Martin & Fedio, 1983; Sailor et al., 2004). Similarly, discourse breakdowns are common from the earliest stages of dementia (Bayles et al., 2018; Mahendra et al., 2018) with consistent evidence of empty speech (Nicholas et al., 1985), impaired cohesion (i.e., more wordiness and reduced relevant ideas conveyed), frequent use of tangential utterances, more sentence fragments and incomplete ideas (Ripich & Terrell, 1988; Tomoeda & Bayles, 1993), and reduced sentence comprehension (Small et al., 1997).

In the early stages of AD, persons with mild dementia present with several spared abilities, including orientation to self and to other persons, ability to produce fluent sentences, engaging in conversation, and consistently following two- or three-step commands (Hopper et al., 2001). Also, persons with mild AD retain semantic memory (i.e., the ability to describe attributes of an object, define a concept, or sort objects by semantic category), although this deteriorates as dementia severity increases (Bayles et al., 1996; Bayles et al., 1999; Cox et al., 1996). Affected persons gradually become more disoriented to time and place, getting easily confused and experiencing increased communication breakdowns (e.g., repetitive question-asking). In middle stages of AD, affected persons may retain the ability to follow one-step and two-step commands, sustain attention for some time, and make relevant on-topic comments about tangible stimuli during conversation (Ashida, 2000; Mahendra, 2001). In the late stages of AD, cognitive-communicative functioning is severely affected (Bayles et al., 2000), but persons with AD can still attend to pleasant stimuli (e.g., music, sensory stimulation) for brief periods of time. Table 6–2 provides a list of cognitive domains affected in AD and examples of tasks used to assess these domains.

Role of Speech-Language Pathologists With Persons With Dementia and MCI

The American Speech-Language-Hearing Association (ASHA) establishes the scope of practice for SLPs and endorses that SLPs play a key role in the screening, assessment, diagnosis, treatment, and research of dementia-based communication disorders (ASHA, n.d., 2016). The range of professional roles and activities performed by SLPs includes the aforementioned components, client and family education, counseling, case management, advocacy and prevention efforts, and interdisciplinary collaboration to ensure the highest quality of care for persons with dementia. Aligning with this view, the next sections address screening, assessment, and intervention for persons with dementia from the perspective of an SLP.

As we begin to discuss the role of SLPs, readers are invited to reflect on

Table 6–2. Cognitive Domains Affected in AD

Cognitive Domain Affected in AD	Sample Assessment Task/Stimulus
Orientation	Answering questions about time and place e.g., *What year is it?* 　　*What month are we in?* 　　*What is the name of this building we are in?*
Attention	Letter scanning e.g., *Please look at this sheet of paper containing letters of the alphabet. Circle every letter A that you can find.*
Executive function	Clock Drawing Test (CDT), Assessment of Activities of Daily Living (ADLs), or Instrumental ADLs e.g., *CDT: Please draw a clock with the arms indicating the time is ten after eleven.* 　　*ADL Assessment: Show me how you make a pot of coffee.*
Working memory	Forward or Backward Digit Span Tasks e.g., *Repeat these numbers after me in the same order: 8, 2, 7, 4*
Episodic memory	Story or Word List Recall e.g., *I am going to tell you a short story. When I'm done, I'd like you to tell it back to me.*
Semantic memory	Similarities and Differences Task e.g., *How are an apple and a banana alike?* 　　*How are an apple and a banana different from each other?*
Language	Confrontation Naming Tasks e.g., *Please name these pictures.* Generative or Category Naming Tasks e.g., *Name as many animals as you can, in one minute.* Object Description e.g., *Describe this object for me, in as much detail as possible.* Discourse e.g., *Conversation Analysis*
Visuospatial function	Figure Copying e.g., *I'd like you to copy this picture.*

shared core values as practitioners when serving diverse persons, families, and communities affected by dementia. These values are inspired by the ASHA Code of Ethics (ASHA, 2015); the Speech-Language Pathology Scope of Practice (ASHA, 2016); the International Classification of Functioning, Disability, and Health (ICF model; WHO, 2001); and deep respect for the rights and dignity of persons with dementia. Whereas SLPs pride themselves on developing and using evidence-based practices (EBPs), we must commit equally to expanding and adapting existing EBPs to better represent our diverse clients and underrepresented communities. Further, our commitment to EBP must be balanced by a strong understanding of community-engaged clinical work (Wong et al., 2022) and implementing culturally and linguistically responsive practices (Hyter & Salas-Provance, 2021).

Screening and Assessment of Persons With Dementia and MCI

Screening

The purpose of brief screenings, prior to or as part of a comprehensive assessment, is to help clinicians in identifying comorbidities (e.g., hearing impairment, depression), obtain information that guides the nature and type of subsequent evaluations, and determine the need for additional referrals (e.g., for neuropsychological or audiological testing). For persons with suspected dementia or MCI, screenings include the following components:

Review of Medical History

Medical records are reviewed to identify a client's prior and current health conditions, active diagnoses, list of medications, recent medical history, psychosocial history, and any report of cognitive-communicative impairments or developmental differences (e.g., dyslexia, attention-deficit/hyperactivity disorder [ADHD], stuttering). Information from medical records, observations, client self-report, and caregiver or family input allows a clinician to derive a Hachinski Ischemia Score (HIS; Hachinski et al., 1975). Using the HIS allows clinicians to determine the likelihood of vascular dementia (Hachinski et al., 2012). The HIS consists of 13 clinical features determined to be present or absent based on a client's medical history. Research studies (Hachinski et al., 1975; Moroney et al., 1997) have validated that a score of 4 or below fits a likely profile of AD, whereas a score of 7 or greater likely suggests VaD or mixed dementia (i.e., AD and VaD).

Sensory Impairments Affecting Hearing and Vision

Sensory impairments of hearing and vision are very prevalent in older adults (Desai et al., 2001; Yueh et al., 2003), and such impairments easily confound the reliability and validity of test results. For example, adults with age-related hearing loss often underperform on some cognitive tests, and this may lead to a spurious dementia diagnosis (Cacciatore et al., 1999; Weinstein, 2019). Recent research has revealed that sensory function is an important modulator of cognitive performance in middle and old age. As one example, hearing loss is now recognized as a potent, midlife modifiable risk factor that greatly predicts the likelihood of cognitive decline and dementia (Livingston et al., 2017; Weinstein, 2019). Thus, clinicians are advised to embed hearing screenings into assessment protocols for older adults with suspected or confirmed dementia. Such hearing screenings should include self-report or informant report of hearing loss (Vassilaki et al., 2019), otoscopy, pure-tone audiometric hearing screening, hearing aid inspection (as needed), and speech discrimination screening (McDonough et al., 2021).

Regarding visual impairments, many screening measures and comprehensive tests that SLPs routinely use require clients to identify objects, describe pictures, read words or sentences, and copy figures. Persons with age-related visual impairments such as cataracts, diabetic retinopathy, and macular degeneration may perform poorly on such tasks. To reliably assess cognitive impairments in MCI or dementia, it is necessary to rule out visual impairments by screening tasks that may include letter/number cancellation, literacy screening, and visual agnosia screening. One test that contains such screening tasks is the Arizona Battery for Cognitive-Communication Disorders (ABCD-2; Bayles & Tomoeda, 2019).

Depression

Depression is common among persons with dementia or MCI and can negatively influence cognitive function. For instance, depression worsens client well-being and motivation, often associated with social withdrawal and loss of interest in daily activities. Thus, depression can magnify cognitive and ADL impairments associated with dementia or MCI and adversely impact client participation in assessment and treatment. Whereas the comprehensive treatment of depression falls outside the SLP scope of practice, SLPs can screen for depression and facilitate timely referrals for further management. SLPs may use any one of multiple tools to screen for depression—including the Geriatric Depression Scale–Short Form or GDS-15 (Sheikh & Yesavage, 1986), the Beck Depression Inventory (BDI-II; Beck et al., 1996), and the Patient Health Questionnaire (PHQ-9; Kroenke et al., 2001). Depending on the clinical setting, SLPs may need to consult with psychologists, counselors, neuropsychologists, social workers, and nurse practitioners to manage screening and referrals for depression.

Cognitive Function

Given that clear evidence for modest or significant cognitive decline is required for a *DSM-5* and *DSM-5-TR* supported diagnosis of mild or major NCD, screening for cognitive impairment is an essential first step toward identifying MCI or dementia. Some of the most widely used tools for screening cognitive function are the Mini-Mental State Examination (MMSE; Folstein et al., 1975), the Veterans Affairs Medical Center Saint Louis University Mental Status Exam (SLUMS; Tariq et al., 2006), the Montreal Cognitive Assessment (MoCA©; Nasreddine et al., 2005), and the Clock Drawing Test (CDT; Agrell & Dehun, 1998; Sunderland et al., 1989).

The MMSE is among the most well-known general screening measures of cognitive status. It can be administered quickly within 10 minutes and has 11 items that result in a maximum possible score of 30 points. It has high sensitivity and specificity, particularly when population norms are used to correct scores for age and the number of years of education (Crum et al., 1993; Harvan & Cotter, 2006). This test was updated in 2001 (Folstein et al., 2001) and is now available in Brief, Standard, and Extended versions (adding Story Memory and Processing Speed tasks) and as a mobile app for iPhone®/iPad® and Android™ devices. Importantly, the MMSE-2 can now be ordered in multiple languages, including three Spanish versions, Chinese, Russian, Hindi, French, and others.

Because the MMSE lacks sensitivity for detecting MCI (Arevalo-Rodriguez et al., 2015), clinicians and researchers increasingly prefer the SLUMS or the MoCA©. The SLUMS features 11 items in a 30-point test and improves on the MMSE by including measures of forward and backward digit span, story recall, and clock drawing. Further, the SLUMS provides education-corrected scores.

The MoCA© is another 30-point test comprising 12 items covering eight domains and has the advantage of being specifically developed to distinguish between healthy aging, MCI, and AD based on obtained scores. This test makes substantial improvements over the MMSE by being more sensitive to detecting MCI and distinguishing it from early AD as well as healthy aging (Wang et al., 2022). Further, the MoCA© features availability in many languages (including versions for participants who are blind, hearing impaired, or illiterate), alternate forms, an electronic version (the eMoCA©), an app, and a 5-minute mini-MoCA© version. The MoCA© provides reliable screening of attention, executive function, episodic memory, and semantic memory with proper training and certification for clinicians, available via their website (https://mocacognition.com/).

While performance across the MMSE, MoCA©, and SLUMS is strongly and positively correlated with one another (Cao et al., 2012; Stewart et al., 2012), scores are not comparable between tests. In other words, it would be inappropriate to equate a score of 20 on the MMSE with a score of 20 on the SLUMS or MoCA©. These tests are currently available in multiple languages and dialects with additional translations and adaptations in continuous development (Steis & Schrauf, 2009). Table 6–3 compares the MMSE, MoCA©, and SLUMS to assist readers in comparing these three screening tools.

Finally, the CDT requires clients to draw an analog clock showing a specific time or to draw the face of a clock and its hands given a circle already drawn. Some version of a CDT appears on the MoCA© and the SLUMS. Performance on the CDT worsens as dementia severity increases and can be used to distinguish healthy aging from mild, moderate, or severe dementia. The CDT has low sensitivity for distinguishing very mild dementia from healthy aging, yet has improved sensitivity and specificity when used in conjunction with age- and education-corrected MMSE scores (Powlishta et al., 2002). In summary, these screening tools also may serve as

Table 6–3. Comparing MCI and Dementia Screening Tools: MMSE, MoCA©, and SLUMS

Mini Mental State Examination (MMSE)	Montreal Cognitive Assessment (MoCA©)	Saint Louis University Mental Status Exam (SLUMS)
Takes about 10 minutes to administer	Takes about 15 minutes to administer	Takes about 7 minutes to administer
Items address orientation to time and place, registration, attention, calculation, recall, and language	Items address orientation to time and place, attention, short-term memory, visuospatial abilities, executive functions, concentration and working memory, and language	Items address orientation to time and place, registration, attention, immediate and delayed recall, calculation, digit span, visuospatial abilities, and executive functions
Available in 75 languages/dialects	Available in nearly 100 languages	Available in 23 languages/dialects
Written instructions normally accompany test forms for training purposes	One-hour training and certification for test administration through MoCA© website	Written and video instructions for test administration available on SLUMS website
Lacks sensitivity for detecting mild cognitive impairment, but highly sensitive and specific for detecting dementia when scores are adjusted for age and years of education	Developed to distinguish between healthy aging and mild, moderate, and severe cognitive impairment	Provides education-corrected scores associated with normal performance, mild neurocognitive disorder, and dementia

one key component of a comprehensive evaluation of cognitive-communicative function in MCI or dementia.

Assessment

Evidence-based assessment for persons with dementia and MCI should be informed by federal mandates under the Nursing Home Reform Act (part of the Omnibus Budget Reconciliation Act [OBRA], 1987), the Patient Protection and Affordable Care Act (PPACA, 2010) and its related Elder Justice Act, the Speech-Language Pathology Scope of Practice (ASHA, 2016), information presented by ASHA on SLP roles in serving persons with dementia via their Practice Portal (ASHA, n.d.), and the International Classification of Functioning, Disability and Health

(ICF) model—a conceptual framework put forward by WHO in 2001. This ICF model suggests that a chronic health condition, like dementia, affects a person's Body Functions and Structures (i.e., anatomical/physiological or psychological functioning), Activities (i.e., ability to perform specific tasks), and Participation (i.e., ability to participate fully in life roles). For instance, a person with dementia is unable to recall a short story on a standardized test (Body Functions and Structures), consequently being unable to remember what is said (Activity), thus being restricted from participating effectively in social conversations (Participation). Beyond these three levels, per the ICF model, personal and environmental factors are strong determinants of how dementia impacts each affected person (Hopper, 2007). The critical contribution of the ICF model is that it gives clinicians a foundation to conceptualize assessment from multiple perspectives (i.e., at distinct levels of Body Functions and Structures, Activity, and Participation) while integrating published evidence, clinician expertise, and client preferences.

The OBRA mandate influences assessment practices in all Medicare-certified long-term care facilities, requiring an initial assessment of resident functional status—the Minimum Data Set (Centers for Medicare & Medicaid Services, 2001), within 14 days for all newly admitted residents and subsequent, regular quarterly assessments in the event of a change in a resident's functioning (i.e., decline or improvement). The Patient Protection and Affordable Care Act (PPACA or ACA) also has added a Medicare benefit via an Annual Wellness Visit, which now requires an assessment to detect cognitive impairment (Cordell et al., 2013) beyond routine checks of medical history, physical and ADL status, medication review, and consideration of necessary referrals. These federal mandates strongly suggest that clinicians must be knowledgeable and skilled about screening and assessment methods for persons with MCI or dementia, to contribute to these mandated evaluations.

As suggested previously, any measures useful in screening for MCI and dementia are valid components of a comprehensive evaluation. There is widespread consensus that the objectives of a comprehensive evaluation of a person with dementia are (Aguirre et al., 2013; Bayles et al., 2018; Hickey & Bourgeois, 2018; Mahendra & Apple, 2007; Mahendra & Hopper, 2022):

1. Identifying early the presence of cognitive communication impairment in dementia and MCI
2. Documenting impaired and spared cognitive and communicative abilities
3. Completing a culturally valid and linguistically appropriate assessment of client functioning
4. Establishing a baseline of cognitive-communicative function, prior to initiating intervention
5. Assessing personal and environmental factors that influence a particular client or family
6. Providing information and resources about dementia or MCI and counseling family members about expected symptom progression
7. Using dynamic assessment approaches or structured therapy trials to determine client candi-

dacy for particular interventions (Mahendra & Hopper, 2022) or need for stimulus presentation in an alternate modality (Mahendra et al., 2005)

With these objectives in mind, presented next are selected assessment measures that are useful for SLPs assessing persons with dementia. This is not an exhaustive review of all available assessment measures but rather provides direction to clinicians in selecting assessment measures.

Standardized Tests for Profiling Performance Across Cognitive Domains

Many existing standardized tests allow SLPs to obtain a profile of client functioning across cognitive domains such as attention, memory, language, visuospatial ability, and executive function. These tests allow an immediate understanding of most affected versus least affected domains for a particular client. Examples of tests in this category include the Repeatable Battery for the Assessment of Neuropsychological Status (RBANS; Randolph et al., 1998), the Dementia Rating Scale–Second Edition (DRS-2; Mattis et al., 1991), and the Cognitive Linguistic Quick Test (CLQT [Helm-Estabrooks, 2001]; CLQT+ [Helm-Estabrooks, 2017]).

The RBANS (Randolph et al., 1998) and the RBANS® Update (Randolph, 2012) were specifically developed to provide a stand-alone test for detecting and profiling dementia in older adults, to serve as a screening neuropsychological test when a full-length battery is inappropriate, and to provide multiple parallel forms to allow reliable retest-ing while controlling for practice effects (Randolph et al., 1998). This test enables the assessment of immediate memory, visuospatial/constructional ability, language, attention, and delayed memory using 12 subtests. It provides norms for persons aged 12 through 89 years, with index scores, percentile ranks, and a total scale score. The RBANS also provides group data for multiple dementia types (e.g., AD, VaD, HAND) and other neurogenic (e.g., head injury) and psychiatric causes (e.g., depression, schizophrenia) of cognitive impairment. The RBANS has been validated in multiple studies for use with persons with MCI and AD (Duff et al., 2008), as well as for assessing community-dwelling healthy older adults. Further, performance on the RBANS reliably predicts functional limitations in persons with MCI and dementia (Freilich & Hyer, 2007; Hobson et al., 2010). Other advantages of the RBANS include availability of two parallel forms in Spanish and options for web-based administration and scoring.

Next, the DRS-2 was designed particularly for persons with dementia and assesses client performance on five subscales—Attention, Initiation/Perseveration, Construction, Conceptualization, and Memory. This test provides age and education corrections for the total DRS-2 score and also has parallel forms to allow retesting without confounding learning effects from repeated test administrations.

Finally, the CLQT+ (Helm-Estabrooks, 2017) is a criterion-referenced test that allows clinicians to assess attention, memory, executive function, language, and visuospatial function in persons with dementia, TBI, or stroke. This test provides norms for persons aged 18 through 89 years, with test scores yielding a composite severity rating ranging from performance within functional limits through severe impairment. Particular advantages of the CLQT and CLQT+ are the availability of test materials in Spanish, a traditional test version (10 subtests), and an aphasia-friendly version (with an added semantic comprehension task).

Standardized Tests for In-Depth Assessment of Select Cognitive Domains

Tests in this group allow SLPs to assess one or two domains in more depth. For instance, if a clinician wishes to know much more about a client's cognitive-communicative functioning, the Arizona Battery for Cognitive-Communication Disorders (ABCD-2; Bayles & Tomoeda, 2019) or the Western Aphasia Battery–Revised (WAB-R; Kertesz, 2006) may be appropriate for selection. The original ABCD (Bayles & Tomoeda, 1993) was among the first comprehensive tests of linguistic communication designed for persons with mild AD. This test includes vision, literacy, and hearing screening subtests along with 14 distinct subtests to assess linguistic expression and comprehension, verbal episodic memory, semantic memory, visuospatial construction, and mental status. The ABCD provides performance data on healthy young and older participants, persons with mild and moderate dementia, and persons with PD with and without dementia. The second edition (ABCD-2) features a new standardization sample including people with a variety of NCDs and expanded norms and data from persons with MCI.

The WAB-R is a widely used, robust, and validated tool for evaluating auditory comprehension, speech and language production, repetition, and naming for persons with dementia and those with PPA (Henry & Grasso, 2018). It also allows for the assessment of reading comprehension, written language production, motor speech production, and nonverbal cognition (e.g., Raven's Progressive Matrices). A shorter, bedside screening version is also available.

Standardized Tests for Functional Assessment of Select Cognitive Domains

Tests in this category are unique in their focus on functional cognition, everyday communication, and performance on real-life activities. Given the progressive nature of dementia, it is imperative that interventions focus on functional tasks and behaviors that optimize client functioning in everyday situations and routines. Thus, tests in this category are extremely useful in honing in on person-centered intervention goals and for informing the selection of specific therapeutic techniques. Two examples of tests useful for the assessment of functional communication are the Communication Activities for Daily Living–Third Edition (CADL-3; Holland et al., 2018) and the Functional Linguistic Communication Inventory (FLCI; Bayles & Tomoeda, 1994).

The CADL-3 has been recently revised and was developed initially for assessing functional communication in persons with aphasia. Previous versions of the test have been validated for assessing functional communication in persons with mild to moderate dementia (Fromm & Holland, 1989). The

CADL-3 is normed on a mixed group of adults with stroke, TBI, dementia, and PPA. This test contains 50 test items that assess communication activities in seven areas: reading-writing-number use, social interaction, divergent communication, contextual communication, nonverbal communication, sequential relationships, and comprehension of humor and metaphor. Unique to the CADL-3 is the use of real-life scenarios and situations for sampling functional communication strategies used by persons with neurogenic communication disorders. For example, one item requires the client to read a sample prescription medication label and then communicate information about the prescribed medication dose and schedule. Another item requires a person to indicate how they would place a 9-1-1 call in the event of a home fire.

The FLCI was designed to assess functional communication in persons with moderate or greater dementia severity. It contains 10 subtests that assess the ability of a client with dementia to greet someone, name objects, answer questions, write, comprehend signs (e.g., an exit door or restroom sign), match objects to pictures, read and comprehend words, reminisce, follow commands, use gestures, and engage in conversation. The updated second edition (FLCI-2; Bayles & Tomoeda, 2020) features a new standardization sample including people with VaD and mixed dementia, in addition to people with AD, to further extend its clinical utility.

Similarly, in the vein of functional assessment of memory, the Rivermead Behavioral Memory Test–Third Edition (RBMT-3; Wilson et al., 2008) is widely used for assessing everyday memory performance. The RBMT-3 is an ecolog-ically valid, efficient test that includes 14 subtests that assess visual and verbal memory, immediate and delayed recall and recognition, prospective memory (e.g., setting an alarm to remember to do something), and the ability to learn new information (e.g., a story, a route around a room). This test was developed in the United Kingdom and features four parallel forms, a UK and North American version of test stimuli, and norms from typical individuals aged 16 to 96 years and from persons with brain injury.

Nonstandardized Assessment Using Subtests of Comprehensive Tests

Depending on dementia severity, time allocated for client evaluation, and the intended purpose of evaluation, clinicians can always use subtests of any aforementioned test as a component of a comprehensive evaluation. For example, the Story Recall subtest on the ABCD-2 is clinically useful for establishing whether a client is having episodic memory impairments in line with those seen in typical aging or more consistent with AD. Similarly, the RBANS-Update has a forward and backward digit span subtest that offers a precise way to assess working memory.

Other Assessment Options—Beyond Routine Standardized Testing

Standardized testing has its pros and cons, with one disadvantage being that standardized tests are often normed on predominantly White, English-speaking, and educated adults. This can make it challenging to confidently use standardized tests when a particular client is not represented in the normative sample either because of their race/ethnicity, language(s) spoken, or their level of education. Standardized testing is often complemented by the use of naturalistic observation across contexts and activities, interviews with professional or personal caregivers, careful assessment of the environment, and using rating scales for quantitative or qualitative measurement of behaviors. For example, clinicians may use rating scales to assess affect and engagement of clients participating in therapeutic or recreational activities. One well-known scale is the Observed Emotion Rating Scale (Lawton et al., 1999). Another important tool is the Environment and Communication Toolkit (ECAT) for Dementia Care (Brush et al., 2012). The ECAT was developed as an assessment protocol to evaluate client performance using yes/no questions, to assess the environment and barriers in it, and to select and customize interventions for persons with dementia. The ECAT provides clinicians with over 300 specific recommendations for interventions and environmental modifications for reducing communication or behavior problems that persons with dementia encounter while completing ADLs. With this backdrop of conceptual understanding of dementia, screening, and assessment methods, we turn to intervention in the final section of this chapter.

Interventions for Persons With Dementia

Two dichotomies deserve mention when categorizing interventions for persons with dementia. The first dichotomy is between pharmacological and nonpharmacological interventions. SLPs do not make decisions about pharmacological interventions for dementia. However, a thorough evidence-based assessment can be invaluable in establishing a dementia diagnosis and related severity of cognitive impairment. This can help initiate appropriate pharmacological management, which may be used in conjunction with nonpharmacological interventions. Nonpharmacological interventions are typically directed toward compensating for cognitive-communicative impairments resulting from dementia (e.g., using a scheduling app to provide reminders and notifications about appointments), managing behavioral problems (e.g., reducing disruptive vocalization or repetitive questions), and enhancing communication, affect, and quality of life. A subgroup of nonpharmacological interventions is aimed at supporting the well-being and quality of life of persons affected by dementia, as well as their family members. Such interventions frequently include education, counseling, caregiver training, and respite services.

A second dichotomy is between direct and indirect interventions (Hopper, 2001; Mahendra, 2001; Mahendra & Hopper, 2022). Direct interventions are those in which persons with dementia themselves participate in compensatory programs or strategy instruction. An example of a direct intervention is applying spaced retrieval training to teach a client to use a memory aid for recalling important information or procedures (e.g., timing of meals or a safe swallowing strategy). Indirect interventions take the form of clinicians providing training to professional and personal caregivers, modifying the physical or social environment to ease demands on cognitive function, and developing stimulating therapeutic activities in collaboration with others (Hickey & Bourgeois, 2018; Hopper, 2001). As one effective example of an intervention implemented by care providers, McGilton et al. (2017) explored the effectiveness of personalized communication plans tailored to the needs of residents with dementia. They developed and tested a person-centered communication intervention based on adapting the Aphasia Framework for Outcome Measurement (Kagan, 1998). Their intervention included (a) individualized communication plans, (b) a training workshop designed to inform caregivers about strategies for supporting communication and instruction on applying strategies residents, and (c) mentoring staff to support caregivers in implementing these strategies. They reported positive outcomes for residents with dementia and for care providers, documenting the value of this model for designing and implementing person-centered communication interventions in long-term care settings. Similar to pharmacological and nonpharmacological interventions, direct and indirect interventions co-occur, or some people may opt for one over another.

Given the vast literature on direct and indirect interventions, it is not possible to exhaustively review all interventions SLPs can consider for persons with dementia. A sound place to begin thinking about interventions is to consider key evidence-based features of interventions that have proven efficacious for persons with dementia. Based on published research (Aguirre et al.,

2013; Bayles et al., 2018; Hickey & Bourgeois, 2018; Hill et al., 2011; Hopper et al., 2013; Mahendra et al., 2011), some of these core features include providing persons with dementia:

1. Repeated and rich presentation of target information
2. Contexts for learning by doing and multiple opportunities to practice generating target responses
3. Ways to capitalize on relatively spared cognitive capacities (such as sustained attention)
4. Cognitive stimulation to activate experience-dependent neuroplasticity
5. Task formats that reduce the likelihood of errors during initial learning and increase the chance of early success
6. Exposure to personally meaningful, tangible sensory stimuli
7. Structured cues or cueing hierarchies that support information retrieval
8. Opportunities for creative and symbolic activity (e.g., using art, music, gardening)
9. Experiences that offer community engagement, intergenerational programming, and regular physical activity

Table 6–4 lists these core features with examples of direct intervention techniques. This section ends with providing readers pertinent information on select intervention approaches of particular significance for SLPs. These approaches were selected based on availability of empirical evidence for their efficacy, particular utility for dementia, and their proven success

Table 6–4. Key Features of Successful Interventions for Dementia, With Examples

Features of Successful Interventions	Sample Intervention
1. Repeated presentation and spaced recall of target information	*Spaced retrieval training* *Computer-assisted cognitive training* *Memory books/wallets/aids* *Spaced retrieval training*
2. Provide contexts for learning by doing and multiple opportunities to generate target responses	*Computer-assisted cognitive training* *Montessori-based interventions*
3. Task formats that reduce error likelihood during initial learning	*Environmental modifications* *Graphic cuing systems* *Technology-assisted interventions (e.g., automated coaching systems)*
4. Capitalize on relatively spared sustained attention during intervention	*Montessori-based interventions* *Music-based interventions* *Physical exercise interventions*
5. Exposure to meaningful sensory stimuli	*Reminiscence therapy* *Simulated presence therapy* *Music-based or art-based interventions*
6. Opportunities for meaningful social engagement	*Reminiscence/conversation groups* *Intergenerational programming*

for facilitating functional cognition, enhancing communication, and social engagement in persons with dementia. The exemplar approaches discussed next include spaced retrieval training, memory books/memory wallets, and interventions that utilize reminiscence and sensory stimulation.

Spaced Retrieval Training (SRT)

First described by Landauer and Bjork (1978) as a technique to improve episodic learning of information in young adults, spaced retrieval training (SRT) is a shaping paradigm for facilitating recall of information or procedures. Camp (1989) modified and adapted SRT for persons with AD, and since then, the technique has been used successfully with mild and moderate dementia. Spaced retrieval training (Hopper et al., 2005; Lee et al., 2009; Mahendra, 2011) involves teaching new facts or a new motor procedure to a person with dementia, who then practices recalling the information or procedure immediately and over gradually increasing lengths of time. Time intervals after a successful recall attempt are doubled while those after a recall failure are maintained or reduced to support successful retrieval. In this way, persons with dementia can learn and recall functional information (e.g., a room number, meal schedule) or skills (e.g., a safe swallowing strategy, compensatory maneuver) over extended time. Such functional learning optimizes client functioning, independence, and safety and reduces the need for one-on-one assistance.

Spaced retrieval training has been hugely successful for persons with memory disorders (Schacter et al., 1985), TBI (Bourgeois et al., 2007), and dementia (Brush & Camp, 1998; Hopper et al., 2005; Hopper et al., 2009; Hopper et al., 2013; Mahendra, 2011). Types of information and skills trained in dementia vary from teaching names of relevant people (Cherry et al., 2010; Hopper et al., 2009; Mahendra, 2011), prospective memory tasks (Ozgis et al., 2009), safe swallow strategies (Brush & Camp, 1998), communicative strategies, and use of memory aids (Bourgeois et al., 2003). For a recent evidence-based systematic review on cognitive interventions for dementia that includes spaced retrieval training, readers are directed to the work of Hopper and colleagues (2013).

Spaced retrieval training is efficacious because it involves repeated presentation of target information and extensive opportunities to practice retrieving target information while extending the time interval over which recall is successfully maintained. Incidentally, by requiring successful recall prior to lengthening a retention interval, SRT utilizes the principle of errorless learning (Baddeley, 1992). This type of learning is likely superior to trial-and-error learning for persons with dementia because it discourages guessing, constrains response choices, and restricts the number of errors possible during initial learning. Reducing errors during early learning greatly advantages information or skill acquisition for persons with dementia because it renders the learning more stable, without the confound of intervening errors that can derail learning (Clare & Jones, 2008). Hopper and colleagues (2005) have suggested that persons with mild to moderately severe dementia, episodic memory impairments, and the ability to sustain attention to structured learning tasks are suitable candidates for SRT. It is key for clinicians to think about SRT as an effective modality in which to nest intervention for goals ranging from enhancing on-topic communication, retaining a safety strategy, supporting dysphagia therapy, or learning to use a low-tech augmentative alternative communication device or memory aid. Currently, SRT can now be effectively carried out using the spaced retrieval training therapy app from Tactus Therapy Solutions (https://tactustherapy.com/). Next, we talk about the use of memory books and wallets for persons with dementia.

Memory Books/Memory Wallets

Memory aids such as memory books and memory wallets are examples of low-tech supports that can enhance cognitive-communicative function, social engagement, and quality of life for persons with dementia by facilitating orientation, increasing meaningful and on-topic conversations (Bourgeois, 1990), turn-taking, and fruitful exchanges of information with caregivers (Bourgeois, 1992; Hoerster et al., 2001). Further, using memory books and wallets can effectively reduce negative behaviors (Bourgeois, 2013; Bourgeois et al., 1997) stemming from episodic memory loss and resulting confusion (e.g., disruptive vocalizations, repeating the same question). A memory book or wallet usually consists of a collection of relevant information, supported by salient and accessible visual cues (e.g., large-font text, pictures, pictographs, or photographs). A memory wallet is designed to be a smaller, portable version of a memory book that can be easily carried by a client and integrated into any communicative situation or activity routine.

Memory books and wallets utilize previously familiar information and clear visual supports (e.g., pictures, pictographs, photos) to prime personally relevant facts and to promote expression of needs and preferences to communication partners. Such memory aids reduce the burden on a fragile episodic memory, yet simultaneously engage spared language abilities while fostering enhanced engagement and independence during communication. Memory books and wallets are most suitable for persons with mild to moderate dementia who can read and process visual information and have the desire to learn a functional strategy for supporting communication. For specific ideas and adaptations to design versatile memory aids, Bourgeois (2013) provides an excellent guide on developing memory books and other graphic cuing systems.

Interventions Utilizing Reminiscence and Sensory Stimulation

There are several interventions that are successfully used for persons with dementia and capitalize on spared sensory processing, benefit of tangible stimuli, and the therapeutic effects of conversation and socialization. Such beneficial interventions include reminiscence therapy (RT), music-based interventions, and Montessori-based dementia programming (Camp, 1999; Orsulic-Jeras et al., 2000). RT stimulates recall through a structured review of past events and memories. Reminiscing about the past with tangible sensory stimuli (e.g., photo albums, souvenirs from a memorable vacation) offers persons with dementia an opportunity to have social connection and conversation. As an intervention, RT is personally meaningful and also appropriate for seniors from racially and linguistically diverse backgrounds (Harris, 1997). RT has been shown to have positive outcomes on communication, quality of life, and engagement of persons with dementia (Kim et al., 2006; Saragih et al., 2022) and on staff perceptions of the communication ability of persons with dementia (Hopper et al., 2007). Further, RT helps to decrease depressive and neuropsychiatric symptoms (Saragih et al., 2022) among persons with dementia. Group RT is common in activity programming for persons with dementia, with the goal being to engage participants in on-topic and shared conversation on varied topics (e.g., famous events, personal milestones).

Music also is a potent stimulus for reminiscence and for facilitating communication in persons with dementia (Ashida, 2000; Brotons & Koger, 2000). A growing body of research documents that music-based interventions such as group music therapy and choral singing may improve cognitive function and quality of life for people living with dementia (Moreno-Morales, et al., 2020). Further, music helps to reduce negative affect and anxiety (Hofbauer et al., 2022) while improving emotional well-being for persons living with dementia (van der Steen et al., 2018).

Finally, Montessori-based interventions (Camp, 1999; Mahendra et al., 2006) benefit persons with dementia by providing a stimulating, learning-by-doing environment in which a person works independently at their own pace. Montessori methods use the following features for designing functional interventions for persons with dementia: (a) breaking down tasks into component steps, (b) using guided repetition and cuing to support task completion, (c) progressing through tasks sequentially, and (d) moving from tasks based on simple, concrete concepts to those involving more complex, abstract concepts. Montessori-based interventions have been reported to enhance affect, improve motivation and task engagement, reduce agitation (Vance & Johns, 2002), and benefit functional cognition in dementia (Mahendra et al., 2006; Vance & Porter, 2000). A clear advantage of Montessori activities is that functional and recreational activities can be selected for persons with mild, moderate, or severe dementia. For example, a client with mild dementia can complete a Color Tiles activity (Vance & Johns, 2002), which requires a person to arrange tiles in a sequence ranging from lightest to darkest. This activity relies on seriation, and successful completion allows progression to an everyday task like sorting laundry into light and dark clothing. Similarly, a person with moderate to moderately severe dementia can practice pouring beans, rice, or other material into containers of different sizes and shapes. Successful performance on these pouring tasks can then be utilized by engaging residents with pouring drinks in the dining room. A person with severe dementia could engage in a simpler sensorimotor activity like a Discovery Bowl, in which participants search for colorful objects such as three-dimensional shapes, hidden in a bowl of rice.

Future Directions

As the population in the United States and the rest of the world ages rapidly, changes are needed in health care legislation (e.g., the National Alzheimer's Project Act in the United States), service delivery mechanisms (e.g., the Affordable Care Act in the United States), and large-scale investment in a public health approach for focused screening, assessment, and intervention for and prevention of dementia and MCI (e.g., Building Our Largest Dementia [BOLD] Infrastructure for Alzheimer's Act, 2018), expressed in Public Law 115–406. Technology is increasingly shaping the approach to research and development of cognitive and behavioral interventions, with many exciting emerging developments relative to the design of smart homes, deployment of sensor technology, use of mobile health networks, automated coaching systems, therapy apps (e.g., Constant Therapy®), telerehabilitation, and self-administered computer programs for improving memory and communication. Further, given the implications of the dementia epidemic facing our country and the globe, urgent emphasis is needed on expanding didactic and clinical training in geriatrics and dementia within the SLP and audiology curriculum. Finally, training the next generation of providers must be infused with rich opportunities for service learning, interprofessional education and practice, and community-engaged education and outreach to diverse populations.

Case Study

Background Information and Chart Review

Mrs. V is a 78-year-old, bilingual, Latina woman whose first language was Spanish and who learned English as a young adult after moving to the United States. She has lived in an assisted living unit (within a continuum-of-care facility) in the San Francisco Bay Area for 3 years. She worked as a nanny for 24 years, prior to retiring. Her medical history was significant for hypertension and coronary artery disease, and a diagnosis of MCI made at the time of admission to her current facility. Her MCI diagnosis was made based on the findings of an interdisciplinary team, using the *DSM-5-TR* criteria and a neuroimaging-supported diagnosis. Mrs. V is on the following

medications—daily low-dose aspirin, a beta-blocker to treat her blood pressure and lower her heart rate, and a statin to lower cholesterol. Her older sister (now deceased) had dementia due to AD. She has one daughter, who lives nearby and is actively involved in her mother's care. Mrs. V was referred to the SLP by the charge nurse requesting a comprehensive assessment after observing disorientation, worsening memory, communication breakdowns, frequent expressions of boredom (e.g., "I have nothing to do"), confusion about her daily schedule (e.g., "I don't know what's next"), and frustration with being unable to use her cellphone independently to call her daughter. She also is frustrated with food choices and not being able to watch TV shows in Spanish (e.g., on Telemundo).

Person-Centered Assessment Approach

In implementing a person-centered assessment (Hopper et al., 2015) for Mrs. V., the SLP collaborated with a trained bilingual Spanish-English interpreter and conducted:

a. Otoscopy and an audiometric hearing screening (to check for hearing loss)
b. An interview to understand her concerns while examining conversational interaction and insight into her cognitive functioning (this interview was also conducted via Zoom [https://zoom.us/] with her daughter to obtain information about her observations and any concerns). In the context of this

interview, a language history and use questionnaire was completed with a trained interpreter assisting the SLP. This interview revealed that Mrs. V loved to talk to others, cook, and sing. She shared that her favorite activities include gardening and helping to make meals, exclaiming *"soy una gran cocinera"* (translated as "I'm a great cook"). She had limited insight about her worsening memory or repetitive discourse. She fluidly switched from English to Spanish and often used phrases and exclamations in Spanish during her responses. Responses in her questionnaire indicated that she currently speaks more Spanish now than English since moving into the assisted living facility.

c. Brief, standardized assessment using the MoCA© (to establish an index of the severity of cognitive impairment)—at Mrs. V's preference, this was completed in Spanish and scored with the interpreter's assistance.

d. Nonstandardized assessment of language and communicative function in English using select subtests from the ABCD-2 (i.e., Immediate and Delayed Story Recall, Object Naming, Object Description, Reading Comprehension). The Object Naming Test also was completed in Spanish to compare her performance in English versus Spanish on the same task. She performed significantly better on the Object Naming in Spanish than in English.

e. Nonstandardized assessment using sections of the ECAT, pertinent for evaluation of Mrs. V's environment within her assisted living unit.

f. Brief observation of Mrs. V in her room and during an art activity session to assess participation in ADLs.

Results obtained from these tasks are summarized in the chart below.

Short-Term and Long-Term Goals

Based on these results, long-term and short-term goals are selected:

Long-Term Goal: Mrs. V will enhance her social and communicative participation by engaging in stimulating recreational activities, social interaction, and communication with family, independently or with minimal cueing.

Short-Term Goal 1: Mrs. V's room environment will be modified to enhance her orientation to time, place, and her daily schedule using an accessible print calendar and a large-font, activity schedule (in her room and also attached to her walker).

Short-Term Goal 2: Mrs. V will be trained using SRT to use graphic cue cards (located next to her phone and also adhered to the back of her phone), listing the sequence of steps (with pictographs) so she could call her daughter.

Short-Term Goal 3: Mrs. V will be taught to use a memory wallet (with photographic stimuli and text in English and Spanish) to initiate

Test/Measure	Result Obtained
Otoscopy and Audiometric Hearing Screen	Outcome: *Pass*
Interview	– Client primary concerns: Boredom, difficulty navigating schedule; difficulty using cell phone to call daughter
	– Limited insight into altered cognition
	– Preferred activities and conversation topics were identified
MoCA (in Spanish)	Score: 16/30 (consistent with mild dementia)
ABCD-2	
Immediate Story Recall	Score: 7/17
Delayed Story Recall	Score: 1/17
Following Commands	Score: 9/9
Object Naming	Score: 11/20 (English) 16/20 (Spanish)
Object Description	Score: 4/10
Reading Comprehension	Score: 14/15
ECAT	
Evaluating Orientation Cues in Environment	Intervention needed
Evaluating Appliance Use (phone, iPad, TV)	Intervention needed
Evaluating Social Environment	Intervention needed
Client Observation	– Mrs. V enjoyed social interaction
	– Mrs. V code-switched effectively between English and Spanish
	– Mrs. V was easily frustrated with art activity
	• Insufficient dementia-friendly instructions
	• Difficult to hear facilitator instructions
	• No graphic cues were used to support task completion

conversation about her life and family.

Short-Term Goal 4: Mrs. V will be verbally encouraged (by staff and family) to attend at least one social activity daily.

Additionally, the SLP may collaborate with recreational therapy or activities staff to create opportunities for Mrs. V to engage in therapeutic gardening or flower arranging given that these were some of her cherished activities. Also, given her lifetime habit of enjoying cooking, Mrs. V could be encouraged to assist with dining room duties, such as serving dessert or cutting up fruit, and to cook under supervision in the rehab kitchen. Mrs. V was seen for twelve 45-minute sessions over 4 weeks to address these goals using a combination of SRT and tangible memory aids. The SRT was implemented to sequentially teach Mrs. V to use her memory wallet to initiate biographical conversations and to use her cell phone to call her daughter. In collaboration with her daughter, Mrs. V was provided with an iPad on which she could access Spanish TV shows via a desktop application. The iPad was selected as an appropriate device for Mrs. V, based on information shared by her family about her independent use of and familiarity with using an iPad for reading the news and watching shows.

The first procedure training involved asking Mrs. V, "What can you use to share information about your family?" Mrs. V was to answer, "I can use my memory wallet," followed by using the wallet to share at least one piece of information. To begin a trial, the tar-

get question was presented verbally in the same form, followed by stating the correct response and modeling how to use the memory wallet to share information. One minute later, Mrs. V was asked the target question. If she did not recall the answer, the clinician provided the answer and had Mrs. V repeat it. Then, she was asked the same question again 1 minute later, and if she answered accurately this time and used the wallet, this question was repeated after 2 minutes (i.e., the recall interval was doubled after every successful recall). In this way, her intentional recall of using her individualized memory wallet was extended over a full therapy session. When she successfully recalled that she could use her memory wallet in conversation beyond a 32-minute recall interval, maintained over two consecutive sessions, she was encouraged to practice sharing details from the wallet to begin a conversation. She maintained her ability to use her memory wallet, over the remainder of therapy, with a gradual increase in the number of facts she shared using this memory wallet.

Subsequently, SRT was used to teach Mrs. V a second procedure in response to the prompt, "Show me how you would make a call to your daughter." Mrs. V had to show four sequential steps on her iPhone—namely, to press the green phone icon 📞, press the Contacts icon 👥, press the name *Liliana* (daughter's name), then press 📞 to make the call. During initial training, she was only asked to point to the final icon (so as not to call her daughter on each trial). Repeated SRT shaping trials were conducted until Mrs. V was able to recall this sequence of four steps over the duration of a therapy session and called her daughter successfully at the end of the session with minimal assistance from the clinician. One of the advantages of SRT is that it can be nested within other therapy goals for a client. For instance, if a client is recalling information over a 16-minute interstimulus interval, the clinician can address other therapy goals (i.e., learning to read and review her activity schedule) or carry out language stimulation activities or games.

References

Agrell, B., & Dehun, O. (1998). Review: The Clock Drawing Test. *Age and Ageing, 27,* 399–403.

Aguirre, E., Woods, R. T., Spector, A., & Orrell, M. (2013). Cognitive stimulation for dementia: A systematic review of the evidence of effectiveness from randomized controlled trials. *Ageing Research Reviews, 12*(1), 253–262.

Albert, M. S., DeKosky, S. T., Dickson, D., Dubois, B., Feldman, H. H., Fox, N. C., . . . Phelps, C. H. (2011). The diagnosis of mild cognitive impairment due to Alzheimer's disease: Recommendations from the National Institute on Aging-Alzheimer's Association workgroups on diagnostic guidelines for Alzheimer's disease. *Alzheimer's & Dementia, 7*(3), 270–279.

Alves, J., Magalhães, R., Machado, A., Gonçalves, O. F., Sampaio, A., & Petrosyan, A. (2013). Nonpharmacological cognitive intervention for aging and dementia: Current perspectives. *World Journal of Clinical Cases, 1*(8), 233–241.

Alzheimer's Association. (2022). 2022 Alzheimer's disease facts and figures. *Alzheimer's and Dementia: The Journal of the Alzheimer's Association, 18*(4), 700–789.

American Psychiatric Association. (2013). *Diagnostic and statistical manual of mental disorders* (5th ed.).

American Psychiatric Association. (2022). *Neurocognitive disorders supplement* (5th ed.). https://psychiatryonline.org/pb-assets/dsm/update/DSM-5-TR_Neuro-cognitive-Disorders-Supplement_2022_APA_Publishing.pdf

American Speech-Language-Hearing Association. (n.d.). *Dementia* [Practice portal]. https://www.asha.org/practice-portal/clinical-topics/dementia/

American Speech-Language-Hearing Association. (2015). *Code of ethics* [Ethics]. https://www.asha.org/policy/

American Speech-Language-Hearing Association. (2016). *Scope of practice in speech-language pathology* [Scope of practice]. https://www.asha.org/policy/

Amieva, H., Jacqmin-Gadda, H., Orgogozo, J.-M., Le Carret, N., Helmer, C., Letenneur, L., . . . Dartigues, J.-F. (2005). The 9-year cognitive decline before dementia of the Alzheimer type: A prospective population-based study. *Brain, 128*(5), 1093–1101. https://doi.org/10.1093/brain/awh451

Antinori, A., Arendt, G., Becker, J. T., Brew, B. J., Byrd, D. A., Cherner, M., . . . Wojna, V. E. (2007). Updated research nosology for HIV-associated neurocognitive disorders. *Neurology, 69*(18), 1789–1799.

Arevalo-Rodriguez, I., Smailagic, N., Figuls, M. R. I., Ciapponi, A., Sanchez-Perez, E., Giannakou, A., . . . Cullum, S. (2015). Mini-Mental State Examination (MMSE) for the detection of Alzheimer's disease and other dementias in people with mild cognitive impairment (MCI). *Cochrane Database of Systematic Reviews, 3,* 1–74.

Arkin, S., & Mahendra, N. (2001). Discourse analysis of Alzheimer's patients before and after intervention: Methodology and outcomes. *Aphasiology, 15*(6), 533–569.

Ash, S., McMillan, C., Gross, R. G., Cook, P., Gunawardena, D., Morgan, B., . . . Grossman, M. (2012). Impairments of speech fluency in Lewy body spectrum disorder. *Brain and Language, 120*(3), 290–302.

Ashida, S. (2000). The effect of reminiscence music therapy sessions on changes in depressive symptoms in elderly persons with dementia. *Journal of Music Therapy, 37*(3), 170–182.

Baddeley, A. D. (1992). Implicit memory and errorless learning: A link between cognitive theory and neuropsychological rehabilitation? In L. R. Squire & N. Butters (Eds.), *Neuropsychology of memory* (2nd ed., pp. 309–314). Guilford.

Baddeley, A. D. (2002). The concept of episodic memory. In A. Baddeley & M. A. Conway (Eds.), *Episodic memory: New directions in research* (pp. 1–10). Oxford University Press.

Baddeley, A. D., Baddeley, H. A., Bucks, R. S., & Wilcock, G. K. (2001). Attentional control in Alzheimer's disease. *Brain, 124,* 1492–1508.

Ballard, C., Aarsland, D., Francis, P., & Corbett, A. (2013). Neuropsychiatric symptoms in patients with dementias associated with cortical Lewy bodies: Pathophysiology, clinical features, and pharmacological management. *Drugs & Aging, 30,* 603–611.

Baudic, S., Barba, G. D., Thibaudet, M. C., Smagghe, S., Remy, P., & Traykov, L. (2006). Executive function deficits in early Alzheimer's disease and their relations with episodic memory. *Archives of Clinical Neuropsychology, 21*(1), 15–21.

Baumgart, M., Snyder, H. M., Carrillo, M. C., Fazio, S., Kim, H., & Johns, H. (2015). Summary of the evidence on modifiable risk factors for cognitive decline and dementia: A population-based perspective. *Alzheimers Dementia, 11*(6), 718–726.

Bayles, K. A. (1991). Alzheimer's disease symptoms: Prevalence and order of appearance. *Journal of Applied Gerontology, 10*(4), 419–430.

Bayles, K. A., McCullough, K., & Tomoeda, C. K. (2018). *Cognitive-communication disorders of MCI and dementia* (3rd ed.). Plural Publishing.

Bayles, K. A., & Tomoeda, C. K. (1993). *The Arizona Battery for Communication Disorders of Dementia.* Canyonlands Publishing.

Bayles, K. A., & Tomoeda, C. K. (1994). *Functional Linguistic Communication Inventory.* Canyonlands Publishing.

Bayles, K. A., & Tomoeda, C. K. (2019). *ABCD-2: Arizona Battery for Cognitive-Communication Disorders, Second edition–Complete kit.* Pro-Ed.

Bayles, K. A., & Tomoeda, C. K. (2020). *FLCI-2: Functional Linguistic Communication Inventory, Second edition–Complete kit.* Pro-Ed.

Bayles, K. A., Tomoeda, C. K., & Cruz, R. (1999). Performance of Alzheimer's disease patients in judging word relatedness. *Journal of the International Neuropsychological Society, 5,* 668–675.

Bayles, K. A., Tomoeda, C. K., Cruz, R. F., & Mahendra, N. (2000). Communication abilities of individuals with late-stage Alzheimer disease. *Alzheimer Disease and Associated Disorders, 14*(3), 176–181.

Bayles, K. A., Tomoeda, C. K., & Rein, J. A. (1996). Phrase repetition in Alzheimer's disease: Effect of meaning and length. *Brain and Language, 54*(2), 246–261.

Beck, A. T., Steer, R. A., & Brown, G. K. (1996). *Beck Depression Inventory (BDI®-II).* San Psychological Corporation.

Bir, S. C., Khan, M. W., Javalkar, V., Toledo, E. G., & Kelley, R. E. (2021). Emerging concepts in vascular dementia: A review. *Journal of Stroke and Cerebrovascular Diseases, 30*(8), 105864.

Bourgeois, M. S. (1990). Enhancing conversation skills in patients with Alzheimer's disease using a prosthetic memory aid. *Journal of Applied Behavior Analysis, 23*(1), 29–42.

Bourgeois, M. S. (1992). Evaluating memory wallets in conversations with patients with dementia. *Journal of Speech and Hearing Research, 35,* 1344–1357.

Bourgeois, M. S. (2013). *Memory and communication aids for people with dementia.* Health Professions Press.

Bourgeois, M. S., Burgio, L. D., Schultz, R., Beach, S., & Palmer, B. (1997). Modifying repetitive verbalizations of community-dwelling patients with Alzheimer's disease. *Gerontologist*, *37*(1), 30–39.

Bourgeois, M. S., Camp, C. J., Rose, M., White, B., Malone, M., Carr, J., & Rovine, M. (2003). A comparison of training strategies to enhance use of external aids by persons with dementia. *Journal of Communication Disorders*, *36*, 361–378.

Bourgeois, M. S., Lenius, K., Turkstra, L., & Camp, C. (2007). The effects of cognitive teletherapy on reported everyday memory behaviors of persons with chronic traumatic brain injury. *Brain Injury*, *21*(12), 1245–1257.

Brotons, M., & Koger, S. M. (2000). The impact of music therapy on language functioning in dementia. *Journal of Music Therapy*, *37*(3), 183–195.

Brush, J., Calkins, M., Bruce, C., & Sanford, J. (2012). *Environment and Communication Assessment Toolkit (ECAT) for dementia care*. Health Professions Press.

Brush, J., & Camp, C. (1998). *A therapy technique for improving memory: Spaced Retrieval*. Menorah Park Center for the Aging.

Buckner, R. L., Snyder, A. Z., Shannon, B. J., LaRossa, G., Sachs, R., Fotenos, A. F., . . . Mintun, M. A. (2005). Molecular, structural, and functional characterization of Alzheimer's disease: Evidence for a relationship between default activity, amyloid, and memory. *Journal of Neuroscience*, *25*(34), 7709–7717.

Building Our Largest Dementia (BOLD) Infrastructure Act, U.S.C. § S. 2076. (2018). https://uscode.house.gov/statutes/pl/115/406.pdf

Cacciatore, F., Napoli, C., Abete, P., Marciano, E., Triassi, M., & Rengo, F. (1999). Quality of life determinants and hearing function in an elderly population: Observatorio Geriatrico Campano Study Group. *Gerontology*, *45*, 323–328.

Cairns, N. J., Bigio, E. H., Mackenzie, I. R. A., Neumann, M., Lee, V. M.-Y., Hatan-paa, K. J., . . . Mann, D. M. A. (2007). Neuropathologic diagnostic and nosologic criteria for frontotemporal lobar degeneration: Consensus of the Consortium for Frontotemporal Lobar Degeneration. *Acta Neuropathologica*, *114*(1), 5–22. https://doi.org/10.1007/s00401-007-0237-2

Camp, C. J. (1989). Facilitation in learning of Alzheimer's disease. In G. Gilmore, P. Whitehouse, & M. Wykle (Eds.), *Memory and aging: Theory, research, and practice* (pp. 212–225). Springer.

Camp, C. J. (1999). *Montessori-based activities for persons with dementia* (Vol. 1). Menorah Park Center for Senior Living.

Cao, L., Hai, S., Lin, X., Shu, D., Wang, S., Yue, J., . . . Dong, B. (2012). Comparison of the Saint Louis University Mental Status Examination, the Mini-Mental State Examination, and the Montreal Cognitive Assessment in Detection of Cognitive Impairment in Chinese elderly from the geriatric department. *Journal of the American Medical Directors Association*, *13*(7), 626–629.

Centers for Medicare & Medicaid Services. (2001). Transmittal AB-01135. Medical review of services for patients with dementia. https://www.cms.gov/Regulations-and-Guidance/Guidance/Transmittals/downloads/ab01135.pdf

Cherry, K. E., Walvoord, A. G., & Hawley, J. S. (2010). Spaced retrieval enhances memory for a name-face-occupation association in older adults with probable Alzheimer's disease. *Journal of General Psychology*, *171*(2), 168–181.

Clare, L., & Jones, R. S. P. (2008). Errorless learning in the rehabilitation of memory impairment: A critical review. *Neuropsychology Review*, *18*, 1–23.

Clark, L. J., Gatz, M., Zheng, L., Chen, Y.-L., McCleary, C., & Mack, W. J. (2009). Longitudinal verbal fluency in normal aging, preclinical and prevalent Alzheimer's disease. *American Journal of Alzheimer's Disease and Other Dementias*, *24*(6), 461–468.

Collette, F., Delrue, G., Van Der Linden, M., & Salmon, E. (2001). The relationships between executive dysfunction and frontal hypometabolism in Alzheimer's disease. *Brain and Cognition, 47*, 272–275.

Cordell, C. B., Borson, S., Boustani, M., Chodosh, J., Reuben, D., Verghese, J., . . . Fried, L. B. (2013). Alzheimer's Association recommendations for operationalizing the detection of cognitive impairment during the Medicare Annual Wellness Visit in a primary care setting. *Alzheimer's & Dementia, 9*(2), 141–150.

Cox, D. M., Bayles, K. A., & Trosset, M. W. (1996). Category and attribute knowledge deterioration in Alzheimer's disease. *Brain and Language, 52*(3), 536–550.

Crum, R. M., Anthony, J. C., Bassett, S. S., & Folstein, M. F. (1993). Population-based norms for the Mini-Mental State Examination by age and education level. *Journal of the American Medical Association, 269*(18), 2386–2391.

Deramecourt, V., Lebert, F., Debachy, B., Mackowiak-Cordoliani, M. A., Bombois, S., Kerdraon, O., . . . Pasquier, F. (2010). Prediction of pathology in primary progressive language and speech disorders. *Neurology, 74*(1), 42–49.

Desai, M., Pratt, L. A., Lentzner, H., & Robinson, K. N. (2001). *Trends in vision and hearing among older Americans.* National Center for Health Statistics.

Dickerson, B. C., & Eichenbaum, H. (2010). The episodic memory system: Neurocircuitry and disorders. *Neuropsychopharmacology, 35*(1), 86–104.

Duff, K., Humphreys-Clark, J., O'Bryant, S., Mold, J., Schiffer, R., & Sutker, P. (2008). Utility of the RBANS in detecting cognitive impairment associated with Alzheimer's disease: Sensitivity, specificity, and positive and negative predictive powers. *Archives of Clinical Neuropsychology, 23*(5), 603–612.

Elzaguirre, N. O., Rementeria, G. P., Gonzalez-Torres, M., & Gaviria, M. (2017). Updates in vascular dementia. *Heart and Mind, 1*, 22–35.

Europa, E., Iaccarino, L., Perry, D. C., Weis, E., Welch, A. E., Rabinovici, G. D., . . . Henry, M. L. (2020). Diagnostic assessment in primary progressive aphasia: An illustrative case example. *American Journal of Speech-Language Pathology, 29*(4), 1833–1849.

Foldi, N. S., Lobosco, J. J., & Schaefer, L. A. (2002). The effect of attentional dysfunction in Alzheimer's disease: Theoretical and practical implications. *Seminars in Speech and Language, 23*(2), 139–150.

Folstein, M. F., Folstein, S. E., & Fanjiang, G. (2001). *Mini-Mental State Examination: Clinical guide.* Psychological Assessment Resources.

Folstein, M. F., Folstein, S. E., & McHugh, P. R. (1975). Mini-Mental State: A practical method for grading the cognitive state of patients for the clinician. *Journal of Psychiatric Research, 12*, 189–198.

Freilich, B. M., & Hyer, L. A. (2007). Relation of the Repeatable Battery for Assessment of Neuropsychological Status (RBANS) to measures of daily functioning in dementia. *Psychological Reports, 101*(1), 119–129.

Fromm, D., & Holland, A. L. (1989). Functional communication in Alzheimer's disease. *Journal of Speech and Hearing Disorders, 54*, 535–540.

Ganguli, M., Blacker, D., Blazer, D. G., Grant, I., Jeste, D. V., Paulsen, J. S., . . . Sachdev, P. S. (2011). Classification of neurocognitive disorders in DSM-5: A work in progress. *The American Journal of Geriatric Psychiatry, 19*(3), 205–210.

Ganguli, M., Tangalos, E. G., Cummings, J. L., & DeKosky, S. T. (2001). Practice parameter: Early detection of dementia: Mild cognitive impairment (an evidence-based review). Report of the Quality Standards Subcommittee of the American Academy of Neurology. *Neurology, 56*, 1133–1142.

Geraudie, A., Battista, P., García, A. M., Allen, I. E., Miller, Z. A., Gorno-Tempini, M. L., & Montembeault, M. (2021). Speech and language impairments in behavioral variant frontotemporal dementia: A systematic review. *Neuroscience & Biobehavioral Reviews, 131,* 1076–1095.

Gorno-Tempini, M. L., Dronkers, N. F., Rankin, K. P., Ogar, J. M., Phengrasamy, L., Rosen, H. J., . . . Miller, B. L. (2004). Cognition and anatomy in three variants of primary progressive aphasia. *Annals of Neurology, 55*(3), 335–346.

Gorno-Tempini, M. L., Hillis, A. E., Weintraub, S., Kertesz, A., Mendez, M., Cappa, S. F., . . . Grossman, M. (2011). Classification of primary progressive aphasia and its variants. *Neurology, 76*(11), 1006–1014.

Grabowski, T. J., & Damasio, A. R. (2004). Definition, clinical features, and neuroanatomical basis of dementia. In M. Esiri, V. Lee, & J. Trojanowski (Eds.), *Neuropathology of dementia* (2nd ed., pp. 1–10). Cambridge University Press.

Hachinski, V. C., Iliff, L. D., Zilhka, E., Du Boulay, G. H., McAllister, V. L., Marshall, J., . . . Symon, L. (1975). Cerebral blood flow in dementia. *Archives of Neurology, 32*(9), 632–637.

Hachinski, V. C., Oveisgharan, S., Romney, K., & Shankle, W. R. (2012). Optimizing the Hachinski Ischemia Scale. *Archives of Neurology, 69*(2), 169–175.

Hanson, J. C., & Lippa, C. F. (2009). Lewy body dementia. *International Review of Neurobiology, 84,* 215–228.

Harris, J. (1997). Reminiscence: A culturally and developmentally appropriate language intervention for older adults. *American Journal of Speech-Language Pathology, 6*(3), 19–26.

Harvan, J. R., & Cotter, V. (2006). An evaluation of dementia screening in the primary care setting. *Journal of the American Academy of Nurse Practitioners, 18*(8), 351–360.

Heaton, R. K., Clifford, D. B., Franklin, D. R., Woods, S. P., Ake, C., Vaida, F., . . . Grant, I. (2010). HIV-associated neurocognitive disorders persist in the era of potent antiretroviral therapy: CHARTER Study. *Neurology, 75*(23), 2087–2096.

Helm-Estabrooks, N. (2001). *Cognitive Linguistic Quick Test (CLQT).* Pearson.

Helm-Estabrooks, N. (2017). *Cognitive Linguistic Quick Test-Plus (CLQT™+).* Pearson.

Henry, M. L., & Grasso, S. M. (2018). Assessment of individuals with primary progressive aphasia. *Seminars in Speech and Language, 39,* 231–241.

Hickey, E. L., & Bourgeois, M. S. (2018). *Dementia: Person-centered assessment and intervention.* Routledge.

Hill, N. L., Kolanowski, A. M., & Gill, D. J. (2011). Plasticity in early Alzheimer's disease: An opportunity for intervention. *Topics in Geriatric Rehabilitation, 27*(4), 257–267.

Hobson, V. L., Hall, J. R., Humphreys-Clark, J. D., Schrimsher, G. W., & O'Bryant, S. E. (2010). Identifying functional impairment with scores from the Repeatable Battery for the Assessment of Neuropsychological Status (RBANS). *International Journal of Geriatric Psychiatry, 25*(2), 525–530.

Hoerster, L., Hickey, E., & Bourgeois, M. (2001). Effects of memory aids on conversations between nursing home residents with dementia and nursing assistants. *Neuropsychological Rehabilitation, 11,* 399–427.

Hofbauer, L. M., Ross, F. D., & Rodriguez, F. S. (2022). Music-based interventions for community-dwelling people with dementia: A systematic review. *Health and Social Care in the Community, 30*(6), 2186–2201.

Holland, A. L., Fromm, D., & Wozniak, L. (2018). *Communication Activities of Daily Living–Third edition (CADL 3).* Pro-Ed.

Hopper, T. (2001). Indirect interventions to facilitate communication in Alzheimer's disease. *Seminars in Speech and Language, 22*(4), 305–315.

Hopper, T. (2007). The ICF and dementia. *Seminars in Speech and Language, 28,* 273–282.

Hopper, T., Bayles, K. A., & Kim, E. (2001). Retained neuropsychological abilities of individuals with Alzheimer's disease. *Seminars in Speech & Language, 22*(4), 261–273.

Hopper, T., Bourgeois, M., Pimentel, J., Qualls, C. D., Hickey, E., Frymark, T., & Schooling, T. (2013). An evidence-based systematic review on cognitive interventions for individuals with dementia. *American Journal of Speech-Language Pathology, 22*, 126–145.

Hopper, T., Cleary, S., Baumback, N., & Fragomeni, A. (2007). Table fellowship: Mealtime as a context for conversation with individuals who have dementia. *Alzheimer's Care Quarterly, 8*(1), 34–42.

Hopper, T., Douglas, N., & Khayum, B. (2015). Direct and indirect interventions for cognitive-communication disorders of dementia. *Perspectives on Neurophysiology and Neurogenic Speech and Language Disorders, 25*(4), 142–157.

Hopper, T., Drefs, S., Bayles, K., Tomoeda, C. K., & Dinu, I. (2009). The effects of modified spaced-retrieval training on learning and retention of face-name associations by individuals with dementia. *Neuropsychological Rehabilitation, 5*, 1–22.

Hopper, T., Mahendra, N., Kim, E., Azuma, T., Bayles, K. A., Cleary, S., & Tomoeda, C. K. (2005). Evidence-based practice recommendations for individuals working with dementia: Spaced retrieval training. *Journal of Medical Speech-Language Pathology, 13*(4), xxvii–xxxiv.

Huey, E. D., Manly J. J., Tang, M. X., Schupf, N., Brickman, A. M., Manoochehri, M., . . . Mayeux, R. (2013). Course and etiology of dysexecutive MCI in a community sample. *Alzheimer's & Dementia, 9*, 632–639.

Hyter, Y. D., & Salas-Provance, M. B. (2021). *Culturally responsive practices in speech, language, and hearing sciences* (2nd ed.). Plural Publishing.

Jack, C. R., Wiste, H. J., Vemuri, P., Weigand, S. D., Senjem, M. L., Zeng, G., . . . Knopman, D. S. (2010). Brain beta-amyloid measures and magnetic resonance imaging atrophy both predict time-to-progression from mild cognitive impairment to Alzheimer's disease. *Brain, 133*, 3336–3348.

Josephs, K. A., Whitwell, J. L., Duffy, J. R., Vanvoorst, W. A., Strand, E. A., Hu, W. T., . . . Petersen, R. C. (2008). Progressive aphasia secondary to Alzheimer disease vs FTLD pathology. *Neurology, 70*(1), 25–34.

Kagan, A. (1998). Supported conversation for adults with aphasia: Methods and resources for training conversation partners. *Aphasiology, 12*(9), 816–830.

Kapasi, A., DeCarli, C., & Schneider, J. A. (2017). Impact of multiple pathologies on the threshold for clinically overt dementia. *Acta Neuropathologica, 134*(2), 171–186.

Kertesz, A. (2006). *Western Aphasia Battery–Revised.* Pearson.

Kim, E., Cleary, S., Hopper, T., Bayles, K., Mahendra, N., Azuma, T., & Rackley, A. (2006). Evidence-based practice recommendations for working with individuals with dementia: Group reminiscence therapy. *Journal of Medical Speech-Language Pathology, 14*(3), xxiii–xxxiv.

Kirova, A.-M., Bays, R. B., & Lagalwar, S. (2015). Working memory and executive function decline across normal aging, mild cognitive impairment, and Alzheimer's disease. *BioMed Research International, 2015*, e748212.

Kopstein, M., & Mohlman, D. J. (2022). *HIV-1 encephalopathy and AIDS dementia complex.* StatPearls Publishing. https://www.ncbi.nlm.nih.gov/books/NBK507700/

Kornblith, E., Bahorik, A., Boscardin, W. J., Xia, F., Barnes, D. E., & Yaffe, K. (2022). Association of race and ethnicity with incidence of dementia among older adults. *Journal of the American Medical Association, 327*(15), 1488–1495.

Kroenke, K., Spitzer, R. L., & Williams, J. B. (2001). The PHQ-9: Validity of a brief depression severity measure. *Journal of General Internal Medicine, 16*(9), 606–661.

Landauer, T. K., & Bjork, R. A. (1978). Optimum rehearsal patterns and name learning. In M. M. Grunenberg, P. S. Morris, & R. N. Sykes (Eds.), *Practice aspects of memory* (pp. 625–632). Academic Press.

Lawton, M. P., Van Haitsma, K., & Klapper, J. A. (1999). *Observed Emotion Rating Scale.* https://www.abramson center .org/media/1199/observed-emotion-rating-scale.pdf

Lee, S., Kim, D., & Lee, H. (2022). Examine race/ethnicity disparities in perception, intention, and screening of dementia in a community setting: Scoping review. *International Journal of Environmental Research and Public Health, 19*(14), Article 14.

Lee, S. B., Park, C. S., Jeong, J. W., Choe, J. Y., Hwang, Y. J., Park, C.-A., . . . Kim, K. W. (2009). Effects of spaced retrieval training (SRT) on cognitive function in Alzheimer's disease (AD) patients. *Archives of Gerontology and Geriatrics, 49*(2), 289–293.

Liu, C.-C., Kanekiyo, T., Xu, H., & Bu, G. (2013). Apolipoprotein E and Alzheimer disease: Risk, mechanisms, and therapy. *Nature Reviews Neurology, 9*(2), 106–118.

Livingston, G., Sommerlad, A., Orgeta, V., Costafreda, S. G., Huntley, J., Ames, D., . . . Mukadam, N. (2017). Dementia prevention, intervention, and care. *The Lancet, 390*(10113), 2673–2734.

Mahendra, N. (2001). Direct interventions for improving the performance of individuals with Alzheimer's disease. *Seminars in Speech & Language, 22*(4), 289–302.

Mahendra, N. (2011). Computer-assisted spaced retrieval training of faces and names for persons with dementia. *Nonpharmacological Therapies in Dementia, 1*(3), 217–238.

Mahendra, N. (2012). The logopenic variant of primary progressive aphasia: Effects on linguistic communication. *Perspectives on Gerontology, 17*(2), 50–59.

Mahendra, N., & Apple, A. (2007). Human memory systems: A framework for understanding dementia. *The ASHA Leader, 12*(16), 8–11.

Mahendra, N., Bayles, K. A., & Harris, F. P. (2005). Effect of presentation modality on immediate and delayed recall in individuals with Alzheimer's disease. *American Journal of Speech-Language Pathology, 14*(2), 144–155.

Mahendra, N., & Engineer, N. (2009). Effects of vascular dementia on cognition and linguistic communication: A case study. *Perspectives on Neurophysiology and Neurogenic Speech and Language Disorders, 19*(4), 107–116.

Mahendra, N., Hickey, E., & Bourgeois, M. S. (2018). Cognitive-communicative characteristics: Profiling types of dementia. In E. Hickey & M. S. Bourgeois (Eds.), *Dementia: Person-centered assessment and intervention* (pp. 42–80). Routledge.

Mahendra, N., & Hopper, T. (2022). Dementia and related cognitive disorders. In I. Papathanasiou, & P. Coppens (Eds.), *Aphasia and related neurogenic communication disorders* (3rd ed., pp. 503–542). Jones and Bartlett Learning.

Mahendra, N., Hopper, T., Bayles, K., Azuma, T., Cleary, S., & Kim, E. (2006). Evidence-based practice recommendations for working with individuals with dementia: Montessori-based interventions. *Journal of Medical Speech Language Pathology, 14*(1), xv–xxv.

Mahendra, N., Scullion, A., & Hamerschlag, C. (2011). Cognitive-linguistic interventions for persons with dementia: A practitioner's guide to three evidence-based techniques. *Topics in Geriatric Rehabilitation, 27*(4), 1–12.

Mariani, E., Monastero, R., & Meocci, P. (2007). Mild cognitive impairment: A systematic review. *Journal of Alzheimer's Disease, 12*, 22–35.

Martin, A., & Fedio, P. (1983). Word production and comprehension in Alzheimer's disease: The breakdown of semantic knowledge. *Brain and Language, 19*, 124–141.

Martyr, A., & Clare, L. (2012). Executive function and activities of daily living in Alzheimer's disease: A correlational metaanalysis. *Dementia and Geriatric Cognitive Disorders, 33*(2–3), 189–203.

Mattis, S., Jurica, P., & Leitten, C. (1991). *Dementia Rating Scale (DRS-2)*. Psychological Assessment Resources.

Mayeda, E. R., Glymour, M. M., Quesenberry, C. P., & Whitmer, R. A. (2016). Inequalities in dementia incidence between six racial and ethnic groups over 14 years. *Alzheimer's & Dementia, 12*(3), 216–224.

McDonough, A., Dookhy, J., McHale, C., Sharkey, J., Fox, S., & Kennelly, S. P. (2021). Embedding audiological screening within memory clinic care pathway for individuals at risk of cognitive decline—Patient perspectives. *BMC Geriatrics, 21*, 691. https://doi.org/10.1186/s12877-021-02701-0

McGilton, K. S., Rochon, E., Sidani, S., Shaw, A., Ben-David, B. M., Saragosa, M., . . . Pichora-Fuller, M. K. (2017). Can we help care providers communicate more effectively with persons having dementia living in long-term care homes? *American Journal of Alzheimer's Disease & Other Dementias, 32*(1), 41–50.

McKeith, I., Taylor, J. P., Thomas, A., Donaghy, P., & Kane, J. (2016). Revisiting DLB diagnosis: A consideration of prodromal DLB and of the diagnostic overlap with Alzheimer disease. *Journal of Geriatric Psychiatry & Neurology, 29*(5), 249–253.

McKhann, G. M., Knopman, D. S., Chertkow, H., Hyman, B. T., Jack, C. R., Kawas, C. H., . . . Phelps, C. H. (2011). The diagnosis of dementia due to Alzheimer's disease: Recommendations from the National Institute on Aging-Alzheimer's Association workgroups on diagnostic guidelines for Alzheimer's disease. *Alzheimer's & Dementia, 7*(3), 263–269.

Mehta, K., & Yeo, G. (2016). Systematic review of dementia prevalence and incidence in US race/ethnic populations. *Alzheimer's and Dementia, 13*(1), 72–83.

Mesulam, M., Wicklund, A., Johnson, N., Rogalski, E., Léger, G. C., Rademaker, A., . . . Bigio, E. H. (2008). Alzheimer and frontotemporal pathology in subsets of primary progressive aphasia. *Annals of Neurology, 63*(6), 709–719.

Mitchell, A. J., & Shiri-Feshki, M. (2009). Rate of progression of mild cognitive impairment to dementia: Meta-analysis of 41 robust inception cohort studies. *Acta Psychiatrica Scandinavica, 119*, 252–265.

Moreno-Morales, C., Calero, R., Moreno-Morales, P., & Pintado, C. (2020). Music therapy in the treatment of dementia: A systematic review and meta-analysis. *Frontiers in Medicine, 19*, 7–160.

Moroney, J. T., Bagiella, E., Desmond, D. W., Hachinski, V. C., Mölsä, P. K., Gustafson, L., . . . Tatemichi, T. K. (1997). Meta-analysis of the Hachinski Ischemic Score in pathologically verified dementias. *Neurology, 49*(4), 1096–1105.

Nasreddine, Z. S., Phillips, N. A., Bédirian, V., Charbonneau, S., Whitehead, V., Collin, I., . . . Chertkow, H. (2005). The Montreal Cognitive Assessment, MoCA: A brief screening tool for mild cognitive impairment. *Journal of the American Geriatrics Society, 53*(4), 695–699.

National Institute on Aging. (2012). *Frontotemporal disorders information for patients, families and caregivers*. https://www.nia.nih.gov/research/alzheimers-dementia-outreach-recruitment-engagement-re sources/frontotemporal-disorders

National Institute on Aging. (2022). *What are frontotemporal disorders?* https://www.nia.nih.gov/health/what-are-frontotemporal-disorders

Nicholas, M., Obler, L., Albert, M., & Helm-Estabrooks, N. (1985). Empty speech in Alzheimer's disease and fluent aphasia. *Journal of Speech and Hearing Research, 28*, 405–410.

Novak, P., Chu, J., Ali, M. M., & Chen, J. (2020). Racial and ethnic disparities in serious psychological distress among those with Alzheimer's disease and related dementias. *American Journal of Geriatric Psychiatry, 28*(4), 478–490.

Omnibus Budget Reconciliation Act of 1987, Public Law 100-203 (101 Stat. 1330). (1987).

Orsulic-Jeras, S., Schneider, N., & Camp, C. (2000). Special feature: Montessori activities for long-term care residents with dementia. *Topics in Geriatric Rehabilitation, 16*(1), 78–91.

Ozgis, S., Rendell, P. G., & Henry, J. D. (2009). Spaced retrieval significantly improves prospective memory performance of cognitively impaired older adults. *Gerontology, 55*, 229–232.

Patient Protection and Affordable Care Act. (2010). *The Patient Protection and Affordable Care Act: Detailed summary.* https://www.dpc.senate.gov/healthreformbill/healthbill04.pdf

Petersen, R., & Negash, C. (2008). Mild cognitive impairment: An overview. *CNS Spectrums, 13*(1), 45–53.

Petersen, R. C. (2004). Mild cognitive impairment as a diagnostic entity. *Journal of Internal Medicine, 256*, 183–194.

Petersen, R. C. (2016). Mild cognitive impairment. *Continuum, 22*(2), 404–418.

Petersen, R. C., Lopez, O., Armstrong, M. J., Getchius, T. S. D., Ganguli, M., Gloss, D., . . . Rae-Grant, A. (2018). Practice guideline update summary: Mild cognitive impairment: Report of the Guideline Development, Dissemination, and Implementation Subcommittee of the American Academy of Neurology. *Neurology, 90*(3), 126–135.

Powlishta, K. K., Von Dras, D. D., Stanford, A., Carr, B. B., Tsering, C., Miller, J. P., & Morris, J. C. (2002). The Clock Drawing Test is a poor screen for very mild dementia. *Neurology, 59*, 898–903.

Randolph, C. (1997). Differentiating vascular dementia from Alzheimer's disease: The role of neuropsychological testing. *Clinical Geriatrics, 5*(8), 77–84.

Randolph, C. (2012). *Repeatable Battery for the Assessment of Neuropsychological Status update.* Pearson.

Randolph, C., Tierney, M., Mohr, E., & Chase, T. (1998). The Repeatable Battery for the Assessment of Neuropsychological Status (RBANS™): Preliminary clinical validity. *Journal of Clinical and Experimental Neuropsychology, 20*, 310–319.

Ripich, D. N., & Terrell, B. (1988). Patterns of discourse cohesion and coherence in Alzheimer's disease. *Journal of Speech and Hearing Disorders, 53*, 8–15.

Rohrer, J. D., Rossor, M. N., & Warren, J. D. (2012). Alzheimer's pathology in primary progressive aphasia. *Neurobiology of Aging, 33*(4), 744–752.

Román, G. C. (2005). Clinical forms of vascular dementia. In R. H. Paul, R. Cohen, B. R. Ott, & S. Salloway (Eds.), *Vascular dementia: Cerebrovascular mechanisms and clinical management* (pp. 7–21). Humana Press.

Sailor, K., Antoine, M., Diaz, M., Kuslansky, G., & Kluger, A. (2004). The effects of Alzheimer's disease on item output in verbal fluency tasks. *Neuropsychology, 18*(2), 306–314.

Salmon, D. P., & Bondi, M. W. (2009). Neuropsychological assessment of dementia. *Annual Review of Psychology, 60*, 257–282.

Saragih, I. D., Tonapa, S. I., Yao, C.-T., Saragih, I. S., & Lee, B.-O. (2022). Effects of reminiscence therapy in people with dementia: A systematic review and meta-analysis. *Journal of Psychiatric and Mental Health Nursing, 29*, 883–903.

Schacter, D. L., Rich, S. A., & Stampp, M. S. (1985). Remediation of memory disorders: Experimental evaluation of the spaced retrieval technique. *Journal of Clinical and Experimental Neuropsychology, 7*(1), 79–96.

Schneider, J. A., Arvanitakis, Z., Bang, W., & Bennett, D. A. (2007). Mixed brain pathologies account for most dementia cases in community-dwelling older persons. *Neurology, 69*, 2197–2204.

Schneider, J. A., Arvanitakis, Z., Yu, L., Boyle, P. A., Leurgans, S. E., & Bennett, D. A. (2012). Cognitive impairment, decline and fluctuations in older community-dwelling subjects with Lewy bodies. *Brain, 135*(10), 3005–3014.

Sheikh, J. I., & Yesavage, J. A. (1986). Geriatric Depression Scale (GDS): Recent evidence and development of a shorter version. *Clinical Gerontologist, 5*(1–2), 165–173.

Sieben, A., Van Langenhove, T., Engelborghs, S., Martin, J.-J., Boon, P., Cras, P., . . . Cruts, M. (2012). The genetics and neuropathology of frontotemporal lobar degeneration. *Acta Neuropathologica, 124*(3), 353–372.

Small, J., Kemper, S., & Lyons, K. (1997). Sentence comprehension in Alzheimer's disease: Effects of grammatical complexity, speech rate and repetition. *Psychology & Aging, 12*, 3–11.

Spinelli, E. G., Mandelli, M. L., Miller, Z. A., Santos-Santos, M. A., Wilson, S. M., Agosta, F., . . . Gorno-Tempini, M. L. (2017). Typical and atypical pathology in primary progressive aphasia variants. *Annals of Neurology., 81*(3), 430–443.

Squire, L. R., & Zola-Morgan, S. (1991). The medial temporal lobe memory system. *Science, 253*, 1380–1386.

Steis, M. R., & Schrauf, R. W. (2009). A review of translations and adaptations of the Mini-Mental State Examination in languages other than English and Spanish. *Research in Gerontological Nursing, 2*(3), 214–224.

Stewart, S., O'Riley, A., Edelstein, B., & Gould, C. (2012). A preliminary comparison of three cognitive screening instruments in long term care: The MMSE, SLUMS, and MoCA. *Clinical Gerontologist, 35*(1), 57–75.

Sunderland, T., Hill, J. L., Mellow, A. M., Lawlor, B. A., Gundersheimer, J., Newhouse, P.A., & Grafman, J.H. (1989). Clock drawing in Alzheimer's disease: A novel measure of dementia severity.

Journal of the American Geriatrics Society, 37(8), 725–729.

Tariq, S. H., Tumosa, N., Chibnall, J. T., Perry, M. H., & Morley, J. E. (2006). Comparison of the Saint Louis University Mental Status Examination and the Mini-Mental State Examination for detecting dementia and mild neurocognitive disorder: A pilot study. *American Journal of Geriatric Psychiatry, 14*, 900–910.

Tomoeda, C. K., & Bayles, K. A. (1993). Longitudinal effects of AD on discourse production. *Alzheimer Disease and Associated Disorders, 7*(4), 223–236.

Tulving, E. (1983). *Elements of episodic memory.* Oxford University Press.

United Nations. (2019). *World Population Prospects 2019: Highlights.* https://population.un.org/wpp/publications/files/wpp2019_highlights.pdf

United States Census Bureau. (2020). *65 and older population grows rapidly as baby boomers age.* https://www.census.gov/newsroom/press-releases/2020/65-older-population-grows.html

Vance, D. E., & Johns, R. N. (2002). Montessori improved cognitive domains in adults with Alzheimer's disease. *Physical and Occupational Therapy in Geriatrics, 20*(3–4), 19–36.

Vance, D. E., & Porter R. (2000). Montessori methods yield cognitive gains in Alzheimer's daycares. *Activities Adaptation Aging, 24*(3), 1–21.

van der Steen, J. T., Smaling, H. J. A., van der Wouden, J. C., Bruinsma, M. S., Scholten, R. J. P. M., & Vink, A. C. (2018). Music-based therapeutic interventions for persons with dementia. *Cochrane Database of Systematic Reviews, 7*, 1–99. https://doi.org/10.1002/14651858.CD003477.pub4

Vassilaki, M., Aakre, J. A., Knopman, D. S., Kremers, W. K., Mielke, M. M., Geda, Y. E., . . . Petersen, R. C. (2019). Informant-based hearing difficulties and the risk for mild cognitive impairment and dementia. *Age and Ageing, 48*(6), 888–894.

Wang, X., Li, F., Gao, Q., Jiang, Z., Abudusaimati, X., Yao, J., & Zhu, H. (2022). Evaluation of the accuracy of cognitive screening tests in detecting dementia associated with Alzheimer's disease: A hierarchical Bayesian latent class meta-analysis. *Journal of Alzheimer's Disease*, *87*(1), 285–304. https://doi.org/10.3233/JAD-215394

Weinstein, B. E. (2019). The cost of age-related hearing loss: To treat or not to treat? *Speech, Language and Hearing*, *22*(1), 9–15. https://doi.org/10.1080/2050571X.2018.1533622

Wilson, B. A., Greenfield, E., Clare, L., Baddeley, A., Cockburn, J., Watson, P., Tate, R., Sopena, S., & Nannery, R. (2008). *The Rivermead Behavioural Memory Test, 3rd edition (RBMT-3)*. Pearson Assessment.

Wong, J. A., Min, D. K., Kranick, J., Ushasri, H., Trinh-Shevrin, C., & Kwon, S. C. (2022). Exploring community knowledge, attitudes and perceptions of Alzheimer's disease/Alzheimer's disease-related dementias and healthy ageing in Asian American, Native Hawaiian and Pacific Islanders. *Health & Social Care in the Community*, *30*, e5946–e5958.

World Health Organization. (2001). *International classification of functioning, disability and health*.

World Health Organization. (2017). *Global action plan on the public health response to dementia 2017–2025*.

World Health Organization. (2019). *Risk reduction of cognitive decline and dementia: WHO guidelines*. https://www.who.int/publications/i/item/9789241550543

World Health Organization. (2022). *Fact sheet on dementia*. https://www.who.int/news-room/fact-sheets/detail/dementia

Yueh, B., Shapiro, N., MacLean, C. H., & Shekelle, P. G. (2003). Screening and management of adult hearing loss in primary care: Scientific review. *Journal of the American Medical Association*, *289*, 1976–1985.

7

Cognitive Communication Disorders Associated With Mild Traumatic Brain Injury (Concussion)

Kathryn Y. Hardin and Catherine Wiseman-Hakes

Chapter Learning Objectives

After reading this chapter you will be able to:

1. Describe the trajectory of uncomplicated recovery from acute mild traumatic brain injury (mTBI) as compared to persistent symptomatology and describe how these timelines influence SLP clinical decision-making.

2. Identify communities with mTBI and experience of intersectionalities and how these intersectionalities may impact clinical care for mTBI.

3. Define the concussion phenotypes and describe their use in speech-language pathology (SLP) assessment and interprofessional teaming.

4. Describe the cognitive communication behaviors that may occur after mTBI in order to create an intervention plan.

5. Describe the four types of assessment tools used in mTBI SLP evaluations and how the use of patient-reported outcome measures facilitates patient-centered practices.

6. Explain the overarching SLP intervention principles applicable to all patients with mTBI.

Introduction to Mild TBI

Mild traumatic brain injury (mTBI), also referred to as concussion, is a significant public health concern for adults, children, and active-duty/veteran populations (Soble et al., 2018). Millions of individuals sustain mTBI or concussions worldwide (Dewan et al., 2018; Haarbauer-Krupa et al., 2018; Hunt et al., 2016). Those with concussion/mTBI experience a constellation of symptoms, including changes in cognitive, physical, and psychological functioning, likely representing the effects of neural injury that is typically but not always transient. While some recover relatively quickly, for a significant subset, postinjury symptomology lasts for months or even years (Makdissi et al., 2013). With the increase in awareness and supporting evidence, what was once thought primarily to be a temporary concern is now understood to be a significant problem and life disruptor for many individuals long term (Gaudette et al., 2022; Madhok et al., 2022). This common condition affects all ages, including young children, healthy youth, and the elderly. Individuals describe marked changes in sense of self post-mTBI as well as decreased job and/or academic performance, social engagement, financial stability, and overall quality of life (Iadevaia et al., 2015; Snell et al., 2017; Stergiou-Kita et al., 2016; Wäljas et al., 2015). Furthermore, evidence suggests that 17% of adults did not return to work at 1 year postinjury, and over one-fifth report decreases in annual income (Gaudette et al., 2022). Finally, there remain countless that are undiagnosed as a result of a confluence of under awareness, underreporting, underdiagnosis, and misdiagnosis (Helgeson, 2010). For these reasons, completing a careful assessment of symptoms as soon as possible following injury is important for initial diagnosis, especially when the patient may experience alteration of consciousness and be unable to recall what happened at the time of the injury.

The significant increase in mTBI awareness and potential long-term effects has led to a need for well-trained speech-language pathologists (SLPs) in both educational and medical settings. This chapter will provide a review of the most current research and evidence-based recommendations for evaluating and treating cognitive communication deficits following mTBI. A teachable moment case study is used to illustrate clinical challenges, and supporting resources are made available for additional learning. Due to the high incidence of mTBI associated with military service, the Veteran Affairs/Department of Defense (VA/DoD) has created many clinical recommendations that can be applied to both military and civilian care. While information about service-members and veterans can be found throughout the chapter, the reader will find a special section devoted to service-members and veterans, with extended information specifically regarding military injury in Appendix 7–A. In addition, readers may consider an external resource supported by the American Speech-Language-Hearing Association (ASHA) as in 2022, ASHA joined the national Concussion Awareness Now (CAN) network providing no-cost interprofessional education resources for patients and providers (https://concussionawarenessnow.org).

mTBI Terminology and Timelines

MTBI diagnoses are based on the initial signs and symptoms at the time of the event and that these symptoms are based on physiological disruption within the brain. Diagnosis of mTBI is based on the presence of one or more of the following criteria: (a) change in neurologic function such as possible loss of consciousness, altered mental status, amnesia, or confusion; (b) loss of consciousness (LOC) <30 minutes; (c) Glasgow Coma Scale score of 13 to 15; and (d) posttraumatic amnesia (PTA) <24 hours. In 2023, the American Congress of Rehabilitation Medicine (ACRM) updated and unified their definition of mTBI/concussion, as there are many operationalized definitions found in the literature causing significant confusion for patients and providers. (Silverberg et al., 2021; Silverberg et al., 2023). ACRM reports that "mild TBI" and "concussion" can be used synonymously and interchangeably for the majority of individuals. The terms "concussion" and "mTBI" can be used when structural changes on standard imaging techniques are not present, which is true for most injuries. For injuries where the above criteria are met and positive structural neuroimaging findings exist, "complicated mTBI" should be used. It is paramount that clinicians and clients use mutually shared terminology to avoid confusion in the clinic environment.

There is additional confusion regarding the slowed recovery timeline for the many individuals, often referred to as "protracted" or "incomplete" recovery. The idea of "recovery" after mTBI typically refers to returning to baseline levels of performance in daily activity, an important distinction as research indicates that there may continue to be changes in cellular performance even after an individual feels well. Historically, mTBI was considered transient and symptoms were expected to resolve within 14 days for adults, and in some cases, those with persistent symptoms were labeled "malingering." More recent research indicates that 73% of adults seen in the emergency department with concussion had not functionally recovered within 2 weeks and that 56% of them still had persistent symptoms 6 months postinjury (Madhok et al., 2022). Keeping in mind that as many individuals do not seek critical care, it is conservatively estimated that between 10% and 40% of individuals are living with the long-term persistent symptoms of mTBI (Makdissi et al., 2013). Over time, persistent symptoms are increasingly influenced by co-occurring psychological, social, and environmental factors (Soble et al., 2018).

Terminology for persistent symptoms is also in a period of recalibration, resulting from better understanding mTBI recovery profiles. The field is working to unify the concept of protracted recovery for patients experiencing symptoms 30 days postinjury. Historically, SLPs may have seen the terms "postconcussive symptoms," or "postconcussion syndrome" (PCS), but current preferred terms refer to "persistent" or "prolonged" symptoms or that individuals may experience "incomplete recovery" after mTBI. Individuals seen in SLP outpatient settings are likely those who are experiencing a more protracted recovery profile, and the roles of the SLP will almost certainly shift depending on the time since injury for the client (Hardin et al., 2021). Clinically, SLPs should now recognize that having persistent symptoms is a common occurrence (Madhok et al., 2022) and must be prepared for referrals and literature searches with varying terminology during this time of transition.

Etiologies and Epidemiology mTBI

An estimated 69 million individuals sustain TBI every year worldwide, with approximately 90% of them being mild (Dewan et al., 2018). In the United States, millions of children and adults sustain mTBI every year, though the exact incidence of mTBI remains hard to capture, as the primary problem associated with estimating the incidence of mTBI is that the "mild" nature of the injury directly impacts when and if an individual pursues medical care.

There are three main categories of mTBI: sport-related, mixed-mechanism, and military-related mTBI. Sport-related concussion typically refers to mTBI sustained in athletic training or competition and, depending on the level of sport, may imply individuals with a generally healthy physical condition. Mixed-mechanism is a catchall category that describes traumatic mTBI cases identified from hospital emergency departments and includes falls, motor vehicle accidents, assaults, and other related causalities. While sports-related injuries receive significant media attention, for many groups, such as college students, mixed-mechanism mTBI is far more common (Breck et al., 2019). This is clinically important as recovery times are often longer for mixed-mechanism injuries over sport-related ones (Seiger et al., 2015). Military-related mTBI has numerous causalities, including blast waves or blunt-force trauma, and they can both occur in combat or in the daily operations of a military professional. As with mixed-mechanism injuries, military-related injuries may co-occur with psychological stressors, contributing to greater levels of disability (MacDon-

ald, Johnson, Wierzechoski, et al., 2014; Soble et al., 2018). Learn more about the blast injuries in Appendix 7–A.

Individuals seen in emergency rooms typically have experienced falls (44%) with mixed mechanisms of falls, assault, and motor vehicle accidents combined for nearly 70%. Most injuries seen in the emergency department occur in young children (<4 years), males aged 16 to 24, and women over 65 years (Cancelliere et al., 2017). A known problem with this data set from the Centers for Disease Control and Prevention (CDC) is that millions of people with mTBIs are either treated outside of emergency settings or receive no medical care at all (Taylor et al., 2017). It has been estimated that 50% of individuals with a history of mTBI never receive medical care, whether that is related to geographic access problems, financial constraints with medical care, or rapid recovery of symptoms (Voss et al., 2015). For children, Haarbauer-Krupa et al. (2018) found that families relied on frontline practitioners such as pediatricians (53.4%) or specialty clinics (27%), rather than emergency department/urgent care (16.6%). Limitations in incidence reporting directly impact patients receiving adequate rehabilitative services.

Physiology and Imaging in mTBI

Neurophysiology of Concussion

Giza and Hovda (2001) published a pivotal paper reporting neurophysiological changes of concussion in animal models, essentially creating impact injuries that are similar to sport-related concussion. Understanding the cellular function after injury can be a valuable teaching tool to help explain symptoms and dysfunction with patients. Early on, there is a significant disruption in the ionic balance of the neurons, with potassium rushing out of the cells, while sodium and calcium flood into the cells. At the same time, excess amounts of the neurotransmitter glutamate are released. Dysfunction in the sodium-potassium pump and too much glutamate ultimately result in toxic synapses and slowed communication between neurons. Shortly after injury, the brain temporarily goes into a "hyperactive" state, requiring lots of energy and resources quickly, followed by an extended 7- to 10-day decrease in cerebral blood flow and hypometabolism. This period of hypoactivity has been found to be even longer in adolescence (Grady et al., 2012). These immediate physiologic changes result in many of the acute symptoms associated with mTBI, such as slow processing and motor changes.

In addition to impairments in cellular communication, microstructural changes occur. Diffuse axonal injury remains a hallmark of mTBI, with axons being stretched or broken as a result of the linear and rotational forces on the cells. This impaired synaptic communication can result in increased dysfunction in the frontal lobe, cerebellum, and corpus callosum (Choe & Giza, 2015). Unmyelinated cells are particularly susceptible to damage as they lack the structural support provided by the myelin. It has been hypothesized that one reason for greater deficits in children postinjury is related to their

incomplete myelination (Dennis et al., 2017). Some researchers have argued that in addition to the diffuse axonal injury model of mTBI, changes in thalamic structure and function may also occur (Grossman & Inglese, 2016). The thalamus acts as a central relay station for sensory gating and processing and has cortical projections tied to many cognitive functions, including language and working memory (Chien et al., 2017).

Edema, or inflammation, postinjury can also occur. This is important as ongoing research indicates that neurophysiologic functioning at the cellular level may remain impaired after behavioral functioning has returned to baseline (Kamins et al., 2017). The extent to which the neurological system remains vulnerable to repeated injury during the acute phase of recovery from mTBI, or if an increased vulnerability exists, remains unknown. Most of what is known about cumulative effects of TBI comes from civilian athletes (Soble et al., 2018), and while media attention has highlighted catastrophic outcomes for adolescent and professional athletes, this research remains in its infancy.

Clinical Neuroimaging for mTBI

In the acute stage of traumatic brain injury, computed tomography (CT) and conventional magnetic resonance imaging (MRI) are used to rule out severe complications such as skull fracture, intracranial hemorrhage, and brain edema. In mTBI, conventional CT and MRI are insensitive to more subtle changes in the brain such as diffuse axonal injury (Shenton et al., 2012) and do not provide relevant information to long-term prognosis (Iverson, 2005; Le & Gean, 2009). Therefore, neuroimaging is not recommended as part of a routine evaluation following mTBI, even in emergency medicine; however, neuroimaging may be recommended for individuals with clinical red flags: declining levels of consciousness, focal neurological deficits, failure to recognize people, disorientation, seizures, worsening headache, and repeated vomiting. Research using functional neuroimaging techniques, including diffusion tensor imaging (DTI), functional magnetic resonance imaging (fMRI), positron emission tomography (PET), single-photon emission computed tomography (SPECT), and electroencephalography (EEG), have identified physiological abnormalities associated with mTBI. It is important for clinicians to note that there are no current or definitive biomarkers, neuroimaging procedures, or neuropsychological tests that can determine a remote event resulted in a mTBI (Vanderploeg et al., 2012).

Neurobiopsychosocial Modeling

A neurobiopsychosocial model of acute and persistent symptoms in concussion accounts for the unique variables that impact one's overall success postinjury (McCrea & Manley, 2018), meaning that it is critical to consider the neurologic, biologic, psychological, and social factors when treating mTBI. These factors influence susceptibility to injury, care at the time of injury, and probability for persistent symptoms. Clinicians must consider an individual's perceptions of illness, wellness, and mTBI itself, as well as external variables such as media attention, workplace environments, school support systems, and early parent education as each has been shown to impact clinical outcomes (Mah et al., 2018; Snell et al., 2016).

Modifiers for ongoing symptoms include preinjury factors, including lower education, female sex, youth/adolescents, previous TBI or other neurologic events, history of learning disability, attention-deficit disorder, personal or family histories of migraine/behavioral health, positive neuroimaging, and hospitalization. Wäljas et al. (2015) concluded, "The manifestation of post-concussion symptoms likely represents the cumulative effect of multiple variables, such as genetics, mental health history, current life stress, general medical problems, chronic pain, depression, and substance abuse" (p. 544). There are also peri-injury factors to consider, such as context and mechanism of injury, and postinjury factors, including emerging psychiatric diagnoses (Carroll et al., 2004; Cooper et al., 2011).

Adolescents may be more vulnerable to ongoing symptoms for a number of reasons. This is a period of rapid developmental changes in the brain, particularly in anterior (frontal) regions known to be vulnerable to injury. Additionally, adolescents may be more likely than children to sustain an mTBI through mechanisms with greater mechanical force such as collision sports, motor vehicle collisions, and assaults, which can result in more severe injuries and prolonged recovery (Chadwick et al., 2022).

Sex is another significant factor regarding concussion prevalence, with females having a higher prevalence than males. In high-contact, high-collision sports, females are at greater risk for sustaining mTBI, and previously, when females presented with greater symptom scores, this was assumed to be solely a socialized sex and (female) gender-specific response. However, female brains are physiologically more vulnerable to diffuse axonal injury (DAI) (Rubin et al., 2018; Sollmann et al., 2018). As female axons are generally smaller with fewer axonal support microtubules, when a female axon is exposed to the same force as a male axon, the female axon is more likely to be more damaged (Dolle et al., 2018). Further, data from imaging studies identified that females who had sustained a concussion had greater changes in communication between brain regions that specifically support goal-directed behavior. In contrast, males who had sustained a concussion tended to experience changes in communication between the brain regions that guide behavior based on cues from the internal or external environment (Shafi et al., 2020). Additionally, females typically, though not always, have less neck strength and a smaller neck size compared to males, and weaker neck muscles have been associated with more head acceleration during an impact (Honda et al., 2018). Physiologic, metabolic, and neuroanatomic sex differences, as well as differences in levels of sex hormones, also may account for sex differences in the brain's response to injury (Chadwick et al., 2022).

There is also an increasing body of evidence that female symptoms appear to be more persistent and cognitive deficits more pronounced than those in males, which may be multifactorial

(Tator et al., 2016). Females and males often differ in how they have been socialized to report symptoms, which may lead to sex differences in reported symptom prolongation. There is also a greater incidence of sleep disturbances postinjury among females, which is known to exacerbate other symptoms such as pain and mood (Wiseman-Hakes, Foster, et al., 2022). Moreover, females tend to report higher levels of anxiety and depression compared with males in uninjured samples, and this is also reflected in those who have sustained a concussion (Chadwick et al., 2022).

mTBI Intersectionalities Including Race and Ethnicity

While considerable attention has been paid to the management of mTBI among specific populations, particularly athletes and veterans, there remains a paucity of evidence regarding mTBI among populations with lower sociodemographic and socioeconomic status as well as communities that are considered marginalized or underserved. Among all these communities, mTBI prevalence is high, and these groups often lack attention from medical professionals, including SLPs. Moreover, many individuals from these communities have sustained multiple injuries, often from a young age. We are using the term "intersectionality" to describe the interconnectivity of factors that as they interact create interdependent systems of disadvantage. This term was first introduced by Kimberlé Crenshaw as "a metaphor for understanding the ways that multiple forms of inequality or disadvantage sometimes compound themselves and create obstacles that are often not understood among conventional ways of thinking" (Carbado et al., 2013).

Each factor has importance as a standalone consideration, but when combined, the impacts on individual lives are multiplicative. Specifically, when considering intersectionalities in mTBI, we refer to individuals from the following communities: survivors of domestic, intimate partner, and/or gender-based violence; those who are or have been precariously housed; those who have been involved with the criminal justice system; refugees/asylum seekers, particularly from war-torn countries; and many groups considered as racialized, including those from racial/ethnic minorities.

Race, ethnicity, and social determinants of health are directly related to health-related mTBI outcomes, with Black, Indigenous, and People of Color (BIPOC) having poorer longitudinal outcomes (Schneider et al., 2022). These decreased outcomes for BIPOC individuals are multifactorial: inaccurate diagnoses, dismissive medical practices including lack of rehabilitation referrals, limited access to care and rehabilitation, and decreased health literacy (Brenner et al., 2020; Gao et al., 2018). American BIPOC children and young adults (age ≤19) were less likely to visit the emergency department following mTBI and less likely to be provided with care for pain (Wallace & Mannix, 2021), while Hispanic adults were less likely to be given a CT scan postinjury (Lempke et al., 2022). In Alaska, Canada, Australia, and New Zealand, the prevalence of concussion among Indigenous communities is considerably higher than the general population. Unsurprisingly, when multiple marginalization factors are present, longitudinal outcomes such as employment become significantly worse (Garduño-Ortega et al., 2022).

There are important intersectionalities within these marginalized and underserved communities that are both risk factors for injury as well as barriers for accessing care. Among these groups/communities, the etiology of the mTBI(s) is often violence related and co-occurring with emotional and psychological trauma (Wallace & Mannix 2021; Wiseman-Hakes, Albin, et al., 2022). Further, the sequelae of concussion may be superimposed upon preexisting language and literacy impairments, as well as mental health challenges, experience of adverse childhood events (ACES), and limited or reduced access to the social determinants of health (Wiseman-Hakes, Albin, et al., 2022; Wiseman-Hakes et al., 2023). Symptoms of concussion, especially persistent symptoms, may be misattributed to mental health or other preexisting conditions, especially for these communities.

SLPs have a unique and important role in the screening, identification, and management of concussion related cognitive communication challenges with individuals from these communities, validating the presence of these symptoms, and that they can have a significant impact on daily functioning. Further, given the high prevalence of comorbid trauma and history of trauma, it is imperative that SLPs working with these communities have training in trauma-informed care and culturally sensitive practice. Taking the time to build trust, as well as an understanding of the concepts of "assessment with a purpose" (see "Assessment Modeling" for further details), is critical. Many individuals from these communities are historically underserved and marginalized, and thus, conducting assessments without a clear rationale of how they will help the individual or inform treatment can cause further harm and stigma (Wiseman-Hakes, Albin, et al., 2022). See "A Teachable Moment" at the end of the chapter for a real-world example of intersectionality in the SLP workload. Readers are invited to learn more about intersectionalities in Chapter 9 of this text.

Clinical Phenotypes Associated With Concussion

Symptoms of both acute and persistent mTBI can be wide-ranging and variable across individuals. Clinicians must be aware of how mTBI is manifesting for an individual, rather than assuming that all symptoms will be present. Physical symptoms can include headaches, changes in sleep, dizziness, balance problems, fatigue, vision changes/light sensitivity, phonophobia, and auditory processing deficits. Emotional symptoms can involve irritability, anxiety, depression, and mood swings. Cognitive symptoms include trouble concentrating, attention problems, poor memory, slowed thinking, and communication changes.

One of the most important recent changes for SLPs is the advancement of clinical phenotypes in the areas of concussion. It was previously thought that physical, cognitive, and emotional symptoms were inextricably overlapping, which could lead to inadequate or inappropriate interventions depending on symptomatology. For example, when one is in pain, they often have more trouble thinking and irritability, and this is indeed true; however, more recent research has found that there are distinct phenotypes or groupings of characteristics associated with mTBI for adults and children (Lumba-Brown et al., 2020; Lyon et al., 2022). These phenotypes are critical to SLPs as they help to guide our clinical decision-making and ensure adequate referrals are met.

The five phenotypes associated with mTBI are cognitive, ocular-motor, headache/migraine, vestibular, and anxiety/mood (Lumba-Brown et al., 2020). There may be an additional pediatric phenotype, where a distinct fatigue subtype has been considered rather than infused into other phenotypes (Lyons et al., 2022). Patients can present with multiple phenotypes concurrently, and SLPs must consider each one distinctly. Free screening measures, such as the Concussion Clinical Screen Profile (Kontos et al., 2020), can assist clinicians with phenotype identification.

Cognitive

The cognitive phenotype is the most common presentation in adults, and specific cognitive symptomatology will be explored in detail under the "Cognitive Communication Associated With mTBI" section. In brief, clients report dysfunction with attention, processing speed, working memory, new learning (encoding, storage, and retrieval), and/or executive functioning (Lumba-Brown et al., 2020). Each of these behaviors can drive changes in cognitive-communicative function. Presence of cognitive dysfunction can be detected by comparing preinjury functioning to postinjury testing, when available (< 1 *SD*), or importantly, based on the patient's self-report of significant change in functionality (Lumba-Brown et al., 2020) that supports the American Psychological Association (APA)/ASHA joint statement of Mashima and colleagues (2019). The commonality of the cognitive phenotype reinforces the importance of SLPs in the assessment and intervention of mTBI, which may require SLPs to educate interprofessional colleagues on our roles in mTBI clinical care.

Headache/Migraine

Headache pain remains the most common symptom post-mTBI in adults and children and one that often persists the longest (Lumba-Brown et al., 2020; Stillman et al., 2016), and having a preexisting history of headaches increases one's risk for the headache phenotype. One study of 95 soldiers with histories of mTBI identified 166 distinct types of postconcussive headaches and posttraumatic headache symptoms, and presence of headaches has been tied to poor performance on neurocognitive testing (Finkel et al., 2017; Kontos et al., 2016). The prevalence of headache pain is 90% (Lew et al., 2006) with the most common types categorized as tension, migraine, and a combination of migraine and tension type. In addition to headache pain, hypersensitivity to noise, light, and smells can be tied into this phenotype. Clinicians should be aware that the headache/migraine

phenotype was the most prevalent subtype in children (Lumba-Brown et al., 2020).

Ocular-Motor

In mTBI, impairments in the visual system are well documented and negatively impact accessing and interpreting visual information. Impairments in ocular-motor functioning are extremely common post-mTBI, and it is estimated that as many as 90% of patients present with some form of dysfunction (Thiagarajan et al., 2011). Common impairments occur in convergence and tracking side to side and somewhat rarer occurrences such as a fourth cranial nerve palsy and double vision. Hypersensitivity to light (photophobia) is an additional consideration, and this common experience led in part to the early, erroneous treatment recommendations that individuals should spend extended time in the darkness and persistently wear sunglasses to decrease overall symptom presence. Newer research indicated that these strategies may have had harmful effects (Silverberg & Iverson, 2013). Successful interventions for ocular-motor dysfunction are often paired with vestibular therapies, known as visual-vestibular therapy (Thiagarajan & Ciuffreda, 2015).

These ocular-motor disruptions directly impact daily skills, including reading and related academic/work activities, and symptom exacerbation can result in headaches, nausea, and vomiting. Ocular-motor dysfunction has been reported as a primary limiting factor in successful return to work (Capó-Aponte et al., 2017; Swanson et al., 2017), and students report challenges changing visual focus from a teacher in the front of the classroom to near-point computer work or notetaking. SLPs must consider visual disturbances as a primary problem when patients complain of changes in reading and work success post-mTBI, as well as the potential negative influences on cognitive assessments targeting reading or visual modalities.

Vestibular

The vestibular phenotype is characterized by dizziness, vertigo, disequilibrium (unsteadiness or imbalance), and lightheadedness. Postconcussive dizziness or imbalance post-mTBI has been linked to white matter abnormalities, diffuse axonal injury in the brain, and central and peripheral vestibular damage, such as inner ear damage from blast exposure (Akin et al., 2017; Lau et al., 2011). Estimates are that between 30% and 65% of people with TBI suffer from dizziness and disequilibrium, and these symptoms are provoked with the dynamic assessment of moving the head side to side or up and down (Akin et al., 2017). Management for persistent vestibular dysfunction requires an examination of hearing, balance, coordination, and vision that may be performed by a variety of specialists, including physical therapy (PT), occupational therapy (OT), neurology, otolaryngology, audiology, and ophthalmology or optometry. Functionally, patients often complain that the repeated head movements up and down as occur in a classroom or at a computer may result in feelings of

nausea or seasickness. As noted above, visual-vestibular intervention has become a mainstay of mTBI rehabilitation, now often within the first week postinjury.

Anxiety/Mood Phenotype and Posttraumatic Stress

Changes in behavioral health and emotional regulation are both acute and persistent factors in mTBI, most commonly manifested as feeling more emotional, anxious, nervous, irritable, sad or depressed, hypervigilant to one's environment, and ruminating thoughts. Preexisting concerns related to behavioral health are a key area of assessment for all individuals regardless of age or mechanism of injury, as are an evaluation of current life stressors. Persistent symptomatology can be tied to behavioral health, even if an individual has not had preexisting behavioral health needs. When someone continues to try to function in the face of persistent physical and cognitive deficits, emotional deficits may manifest themselves as an aftereffect of the TBI. Individuals with anxiety/mood phenotype often have significant sleep dysfunction, and it has been found that inactivity post-mTBI can trigger the anxiety/ mood phenotype (Lumba-Brown et al., 2020). This reinforces the importance of active rehabilitation over models of extended rest, as well as the red flag that if patients are reporting decreases in function over time that a referral to behavioral health should be considered.

Posttraumatic stress (PTS; or posttraumatic stress disorder [PTSD]) can also occur in conjunction with an mTBI.

Briefly, PTSD requires that an individual experience directly or be personally impacted by a stressful event. In response to this event, an individual may reexperience this event or be emotionally triggered by situations in daily life. Subsequently, an individual often avoids those triggers and becomes increasingly isolated. These behaviors are caused by the physiological response to the traumatic event, but additional behaviors such as sleep disorders, aggression, and cognitive dysfunction can become worse over time. Some symptoms of PTSD overlap with symptoms of mTBI, such as slowed processing speed, decreased memory and attention, and changes in executive function, while others such as intrusive dreams are not characteristics of mTBI. When treating patients with mTBI and PTSD, it is not the clinician's responsibility or goal to tease out mTBI from PTSD but rather treat the cognitive communication needs, regardless of causality (Mashima et al., 2019). Clinicians must consider referrals to behavioral health in addition to following trauma-informed treatment principles of care.

Additional Consideration: Sleep and Wakefulness

While not a distinct phenotype, changes in sleep and daytime wakefulness are a common occurrence after mTBI. In the acute stage (defined as within 7 days of injury), the majority of individuals regardless of sex or age, experience an increased sleep need characterized by hypersomnia and daytime sleepiness (Wiseman-Hakes et al., 2021). Females report a greater severity of sleep disturbance than males, but both sexes experience an immediate change in sleep in response to the injury. For many individuals, their sleep returns to "normal" (i.e., consistent with their preinjury sleep) by approximately 4 months postinjury, but longer-term sleep disturbances are also associated with prolonged recovery (Fisher et al., 2023; Ludwig et al., 2020; Wiseman-Hakes et al., 2021). This is not surprising as sleep is critical for neurorecovery, neuroplasticity, memory consolidation, and new learning. Further, sleep disturbances can develop acutely following injury or emerge later during recovery and can persist for years after the initial injury if not diagnosed and treated. Chronic insomnia, an inability to initiate or maintain sleep and/or early morning awakening, is present in 46% and 41% of people 6 months and 1 year after mTBI, respectively (Toccalino et al., 2021). Further, the prevalence of medically diagnosed sleep disorders that develop postinjury ranges by disorder, including insomnia (~30%), circadian rhythm sleep disorder (~26%), and sleep apnea (~25%) (Wickwire et al., 2016; Zalai et al., 2020). This is important from a clinical perspective as many of the prolonged symptoms are bidirectional (e.g., disturbed sleep can both cause and be caused by headaches, pain in general, mood disturbances, and irritability). Further, sleep disorders postinjury have been found to exacerbate cognitive communication disorders and new learning (Morrow et al., 2023; Wiseman-Hakes et al., 2011). As sleep (and wakefulness) disturbances are modifiable and treatable factors, SLPs should inquire about sleep patterns and daytime wakefulness and refer for assessment as indicated.

Long-Term Effects of mTBI and Chronic Traumatic Encephalopathy

The chronic effects of mTBI and possible changes in daily function have received considerable media attention, and at this point, the unknowns related to serial mTBI remain greater than facts. The research into chronic effects of serial mTBI remains in its infancy, with minimal longitudinal research available. For nearly a century, clinicians have been concerned about repetitive head trauma accompanying long-term effects on functioning. The notion of being "punch drunk" was first reported in boxers in the 1920s, referring to broad changes in cognition after serial head injury (Martland, 1928). Subsequent references to dementia pugilistica and chronic traumatic encephalopathy (CTE) expanded on these cases (Critchley, 1949; Millspaugh, 1937). More recently, neuropsychological assessments and postmortem neuropathological findings of retired professional football players reignited interests in these potentially chronic conditions (Guskiewicz et al., 2003; Omalu et al., 2011), and CTE has been reported in retired athletes, veterans, and civilians (Mez et al., 2017). Researchers today are considering the potential impacts to long-term functioning from diagnosable mTBI as well as repeated subconcussive blows, hits to the head that do not cross the threshold into a concussive event (McAllister et al., 2014; Talavage et al., 2014).

It is well documented that repeated hits to the head may have significant aftereffects and that those aftereffects can be exponentially impactful (Jordan,

2000). Patients commonly cite how life becomes increasingly difficult after a third or fourth TBI. The increase in public awareness evolving from media coverage, stimulated by reports of CTE, marked by neuropsychiatric features including dementia, parkinsonism, depression, agitation, psychosis, and aggression, has become recognized as a potential late outcome of repetitive TBI (DeKosky et al., 2013). The incidence, prevalence, and the role of genetic factors remain uncertain, and the contribution of age, gender, stress, and alcohol and substance abuse to the development of CTE is undetermined (Stein et al., 2014). It is also critical to remember that these changes in function may or may not be related to CTE, which, despite significant media attention, remains rare (Willer et al., 2018). Moderate-to-severe TBI has been associated with progressive neurologic conditions such as Alzheimer's disease, Parkinson's disease, and amyotrophic lateral sclerosis, and research is emerging at this point as to if/how this research may apply in mTBI (Baker et al., 2018; DeKosky et al., 2018).

Proceeding with caution regarding possible long-term effects from serial mTBI, it is important that SLPs be aware of the current (2023) literature based on CTE. CTE is presumed to be a condition where hyperphosphorylated tau protein accumulates in the brain and causes progressive deterioration of neurologic function, resulting in dementia. This form of tau protein is a distinct form of tau from the one associated with plaques and tangles in Alzheimer's disease. In CTE, tau accumulates throughout the brain, including within the hippocampus, amygdala, and various cortical areas. Diagnostic criteria of

CTE remain somewhat unsettled and largely based on postmortem evaluation (Bieniek et al., 2021; McKee et al., 2016), with individuals presenting with decreased memory and executive function, aggression, depressed mood, erratic behaviors, and changes in motor function and balance. Behavioral symptoms have been reported to be some of the earlier signs of CTE.

Diagnosis of CTE based on the neuropathological presence of tau remains problematic. In one highly publicized study of deceased football players, brains were analyzed postmortem for the presence of CTE-related tau (Mez et al., 2017). Within the convenience sample, 101 of 102 retired NFL players had CTE pathology and 71% of them were diagnosed as severe. While not designed as a prevalence study, one might incorrectly infer that 99% of retired NFL players will develop CTE. In contrast, a neuropathology group in Winnipeg, Canada, analyzed the brains of 111 "everyday folks" aged 18 to 60 years who were autopsied due to a standard medical process (Noy et al., 2016). Fully 35% of these individuals died with detectable CTE pathology, which may imply that CTE-related tau is a common and unremarkable event for many individuals. These two studies are highlighted to reinforce the infancy of research into CTE and that clinicians should proceed with caution when discussing CTE pathology with patients. Future research and advances in imaging techniques will likely help identify behavioral phenotypes and offer additional guidance regarding assessment and intervention (Iverson et al., 2018).

At this point, it remains unknown what neurobiopsychosocial factors may be associated with these longer-term changes, and it remains incumbent on medical professionals to reiterate these unknowns. As clinicians, it is critical that we have the most current information to guide our assessment and treatment decision-making, and while diagnosis is not within our scope of practice, it is also important that SLPs recognize that the possible impacts of serial mTBI, which are all too common, differ from that of CTE, a rare neurological disease (Randolph, 2014). Additionally, SLPs must be aware of the anxiety and fear that patients may experience regarding perceptions that they will develop CTE, whether or not this seems possible based on medical history. As with other dementia processes, SLPs can have confidence to treat behaviors such as memory loss and communication difficulties but should be cautious regarding CTE as a diagnostic label.

Cognitive Communication Changes Associated With mTBI

Cognitive communication deficits encompass difficulty with any aspect of communication and language that is affected by a disruption of cognition (ASHA, 2005a, 2005b). Deficits in cognitive processes, including attention, perception, memory, organization, and executive function, may impact an individual's behavioral self-regulation, social interaction, and academic and vocational performance. The most frequently described concerns include changes in concentration and attention; processing speed; working memory; executive function; social communication; language, including auditory comprehension, word-finding, and reading skills; and stuttering. Functional impacts of the cognitive domains on communication and daily life can be found in Table 7–1, created by Cornis-Pop and colleagues, reprinted by permission (2012).

Attention

Deficits in concentration and attention post-mTBI are commonly reported (Cicerone, 1996; Ozen et al., 2013). Impairments in arousal are a highly visible but relatively rare sign of acute concussion, with loss of consciousness occurring in less than 10% of individuals. For most, impairments in attention result in more functional impairments such as difficulties maintaining concentration, losing train of thought, and problems focusing on workplace and academic tasks. In terms of persistent symptoms, impairments in both visual and verbal attention have been found (Halterman et al., 2005; Howell et al., 2013). Impairments in sustained attention are also described as being problematic, though the literature base for these changes postconcussion is less robust.

Processing Speed

Objective assessments of processing speed indicated slowing, beginning immediately after injury, and that slowing may continue for an extended period. Impaired reaction time may be the clearest sign of slowed processing speed, with examples of decreased speed of finger tapping or speed of

stick drop (Del Rossi, 2017). In the field of speech-language pathology, SLPs look to processing speed tasks that load more heavily on cognitive resources like computerized response time, cancellation tasks, speeded verbal-response tasks, or complex multistep tasks such as are found in the Functional Assessment of Verbal Reasoning and Executive Strategies (Isaki & Turkstra, 2000; MacDonald, 1998).

Working Memory and New Learning

Immediate impairments in working memory (WM) are nearly universally agreed upon when considering acute concussion (Creed et al., 2011; Milman et al., 2005). Young adolescents and college students have shown deficits in verbal and visual working memory 3 to 5 days after injury, with verbal dysfunction being worse (Covassin et al., 2008; Green et al., 2018). While both verbal and visual WM are compromised long term for at least a subset of individuals post-mTBI, the impact of verbal dysfunction is likely more impactful. Verbal WM directly impacts comprehension of language as well as verbal production (Acheson & MacDonald, 2009), with communication needs shifting rapidly based on conversational interactions. As most individuals live in a highly verbal world, even mild dysfunction in verbal WM will directly impact academic, vocational, and social success.

In mTBI, reports have noted up to 79% of individuals experiencing changes in memory and learning (Hall et al., 2005). Traditional memory deficits have been linked to acute concussion,

Table 7–1. Cognitive Changes in Mild Traumatic Brain Injury (mTBI) and Potential Effects on Function and Communications

Cognitive Domain	Changes Caused by mTBI	Effects on Function and Communication
Attention[a]	Lapses in sustained attention Highly distractible Decreased concentration Poor performance on competing tasks or stimuli	Difficulty responding appropriately to incoming information Difficulty learning new information Difficulty filtering out irrelevant stimuli Difficulty conversing in situations with distractions, background noise, and multiple participants Difficulty managing the demands of high-level activity Difficulty sustaining attention when reading complex and/or lengthy material Difficulty shifting attention as needed Difficulty maintaining or changing topics in conversation Tangential discourse Social avoidance to compensate for sense of overstimulation
Speed of Processing	Slowness in processing information	Delayed responses Difficulty making decisions Difficulty comprehending rapid rate of speech Difficulty staying on topic Long pauses within discourse
Memory	Impaired memory Problems with new learning	Difficulty recalling instructions or messages Difficulty learning new information Difficulty remembering names of individuals, appointments, directions, and/or location of personal effects (e.g., keys, cellular telephones, identification cards, head gear) Difficulty recalling details when reading complex and/or lengthy material Difficulty maintaining topic or remembering purpose of conversation Repetition of ideas, statements, questions, conversations, or stories Failure to use compensatory strategies to improve performance on everyday tasks

Table 7–1. *continued*

Cognitive Domain	Changes Caused by mTBI	Effects on Function and Communication
Executive Function & Social Communication	Disorganized thoughts and actions Ineffective planning Reduced initiation Decreased insight Ineffective reasoning, judgment, and problem solving Decreased mental flexibility Difficulties self-monitoring performance and assessing personal strengths and needs Impulsivity and disinhibition	Lack of coherence in discourse Lack of organization in planning daily activities Difficulty implementing plans and actions Difficulty initiating conversations Problems recognizing and repairing conversational breakdowns Inability to determine the needs of communication partners Difficulty making inferences or drawing conclusions Difficulty assuming another person's perspective Difficulty interpreting the behavior of others Difficulty evaluating validity of information Verbose; lack of conciseness in verbal expression Decreased comprehension of abstract language, humor, and/or indirect requests Difficulty meeting timelines Difficulty formulating realistic goals Difficulty recognizing complexity of tasks and need for simplification Difficulty anticipating consequences of actions Inappropriate comments

[a]Because attention is the foundation of other cognitive processes, problems in attention are likely to result in or compound impairment in other processes, including memory and executive functions.

Source: From "Guest Editorial: Cognitive Communication Rehabilitation for Combat-Related Mild Traumatic Brain Injury," by M. Cornis-Pop, P. A. Mashima, C. R. Roth, D. L. MacLennan, L. M. Picon, C. S. Hammond, . . . E. M. Frank, 2012, *Journal of Rehabilitation Research and Development, 49*(7), xi–xxxii. Copyright 2012 by the U.S. Dept. of Veterans Affairs. Reprinted with permission.

with impairments in verbal memory encoding and learning efficiency (Lezak et al., 2004; Nolin, 2006). This is recognizable on functional tasks outside of traditional memory assessments, including academic learning struggles after mTBI. Delayed recall, comprising storage and retrieval domains, is frequently impaired after mTBI, often related to encoding deficits and/or attention. Episodic memory, such as memory for events, is frequently reported as decreased after injury and can negatively impact people's quality of life (Brunger et al., 2014; Mansfield et al., 2015).

Executive Function

Early on, it was known that executive functions can be impaired after mTBI, and impairments in executive function are routinely cited in qualitative literature (Brooks et al., 1999; Brunger et al., 2014; Stergiou-Kita et al., 2016). Specific deficits noted included planning, organization, emotional regulation, and decision-making, though self-awareness is often considered a strength of the individuals post-mTBI. Changes in executive functioning have been reported in children, adolescents, and adults in acute mTBI and in persistent presentations as well (Howell et al., 2013). Significant changes at all levels of executive function were found when compared with unexposed controls, and the degree of impairment increased with age. Deficits included changes in inhibition, shifting, emotional control, planning/organization, initiation, and task monitoring.

Social Cognition and Social Communication

There is broad overlap between the concepts of social cognition and social communication as both deal directly with "the capacity to attend to, recognize, and interpret interpersonal cues that guide social behavior" (McDonald, 2013, p. 231). All social interactions are interdependent on communication messages between partners, whether intended or not, and hence the unextractable overlap between social cognition and social communication. Social communication skills require rapid evaluation of the context and listener, prior to initiating an appropriate topic, providing sufficient but not excessive relevant details, controlling utterance length to enable others to comment, and use of both verbal and nonverbal methods to convey stated and implied meaning (Burgess & Turkstra, 2010).

Changes in social communication after mTBI are a rapidly growing area of study. Parents and young children with histories of mTBI were found to have less mutual engagement, less success in reading interpersonal cues, poorer communication shifting and flow, and, overall, less successful engagement than interactions with uninjured children (Lalonde et al., 2018). These interactions were also found to be more negative in tone than those with uninjured children. Young children with mTBI were found to have reduced emotional recognition of conversational partners and, at 2 years postinjury, decreased theory of mind (Bellerose et al., 2017; D'Hondt et al., 2017). For adults, Theadom et al. (2019) found that at 4 years postinjury, nearly 25% of individuals had deficits interpreting others' expressions and intentions. Additionally, numerous articles cited changes in social participation, social success, and increased isolation (Childers & Hux, 2016; Finebilt et al., 2016; Snell et al., 2017). Impairments of social communication may result from both cognitive and behavioral changes associated with concussion and comorbid conditions (Cornis-Pop et al., 2012). Persisting irritability and anger may manifest as negative self-talk, verbal abusiveness to others, or physical aggression that can negatively affect social interactions (Raskin & Mateer, 2000). Breakdowns in social communication, originating from chronic emotional and self-esteem problems, can contribute to loss of meaningful relationships and result in social isolation and loneliness (Brooks et al. 1987; Ylvisaker & Feeney, 2001). Additionally, SLPs should be aware that patients may present with alexithymia after mTBI, a condition where an individual struggles to identify physiological feelings within the body and describing those emotions to others (Wood et al., 2014). This disconnect can lead to additional communication breakdowns as one partner may view the emotional state of the other quite differently.

Language Presentation in mTBI

Changes in communication have been largely overlooked in mTBI, though there is an evolving evidence base. Impairments in word finding have the strongest literature, and many other areas have qualitative and emerging quantitative research. Despite a limited evidence base for communication changes in mTBI, changes in functional auditory comprehension, verbal expression, reading, and writing have been documented.

Deficits in auditory comprehension are well documented in moderate-to-severe TBI (Nicholas & Brookshire, 1995), but the presence/absence of auditory comprehension changes in mTBI

remains minimally explored. Changes in auditory functioning such as impairments in speech in noise or changes in timing and perception of pitch likely impact auditory comprehension, the ability to interpret receptive auditory communication. In two studies, adolescents and adults with sport-related concussion (SRC) were consistently slower than healthy controls, were less efficient overall responding, and made more errors (Bialúnska & Salvatore, 2017; Salvatore et al., 2017). A study by Kutas and Federmeier (2000) offers an interesting explanation beyond that of simple slower processing speed for changes in auditory processing. By using EEG, the authors showed a relationship between semantic memory and sentence comprehension, where the semantic memory system is in essence "priming" the language system based on previous experiences. A functional example of this occurs when an individual can predict the end of the sentence, even with unfamiliar conversational partners. Semantic memory is one of several subtypes of declarative memory known to be dysfunctional after TBI, and as such, a decline in semantic memory would likely impact successful priming post-mTBI.

The ability to produce a targeted single word is an inherently complex task, and slowed word finding is a commonly cited communication disorder after mTBI (Barrow et al., 2006; Keightley et al., 2014). In general, speeded conditions for naming tasks are considered to have an increase in overall processing load and are frequently preferred in mTBI assessments of naming and cognition. Slowed naming has been found in confrontational naming tasks for adults with acute and subacute mTBI

(Barrow et al., 2003), and this slowing has been identified longitudinally at 60 days. A pattern has been described in children and young adults aged 10 to 22 years with both acute and subacute injuries (Stockbridge et al., 2018). Decreased categorical fluency has also been found in young adults (Keightley et al., 2014).

Modalities for expressive discourse of conversation and writing have parallel presentations in mTBI. Discourse analysis often targets both microlinguistic factors, which impact quality of information within a single phrase, and macrolinguistic factors, which address clarity and cohesion across sentences and throughout the narrative as a whole. Microlinguistic verbal production does indicate some deficits, including slower production and decreased word variety; however, macrolinguistic areas can be markedly impaired with deficits, including decreased content units, mazing, abandoned utterances, vague language, and irrelevant and tangential content (Berisha et al., 2017; Marini et al., 2011). Barry and Tomes (2015) examined remote autobiographical narratives in asymptomatic college students and found that their personal narratives were more challenging for individuals to remember, as well as lacking in vividness and linguistic complexity. There have been similar, but limited, findings in writing, including micro- and macrolinguistic errors of run-on sentences, fragments, grammatical errors, semantic errors, and agreement errors for both verbs and pronouns (Dinnes & Hux, 2017). The only published cohort research targeting writing intervention post-mTBI indicates improvements in macrolinguistic functioning (Ledbetter et al., 2017).

Decreased reading comprehension is a frequent characteristic post-mTBI. Karlin (2011) described numerous academic impacts of concussion, including decreased reading comprehension of speeded sentences. This is a significant concern when working with school-age/collegiate clients. Oral reading fluency and challenges with paraphrasing have also been found (Sohlberg et al., 2014). Decreased processing speed, visual dysfunction, and changes in memory will likely impact reading comprehension skills, and it is critical for a client's visual functioning to be assessed in order to drive appropriate therapeutic interventions. While additional research is needed on reading and reading comprehension in mTBI, interventions have been found to be effective (Laatsch & Guay, 2005; Sohlberg et al., 2014).

Additional Communication Considerations

Auditory Changes

Changes within the auditory system also occur post-mTBI even without injury to the ear or temporal lobe. Hypersensitivity to noise (hyperacusis) is a common occurrence in all types of mTBI, though also a common symptom in healthy adults (Callahan et al., 2018). Dischinger and colleagues (2009) found that 27% of patients seen in an emergency department reported hyperacusis early on and that noise sensitivity was a significant predictor of ongoing symptoms 3 months postinjury. Similar studies have found hyperacusis to be predictive of severity of symptoms and speed of return to sport and that hypersensitivity can develop over time (Chorney et al., 2017; Landon et al., 2012). Both hypersensitivity to noise and tinnitus impact the overall functioning and quality of life for individuals post-mTBI as their presence likely increases levels of discomfort, fatigue, and cognitive overwhelm, as well as any impact on audiologic function.

Tinnitus and auditory sensitivity can be experienced in isolation, but individuals also report decreased auditory functioning in social situations. Vander Werff (2016), in an excellent review article, reported audiological consequences of mTBI in the WHO International Classification of Functioning, Disability and Health (ICF), including impairments in communication such as understanding speech in noise, conversation, and complex interpersonal interactions. A significant amount of daily interaction can occur in noisy environments such as restaurants, stores, workplaces, athletic facilities, and schools. Decreased functioning in noisy environments (speech in noise) has been found post-mTBI in adults exposed to blast (Gallun et al., 2017) and in 84% of adults with community-acquired mTBI (Hoover et al., 2017). Auditory processing disorder (APD), a condition where the integration and interpretation of sound becomes disordered, is estimated to be as high as 85% to 89% in certain populations post-mTBI (Oleksiak et al., 2012).

Speech Presentation in mTBI

Given the common changes in gross motor function after mTBI, it is not surprising that researchers are looking into speech functioning as well. "Slurred speech," one aspect of dysarthria, is a frequently cited symptom of acute concussion; however, after sideline-type assessments, there are minimal objective longitudinal data describing the ongoing dysarthric symptomatology. The ongoing presence of dysarthric speech patterns can be a sign of a more severe neurological picture, one that implicates focal, multifocal, or diffuse involvement of the central and/or peripheral nervous system (Duffy, 2012) and may warrant neuroimaging to diagnose neuropathology. Recent work has explored speech articulation and changes in vocal acoustics post-mTBI. Daudet and colleagues (2017) evaluated vocal production of alternate motion rates (AMRs), sequential motion rates (SMRs), and polysyllabic words in very acute SRC. Statistical analyses indicated group differences for numerous aspects of temporal performance, including diadochokinetic (DDK) rates and variance, and acoustic performance of pitch, pitch variability, and amplitude and amplitude variability. This remains an area to be further explored in research.

Finally, stuttering has been reported in mTBI. There are four main categories of stuttering: developmental, neurogenic (e.g., palilalia), psychogenic, and medication induced, known as tardive dyskinesia. A fifth diagnosis described by Baumgartner and Duffy (1997) is functional (psychogenic) stuttering in adults with neurologic disease. Overall, adult-onset stuttering remains relatively rare, yet most documented cases are determined to have a psychogenic etiology (Duffy et al., 2012; Roth et al., 2015). The differential diagnosis can be most challenging when occurring with a history of mTBI, complicated by comorbidities of disordered sleep, PTSD, depression, and medications.

Acquired stuttering in mTBI, in the absence of PTSD, is extremely rare (Norman et al., 2013; Norman et al., 2018). For individuals with histories of mTBI and PTSD, ruling out medication-induced stuttering is the first step in differential diagnosis. A review of medications and, if possible, withdrawing a symptom-inducing medication by substituting an alternative without speech effects can quickly determine whether tardive dyskinesia is responsible for the symptoms by observing improvement in the speech symptoms within a day to weeks. Symptoms of neurogenic stuttering (the most commonly occurring is palilalia, as observed in Parkinson's disease) are consistent and predictable. Unlike developmental and functional (psychogenic) stuttering symptoms, the symptoms do not wax and wane. Other motor speech stuttering-like symptoms usually are categorized as apraxia of speech or ataxic dysarthria, both of which are relatively easy to differentially diagnose. Therefore, during the initial speech evaluation or within two to three diagnostic treatment sessions, neurogenic-type stuttering can be confirmed when present.

The presence of developmental stuttering is easily ruled out in the absence of a history of stuttering. Functional stuttering, the fourth category previously called psychogenic, is probably the most challenging form of stuttering to diagnose, for no two patients present the same pattern of speech behaviors. Although the speech behaviors in functional stuttering can sometimes resemble developmental stuttering characteristics, many more speech behaviors differentiate acquired stuttering from developmental stuttering (Duffy et al., 2012; Roth et al., 2015). Diagnosis is usually made based on exclusion of the other types. Finally, the confirmation of diagnosis is based on symptom resolution through systematic symptomatic treatment that should include behavioral health.

Military medicine cites multiple examples of functional stuttering post-mTBI in conjunction with PTSD (Mattingly, 2015; Norman et al., 2018; Roth et al., 2015), though authors are cautious to state that neurogenic stuttering should not be ruled out as a possibility, in part due to complexities associated with diagnosis (Norman et al., 2013). While there have been case reports of neurogenic stuttering in the mTBI literature (Rose et al., 2021; Toldi & Jones, 2021), it does seem that true neurogenic stuttering post-mTBI is a rare occurrence. SLPs need to keep in mind, when evaluating a patient with a history of a neurologic event, that it is less likely that sudden onset of stuttering is neurogenic and more likely that it is functional in the presence of neurologic disease or etiology—the fifth diagnostic category of stuttering. The functional nature of it, however, does not discount the importance or physiological nature of the behaviors. When encountering functional communication disorders or any kind, clinicians should engage with interdisciplinary teams experienced in functional movement disorders and refer to published guidelines to ensure best practices for our patients (Baker et al., 2021).

SLP Assessment in mTBI

Assessment Modeling

The typical diagnosis made by SLPs after mTBI is cognitive communication disorder, and this will be the frame for the assessment section. As noted above, clinicians should listen for signs/symptoms of other possible communication needs and modify their evaluations appropriately. The cognitive communication assessment serves to identify and describe underlying strengths and weaknesses of cognitive, language, and social skills; the effects of cognitive communication impairments on the individual's capabilities and performance in everyday contexts; and participation. The outcomes of assessment provide diagnosis and clinical description of the cognitive communication disorder, prognosis, recommendations for intervention and support, and referral for other assessments or services (ASHA, 2004).

SLPs report continuing to struggle with assessments in mTBI. This likely occurs as objective, standardized assessments were not typically designed for milder presentations of cognitive communication disorders, and many tests do not have normative samples inclusive of their local racial, ethnic, linguistic, dialectical, or geographic communities. When available measures are known to be insensitive, clinicians may inadvertently underdiagnose disorders or be dismissive of patient concerns. Mashima and colleagues, in a joint paper published by ASHA and the APA, offer specific recommendations to clinicians to rectify this situation (Mashima et al., 2019). The authors' key recommendation is that, given the poor sensitivity and specificity of cognitive assessments in mTBI, when patients with a history of mTBI report cognitive dysfunction, SLPs should proceed with providing services, even in the absence of documented findings. This parallels the assessment structure regarding the Cognitive Phenotype (Lumba-Brown et al., 2020). In order to meet these recommendations, a successful mTBI evaluation will typically incorporate four elements: (a) patient (and family) interview, (b) patient-reported outcome measure, (c) patient-reported symptom scale, and, frequently, (d) brief measures assessing cognitive communication functioning.

Assessment structures in mTBI are variable depending on how recently an individual was injured (Hardin et al., 2021). In acute injury, fatigue is particularly pronounced, and clinicians must consider energy management and cognitive overwhelm in their evaluation planning. Similarly, visual impairments may directly impact test performance of visually heavy assessments. Evaluations after acute injury are often brief and primarily focused on an interview for gathering information and a symptom checklist with limited additional testing. As many cognitive symptoms resolve relatively quickly in the acute phase, a more comprehensive evaluation is often deferred until 1 month postinjury. For persistent symptoms, a more comprehensive assessment battery may be considered; however, for patients who have had previous protracted recovery, earlier assessment and intervention may be warranted.

If a patient has had recent neuropsychological assessment for this injury (within 6 months), the SLP should reference the previous evaluation, ensuring that redundant testing is not completed across disciplines.

Interview

In mTBI, a significant amount of evaluation time is spent in the collaborative interview. The Modified Delphi panel of SLPs with expertise in mTBI recommends three specific goals for mTBI assessment, identifying patient goals, patient needs, and patient knowledge gaps (Hardin et al., 2021). Most patients will have familiarity with concussion but this does not mean that their knowledge base reflects the current mTBI evidence base; therefore, it is important to understand and incorporate educational topics to update the patient and families' knowledge base. Given that standardized measures often lack sensitivity and specificity in mTBI and that patients are often highly symptomatic, including headaches and visual dysfunction, the patient and family report are of paramount importance. In addition to typical aspects of an interview, such as medical and mTBI histories, symptoms, cognitive communication status, chief concerns, functional levels, and an informal language sample, there are additional considerations for mTBI.

The members of the Modified Delphi panel unanimously agree that patient-centric contextual factors that serve as barriers to or facilitators of successful communication must be explored (Hardin et al., 2021; WHO, 2001). SLPs should evaluate:

- **Personal factors** (knowledge/opinions about mTBI, use of strategies and skills, stressors)
- **Personal expectations** (e.g., thoughts about recovery, motivation)
- **Personal beliefs** (self-advocacy, empowerment, work/academic activities, and performance)
- **Environmental factors** (concussion attitudes and beliefs of teachers, coworkers, supervisors, friends, and family members)

Two examples of interview structures include a problem-focused interview and a patient-centered interview. Krug and Turkstra (2015) describe a problem-focused interview they developed for use in a college concussion clinic. Their interview includes four components: a detailed history to evaluate risk factors for persistent symptoms, assessment of cognitive-communicative complaints, assessment of academic needs and environmental demands, and assessment of client-generated compensations and strategies that the student attempted to use and/or used on an ongoing basis. The traditional structured interview often includes a combination of open- and closed-ended questions that gather information about the injury, symptoms, education and work history, medications, and so on. In a patient-centered interview, described by the Working Group to Develop a Clinician's Guide to Cognitive Rehabilitation in mTBI (2016), the patient is asked to share their story, and the interview is guided by what the patient describes; therefore, it is less structured. If the individuals have previously offered their story to other providers, they may not want to retell it. In this case, a patient-centered, semistructured interview can be used to gather the patients' background information. While listening to the story, the clinician periodically asks to summarize their understandings, notably about any triggers or trauma that led to change in the patient's function; other symptoms and events that may be contributing to or maintaining symptoms; services received, noting benefits gained and unhelpful strategies; and how symptoms have impacted the patient's work and personal life. All interview structures should again follow the principles of trauma-informed practices.

Symptom Checklist

Postconcussion symptom checklists are the gold standard used to document and track a client's symptoms (Krug & Turkstra, 2015). As the gold standard, a symptom checklist should be administered as part of the initial patient intake process and is often intermittently readministered during therapy as one form of outcome measure. It has been found that when patients are asked too frequently about symptoms, symptom scores actually increase. (Therefore, SLPs may frequently ask about burdensome symptoms at every session, but full symptom assessments should not be completed as regularly.) There are numerous free mTBI symptom tracking scales, with little variation between them. Each tool measures between 20 and 30 symptoms, which were noted above in the section on phenotypes. While any validated symptom measure is acceptable (see Table 7–1), there are two options with additional considerations. The Concussion Clinical

Profile Screening (CP Screen; Kontos et al., 2020) was designed to generate the five clinical phenotypes described above by Lumba-Brown et al. (2020), providing strong support for cognitive communication needs as well as referral recommendations. The Acute Concussion Evaluation (ACE; Gioia & Collins, 2006) provides a binary scale (symptoms present/absent) rather than a graduated severity scale. Anecdotally, clinicians report that this can be more efficient for patients to complete and allows clinicians to quickly assess symptom presence.

Patient-Reported Outcome Measures

The use of a patient-reported outcome measure (PROM) is critical to capturing the patient's perceptions of the burden or impacts of their injury/dysfunction. As SLPs know, the diagnosis of a "mild" injury does not necessarily tie to the level of disruption experienced in daily life, and improving quality of life is at the core of our clinical service delivery. PROMs are becoming increasingly important in acquired neurogenic disorders as they offer insight into a patient's lived experience free of judgment by the clinician (Cohen & Hula, 2020; Cohen et al., 2021). PROMs can vary in length, and some tools, such as the TBI-QOL (Traumatic Brain Injury–Quality of Life), have short forms with only 4 to 10 items, providing patient-centered insights very efficiently. These measures tie directly into the WHO model of functioning with mTBI-appropriate tools that cover varying activity domains related to communication, cognition, and life participation and fill a gap in clinical assessment. PROMs are also valuable as clinical outcome measures, reflecting the patient's perceptions of changes in their own levels of functionality, which may reflect more clinically meaningful change than other external measures. Measurement of functional outcomes is important for demonstrating the effectiveness and efficacy of cognitive communication therapy with mTBI.

Many PROMs (Table 7–2) have been created by the National Institutes of Health (NIH) and are available free of charge. SLPs should select PROMs based on the goals of the patient and clinician. For example, clinicians may choose PROMs targeting activity, participation, and overall quality of life, rather than domains more related to body structure and function. After reviewing patient responses, SLPs can more deeply probe items that indicate significant burden or distress in order to incorporate these aspects into intervention. In practice, SLPs may choose to administer the TBI-QOL Ability to Participate in Social Roles and Activities as well as the Satisfaction With Participation in Social Roles and Activities, as these may yield differing aspects of burden and potential therapy targets. The TBI-QOL short forms and item banks are available free of charge by sending an email request to TBI-QOL@ udel.edu, or through the NIH Toolbox/PROMIS iPad applications. While there may be other PROMs appropriate for mTBI, tools identified in Table 7–2 have items tied directly to cognitive communication functioning and have been studied and recommended for individuals with mTBI (Cohen et al., 2022; Lange et al., 2016; Tulsky et al., 2016).

Subjective Measurement Selection

In addition to the administration of PROMs and a symptom checklist, there are subjective measures that can be highly informative in an mTBI evaluation. These measures are different from PROMs, in that, while both use self-report of the patient, these subjective measures are tied to levels of body structure and function, activity, and participation without including impacts or burden of the dysfunction. Some subjective measures do not have an easily accessible objective counterpart, such as the Functional Hearing Questionnaire (FHQ; Saunders et al., 2015), which considers auditory processing, or the LaTrobe Communication Questionnaire (LCQ; Douglas et al., 2000), which examines social communication. Similarly, measures such as the LCQ and the Behavior Rating of Executive Function (BRIEF; Gioia et al., 2002), include both Self and Informant report versions. Comparing perceptions of the patient, family members and even teachers for those with persistent symptoms can offer important insights into daily levels of function as well as gauging if the patient and family are viewing dysfunction in a similar way. (If they are not, this is an important topic to address with some counseling.) Subjective measures can often be completed in advance with a link or access to an electronic health record. This can be more efficient for the patient and offers the clinician some insights into the patient's functioning prior to beginning the evaluation.

Table 7–2 lists subjective and objective measures generated by experts within the mTBI-SLP community (Cornis-Pop et al., 2012; Hardin & Kelly,

Table 7–2. Four Domains of Assessment Measures With Exemplars Used in mTBI Research and Clinical Practice

mTBI Symptom Self-Report Checklists
Acute Concussion Evaluation (ACE; Gioia & Collins, 2006)±
Concussion Clinical Profile Screening (CP Screen; Kontos et al., 2020)
Neurobehavioral Symptom Inventory (NSI; Cicerone & Kalmar, 1995)
Post-Concussion Scale (PCS; Lovell et al., 2006)
Rivermead Post-Concussion Symptoms Questionnaire (RPQ; King et al., 1995)
Sports Concussion Assessment Tool 5 (SCAT5, symptom scale; Echemendía et al., 2017)

Patient-Reported Outcome Measures (PROMs)
WHO Participation Level/QOL:
QOLIBRI Quality of Life after Brain Injury (Von Steinbüchel et al., 2010)
CD-RISC Connor-Davidson Resilience Scale (Campbell-Sills & Stein, 2007)
TBI-QOL Ability to Participate in Social Roles and Activities (Heinenmann et al., 2020)
TBI-QOL Satisfaction With Social Roles and Activities (Heinenmann et al., 2020)
TBI-QOL Resilience (Vos et al., 2019)
WHO Activity Level:
TBI-QOL Communication (Cohen et al., 2019)
TBI-QOL Executive Function (Carlozzi et al., 2019)
TBI-QOL Cognition–General (Carlozzi et al., 2019)

Subjective Cognitive-Communication Measures
Cognitive Domains:
Behavior Rating of Executive Function (BRIEF, any version; Gioia et al., 2002)*±
Communication Domains:
Functional Hearing Questionnaire (Saunders et al., 2015)
LaTrobe Communication Questionnaire Self & Informant Report (Douglas et al., 2000)
Participation Domains:
College Survey for Students With Brain Injury (CSS-BI; Kennedy et al., 2014)
Learning and Service Strategy Inventory (Weinstein et al., 1987)±
Authentic Patient Activity Samples (e.g., patient emails, texts, unedited academic writings, etc.)

continues

Table 7–2. *continued*

Objective Cognitive-Communication Measures
Cognitive Screening:
RBANS (Randolph, 2012)*
Attention/Processing Speed:
Speed & Capacity of Language Processing (SCOLP; Baddeley et al., 1992)
Test of Everyday Attention (TEA/TEA-CH; Robertson et al., 1994)±
WJ III/IV Cognition: IV Subtests 4, 17 (Woodcock et al., 2011; Schrank et al., 2014)
Memory:
Rivermead Behavioral Memory Test–Third Edition (RBMT3; Wilson et al., 2008)
Wechsler Memory Scale IV (WMS-IV; Wechsler, 2009)
Executive Function:
FAVRES/SFAVRES Subtests 2, 4 (McDonald, 1998, 2013)+±
Delis Kaplan Executive Function System (Delis 2000)±
Naming:
Controlled Oral Word Association (COWA) (FAS & Animals) (Tombaugh et al., 1999)
WJ III/IV Oral Language: IV Subtests 4, 8 (Schrank et al., 2014)±
Reading:
Gray Oral Reading Tests (Gray, 1992)±
Speed & Capacity of Language Processing (SCOLP; Baddeley et al., 1992)
Writing:
FAVRES/SFAVRES Subtest 4 (McDonald, 1998, 2013)+±

Note: * = available in Spanish; + = available in French; ± = appropriate for pediatrics. RBANS = Repeatable Battery for the Assessment of Neuropsychological Symptoms; FAVRES = Functional Assessment of Verbal Reasoning & Executive Strategies; SFAVRES = Functional Assessment of Verbal Reasoning & Executive Strategies–Student Version; WJ = Woodcock Johnson Tests.

2019; Hardin et al., 2021). This list is not meant to be comprehensive or exclusive. Few of the normative tests used by speech-language pathologists in the evaluation of postconcussive cognitive communication deficits have been standardized on people with mTBI, and even then, the normative samples are rarely reflective of the broad U.S. population.

Objective Standardized Measures

For the many patients with a history of mTBI, an interview and patient reports (PROMs, symptom checklist, subjective measures) may provide sufficient information to identify treatment goals and strategies. Formal standardized cognitive testing may not be necessary in certain cases for the clinician to design and implement an appropriate rehabilitation plan; however, formal assessment may be required for administrative reasons, such as insurance coverage or documenting functional limitations. Given that normative testing is decontextualized and may be culturally biased, objective findings may not match the patients' complaints. The clinician should never dispute the patient's complaints of cognitive problems; they should be accepted as a valid reflection of daily life. Rationales for engaging in some formalized, normative testing include:

- Identify cognitive strengths. Formal testing may be useful in identifying specific cognitive strengths that can be applied in a rehabilitation program. For example, good attention and concentration can help facilitate learning and memory, or strong visual skills may compensate for verbal challenges.
- Document levels of functionality on standardized measures. At times, testing must be administered as one element of an evaluation, as may be required for insurance authorization or workers' compensation. It is important to note that goals and outcome measures should not be tied to standardized testing.

- Plan vocational/educational supports. Formal standardized testing may be important in vocational planning or return-to-school decisions, and in some cases, it may be necessary to document a need for accommodations.
- Rule in or out other diagnoses. Many times, individuals have a history of mTBI, which is present in their medical history, but could in fact need services for other types of dysfunction.
- Education and feedback. Occasionally, patients may believe that they have significant cognitive impairments or even CTE reflecting underlying brain damage. Strong performance on standardized testing can provide an educational platform on how the brain can perform in areas an individual believed to be "damaged". Positive, supportive feedback from the clinician is important in minimizing disability beliefs. (Clinician's Guide to Cognitive Rehabilitation in mTBI, 2016)

As noted above, the amount formalized testing should be limited in the acute phases, based on the patient's level of symptomatology. Many clinicians have had the experience in mTBI where a patient is fine one minute in an assessment and rapidly decompensates. Not only can this experience leave a patient feeling exhausted and demoralized, but it also puts the emerging therapeutic relationship at risk. In mTBI standardized assessment, typically "less is more" in battery construction. SLPs should prioritize speeded measures, as these tests are often the most sensitive in mTBI to dysfunction (e.g., naming animals in a minute, cancellation measures, or timed subtests from the FAVRES). Many speeded measures are brief, which allows clinicians to obtain data points without overly taxing a patient. For many patients, administering between one and three objective measures will be sufficient for insurance reimbursement and any needed formal documentation.

[Note: Teletherapy evaluations for mTBI can be highly successful; however, timed assessments of processing speed have been shown to be less reliable when administered virtually. This is particularly important in mTBI. As a result, clinicians should consider increasing the size of their confidence intervals and be sure to include that the tool was administered in a nonstandardized fashion (Wright et al., 2020). Brearly et al. (2017) found that telepractice can be effective for verbal naming, digit span, and list learning, three measures commonly used by SLPs in cognitive communication assessment, with reliable high-speed connectivity.]

Intervention Modeling: Interprofessional Teaming, Roles, and Active Therapy

The past decade has seen marked changes in mTBI/concussion research and care. As researchers continue to define mTBI and accompanying clinical phenotypes, cognitive communication rehabilitation specifically for mTBI remains in its infancy and continues to evolve rapidly. As expanded below, SLPs may provide different aspects of care for patients in the acute stages postinjury versus those with persistent

symptoms; however, there are unifying elements at all stages of clinical care.

Interdisciplinary care is recommended to address the breadth of symptoms post-mTBI (Collins et al., 2016), with a team comprising medicine, PT, behavioral health, and cognitive therapy, most commonly provided by SLP. These mTBI guidelines are in concert with the NIH Consensus Panel on TBI (1999), but implementation of revised practice guidelines can be slow to be adopted in mTBI and other areas of clinical care (Cranney et al., 2001; Lebrun et al., 2013), and SLPs remain underutilized in some care teams (Vargo et al., 2016). It remains important that SLPs educate our interprofessional colleagues on the presence of potential cognitive communication deficits and our roles in rehabilitation (Morrow et al., 2023).

SLPs can adopt varying interprofessional roles depending on their patient population, health care models, and personal expertise. Clinicians should expect to see patients with mTBI in acute care, acute rehabilitation, outpatient clinics, private practice, and within the school systems. With aging populations, clinicians can also expect to see geriatric residents in long-term care facilities after events such as falls. In acute care, SLPs may be called on to follow up with individuals seen and discharged from the emergency department or to evaluate cognitive communication for patients with polytrauma injuries. In some clinics, such as collegiate health care, SLPs may be called on to provide immediate support and academic accommodations to continue student success. Many SLPs working in outpatient care and private practice see increases in their caseloads when symptoms have become persistent. (It is unclear if earlier intervention would have prevented or shortened the duration of persistent symptoms for some individuals.)

Clinicians must be aware of limitations in both internal and external evidence bases. At a conceptual level, care for mTBI has shifted significantly with a move away from cocooned, quiet rest after injury to a model of active rehabilitation (Schneider et al., 2017). Intervention practices supporting prolonged inactivity have been shown to be harmful and are outdated, although anecdotal evidence supports that ongoing "rest" models continue to be applied despite clear changes in guidelines. For patients seen only in emergency care or medical office visits, SLPs should recommend that a gradual return to functional activities has started within 48 hours. A similar return to activity should begin as patients are discharged from inpatient care. Models of active intervention apply to both adult and pediatric populations.

Principles of mTBI Rehabilitative Care

Collaborative Coaching

In many ways, the person most responsible for interventional success in mTBI is the patient themselves, as individuals participate in their preinjury lives (e.g., work activities, academics, family care responsibilities, errands). Clinicians work with a patient to identify goals and create a structure to accomplish them, but it falls upon the patient to implement those recommendations. Cognitive-communicative intervention

involves a collaborative effort between a motivated patient and a dedicated clinician who together form a therapeutic alliance or partnership that is based on trust and credibility among the clinician, the patient, and their family (Cornis-Pop et al., 2012). The clinician actively listens to the patient to understand the concerns and impact of the patient's impairments on quality of life. Once a shared trust and clinician credibility are established with the patient, the clinician can facilitate and support the patient to gradually regain functional skills. A strong therapeutic working alliance can positively influence outcomes in postacute TBI rehabilitation (Schonberger et al., 2007; Sherer et al., 2009), as can models of collaborative coaching (Kennedy, 2011; Ylvisaker, 2006).

Education

The first step in an mTBI intervention program is to provide education and validation of symptoms (Kay et al., 1992; Kurowski et al., 2016; Rosenthal, 1993; Sohlberg, 2000). TBI education begins with an interview and continues with the individual's participation in functional goal setting. Education should focus on assisting the individual in understanding the relationship between the acute event that caused their mTBI and its consequences, the history of mTBI including the typical recovery process, the interplay of co-occurring symptoms, and strategies that may assist with compensating and facilitating improved performance to maximize successes and minimize frustration and stress until symptoms resolve. Recovery is facilitated by conveying a positive prognosis that rapid and full recovery is very likely and that patients can help themselves by returning to modulated physical and cognitive activity within 1 to 2 days following injury.

The Modified Delphi Panel recommends that education focuses on (a) empowering, (b) engaging, and (c) informing the patient (Hardin et al., 2021). In addition, clinicians often help patients to "connect the dots" between physiological changes and their subsequent functional impacts. For example, an SLP may need to be explicit in explaining how changes in visual tracking directly influence reading success and reading comprehension. Education also includes validating how additional medical factors, such as a history of learning disabilities (LD) or attention-deficit/hyperactivity disorder, could slow recovery and that these are understood in mTBI models.

Counseling

Counseling is inherently a component of cognitive communication rehabilitation and includes a patient-centered approach that engages the patient's participation in goal setting and integrates goal-directed counseling for eliciting behavior change. Support takes the form of active listening and conveying empathy, optimism, and encouragement. Providing reassurance and instilling the expectation of recovery (within weeks to months) is key to the recovery process and, therefore, should be communicated on a regular basis. Patients experiencing a first mTBI should also be counseled that the goal and expectation should be functional recovery, addressing any misconceptions regarding chronic traumatic encephalopathy. The Demands and Capacities (DC) model (Adams, 1990), frequently referred to in stuttering, can be applied in concussion. Based on the premise that each person has a finite resource (capacity) of cognitive abilities, the presence of comorbidities of pain, disordered sleep, sensory deficits, and psychosocial-emotional changes represents demands or factors that deplete the individual's finite capacity. Thus, reducing comorbidities through interdisciplinary interventions should enhance the individual's cognitive communication functioning. The DC model may assist the patient in acknowledging the benefit of focusing interventions on the comorbidities either before initiating or in conjunction with their cognitive communication rehabilitation.

Motivational interviewing (MI; Miller & Rollnick, 2012) is a method of communication designed to facilitate moving individuals in the direction of change. MI can be used for engaging the patient to explore areas of concern and ways their difficulties are impacting performance at work, at school, or in the home. This process leads to defining functional goals that provide the focus for rehabilitation. MI is used to elicit patients' motivation to change, not telling why or how they are to change, and in this way the clinician conveys respect for patients' autonomy to decide to change. A clinician's goal is to LURE the patient: Listen carefully so we can Understand our client's motivation. Resist the urge to fix it, and Empower our clients (Cook et al., 2020). The clinician follows the patient's lead in the conversation and can use the following mnemonic to remember strategies used in MI, "OARS":

- Open-ended questions (e.g., "How do memory challenges affect you at work?")
- Affirmations (e.g., "So, you forgot your appointment this morning, but it sounds like you remembered all your appointments yesterday. You must feel good about that.")
- Reflections (e.g., "Paper schedules get lost easily.")
- Summaries (e.g., "It sounds like you are having difficulty remembering your schedule because the papers keep getting lost. You would like to have your appointments in your smartphone, so you will remember and attend them more consistently.")

Affirmations and reflections are statements that reassure the patient that they are being heard and understood and can yield specific information that may help in formulating treatment goals. Summaries of the patient's comments can be used to tie together information within an interview and to highlight and focus information for identifying goals and strategies. MI is a core clinical strategy, not only in mTBI but in many areas of habilitation and rehabilitation.

Modifications and Accommodations

Maintaining communications with the patient's family members, employers, teachers, and peers is an essential component of cognitive communication intervention. The inclusion of the patient's support team in their rehabilitation process facilitates a greater understanding of the challenges and needs of the individual as they reenter the community. Working with family members or caregivers may include recommending strategies for modifying the environment to remove communication barriers and for enhancing community participation. Typically, SLPs can write these recommendations independently (without the co-sign of a physician), although some systems may require the signature of doctoral-level clinician.

Early modifications may reflect total time engaged in an activity, for example, temporarily decreasing the hours at work or decreasing the homework assignments early on. Modifications may take the form of making adaptations to the patient's home or work environment such as adjusting the lighting or reducing noise. The patient may find it best to work in a space with fewer distractions rather than working in a large open space with many people and few barriers. Over time, modifications and accommodations may reflect extended exam/quiz time for students or restructuring an environment to compensate for memory deficits, such as increasing scheduling reminders or establishing a set location for important personal items that go back and forth between home and work (e.g., keys, phone, wallet).

Outcomes and Goal Setting

The structure of goals and outcomes is parallel across time points in mTBI intervention, and given the nature of the injury, all goals must be inherently functional for the patient's daily life. Tracking outcomes should be a priority for SLPs as many of our clinical interventions have limited evidence bases. By tracking outcomes with standardized measures, SLPs can further build a database supporting therapeutic intervention and the roles of SLPs in mTBI clinical care (Cornis-Pop et al., 2012; Helmick & Members of the Consensus Conference, 2010). The use of collaborative Goal Attainment Scaling (GAS) goals and PROMs ensures that the outcomes are directly relevant to the patient, and clinicians can also choose targets such as community participation or social skills assessments. Data tracking functional outcomes can seem more challenging than decontextualized in-clinic targets, but SLPs should be empowered to consider various data-capture methodologies. Options for clinicians include using patient logs, self-reports of progress and outcomes, journaling, weekly feedback forms, and review of calendars or smartphone applications. Clinicians at times opt for outcome measures such as job/school attendance or performance; however, more contemporary research indicates that these dichotomized measures may not reflect the lived experience of the patient. For example, when an adult may have returned to work full-time, many report having to work harder to be successful (Mansfield et al., 2015; Silverberg et al., 2018). Similarly, college students with mTBI report changing to less complex majors postinjury, reflecting a persistent change in function (Kennedy et al., 2008). GAS goals can effectively measure soft signs, such as effort, in functionally relevant tasks.

GAS is a flexible system of measuring objective, measurable, and time-based outcome goals, based on a 5-point scale. During the process of establishing the treatment goals, the patient and clinician agree on the anticipated frequency and duration of therapy. The process of collaboration in the treatment planning and goal setting engages the patient in the therapy process, facilitates realistic goal setting, and establishes a shared responsibility in the therapeutic outcome. The implementation of GAS in establishing treatment goals is an effective way to ensure the patient sets the direction for their therapy (Hardin et al., 2021; Mashima et al., 2019). GAS ensures that goals are functional for the patient's daily needs, rather than addressing decontextualized "clinic-only" targets. An example of GAS treatment goals could be maintaining sustained attention with background distraction, reviewing a daily schedule application multiple times over the course of a day, using notetaking strategies for reading material of extended lengths, expanding initiation attempts in group settings, or maintaining productive hours at work with limited excess effort. The 5-point GAS scale has been found to be a valuable procedure for ensuring that treatment is goal directed and for guiding social reinforcement in behavioral treatment in both mental health and rehabilitation settings (Malec et al., 1991). Clinicians may select a 5-point scale ranging from −2, −1, 0, +1, +2, or 1 to 5 depending on personal preference. After the patient and clinician establish a baseline level of functioning, a 5-point equidistant scale is created, with the current level of functioning at Level 2 (Level 1 would be a decrease in functionality). The end of therapy target is at a Level 3, and each week the patient is reminded of where they are in terms of progress to ensure the appropriateness of the goal and maintain motivation to complete the goal. Clients can always surpass the initial clinical goals, which are Levels 4 and 5. Additional information on the creation of GAS goals in TBI can be found in Finch et al. (2019).

Trauma-Informed Care

A TBI is by nature a "traumatic "injury, and while sports injuries receive much of the popular press, most injuries result from mixed methodologies, which may have more traumatic causalities. Moreover, individuals do not have to have experienced assault or a motor vehicle accident to have either a trauma response or a preexisting trauma history. Initially, we recommend that whenever possible, SLPs complete training in trauma-informed care and to remember that these principles apply in disorders and experiences outside of only mTBI. Clinicians should work to create a clinical environment that is nonthreatening and comfortable (Wiseman-Hakes, Albin, et al., 2022). In doing so, clinicians may have to be mindful of mirrors or bright windows that may feel disruptive. During early sessions when trust building is particularly important, clinicians should prioritize listening, using simple language, and the principles of motivational interviewing. Invitational language invites a client to respond and "can help reduce any dynamics where clients perceive that they must accommodate to or respond to the clinician's demands" (Wiseman-Hakes, Albin, et al., 2022). Similarly, asking a patient for permission to ask questions helps restore power to the patient (Ballan & Freyer, 2021). Interprofessional teaming also is helpful, providing an opportunity to be shared professionally during rounds, rather than asking a client to repeat redundant information. Finally, conducting sessions using a strengths-based approach with compassion and kindness will go a long way to create a safe, therapeutic environment (Wiseman-Hakes, Albin, et al., 2022).

Resilience

An emerging principle in TBI rehabilitation overall is the concept of resilience, which refers to successful adaptation or the ability to "bounce back" after experiencing trauma or other adverse experiences (Neils-Strunjas et al., 2017). Resilience is a multifactorial concept that often includes coping, engaging in positive behaviors after challenges, maintaining a positive outlook, and pursuing goal-directed activities (Neil-Strunjas et al., 2017). Individuals who sustain TBI may have lower resilience than the general U.S. population (Lukow et al., 2015), and in mTBI, resilience has been found as a factor influencing health care outcomes for adolescents, civilian, and veterans (Losoi et al., 2015; Neils-Strunjas et al., 2017; Wade et al., 2022). Individuals with higher levels of resilience may respond more quickly in cognitive communication rehabilitation, and relatedly, for those with low resilience and mTBI, SLPs should consider incorporating resilience activities into therapy. As this is an expanding area of practice (Hardin et al., 2021), clinicians are encouraged to explore resilience further with publications of Neils-Strunjas et al. (2017) and Rothbart and Sohlberg (2021).

Acute mTBI Intervention

In the presence of an acute mTBI, the purpose of an initial visit is to acknowledge symptoms, provide education, and track and facilitate the resolution of symptoms to assist the individual in returning to their preinjury state and initiate intervention. Reduction in both the severity and duration of persisting symptoms has been demonstrated following a brief psychoeducational intervention during the acute postinjury period (Comper et al., 2005) and lifestyle modifications. Therefore, as early as the first visit (evaluation), intervention is initiated through education and symptomatic treatment.

Intervention is best provided in the form of an interdisciplinary team approach to symptomatic treatment of comorbidities to minimize the risk of persisting cognitive communication deficits and to increase the likelihood of full recovery. Specialists on the team are called upon to address sleep hygiene, diet, social communication, recreation and exercise as tolerated, behavioral intervention, and cognitive activity. The specialists involved will vary depending on both patient needs and facility parameters (e.g., specialists available, school-based requirements such as nursing or athletic trainers). Maintaining communication and employing unifying messaging is particularly critical for large TBI teams (Hebert et al., 2020) treating individuals with rapidly changing health presentations. SLPs have unique skills to monitor and modify team lexical choices to enhance patient understanding.

Speech-language pathologists can be called upon to provide education, facilitation, and compensation for symptoms while emphasizing the expectation of recovery and return to work/school. One option for acute intervention are the principles of the SMART trial that, through education, focuses on symptom management, return to activity, maintaining a positive attitude, limiting stress, brief focus strategies for attention and memory, and metacognitive strategy instruction (Kurowski et al., 2016). SMART itself is an application-based program for adolescents, but the principles align with the core content in acute mTBI rehabilitation. In addition to reinforcing the information being communicated by the other team members, treatment goals may include providing strategies for controlling environmental distractors, training strategies for behavioral management of symptoms, reviewing memory strategies, and encouraging the routine use of cognitive tools and strategies (e.g., calendar, notepad, smartphone, and smartwatch). Clinicians should be mindful that these are core principles in concussion rehabilitation, and while evaluating each area, deep intervention should be focused in areas of greater need. Additionally, Wade et al. (2022) found that preinjury coping styles and resilience impacted success in the SMART randomized controlled trial, which reinforces the importance of biopsychological factors in mTBI recovery.

Additional Rehabilitation Considerations for Persistent Cognitive Communication Deficits

Persons reporting persisting cognitive communication difficulties following mTBI should be assessed and treated symptomatically regardless of the time elapsed since injury. Multiple factors, including demographic, medical, psychiatric, and psychosocial-emotional variables, and mTBI comorbidities and their interactions all contribute to ongoing persistent symptoms (Vanderploeg et al., 2009). Regardless of the etiology of the symptoms, interventions should be designed to reduce the level of functional disability caused by cognitive communication symptoms (Cornis-Pop, 2008). There is increasing evidence that improvements may continue years postinjury and be supported through active treatment (Draper & Ponsford, 2008).

A patient-centered approach to rehabilitation is designed by incorporating results of the team members' evaluations into a comprehensive treatment plan with targeted, functional long- and short-term goals that are monitored regularly. The length of time postinjury as well as the cumulative number of mTBIs may influence the rate of change in cognitive communication areas. Similar considerations are true for individuals experiencing posttraumatic stress or other behavioral comorbidities, those who have significant trauma histories (e.g., adverse childhood experiences), and those with significant acute stressors.

Clinical experience with patients with persistent symptoms suggests that a comprehensive approach to rehabilitation, which provides individual- and group-based treatment of cognitive, emotional, and interpersonal skills, within an integrated therapeutic environment addresses the functional impairment and promotes meaningful and satisfactory quality of life, even in the presence of persisting limitations (Cicerone et al., 2008; Cornis-Pop et al., 2012; Helmick & Members of the Consensus Conference, 2010). Clinicians may be interested in a structured cognitive intervention approach, particularly if they are new to mTBI intervention. Twamley and colleagues (2014) developed one of the most widely implemented cognitive rehabilitation interventions that includes both didactics and strategy training. The program is presented in cognitive modules that can be adapted for both individual and group interventions. In a randomized controlled trial, the authors reported improved postconcussive symptoms and prospective memory (Twamley et al., 2014) at completion of the study, and at the 1-year follow-up, there was evidence of continued reduction in symptomatology (Caplan et al., 2015). Often, however, clinicians will choose to target the specific areas of greatest impact for a patient over a structured model. In this case, cognitive rehabilitation can still result in enduring improvements in functionality, as evidenced by longitudinal data collected 5 years after cognitive-rehabilitation intervention (Kennedy et al., 2022), and addresses one or more of the following domains, specific to individual patient complaints: attention, speed of information processing, memory, executive function, and social communication.

Individual Therapy

Cognitive communication treatment is a systematic, functionally oriented program of therapeutic activities that is based on assessment and understanding of a patient's brain-behavioral needs (Cicerone et al., 2000), paired with patient priorities. Interventions include strengthening previously learned patterns of behavior, establishing new patterns through use of internal and external cognitive strategies, and enabling the individual to adapt to the changes in their revised approaches to cognitive-communicative functioning. Increased performance success is reinforced through repetition, learning opportunities, and gradually increasing task stimuli and complexity in a systematic approach.

Systematic instruction (Ehlhardt et al., 2008), founded on the theory that persons with learning challenges benefit most from structured training, is an effective intervention model for cognitive communication impairments of mTBI (Sohlberg et al., 2023). Structured training includes presentation of explicit models and reinforcement of learning when first acquiring new information, use of facilitation and compensatory strategies, structured and guided practice to enhance mastery, and maintenance and generalization across contexts (Sohlberg et al., 2023). Effective treatments incorporate principles of learning theory that enhance neuroplasticity, including intensive, repetitive practice of functional targets with careful consideration of salience, potential for generalization, and personal factors (Sohlberg & Turkstra, 2011). Several studies have examined strategy training that teaches individuals to cope with cognitive difficulties through use of functional adaptive skills, techniques, and use of external aids such as smart devices such as smartphone applications (Huckans et al., 2010; Storzback et al., 2017; Twamley et al., 2014).

Deficit-Specific Treatments

Clinicians working in TBI rehabilitation commonly target specific cognitive or communication targets with their clients: attention, memory, executive functioning, and social communication. As the specifics of these individuals' treatments are covered in the earlier chapters of this text, we have elected to briefly address interventions supported in mTBI, and readers are encouraged to return to the key chapters for additional information. It is also important to note that intervention studies in mTBI continue to increase; however, the intervention literature for moderate-to-severe TBI is more robust than that of mTBI. Therefore, when clinicians have patients with repeated mTBIs accompanied by significant levels of disability or very chronic presentations, the therapeutic literature for moderate TBI may help inform clinicians' intervention planning.

Attention

Metacognitive strategy instruction (MSI) uses direct instruction to facilitate behavioral self-control and to deliberately monitor performance of a task and then to modify the behavior if the performance is less than optimal (Sohlberg et al., 2005). There are numerous examples of MSI within the literature, and each relies on related principles of goal-directed behavior: "Systematic, step-by-step instruction in the use of strategies to facilitate self-regulation of states of mind, task preparation, and task execution" (Sohlberg & Ledbetter, 2016, p. 143). The steps frequently applied in metacognitive skills training for problem-solving deficits are (Sohlberg & Turkstra, 2011):

> 1. Identify a desired goal.
> 2. Anticipate what needs to be done to reach the goal, including identifying challenges and facilitators for goal completion.
> 3. Initiate the task.
> 4. Self-monitor and evaluate progress, modifying task parameters if needed.
> 5. Review what was successful and unsuccessful.

One positive prognostic factor in mTBI is that patients typically have good awareness of their skills and deficits. This intact awareness helps facilitate MSI success, when individuals with more impaired awareness could struggle with these types of interventions. MSI can be applied in numerous ways in SLP intervention, ranging from support recommendations in more structured clinical tasks to direct real-world participation strategies. These same metacognitive strategies are beneficial in addressing executive function deficits as well.

Patient education on attention is also an important contribution. Treatments that focus on strategies to allocate attention resources (e.g., rehearsal, self-pacing, self-talk) and reduce anxiety and frustration related to high-level working memory demands are effective for addressing attention impairments in people with mTBI (Cicerone, 2002). The long-term use of artificial stimulation blockers, such as ear plugs, is typically not recommended as it can make problems such as hypersensitivity to noise more pronounced.

Processing Speed

Individuals with mTBI often describe slowed thinking and concentration problems. Slowing of information processing has been attributed to attention deficits (Gentilinia et al., 1989), memory functioning (Cicerone, 1996), and cognitive communication processes, including encoding information, verbal comprehension, and responding to novel situations (Cornis-Pop et al., 2012). The most effective way of improving processing speed is with medications; however, many patients may not be interested in stimulant/related medications or may not be appropriate candidates. Therefore, clinicians should consider using strategies such as verbal meditation, self-pacing, and self-monitoring of mental effort to allocate attention resources and manage the flow rate of information (Cicerone, 2002; Fasotti et al., 2000). Minimizing distractions, allocating sufficient time to complete tasks, planning for rest breaks, and reducing demands of competing tasks are additional strategies for assisting an individual with slowed information processing. A variety of cognitive assistive technologies may also be of benefit (e.g., smart pen or computer application that audio-records lectures as one takes notes or uses a timer for cuing to take a break). Comorbidities and factors, including poor sleep, PTSD, and other mental health conditions, should be considered in addition to underlying cognitive processes that may impact processing speed (Belanger et al., 2009). Finally, clinicians should be mindful that repeated practice activities facilitate faster response times, as tasks move from being conscious to automatic. Educating patients on the importance of repetition can help ensure home treatment practice.

Computer Brain Games

There has been extensive academic writing on the roles of decontextualized-computer activities, also called "brain games," in mTBI. In addition, many patients have been exposed to mass media advertising for brain training subscriptions that promote improved cognitive functioning in daily activities, such as work and school, and after brain injury. As a result of this advertising, patients may ask SLPs for their opinions on these sites and/or may have subscribed to them independently prior to beginning services. SLPs need to be aware that Federal Trade Commission (FTC) found at least some sites used deceptive advertising by preying on "consumer fears" (e.g., Lumosity) and prohibited future advertising without credible data supporting their claims of improved cognitive function (Federal Trade Commission, 2016).

In mTBI, there have been two published randomized controlled trials (RCTs) of decontextualized computer activities in military-related mTBI (Cooper et al., 2017; Mahncke et al., 2021). The first study is the SCORE clinical trial (Cooper et al., 2017) that compared four 6-week treatment arms: (a) psychoeducation, (b) independent self-administered computer-based cognitive rehabilitation, (c) therapist-directed manualized cognitive rehabilitation (psychoeducation, external aids, cognitive strategies, drills, and generalization tasks), and (d) therapist-directed cognitive rehabilitation integrated with cognitive behavioral therapy (CBT) psychotherapy. In this study, not only did the independent self-administered computer cognitive rehabilitation (Arm 2) not improve cognitive function, but the authors cite that these self-administered or independent computer tasks may in fact "be harmful," specifically noting that "this finding is disconcerting because such independent computerized activities are a frequent treatment recommendation by health care providers" (Vanderploeg et al., 2018, impact statement).

The second RCT was the BRAVE trial, completed with military servicemembers and veterans who sustained mTBI who did not have concurrent PTSD (Mahncke et al., 2021). This study intervention used the "plasticity-based" brain training program BrainHQ (PositScience) 1 hour/day, 5 days/week for 13 weeks in conjunction with weekly technical support. Postintervention, the participants in the experimental training group did improve on a cognitive composite score comprising commonly used SLP assessment measures including the Rey Auditory Verbal Learning Test (RAVLT), trails tests, and digit span. Of critical importance, however, was the lack of participant improvement on any functional outcome measures tied to daily activities (e.g., Timed Instrumental Daily Activities; Mayo-Portland Adaptability Index; Frontal

Systems Behavior Scale). In a commentary on the BRAVE trial, Whyte and Turkstra (2021) note that the improvements in the cognitive composite "are intriguing" (p. 1935) but that these changes did not translate into functional improvements in activity or participation.

In essence, these brain training activities did not generalize into real-world change. It is this lack of generalizability that lies at the heart of why clinicians should avoid decontextualized brain training, and it is not recommended for patients with moderate-to-severe TBI (Ponsford et al., 2023). There are cases where computer activities can result in near transfer of skills, such as realistic driving simulators improving on-road driving skills. If an SLP chooses to use computer rehabilitation, one should be considerate about the overlap of the computer-based tasks and their real-world approximation. Tasks with significant overlap have greater potential to generalize as they likely reflect a more contextualized activity (e.g., driving simulator and driving). When considering computer-based cognitive rehabilitation, Sohlberg et al. (2023) recommend that clinicians:

1. carefully consider the patient's candidacy, such as profile of needs, motivation, and cognitive reserves;
2. ensure that treatment parameters follow the neural plastic intervention principles recommended by Kleim and Jones (2008), such as intensity and functionality; and
3. ensure that the treatment selected is both applicable to the patient's cognitive communication needs and meaningful to the patient themselves.

Technology continues to advance at rapid rates, and recommendations could change in the future; however, our role as rehabilitationists is to facilitate improvements in client-centric activities and participation, and at present, the evidence supports continuing functional tasks in SLP-mTBI clinical care over independent decontextualized brain training activities.

Memory

Helmick and Members of the Consensus Conference (2010) state, "Memory training is the most frequently prescribed form of cognitive rehabilitation" (p. 245). Levin and Goldstein (1986) suggested that the memory problems experienced after a TBI represent difficulty retrieving information because of deficits in the encoding stage of memory as a result of decreased ability to generate semantic associations and visual imagery. Memory interventions are often divided into internal strategies, those that do not require any materials outside the brain and external strategies, which utilize additional materials.

Internal strategies are most effective when individuals have mild-to-moderate memory dysfunction (Veli-konjia et al., 2023) and have been found to be effective in mTBI. Examples of these strategies include visualization, chunking, internal rehearsal, paraphrasing, categorizing, and creating personalized mnemonic devices (Cisneros et al., 2021; O'Neil-Pirozzi et al., 2010; Twamley et al., 2014). Additionally, approaches such as PQRST (Preview, Question, Read, State, Test) and metacognitive strategies have also been found to be effective for mild memory disorders (Velikonjia et al., 2023). Clinical reinforcement and real-world application outside the clinic environment facilitate generalization for our patients.

External strategies have also been found effective in mTBI, and clinicians should always consider incorporating external supports for memory needs. Examples of evidence-based external strategies include notetaking, calendar use, writing things down, and use of smartphones and smartwatches (Tiersky et al., 2005; Twamley et al., 2014). Based on guidance from the Defense and Veterans Brain Injury Center (DVBIC) consensus, "efficacy has been demonstrated for memory training" (Helmick & Members of the Consensus Conference, 2010, p. 245), particularly for patients with mTBI and mild memory impairment. The benefits of training in the use of external memory strategies and devices in functional real-life contexts cannot be underestimated.

Executive Functions

Executive functions comprise those mental capacities necessary for formulating goals, planning steps to achieve them, and carrying out the plans effectively (Lezak, 1982). Deficits in executive functions should be addressed in cognitive communication therapy since they are likely to affect functional activities and participation in everyday life events (Cornis-Pop et al., 2012). A robust literature supports the use of MSI as an intervention for executive function impairments due to mTBI (Cisneros et al., 2021; Hardin et al., 2021; Helmick & Members of the Consensus Conference, 2010; Novakovic-Agopian et al., 2021). Although remediation of executive functions initially often focuses on external strategies and explicit instructions and feedback, it should gradually shift to the internalization of self-regulation strategies through internalized self-instruction and self-monitoring (Cicerone et al., 2005; Kennedy & Coelho, 2005).

Assistive Technology for Cognition

The training in the use of assistive technology for cognition (ATC) to compensate for deficits can be beneficial to the transition of the patients back into the community. Assistive technology includes smart devices (e.g., smartphones, smartwatches, tablets, recording devices, etc.) and applications for the devices that assist with planning, organization, time management, information storage and retrieval, notetaking (manually or voice to text), reminder alarms, accessing new information, navigation, and virtual assistance with placing calls, getting directions, and taking messages. One of the most exciting features of ATC use is that they normalize support systems for the patient when integrated into cognitive rehabilitation.

There is a growing literature documenting the benefits of ATC among individuals with cognitive disabilities (de Joode et al., 2010; Gillespie et al., 2012). Clinicians should be mindful of selecting technology that fits the patient's desires and preferences, rather than those of the SLP. Similarly, clinicians should consider ATC that has a long-term application for the patients, rather than a temporary intervention. When new devices and strategy use are being implemented for cognitive impairments, training is essential for the successful generalization to real-life functioning. In the case of the more complex assistive technology devices, use of spaced retrieval in functional applications may be optimal for training acquiring skills in using the devices and their respective applications.

Social Communication and Group Interventions

Changes in social communication after concussion are an expanding research area. While previously overlooked, clinicians must now be aware that changes in social communication can and do occur after mTBI in adults and children (Bellerose et al., 2017; Theadom et al., 2019). Speech-language pathologists have reported success treating social communication deficits after mTBI in peer-focused groups (Hardin & Kelly, 2019; Schneider & Van Auken, 2018), although there has been little experimental research in this area. Cornis-Pop et al. (2012) suggest that social communication treatment focus on affective-behavioral impairments (e.g., anger and anxiety) and working with family and friends within the individual's circle of support on techniques that facilitate improved communication skills. These strategies would best be implemented through collaboration with a mental health provider.

Looking to the moderate-to-severe TBI literature, Dahlberg and colleagues (2007) demonstrated improved social communication skills in a randomized controlled trial, maintained through a 9-month follow-up, using a curriculum that emphasized self-awareness and self-assessment; individual goal setting; use of the group process to foster interaction, feedback, problem solving, and social support; and generalization of skills through the involvement of family, friends, and weekly assignments completed in the home or community. Ylvisaker and colleagues (2005) suggest the following components of social skills intervention for persons with TBI:

- Educate and train communication partners to interact supportively.
- Select personally important social interactive competencies.
- Provide extensive practice of socially appropriate behaviors.
- Provide situational coaching and training specifically designed to improve social perception and interpretation of others' behaviors and to improve self-monitoring of stress levels, so that individuals can remove themselves from the situation as needed.
- Include situational training.
- Coach the individual to evaluate and reward personal "social successes."

■ Counsel to develop an individual's sense of self that includes positive social interaction strategies.

Many life activities, such as work, school, and spiritual settings, involve group-based activities and teams, and therefore group therapy can be ideal for working with individuals on cognitive-social communication skills. Group treatment within community settings provides a more natural communicative context and should be considered a strategy to facilitate generalization of improved cognitive communication abilities beyond the clinic and into real-life situations. Twamley et al. (2014) developed the Cognitive Symptom Management and Rehabilitation Therapy (CogSMART) program that is effective in training cognitive skills and symptom management and can be delivered in a group or an individual setting. Similar models are continuing to evolve in civilian care as well (Hardin & Kelly, 2019; Schneider & Van Auken, 2018).

In addition to traditional group therapies, individuals may be interested in peer mentorship or SLP-facilitated support groups. Local brain injury chapters may provide support groups for individuals with mTBI, offering a less structured environment to engage in social communication. An alternative to traditional group therapies are the advances in peer-mentorship opportunities. O'Brien et al. (2021) found that symptomatic college students had positive experiences learning from trained peer-mentors on their experiences as a college student with mTBI. Clinicians should be mindful to include aspects of social communication and group functioning in mTBI intervention.

Discharge From Cognitive Communication Treatment

Discharge from cognitive communication treatment begins at the start of therapy with the development of the treatment plan or including the long- and short-term goals, frequency, and duration of treatment. Optimally, discharge is defined by the patient's achievement of their individualized treatment plan. There are no established thresholds on standardized testing that can substitute for clinician judgment and patient goals, perceptions, and preferences (Cornis-Pop et al., 2012). When a patient completes therapy by achieving their goals, recommendations are provided to facilitate a smooth transition back to work or school by including (a) gradual work reentry, (b) flexibility in setting a work schedule that allows for a shortened work schedule or breaks during the day, (c) environmental modifications, and (d) reduced work responsibilities. At the completion of the therapy program, the successful return to the community, whether it be returning to active-duty status or to a civilian position, to school, or to employment, is measured by the patient's successful maintenance at the level of functioning achieved at discharge (Management of Concussion/mTBI Working Group, 2009).

A Teachable Moment

I had my own clinical paradigm shift after meeting a mother, Maria, and her early elementary-aged daughter Neveah, about 5 years into my clinical career. They had been together in a car accident about a year before, both sustaining mild TBIs with persistent symptoms. We met after they had driven over 90 miles in a white-out blizzard to attend Maria's outpatient speech evaluation with me. At first, I was both shocked and saddened by her choice to drive, given the storm severity, and felt that this choice must have reflected her cognitive communication dysfunction. Moreover, it wasn't really an appropriate appointment to bring a child. I soon learned, however, that Maria and Neveah came together because they were "couch surfing," having no stable housing and nowhere safe for Neveah to stay.

In addition to the car accident, Maria was a survivor of TBI from intimate partner violence (IPV), and Maria protected herself and her daughter by fleeing that unsafe environment, in turn leading to their precarious housing. Neveah had not enrolled in school that year given their unstable housing, and Maria remained unemployed in order to homeschool Neveah with a second-grade workbook, like you could find at Costco. Maria had preexisting limited health care literacy and when partnered with TBIs and a cognitive communication disorder, she became frustrated and overwhelmed trying to access any care. Maria had been trying unsuccessfully for months to find services for them, putting Neveah on extended waiting lists for publicly funded evaluations. (Given her limited health literacy, Maria didn't know that Neveah would have received free services at school, if she'd been enrolled.) This is why, even when confronted with a blizzard, Maria made certain that they would attend that appointment on time, no matter the challenges of getting there.

Our evaluation was unconventional. This family needed acute functional support, not a standardized speech-language-cognitive evaluation. Moreover, it didn't make sense for Maria to become my patient (these were the days before telehealth), and our clinic did not provide pediatric services. My supervisor agreed that I could help to case manage remotely for this family over the next several weeks. We contacted possible TBI teams in Neveah's school districts, facilitating a direct referral for services, and those professionals assisted us in finding the best local school for her needs. I acted as Maria's advocate, facilitating local rehab appointments, bypassing much of the high-level language comprehension required to begin outpatient services, and connecting her with resources for survivors of IPV. As a result of our teaming, Neveah started school and Maria acquired low-cost stable housing.

In retrospect, driving to Boulder, Colorado, was perhaps the best decision Maria could have made at that moment. You might have rescheduled the appointment, without thinking twice about it, just like every other patient I had that day—I know that I would have. But for Maria, who had faced closed door after closed door, on that snowy afternoon, she had access to care and would not let that opportunity slip away. And she brought Neveah, because she (correctly) guessed that we would find a way to help her too. My assumptions about Maria were wrong. We can never know the challenges that our clients face. I initially viewed Maria through a lens of cognitive disability, not through the lens of her formidable strengths, and in doing so I did her a tremendous disservice. Thankfully, she was significantly wiser than her clinician.

K. Hardin

References

Aase, D. M., Babione, J. M., Proescher, E., Greenstein, J. E., DiGangi, J. A., Schroth, C., . . . Phan, K. L. (2018). Impact of PTSD on post-concussive symptoms, neuropsychological functioning, and pain in post 9/11 veterans with mild traumatic brain injury. *Psychiatry Research*, *268*, 460–466. https://doi.org/10.1016/j.psychres.2018.08.019

Acheson, D. J., & MacDonald, M. C. (2009). Verbal working memory and language production: Common approaches to the serial ordering of verbal information. *Psychological Bulletin*, *135*(1), 50–68. https://doi.org/10.1037/a0014411

Adams, M. R. (1990). The Demands and Capacities Model I: Theoretical elaborations. *Journal of Fluency Disorders*, *15*(3), 135–141. https://doi.org/10.1016/0094-730X(90)90014-J

Akin, F. W., Murnane, O. D., Hall, C. D., & Riska, K. M. (2017). Vestibular consequences of mild traumatic brain injury and blast exposure: A review. *Brain Injury*, *31*(9), 1188–1194. https://doi.org/10.1080/02699052.2017.1288928

American Speech-Language-Hearing Association. (2004). *Preferred practice patterns for the profession of speech-language pathology* [Preferred practice patterns]. http://www.asha.org/policy

American Speech-Language-Hearing Association. (2005a). *Knowledge and skills needed by speech-language pathologists providing services to individuals with cognitive communication disorders* [Knowledge and skills]. http://www.http://asha.org/policy

American Speech-Language-Hearing Association. (2005b). *Roles of speech-language pathologists in the identification, diagnosis, and treatment of individuals with cognitive communication disorders* [Position statement]. http://www.asha.org/policy

Anto-Ocrah, M., Oktapodas Feiler, M., Pukall, C., & Pacos-Martinez, A. (2021). Resilience and sexuality after concussion in women. *Sexual Medicine*, *9*(1), 100297. https://doi.org/10.1016/j.esxm.2020.100297

Aubry, M., Cantu, R., Dvorak, J., Graf-Baumann, T., Johnston, K., Kelly, J. P., . . . Concussion in Sport Group. (2002). Summary and agreement statement of the first International Conference on Concussion in Sport, Vienna 2001. Recommendations for the improvement of safety and health of athletes who may suffer concussive injuries. *British Journal of Sports Medicine*, *36*(1), 6–10. https://doi.org/10.1136/bjsm.36.1.6

Baddeley, A., Emslie, H., & Nimmo-Smith, I. (1992). *Speed and Capacity of Language Processing (SCOLP)*. Pearson Education.

Bagalman, E. (2014). *Traumatic brain injury among veterans* (Congressional Report No. R40941). http://www.ncsl.org/documents/statefed/health/TBI_Vets2013.pdf

Baker, J., Barnett, C., Cavalli, L., Dietrich, M., Dixon, L., Duffy, J. R., . . . McWhirter, L. (2021). Management of functional communication, swallowing, cough and related disorders: Consensus recommendations for speech and language therapy. *Journal of Neurology, Neurosurgery, and Psychiatry*, *92*(10), 1112–1125. https://doi.org/10.1136/jnnp-2021-326767

Baker, J. G., Leddy, J. J., Hinds, A. L., Haider, M. N., Shucard, J., Sharma, T., . . . Willer, B. S. (2018). An exploratory study of mild cognitive impairment of retired professional contact sport athletes. *Journal of Head Trauma Rehabilitation*, *33*(5), E16–E23. https://doi.org/10.1097/HTR.0000000000000420

Ballan, M. S., & Freyer, M. (2021). Addressing intimate partner violence with female patients with chronic physical disabilities: The role of physical therapists. *Disability and Rehabilitation*, *43*(10), 1404–1409. https://doi.org/10.1080/09638288.2019.1664648

Barrow, I. M., Collins, J. N., & Britt, L. D. (2006). The influence of an auditory distraction on rapid naming after a mild traumatic brain injury: A longitudinal study. *Journal of Trauma*, *61*(5), 1142–1149. https://doi.org/10.1097/01.ta.0000241238.70269.c1

Barrow, I. M., Hough, M., Rastatter, M. P., Walker, M., Holbert, D., & Rotondo, M. F. (2003). Can within-category naming identify subtle cognitive deficits in the mild traumatic brain-injured patient? *Journal of Trauma*, *54*(5), 888–895; discussion 895. https://doi.org/10.1097/01.TA.0000057150.60668.7C

Barry, N. C., & Tomes, J. L. (2015). Remembering your past: The effects of concussion on autobiographical memory recall. *Journal of Clinical and Experimental Neuropsychology*, *37*(9), 994–1003. https://doi.org/10.1080/13803395.2015.1038981

Baumgartner, J., & Duffy, J. R. (1997). Psychogenic stuttering in adults with and without neurologic disease. *Journal of Medical Speech-Language Pathology*, *5*(2), 75–95.

Belanger, H. G., Kretzmer, T., Yoash-Gantz, R., Pickett, T., & Tupler, L. A. (2009). Cognitive sequelae of blast-related versus other mechanisms of brain trauma. *Journal of the International Neuropsychological Society*, *15*(1), 1–8. https://doi.org/10.1017/S1355617708090036

Belanger, H. G., Vanderploeg, R. D., Curtiss, G., & Warden, D. L. (2007). Recent neuroimaging techniques in mild traumatic brain injury. *Journal of Neuropsychiatry and Clinical Neurosciences*, *19*(1), 5–20. https://doi.org/10.1176/jnp.2007.19.1.5

Bellerose, J., Bernier, A., Beaudoin, C., Gravel, J., & Beauchamp, M. H. (2017). Long-term brain-injury-specific effects following preschool mild TBI: A study of theory of mind. *Neuropsychology*, *31*(3), 229–241. https://doi.org/10.1037/neu0000341

Berisha, V., Wang, S., LaCross, A., Liss, J., & Garcia-Filion, P. (2017). Longitudinal changes in linguistic complexity among professional football players. *Brain and Language*, *169*, 57–63. https://doi.org/10.1016/j.bandl.2017.02.003

Bieniek, K. F., Cairns, N. J., Crary, J. F., Dickson, D. W., Folkerth, R. D., Keene, C. D., . . . TBI/CTE Research Group. (2021). The second NINDS/NIBIB consensus meeting to define neuropathological criteria for the diagnosis of chronic traumatic encephalopathy. *Journal of Neuropathology and Experimental Neurology*, *80*(3), 210–219. https://doi.org/10.1093/jnen/nlab001

Bolzenius, J. D., Roskos, P. T., Salminen, L. E., Paul, R. H., & Bucholz, R. D. (2015).

Cognitive and self-reported psychological outcomes of blast-induced mild traumatic brain injury in veterans: A preliminary study. *Applied Neuropsychology. Adult, 22*(2), 79–87. https://doi.org/10.1080/23279095.2013.845823

Brearly, T. W., Shura, R. D., Martindale, S. L., Lazowski, R. A., Luxton, D. D., Shenal, B. V., & Rowland, J. A. (2017). Neuropsychological test administration by videoconference: A systematic review and meta-analysis. *Neuropsychology Review, 27*(2), 174–186. https://doi.org/10.1007/s11065-017-9349-1

Breck, J., Bohr, A., Poddar, S., McQueen, M. B., & Casault, T. (2019). Characteristics and incidence of concussion among a US collegiate undergraduate population. *JAMA Network Open, 2*(12), e1917626. https://doi.org/10.1001/jamanetworkopen.2019.17626

Brenner, E. K., Grossner, E. C., Johnson, B. N., Bernier, R. A., Soto, J., & Hillary, F. G. (2020). Race and ethnicity considerations in traumatic brain injury research: Incidence, reporting, and outcome. *Brain Injury, 34*(6), 799–808. https://doi.org/10.1080/02699052.2020.1741033

Brooks, J., Fos, L. A., Greve, K. W., & Hammond, J. S. (1999). Assessment of executive function in patients with mild traumatic brain injury. *Journal of Trauma, 46*(1), 159–163. https://doi.org/10.1097/00005373-199901000-00027

Brooks, N., McKinlay, W., Symington, C., Beattie, A., & Campsie, L. (1987). Return to work within the first seven years of severe head injury. *Brain Injury, 1*(1), 5–19. https://doi.org/10.3109/02699058709034439

Brunger, H., Ogden, J., Malia, K., Eldred, C., Terblanche, R., & Mistlin, A. (2014). Adjusting to persistent post-concussive symptoms following mild traumatic brain injury and subsequent psychoeducational intervention: A qualitative analysis in military personnel. *Brain Injury, 28*(1), 71–80. https://doi.org/10.3109/02699052.2013.857788

Burgess, S., & Turkstra, L. S. (2010). Quality of communication life in adolescents with high-functioning autism and Asperger syndrome: A feasibility study. *Language, Speech, and Hearing Services in Schools, 41*(4), 474–487. https://doi.org/10.1044/0161-1461(2010/09-0007)

Callahan, M. L., Binder, L. M., O'Neil, M. E., Zaccari, B., Roost, M. S., Golshan, S., . . . Storzbach, D. (2018). Sensory sensitivity in Operation Enduring Freedom/Operation Iraqi Freedom veterans with and without blast exposure and mild traumatic brain injury. *Applied Neuropsychology. Adult, 25*(2), 126–136. https://doi.org/10.1080/23279095.2016.1261867

Campbell-Sills, L., & Stein, M. B. (2007). Psychometric analysis and refinement of the Connor–Davidson Resilience Scale (CD-RISC): Validation of a 10-item measure of resilience. *Journal of Traumatic Stress, 20*(6), 1019–1028. https://doi.org/10.1002/jts.20271

Cancelliere, C., Coronado, V. G., Taylor, C. A., & Xu, L. (2017). Epidemiology of isolated versus nonisolated mild traumatic brain injury treated in emergency departments in the United States, 2006–2012: Sociodemographic characteristics. *Journal of Head Trauma Rehabilitation, 32*(4), E37–E46. https://doi.org/10.1097/HTR.0000000000000260

Capó-Aponte, J. E., Jorgensen-Wagers, K. L., Sosa, J. A., Walsh, D. V., Goodrich, G. L., Temme, L. A., & Riggs, D. W. (2017). Visual dysfunctions at different stages after blast and non-blast mild traumatic brain injury. *Optometry and Vision Science, 94*(1), 7–15. https://doi.org/10.1097/OPX.0000000000000825

Carbado, D. W., Crenshaw, K. W., Mays, V. M., & Tomlinson, B. (2013). INTERSECTIONALITY: Mapping the movements of a theory. *Du Bois Review: Social Science Research on Race, 10*(2), 303–312. https://doi.org/10.1017/S1742058X13000349

Carlozzi, N. E., Tyner, C. E., Kisala, P. A., Boulton, A. J., Sherer, M., Chiaravalloti, N., & Tulsky, D. S. (2019). Measuring self-reported cognitive function following TBI: Development of the TBI-QOL executive function and cognition-general concerns item banks. *Journal of Head Trauma Rehabilitation, 34*(5), 308–325. https://doi.org/10.1097/HTR.0000000000000520

Carlson, K. F., Kehle, S. M., Meis, L. A., Greer, N., MacDonald, R., Rutks, I., . . . Wilt, T. J. (2011). Prevalence, assessment, and treatment of mild traumatic brain injury and posttraumatic stress disorder: A systematic review of the evidence. *Journal of Head Trauma Rehabilitation, 26*(2), 103–115. https://doi.org/10.1097/HTR.0b013e3181e50ef1

Carlson, K. F., Nelson, D., Orazem, R. J., Nugent, S., Cifu, D. X., & Sayer, N. A. (2010). Psychiatric diagnoses among Iraq and Afghanistan war veterans screened for deployment-related traumatic brain injury. *Journal of Traumatic Stress, 23*(1), 17–24. https://doi.org/10.1002/jts.20483

Centers for Disease Control and Prevention (CDC) & National Center for Injury Prevention and Control. (2003). *Report to Congress on mild traumatic brain injury in the United States: Steps to prevent a serious public health problem.*

Chadwick, L., Sharma, M. J., Madigan, S., Callahan, B. L., & Yeates, K. O. (2022). Classification criteria and rates of persistent postconcussive symptoms in children: A systematic review and meta-analysis. *The Journal of Pediatrics, 246*, 131–137.e2. https://doi.org/10.1016/j.jpeds.2022.03.039

Chien, J. H., Cheng, J. J., & Lenz, F. A. (2016). The thalamus. In P. M. Conn (Ed.), *Conn's translational neuroscience* (pp. 289–297). Academic Press.

Childers, C., & Hux, K. (2016). Invisible injuries: The experiences of college students with histories of mild traumatic brain injury. *Journal of Postsecondary Education and Disability, 29*(4), 389–405.

Choe, M. C., & Giza, C. C. (2015). Diagnosis and management of acute concussion. *Seminars in Neurology, 35*(1), 29–41. https://doi.org/10.1055/s-0035-1544243

Chorney, S. R., Suryadevara, A. C., & Nicholas, B. D. (2017). Audiovestibular symptoms as predictors of prolonged sports related concussion among NCAA athletes. *Laryngoscope, 127*(12), 2850–2853. https://doi.org/10.1002/lary.26564

Cicerone, K. D. (1996). Attention deficits and dual task demands after mild traumatic brain injury. *Brain Injury, 10*(2), 79–89. https://doi.org/10.1080/026990596124566

Cicerone, K. D. (2002). Remediation of "working attention" in mild traumatic brain injury. *Brain Injury, 16*(3), 185–195. https://doi.org/10.1080/02699050110103959

Cicerone, K. D., Dahlberg, C., Kalmar, K., Langenbahn, D. M., Malec, J. F., Bergquist, T. F., . . . Morse, P. A. (2000). Evidence-based cognitive rehabilitation: Recommendations for clinical practice. *Archives of Physical Medicine and Rehabilitation, 81*(12), 1596–1615. https://doi.org/10.1053/apmr.2000.19240

Cicerone, K. D., Dahlberg, C., Malec, J. F., Langenbahn, D. M., Felicetti, T., Kneipp, S., . . . Catanese, J. (2005). Evidence-based cognitive rehabilitation: Updated review of the literature from 1998 through 2002. *Archives of Physical Medicine and Rehabilitation, 86*(8), 1681–1692. https://doi.org/10.1016/j.apmr.2005.03.024

Cicerone, K. D., & Kalmar, K. (1995). Persistent postconcussion syndrome: The structure of subjective complaints after mild traumatic brain injury. *Journal of Head Trauma Rehabilitation, 10*(3), 1–17. https://doi.org/10.1097/00001199-199510030-00002

Cicerone, K. D., Mott, T., Azulay, J., Sharlow-Galella, M. A., Ellmo, W. J., Paradise, S., & Friel, J. C. (2008). A randomized controlled trial of holistic neuropsychologic rehabilitation after traumatic brain injury. *Archives of Physical Medicine and Rehabilitation, 89*(12), 2239–2249. https://doi.org/10.1016/j.apmr.2008.06.017

Cisneros, E., de Guise, E., Belleville, S., & McKerral, M. (2021). A controlled clinical efficacy trial of multimodal cognitive rehabilitation on episodic memory functioning in older adults with traumatic brain injury. *Annals of Physical and Rehabilitation Medicine, 64*(5), 101563. https://doi.org/10.1016/j.rehab.2021.101563

Coelho, C., Ylvisaker, M., & Turkstra, L. S. (2005). Nonstandardized assessment approaches for individuals with traumatic brain injuries. *Seminars in Speech and Language, 26*(4), 223–241. https://doi.org/10.1055/s-2005-922102

Cohen, M. L., Harnish, S. M., Lanzi, A. M., Brello, J., Hula, W. D., Victorson, D., . . . Tulsky, D. S. (2022). Establishing severity levels for patient-reported measures of functional communication, participation, and perceived cognitive function for adults with acquired cognitive and language disorders. *Quality of Life Research, 32*, 1–12. https://doi.org/10.1007/s11136-022-03337-2

Cohen, M. L., & Hula, W. D. (2020). Patient-reported outcomes and evidence-based practice in speech-language pathology. *American Journal of Speech-Language Pathology, 29*(1), 357–370. https://doi.org/10.1044/2019_AJSLP-19-00076

Cohen, M. L., Lanzi, A. M., & Boulton, A. J. (2021). Clinical use of PROMIS, neuroQoL, TBI-QoL, and other patient-reported outcome measures for individual adult clients with cognitive and language disorders. *Seminars in Speech and Language, 42*(3), 192–210. https://doi.org/10.1055/s-0041-1731365

Collins, M. W., Kontos, A. P., Okonkwo, D. O., Almquist, J., Bailes, J., Barisa, M., . . . Zafonte, R. (2016). Statements of agreement from the targeted evaluation and active management (TEAM) approaches to treating concussion meeting held in Pittsburgh, October 15–16, 2015. *Neurosurgery, 79*(6), 912–929. https://doi.org/10.1227/NEU.0000000000001447

Comper, P., Bisschop, S. M., Carnide, N., & Tricco, A. (2005). A systematic review of treatments for mild traumatic brain injury.

Brain Injury, 19(11), 863–880. https://doi.org/10.1080/02699050400025042

Cook, P., Thorne, J., Miering, S., & Sylla, L. (August, 2020). Motivational interviewing for coaching. *Virtual.* Presented at the 2020 National Ryan White Conference.

Cooper, D. B., Bowles, A. O., Kennedy, J. E., Curtiss, G., French, L. M., Tate, D. F., & Vanderploeg, R. D. (2017). Cognitive rehabilitation for military service members with mild traumatic brain injury: A randomized clinical trial. *Journal of Head Trauma Rehabilitation, 32*(3), E1–E15. https://doi.org/10.1097/HTR.0000000000000254

Cooper, D. B., Kennedy, J. E., Cullen, M. A., Critchfield, E., Amador, R. R., & Bowles, A. O. (2011). Association between combat stress and post-concussive symptom reporting in OEF/OIF service members with mild traumatic brain injuries. *Brain Injury, 25*(1), 1–7. https://doi.org/10.3109/02699052.2010.531692

Cornis-Pop, M. (2008). The role of speech language pathologists in the cognitive communication rehabilitation of traumatic brain injury. *California Speech-Language-Hearing Association Magazine, 38*(1), 14–18.

Cornis-Pop, M., Mashima, P. A., Roth, C. R., MacLennan, D. L., Picon, L. M., Hammond, C. S., . . . Frank, E. M. (2012). Guest editorial: Cognitive communication rehabilitation for combat-related mild traumatic brain injury. *Journal of Rehabilitation Research and Development, 49*(7), xi–xxxii. https://doi.org/10.1682/jrrd.2012.03.0048

Covassin, T., Stearne, D., & Elbin, R. III. (2008). Concussion history and postconcussion neurocognitive performance and symptoms in collegiate athletes. *Journal of Athletic Training, 43*(2), 119–124. https://doi.org/10.4085/1062-6050-43.2.119

Cranney, M., Warren, E., Barton, S., Gardner, K., & Walley, T. (2001). Why do GPs not implement evidence-based guidelines? A descriptive study. *Family Practice,*

18(4), 359–363. https://doi.org/10.1093/fampra/18.4.359

Creed, J. A., DiLeonardi, A. M., Fox, D. P., Tessler, A. R., & Raghupathi, R. (2011). Concussive brain trauma in the mouse results in acute cognitive deficits and sustained impairment of axonalunction. *Journal of Neurotrauma, 28*(4), 547–563. https://doi.org/10.1089/neu.2010.1729

Critchley, M. (1949). *Punch-drunk syndromes: The chronic traumatic encephalopathy of boxers. Hommage a Clovis Vincent.* Maloine.

Dahlberg, C. A., Cusick, C. P., Hawley, L. A., Newman, J. K., Morey, C. E., Harrison-Felix, C. L., & Whiteneck, G. G. (2007). Treatment efficacy of social communication skills training after traumatic brain injury: A randomized treatment and deferred treatment controlled trial. *Archives of Physical Medicine and Rehabilitation, 88*(12), 1561–1573. https://doi.org/10.1016/j.apmr.2007.07.033

Daudet, L., Yadav, N., Perez, M., Poellabauer, C., Schneider, S., & Huebner, A. (2017). Portable mTBI assessment using temporal and frequency analysis of speech. *IEEE Journal of Biomedical and Health Informatics, 21*(2), 496–506. https://doi.org/10.1109/JBHI.2016.2633509

de Ceballos, J. P., Turégano-Fuentes, F., Perez-Diaz, D., Sanz-Sanchez, M., Martin-Llorente, C., & Guerrero-Sanz, J. E. (2005). 11 March 2004: The terrorist bomb explosions in Madrid, Spain—An analysis of the logistics, injuries sustained and clinical management of casualties treated at the closest hospital. *Critical Care, 9*(1), 104–111. https://doi.org/10.1186/cc2995

de Joode, E., van Heugten, C., Verhey, F., & van Boxtel, M. (2010). Efficacy and usability of assistive technology for patients with cognitive deficits: A systematic review. *Clinical Rehabilitation, 24*(8), 701–714. https://doi.org/10.1177/0269215510367551

Defense Centers of Excellence. (2013). *Neuroimaging following mild traumatic brain injury in the non-deployed setting. DCoE clinical recommendations.*

DeKosky, S. T., Blennow, K., Ikonomovic, M. D., & Gandy, S. (2013). Acute and chronic traumatic encephalopathies: Pathogenesis and biomarkers. *Nature Reviews. Neurology, 9*(4), 192–200. https://doi.org/10.1038/nrneurol.2013.36

DeKosky, S. T., Jaffee, M., & Bauer, R. (2018). Long-term mortality in NFL professional football players: No significant increase, but questions remain. *JAMA, 319*(8), 773–775. https://doi.org/10.1001/jama.2017.20885

Delis, D. C., Kramer, J. H., Kaplan, E., & Ober, B. A. (2000). *California Verbal Learning Test–Second edition (CVLT-II).* Pearson Education.

Del Rossi, G. (2017). Evaluating the recovery curve for clinically assessed reaction time after concussion. *Journal of Athletic Training, 52*(8), 766–770. https://doi.org/10.4085/1062-6050-52.6.02

Dennis, E. L., Babikian, T., Giza, C. C., Thompson, P. M., & Asarnow, R. F. (2017). Diffusion MRI in pediatric brain injury. *Child's Nervous System, 33*(10), 1683–1692. https://doi.org/10.1007/s00381-017-3522-y

DePalma, R. G., Burris, D. G., Champion, H. R., & Hodgson, M. J. (2005). Blast injuries. *New England Journal of Medicine, 352*(13), 1335–1342. https://doi.org/10.1056/NEJMra042083

Dewan, M. C., Rattani, A., Gupta, S., Baticulon, R. E., Hung, Y. C., Punchak, M., . . . Rosenfeld, J. V. (2018). Estimating the global incidence of traumatic brain injury. *Journal of Neurological Surgery, 130*(4), 1–18.

D'Hondt, F., Lassonde, M., Thebault-Dagher, F., Bernier, A., Gravel, J., Vannasing, P., & Beauchamp, M. H. (2017). Electrophysiological correlates of emotional face processing after mild traumatic brain injury in preschool children. *Cognitive, Affective and Behavioral Neuroscience, 17*(1), 124–142. https://doi.org/10.3758/s13415-016-0467-7

Dinnes, C., & Hux, K. (2017). A multicomponent writing intervention for a college student with mild brain injury. *Communication Disorders Quarterly, 4,* 1–11.

Dischinger, P. C., Ryb, G. E., Kufera, J. A., & Auman, K. M. (2009). Early predictors of postconcussive syndrome in a population of trauma patients with mild traumatic brain injury. *Journal of Trauma, 66*(2), 289–296; discussion 296. https://doi.org/10.1097/TA.0b013e3181961da2

Douglas, J. M., O'Flaherty, C. A., & Snow, P. C. (2000). Measuring perception of communicative ability: The development and evaluation of the La Trobe Communication Questionnaire. *Aphasiology, 14*(3), 251–268. https://doi.org/10.1080/0268 70300401469

Draper, K., & Ponsford, J. (2008). Cognitive functioning ten years following traumatic brain injury and rehabilitation. *Neuropsychology, 22*(5), 618–625. https://doi.org/10.1037/0894-4105.22.5.618

Duffy, J. R. (2012). *Motor speech disorders: Substrates, differential diagnosis, and management* (3rd ed.). Elsevier.

Ehlhardt, L. A., Sohlberg, M. M., Kennedy, M., Coelho, C., Ylvisaker, M., Turkstra, L. S., & Yorkston, K. (2008). Evidence based practice guidelines for instructing individuals with neurogenic memory impairments: What have we learned in the past 20 years? *Neuropsychological Rehabilitation, 18*(3), 300–342. https://doi.org/10.1080/09602010701733190

Elsayed, N. M. (1997). Toxicology of blast overpressure. *Toxicology, 121*(1), 1–15. https://doi.org/10.1016/s0300-483x(97)03651-2

Fasotti, L., Kovacs, F., Eling, P. A. T. M., & Brouwer, W. H. (2000). Time pressure management as a compensatory strategy training after closed head injury. *Neuropsychological Rehabilitation, 10*(1), 47–65. https://doi.org/10.1080/096020100389291

Fausti, S. A., Wilmington, D. J., Gallun, F. J., Myers, P. J., & Henry, J. A. (2009). Auditory and vestibular dysfunction associated with blast-related traumatic brain injury. *Journal of Rehabilitation Research and Development, 46*(6), 797–810. https://doi.org/10.1682/jrrd.2008.09.0118

Federal Trade Commission. (2016). *Lumosity to pay $2 million to settle FTC deceptive advertising charges for its "brain training" program* [Press release]. https://www.ftc.gov/news-events/news/press-releases/2016/01/lumosity-pay-2-million-settle-ftc-deceptive-advertising-charges-its-brain-training-program

Finch, E., Copley, A., McLisky, M., Cornwell, P. L., Fleming, J. M., & Doig, E. (2019). Can goal attainment scaling (GAS) accurately identify changes in social communication impairments following TBI? [Speech]. *Speech, Language and Hearing, 22*(3), 183–194. https://doi.org/10.1080/2050571X.2019.1611220

Finkel, A. G., Ivins, B. J., Yerry, J. A., Klaric, J. S., Scher, A., & Sammy Choi, Y. (2017). Which matters more? A retrospective cohort study of headache characteristics and diagnosis type in soldiers with mTBI/concussion. *Headache: The Journal of Head and Face Pain, 57*(5), 719–728. https://doi.org/10.1111/head.13056

Finkel, M. F. (2006). The neurological consequences of explosives. *Journal of the Neurological Sciences, 249*(1), 63–67. https://doi.org/10.1016/j.jns.2006.06.005

Fisher, M., Wiseman-Hakes, C., Obeid, J., & DeMatteo, C. (2023). Does sleep quality influence recovery outcomes after postconcussive injury in children and adolescents? *Journal of Head Trauma Rehabilitation, 38*(3), 240–248. https://doi.org/10.1097/HTR.0000000000000811

Fulton, J. J., Calhoun, P. S., Wagner, H. R., Schry, A. R., Hair, L. P., Feeling, N., . . . Beckham, J. C. (2015). The prevalence of posttraumatic stress disorder in Operation Enduring Freedom/Operation Iraqi Freedom (OEF/OIF) veterans: A meta-analysis. *Journal of Anxiety Disorders, 31,* 98–107. https://doi.org/10.1016/j.janxdis.2015.02.003

Gallun, F. J., Papesh, M. A., & Lewis, M. S. (2017). Hearing complaints among veterans following traumatic brain injury. *Brain Injury, 31*(9), 1183–1187. https://doi.org/10.1080/02699052.2016.1274781

Gao, S., Kumar, R. G., Wisniewski, S. R., & Fabio, A. (2018). Disparities in health care utilization of adults with traumatic brain injuries are related to insurance, race and ethnicity: A systematic review. *Journal of Head Trauma Rehabilitation, 33*(3), E40–E50. https://doi.org/10.1097/HTR.0000000000000338

Garduño-Ortega, O., Li, H., Smith, M., Yao, L., Wilson, J., Zarate, A., & Bushnik, T. (2022). Assessment of the individual and compounding effects of marginalization factors on injury severity, discharge location, recovery, and employment outcomes at 1 year after traumatic brain injury. *Frontiers in Neurology, 13*, 942001. https://doi.org/10.3389/fneur.2022.942001

Gaudette, É., Seabury, S. A., Temkin, N., Barber, J., DiGiorgio, A. M., Markowitz, A. J., ... TRACK-TBI Investigators. (2022). Employment and economic outcomes of participants with mild traumatic brain injury in the TRACK-TBI study. *JAMA Network Open, 5*(6), e2219444. https://doi.org/10.1001/jamanetworkopen.2022.19444

Gentilinia, M., Nichell, P., & Schoenhube, R. (1989). Assessment of attention in mild head injury. In H. S. Levin, H. M. Eisenberg & A. L. Benton (Eds.), *Mild head injury* (pp. 162–175). Oxford University Press.

Gillespie, A., Best, C., & O'Neill, B. (2012). Cognitive function and assistive technology for cognition: A systematic review. *Journal of the International Neuropsychological Society, 18*(1), 1–19. https://doi.org/10.1017/S1355617711001548

Gioia, G., & Collins, M. (2006). *Acute Concussion Evaluation (ACE): Physician/clinician office version.* http://www.cdc.gov/concussion/head-sup/pdf/ace-a.pdf

Gioia, G. A., Isquith, P. K., Guy, S. C., & Kenworthy, L. (2002). *Behavior Rating Inventory of Executive Function® (BRIEF®).* PAR.

Giza, C. C., & Hovda, D. A. (2001). The neurometabolic cascade of concussion. *Journal of Athletic Training, 36*(3), 228–235.

Gondusky, J. S., & Reiter, M. P. (2005). Protecting military convoys in Iraq: An examination of battle injuries sustained by a mechanized battalion during Operation Iraqi Freedom II. *Military Medicine, 170*(6), 546–549. https://doi.org/10.7205/milmed.170.6.546

Grady, M. F., Master, C. L., & Gioia, G. A. (2012). Concussion pathophysiology: Rationale for physical and cognitive rest. *Pediatric Annals, 41*(9), 377–382. https://doi.org/10.3928/00904481-20120827-12

Gray, J. M., Robertson, I., Pentland, B., & Anderson, S. (1992). Microcomputer based attentional retraining after brain damage: A randomized group controlled trial. *Neuropsychological Rehabilitation, 2*(2), 97–115. https://doi.org/10.1080/09602019208401399

Green, S. L., Keightley, M. L., Lobaugh, N. J., Dawson, D. R., & Mihailidis, A. (2018). Changes in working memory performance in youth following concussion. *Brain Injury, 32*(2), 182–190. https://doi.org/10.1080/02699052.2017.1358396

Grossman, E. J., & Inglese, M. (2016). The role of thalamic damage in mild traumatic brain injury. *Journal of Neurotrauma, 33*(2), 163–167. https://doi.org/10.1089/neu.2015.3965

Guerriero, R., Hawash, K., Pepin, M., Wolff, R., & Meehan III, W. (2015). Younger children recover faster and have less premorbid conditions than adolescents with concussion (I5–5E). *Neurology, 84*(14), I5–I5E.

Guskiewicz, K. M., McCrea, M., Marshall, S. W., Cantu, R. C., Randolph, C., Barr, W., ... Kelly, J. P. (2003). Cumulative effects associated with recurrent concussion in collegiate football players: The NCAA Concussion Study. *JAMA, 290*(19), 2549–

2555. https://doi.org/10.1001/jama.290 .19.2549

Haarbauer-Krupa, J., Arbogast, K. B., Metzger, K. B., Greenspan, A. I., Kessler, R., Curry, A. E., . . . Master, C. L. (2018). Variations in mechanisms of injury for children with concussion. *Journal of Pediatrics*, *197*, 241–248. https://doi .org/10.1016/j.jpeds.2018.01.075

Hall, R. C., Hall, R. C., & Chapman, M. J. (2005). Definition, diagnosis, and forensic implications of postconcussional syndrome. *Psychosomatics*, *46*(3), 195–202. https://doi.org/10.1176/appi.psy.46.3.195

Halterman, C. I., Langan, J., Drew, A., Rodriguez, E., Osternig, L. R., Chou, L. S., & van Donkelaar, P. V. (2006). Tracking the recovery of visuospatial attention deficits in mild traumatic brain injury. *Brain*, *129*(3), 747–753. https://doi .org/10.1093/brain/awh705

Hardin, K. Y., Black, C., Caldbick, K., Kelly, M., Malhotra, A., Tidd, C., . . . Turkstra, L. S. (2021). Current practices among speech-language pathologists for mild traumatic brain injury: A mixed-methods modified Delphi approach. *American Journal of Speech-Language Pathology*, *30*(4), 1625–1655. https://doi.org/10.1044/2021 _AJSLP-20-00311

Hardin, K. Y., & Kelly, J. P. (2019). The role of speech-language pathology in an interdisciplinary care model for persistent symptomatology of mild traumatic brain injury. *Seminars in Speech and Language*, *40*(1), 65–78. https://doi.org/10 .1055/s-0038-1676452

Hebert, J., Babcock, M., Hardin, K. Y., Diefenbach, H., Milo, S., Elliott, G., . . . Filley, C. (2020). Enhancing interdisciplinary care for patients with mild traumatic brain injury (TBI): Implementing shared vocabulary to improve outcomes. *Journal of Head Trauma Rehabilitation*, *35*(2), E179–E180.

Helgeson, S. R. (2010). Identifying brain injury in state juvenile justice correlations, and homeless populations: Challenges and promising practices. *Brain Injury Professional*, *7*(4), 18–20.

Helmick, K., & Members of Consensus Conference. (2010). Cognitive rehabilitation for military personnel with mild traumatic brain injury and chronic postconcussional disorder: Results of April 2009 consensus conference. *NeuroRehabilitation Conference*, *26*(3), 239–255. https:// doi.org/10.3233/NRE-2010-0560

Honda, J., Chang, S. H., & Kim, K. (2018). The effects of vision training, neck musculature strength, and reaction time on concussions in an athletic population. *Journal of Exercise Rehabilitation*, *14*(5), 706–712. https://doi.org/10.12965/jer .1836416.208

Hoover, E. C., Souza, P. E., & Gallun, F. J. (2017). Auditory and cognitive factors associated with speech-in-noise complaints following mild traumatic brain injury. *Journal of the American Academy of Audiology*, *28*(4), 325–339. https://doi .org/10.3766/jaaa.16051

Howell, D., Osternig, L., Van Donkelaar, P., Mayr, U., & Chou, L. S. (2013). Effects of concussion on attention and executive function in adolescents. *Medicine and Science in Sports and Exercise*, *45*(6), 1030–1037. https://doi.org/10.1249/ MSS.0b013e3182814595

Huckans, M., Pavawalla, S., Demadura, T., Kolessar, M., Seelye, A., Roost, N., . . . Storzbach, D. (2010). A pilot study examining effects of group-based cognitive strategy training treatment on self-reported cognitive problems, psychiatric symptoms, functioning, and compensatory strategy use in OIF/OEF combat veterans with persistent mild cognitive disorder and history of traumatic brain injury. *Journal of Rehabilitation Research and Development*, *47*(1), 43–60. https:// doi.org/10.1682/jrrd.2009.02.0019

Hunt, C., Zanetti, K., Kirkham, B., Michalak, A., Masanic, C., Vaidyanath, C., . . . Ouchterlony, D. (2016). Identification of hidden health utilization services and costs in adults awaiting tertiary care following mild traumatic brain injury in Toronto, Ontario, Canada. *Concussion, 1*(4), CNC21. https://doi.org/10.2217/cnc-2016-0009

Iadevaia, C., Roiger, T., & Zwart, M. B. (2015). Qualitative examination of adolescent health-related quality of life at 1 year postconcussion. *Journal of Athletic Training, 50*(11), 1182–1189. https://doi.org/10.4085/1062-6050-50.11.02

Isaki, E., & Turkstra, L. (2000). Communication abilities and work re-entry following traumatic brain injury. *Brain Injury, 14*(5), 441–453. https://doi.org/10.1080/026990500120547

Iverson, G. L. (2005). Outcome from mild traumatic brain injury. *Current Opinion in Psychiatry, 18*(3), 301–317. https://doi.org/10.1097/01.yco.0000165601.29047.ae

Iverson, G. L., Keene, C. D., Perry, G., & Castellani, R. J. (2018). The need to separate chronic traumatic encephalopathy neuropathology from clinical features. *Journal of Alzheimer's Disease, 61*(1), 17–28. https://doi.org/10.3233/JAD-170654

Ivins, B. J., Kane, R., & Schwab, K. A. (2009). Performance on the automated neuropsychological assessment metrics in a nonclinical sample of soldiers screened for mild TBI after returning from Iraq and Afghanistan: A descriptive analysis. *Journal of Head Trauma Rehabilitation, 24*(1), 24–31. https://doi.org/10.1097/HTR.0b013e3181957042

Jordan, B. D. (2000). Chronic traumatic brain injury associated with boxing. *Seminars in Neurology, 20*(2), 179–185. https://doi.org/10.1055/s-2000-9826

Kamins, J., Bigler, E., Covassin, T., Henry, L., Kemp, S., Leddy, J. J., . . . Giza, C. C. (2017). What is the physiological time to recovery after concussion? A systematic review. *British Journal of Sports Medicine, 51*(12), 935–940. https://doi.org/10.1136/bjsports-2016-097464

Karlin, A. M. (2011). Concussion in the pediatric and adolescent population:

Different population, different concerns. *Physical Medicine and Rehabilitation, 3*(10, Suppl. 2), S369–S379.

Kay, T., Newman, B., Cavallo, M., Ezrachi, O., & Resnick, M. (1992). Toward a neuropsychological model of functional disability after mild traumatic brain injury. *Neuropsychology, 6*(4), 371–384. https://doi.org/10.1037/0894-4105.6.4.371

Keightley, M. L., Saluja, R. S., Chen, J. K., Gagnon, I., Leonard, G., Petrides, M., & Ptito, A. (2014). A functional magnetic resonance imaging study of working memory in youth after sports-related concussion: Is it still working? *Journal of Neurotrauma, 31*(5), 437–451. https://doi.org/10.1089/neu.2013.3052

Kennedy, J. E., Cooper, D. B., Curtiss, G., Shelton, J. L., Bowles, A. O., Tate, D. F., . . . Vanderploeg, R. D. (2022). Research Letter: Long-term outcomes following cognitive rehabilitation for mild traumatic brain injury: A 5-year follow-up of a cohort from the SCORE randomized clinical trial. *Journal of Head Trauma Rehabilitation, 37*(6), 390–395. https://doi.org/10.1097/HTR.0000000000000800

Kennedy, M. R., & Coelho, C. (2005). Self-regulation after traumatic brain injury: A framework for intervention of memory and problem solving. *Seminars in Speech and Language, 26*(4), 242–255. https://doi.org/10.1055/s-2005-922103

Kennedy, M. R. T., & Krause, M. O. (2011). Self-regulated learning in a dynamic coaching model for supporting college students with traumatic brain injury: Two case reports. *Journal of Head Trauma Rehabilitation, 26*(3), 212–223. https://doi.org/10.1097/HTR.0b013e318218dd0e

Kennedy, M. R., Krause, M. O., & Turkstra, L. S. (2008). An electronic survey about college experiences after traumatic brain injury. *NeuroRehabilitation, 23*(6), 511–520.

King, N. S. F., Crawford, S., Wenden, F. J., Moss, N. E. G., & Wade, D. T. (1995). The Rivermead Post Concussion Symptoms Questionnaire: A measure of symptoms commonly experienced after head injury and its reliability. *Journal of Neurology, 242*(9), 587–592. https://doi.org/10.1007/BF00868811

Kleim, J. A., & Jones, T. A. (2008). Principles of experience-dependent neural plasticity: Implications for rehabilitation after brain damage. *Journal of Speech, Language, Hearing Research, S1*(1), S225–S239.

Kontos, A. P., Elbin, R. J., Trbovich, A., Womble, M., Said, A., Sumrok, V. F., . . . Collins, M. (2020). Concussion Clinical Profiles Screening (CP screen) tool: Preliminary evidence to inform a multidisciplinary approach. *Neurosurgery, 87*(2), 348–356. https://doi.org/10.1093/neuros/nyz545

Kontos, A. P., Sufrinko, A., Womble, M., & Kegel, N. (2016). Neuropsychological assessment following concussion: An evidence-based review of the role of neuropsychological assessment pre- and post-concussion. *Current Pain and Headache Reports, 20*(6), 38. https://doi.org/10.1007/s11916-016-0571-y

Krug, H., & Turkstra, L. S. (2015). Assessment of cognitive communication disorders in adults with mild traumatic brain injury. *Perspectives on Neurophysiology and Neurogenic Speech and Language Disorders, 25*(1), 17–35. https://doi.org/10.1044/nnsld25.1.17

Kurowski, B. G., Wade, S. L., Dexheimer, J. W., Dyas, J., Zhang, N., & Babcock, L. (2016). Feasibility and potential benefits of a web-based intervention delivered acutely after mild traumatic brain injury in adolescents: A pilot study. *Journal of Head Trauma Rehabilitation, 31*(6), 369–378. https://doi.org/10.1097/HTR.0000000000000180

Kutas, M., & Federmeier, K. D. (2000). Electrophysiology reveals semantic memory use in language comprehension. *Trends in Cognitive Sciences, 4*(12), 463–470. https://doi.org/10.1016/s1364-6613(00)01560-6

Laatsch, L., & Guay, J. (2005). Rehabilitation of reading comprehension fluency in adults with acquired brain injury. *Journal of Cognitive Rehabilitation, 23*, 5–12.

Lalonde, G., Bernier, A., Beaudoin, C., Gravel, J., & Beauchamp, M. H. (2018). Investigating social functioning after early mild TBI: The quality of parent–child interactions. *Journal of Neuropsychology, 12*(1), 1–22. https://doi.org/10.1111/jnp.12104

Landon, J., Shepherd, D., Stuart, S., Theadom, A., & Freundlich, S. (2012). Hearing every footstep: Noise sensitivity in individuals following traumatic brain injury. *Neuropsychological Rehabilitation, 22*(3), 391–407. https://doi.org/10.1080/09602011.2011.652496

Lange, R. T., Brickell, T. A., Bailie, J. M., Tulsky, D. S., & French, L. M. (2016). Clinical utility and psychometric properties of the traumatic Brain Injury Quality of Life Scale (TBI-QOL) in US military service members. *Journal of Head Trauma Rehabilitation, 31*(1), 62–78. https://doi.org/10.1097/HTR.0000000000000149

Lau, B. C., Kontos, A. P., Collins, M. W., Mucha, A., & Lovell, M. R. (2011). Which on-field signs/symptoms predict protracted recovery from sport-related concussion among high school football players? *American Journal of Sports Medicine, 39*(11), 2311–2318. https://doi.org/10.1177/0363546511410655

Lebrun, C. M., Mrazik, M., Prasad, A. S., Tjarks, B. J., Dorman, J. C., Bergeron, M. F., . . . Valentine, V. D. (2013). Sport concussion knowledge base, clinical practices and needs for continuing medical education: A survey of family physicians and cross-border comparison. *British Journal of Sports Medicine, 47*(1), 54–59. https://doi.org/10.1136/bjsports-2012-091480

Ledbetter, A. K., Sohlberg, M. M., Fickas, S. F., Horney, M. A., & McIntosh, K. (2017). Evaluation of a computer-based prompting intervention to improve essay writing in undergraduates with cognitive impairment after acquired brain injury. *Neuropsychological Rehabilitation, 27*, 1–30.

Lempke, L. B., Kerr, Z. Y., Melvin, P., Walton, S. R., Wallace, J. S., Mannix, R. C., . . . Ward, V. L. (2022). Examining racial and ethnic disparities in adult emergency department patient visits for concussion in the United States. *Frontiers in Neurology, 13,* 988088. https://doi.org/10.3389/fneur.2022.988088

Levin, H. S., & Goldstein, F. C. (1986). Organization of verbal memory after severe closed-head injury. *Journal of Clinical and Experimental Neuropsychology, 8*(6), 643–656. https://doi.org/10.1080/01688638608405185

Lew, H. L., Jerger, J. F., Guillory, S. B., & Henry, J. A. (2007). Auditory dysfunction in traumatic brain injury. *Journal of Rehabilitation Research and Development, 44*(7), 921–928. https://doi.org/10.1682/jrrd.2007.09.0140

Lew, H. L., Lin, P. H., Fuh, J. L., Wang, S. J., Clark, D. J., & Walker, W. C. (2006). Characteristics and treatment of headache after traumatic brain injury: A focused review. *American Journal of Physical Medicine and Rehabilitation, 85*(7), 619–627. https://doi.org/10.1097/01.phm.0000223235.09931.c0

Lezak, M. D. (1982). The problem of assessing executive functions. *International Journal of Psychology, 17*(1–4), 281–297. https://doi.org/10.1080/00207598208247445

Lezak, M. D., Howieson, D. B., Loring, D. W., & Fischer, J. S. (2004). *Neuropsychological assessment.* Oxford University Press.

Lindquist, L. K., Love, H. C., & Elbogen, E. B. (2017). Traumatic brain injury in Iraq and Afghanistan veterans: New results from a National Random Sample Study. *Journal of Neuropsychiatry and Clinical Neurosciences, 29*(3), 254–259. https://doi.org/10.1176/appi.neuropsych.16050100

Losoi, H., Silverberg, N. D., Wäljas, M., Turunen, S., Rosti-Otajärvi, E., Helminen, M., . . . Iverson, G. L. (2015). Resilience is associated with outcome from mild traumatic brain injury. *Journal of Neu-*

rotrauma, 32*(13), 942–949. https://doi.org/10.1089/neu.2014.3799

Lucić, M. (1995). Therapy of middle ear injuries caused by explosive devices. *Vojnosanitetski Pregled, 52*(3), 221–224.

Ludwig, R., D'Silva, L., Vaduvathiriyan, P., Rippee, M. A., & Siengsukon, C. (2020). Sleep disturbances in the acute stage of concussion are associated with poorer long-term recovery: A systematic review. *PM and R, 12*(5), 500–511. https://doi.org/10.1002/pmrj.12309

Lukow, H. R., Godwin, E. E., Marwitz, J. H., Mills, A., Hsu, N. H., & Kreutzer, J. S. (2015). Relationship between resilience, adjustment, and psychological functioning after traumatic brain injury: A preliminary report. *Journal of Head Trauma Rehabilitation, 30*(4), 241–248. https://doi.org/10.1097/HTR.0000000000000137

Lumba-Brown, A., Teramoto, M., Bloom, O. J., Brody, D., Chesnutt, J., Clugston, J. R., . . . Ghajar, J. (2020). Concussion guidelines step 2: Evidence for subtype classification. *Neurosurgery, 86*(1), 2–13. https://doi.org/10.1093/neuros/nyz332

Lumba-Brown, A., Yeates, K. O., Sarmiento, K., Breiding, M. J., Haegerich, T. M., Gioia, G. A., . . . Timmons, S. D. (2018). Centers for Disease Control and Prevention guideline on the diagnosis and management of mild traumatic brain injury among children. *JAMA Pediatrics, 172*(11), e182853. https://doi.org/10.1001/jamapediatrics.2018.2853

MacDonald, C. L., Johnson, A. M., Nelson, E. C., Werner, N. J., Fang, R., Flaherty, S. F., & Brody, D. L. (2014). Functional status after blast-plus-impact complex concussive traumatic brain injury in evacuated United States military personnel. *Journal of Neurotrauma, 31*(10), 889–898. https://doi.org/10.1089/neu.2013.3173

MacDonald, C. L., Johnson, A. M., Wierzechowski, L., Kassner, E., Stewart, T., Nelson, E. C., . . . Brody, D. L. (2014). Prospectively assessed clinical outcomes in concussive blast vs nonblast traumatic brain injury among evacuated US military personnel. *JAMA Neurology, 71*(8), 994–1002. https://doi.org/10.1001/jama neurol.2014.1114

MacDonald, S. (1998). *Functional Assessment of Verbal Reasoning and Executive Strategies.* Clinical Publishing.

Madhok, D. Y., Rodriguez, R. M., Barber, J., Temkin, N. R., Markowitz, A. J., Kreitzer, N., . . . TRACK-TBI Investigators. (2022). Outcomes in patients with mild traumatic brain injury without acute intracranial traumatic injury. *JAMA Network Open, 5*(8), e2223245. https://doi.org/10.1001/ jamanetworkopen.2022.23245

Mah, K., Hickling, A., & Reed, N. (2018). Perceptions of mild traumatic brain injury in adults: A scoping review. *Disability and Rehabilitation, 40*(8), 960–973. https://doi.org/10.1080/09638288.2016 .1277402

Makdissi, M., Cantu, R. C., Johnston, K. M., McCrory, P., & Meeuwisse, W. H. (2013). The difficult concussion patient: What is the best approach to investigation and management of persistent (>10 days) postconcussive symptoms? *British Journal of Sports Medicine, 47*(5), 308–313. https://doi.org/10.1136/bjsports-2013-092255

Malec, J. F., Smigielski, J. S., & DePompolo, R. W. (1991). Goal attainment scaling and outcome measurement in postacute brain injury rehabilitation. *Archives of Physical Medicine and Rehabilitation, 72*(2), 138–143.

Management of Concussion/mTBI Working Group. (2009). VA/DoD clinical practice guideline for management of concussion/mild traumatic brain injury. *Journal of Rehabilitation Research and Development, 46*(6), CP1–C68.

Mansfield, E., Stergiou-Kita, M., Cassidy, J. D., Bayley, M., Mantis, S., Kristman, V., . . . Colantonio, A. (2015). Return-to-work challenges following a work-related mild TBI: The injured worker perspective. *Brain Injury, 29*(11), 1362–1369. https:// doi.org/10.3109/02699052.2015.1053524

Marini, A., Galetto, V., Zampieri, E., Vorano, L., Zettin, M., & Carlomagno, S. (2011). Narrative language in traumatic brain injury. *Neuropsychologia, 49*(10), 2904–2910. https://doi.org/10.1016/j.neuro psychologia.2011.06.017

Martin, E. M., Lu, W. C., Helmick, K., French, L., & Warden, D. L. (2008). Traumatic brain injuries sustained in the Afghanistan and Iraq wars. *Journal of Trauma Nursing, 15*(3), 94–99; quiz 100. https://doi.org/10.1097/01.JTN.00003 37149.29549.28

Martland, H. S. (1928). Punch drunk. *JAMA, 91*(15), 1103–1107. https://doi .org/10.1001/jama.1928.02700150029009

Mattingly, E. O. (2015). Dysfluency in a service member with comorbid diagnoses: A case study. *Military Medicine, 180*(1), e157–e159. https://doi.org/10.7205/MIL MED-D-14-00238

Mayorga, M. A. (1997). The pathology of primary blast overpressure injury. *Toxicology, 121*(1), 17–28. https://doi.org/10 .1016/s0300-483x(97)03652-4

McAllister, T. W., Ford, J. C., Flashman, L. A., Maerlender, A., Greenwald, R. M., Beckwith, J. G., . . . Jain, S. (2014). Effect of head impacts on diffusivity measures in a cohort of collegiate contact sport athletes. *Neurology, 82*(1), 63–69. https://doi .org/10.1212/01.wnl.0000438220.16190.42

McCrea, M., & Manley, G. (2018). State of the science on pediatric mild traumatic brain injury: Progress toward clinical translation. *JAMA Pediatrics, 172*(11), e182846. https://doi.org/10.1001/jama pediatrics.2018.2846

McDonald, S. (1998). Communication and language disturbances following traumatic brain injury. In B. Stemmer & H. A. Whitaker (Eds.), *Handbook of neurolinguistics* (pp. 485–494). Academic Press.

McDonald, S. (2013). Impairments in social cognition following severe traumatic brain injury. *Journal of the International Neuropsychological Society, 19*(3), 231–246. https://doi.org/10.1017/S13556177120 01506

McKee, A. C., Cairns, N. J., Dickson, D. W., Folkerth, R. D., Keene, C. D., Litvan, I., . . . TBI/CTE group. (2016). The first NINDS/NIBIB consensus meeting to define europathological criteria for the diagnosis of chronic traumatic encephalopathy. *Acta Neuropathologica*, *131*(1), 75–86. https://doi.org/10.1007/s00401-015-1515-z

Mez, J., Daneshvar, D. H., Kiernan, P. T., Abdolmohammadi, B., Alvarez, V. E., Huber, B. R., . . . McKee, A. C. (2017). Clinicopathological evaluation of chronic traumatic encephalopathy in players of American football. *JAMA*, *318*(4), 360–370. https://doi.org/10.1001/jama.2017.8334

Miller, W. R., Rollnick, S., & ProQuest (Firm). (2012). *Motivational interviewing: Helping people change* (3rd ed.). Guilford.

Millspaugh, J. A. (1937). Dementia pugilistica. *United States Naval Medical Bulletin*, *35*(297), 303.

Milman, A., Rosenberg, A., Weizman, R., & Pick, C. G. (2005). Mild traumatic brain injury induces persistent cognitive deficits and behavioral disturbances in mice. *Journal of Neurotrauma*, *22*(9), 1003–1010. https://doi.org/10.1089/neu.2005.22.1003

Mollayeva, T., El-Khechen-Richandi, G., & Colantonio, A. (2018). Sex and gender considerations in concussion research. *Concussion*, *3*(1), CNC51. https://doi.org/10.2217/cnc-2017-0015

Mooney, G., & Speed, J. (2001). The association between mild traumatic brain injury and psychiatric conditions. *Brain Injury*, *15*(10), 865–877. https://doi.org/10.1080/02699050110065286

Morrow, E. L., Mayberry, L. S., & Duff, M. C. (2023). The growing gap: A study of sleep, encoding, and consolidation of new words in chronic traumatic brain injury. *Neuropsychologia*. Advance online publication. https://doi.org/10.1016/j.neuropsychologia.2023.108518

Neils-Strunjas, J., Paul, D., Clark, A. N., Mudar, R., Duff, M. C., Waldron-Perrine, B., & Bechtold, K. T. (2017). Role of resilience in the rehabilitation of adults with acquired brain injury. *Brain Injury*, *31*(2), 131–139. https://doi.org/10.1080/02699052.2016.1229032

Nelson, N. W., Hoelzle, J. B., Doane, B. M., McGuire, K. A., Ferrier-Auerbach, A. G., Charlesworth, M. J., . . . Sponheim, S. R. (2012). Neuropsychological outcomes of US veterans with report of remote blast-related concussion and current psychopathology. *Journal of the International Neuropsychological Society*, *18*(5), 845–855. https://doi.org/10.1017/S1355617712000616

Nicholas, L. E., & Brookshire, R. H. (1995). Comprehension of spoken narrative discourse by adults with aphasia, right-hemisphere brain damage, or traumatic brain injury. *American Journal of Speech-Language Pathology*, *4*(3), 69–81. https://doi.org/10.1044/1058-0360.0403.69

NIH Consensus Development Panel on Rehabilitation of Persons with Traumatic Brain Injury. (1999). Consensus conference. Rehabilitation of persons with traumatic brain injury. NIH Consensus Development Panel on Rehabilitation of persons with traumatic brain injury. *JAMA*, *282*(10), 974–983. https://doi.org/10.1001/jama.282.10.974

Nolin, P. (2006). Executive memory dysfunctions following mild traumatic brain injury. *Journal of Head Trauma Rehabilitation*, *21*(1), 68–75. https://doi.org/10.1097/00001199-200601000-00007

Norman, R. S., Jaramillo, C. A., Amuan, M., Wells, M. A., Eapen, B. C., & Pugh, M. J. (2013). Traumatic brain injury in veterans of the wars in Iraq and Afghanistan: Communication disorders stratified by severity of brain injury. *Brain Injury*, *27*(13–14), 1623–1630. https://doi.org/10.3109/02699052.2013.834380

Norman, R. S., Jaramillo, C. A., Eapen, B. C., Amuan, M. E., & Pugh, M. J. (2018). Acquired stuttering in veterans of the wars in Iraq and Afghanistan: The role of traumatic brain injury, post-traumatic stress disorder, and medications. *Military Medicine, 183*(11–12), e526–e534. https://doi.org/10.1093/milmed/usy067

Novakovic-Agopian, T., Posecion, L., Kornblith, E., Abrams, G., McQuaid, J. R., Neylan, T. C., . . . Chen, A. J. W. (2021). Goal-Oriented Attention Self-Regulation Training improves executive functioning in veterans with post-traumatic stress disorder and mild traumatic brain injury. *Journal of Neurotrauma, 38*(5), 582–592. https://doi.org/10.1089/neu.2019.6806

Noy, S., Krawitz, S., & Del Bigio, M. R. (2016). Chronic traumatic encephalopathy-like abnormalities in a routine neuropathology service. *Journal of Neuropathology and Experimental Neurology, 75*(12), 1145–1154. https://doi.org/10.1093/jnen/nlw092

O'Brien, K. H., Wallace, T., & Kemp, A. (2021). Student perspectives on the role of peer support following concussion: Development of the SUCCESS peer mentoring program. *American Journal of Speech-Language Pathology, 30*(2S), 933–948. https://doi.org/10.1044/2020_AJSLP-20-00076

Oleksiak, M., Smith, B. M., St Andre, J. R., Caughlan, C. M., & Steiner, M. (2012). Audiological issues and hearing loss among veterans with mild traumatic brain injury. *Journal of Rehabilitation Research and Development, 49*(7), 995–1004. https://doi.org/10.1682/jrrd.2011.01.0001

Omalu, B., Bailes, J., Hamilton, R. L., Kamboh, M. I., Hammers, J., Case, M., & Fitzsimmons, R. (2011). Emerging histomorphologic phenotypes of chronic traumatic encephalopathy in American athletes. *Neurosurgery, 69*(1), 173–183; discussion 183. https://doi.org/10.1227/NEU.0b013e318212bc7b

O'Neil-Pirozzi, T. M., Strangman, G. E., Goldstein, R., Katz, D. I., Savage, C. R., Kelkar, K., . . . Glenn, M. B. (2010). A controlled treatment study of internal memory strategies (I-MEMS) following traumatic brain injury. *Journal of Head Trauma Rehabilitation, 25*(1), 43–51. https://doi.org/10.1097/HTR.0b013e3181bf24b1

Ouellet, M. C., Beaulieu-Bonneau, S., & Morin, C. M. (2015). Sleep-wake disturbances after traumatic brain injury. *Lancet. Neurology, 14*(7), 746–757. https://doi.org/10.1016/S1474-4422(15)00068-X

Owens, B. D., Kragh, J. F., Jr., Wenke, J. C., Macaitis, J., Wade, C. E., & Holcomb, J. B. (2008). Combat wounds in operation Iraqi Freedom and operation Enduring Freedom. *Journal of Trauma, 64*(2), 295–299. https://doi.org/10.1097/TA.0b013e318163b875

Ozen, L. J., Itier, R. J., Preston, F. F., & Fernandes, M. A. (2013). Long-term working memory deficits after concussion: Electrophysiological evidence. *Brain Injury, 27*(11), 1244–1255. https://doi.org/10.3109/02699052.2013.804207

Pennardt, A., & Franke, E. (2021). Blast injury. *Emergency Medical Services,* 278–284.

Phillips, Y. Y. (1986). Primary blast injuries. *Annals of Emergency Medicine, 15*(12), 1446–1450. https://doi.org/10.1016/s0196-0644(86)80940-4

Rabinowitz, A. R., Li, X., McCauley, S. R., Wilde, E. A., Barnes, A., Hanten, G., . . . Levin, H. S. (2015). Prevalence and predictors of poor recovery from mild traumatic brain injury. *Journal of Neurotrauma, 32*(19), 1488–1496. https://doi.org/10.1089/neu.2014.3555

Raikes, A. C., & Schaefer, S. Y. (2016). Sleep quantity and quality during acute concussion: A pilot study. *Sleep, 39*(12), 2141–2147. https://doi.org/10.5665/sleep.6314

Randolph, C. (2012). *RBANS update: Repeatable Battery for the Assessment of Neuropsychological Status.* Pearson Education and PsychCorp.

Randolph, C. (2014). Is chronic traumatic encephalopathy a real disease? *Current Sports Medicine Reports, 13*(1), 33–37. https://doi.org/10.1097/OPX.0000000000000170

Raskin, S. A., & Mateer, C. A. (2000). *Neuropsychological management of mild traumatic brain injury.* Oxford University Press.

Robertson, I. H., Ward, T., Ridgeway, V., & Nimmo-Smith, I. (1994). *Test of Everyday Attention (TEA)*. Pearson Education.

Rose, S. C., Weldy, D. L., Zhukivska, S., & Pommering, T. L. (2021). Acquired stuttering after pediatric concussion. *Acta Neurologica Belgica, 122*(2), 545–546.

Rosenthal, M. (1993). Mild traumatic brain injury syndrome. *Annals of Emergency Medicine, 22*(6), 1048–1051. https://doi.org/10.1016/s0196-0644(05)82749-0

Roth, C. R., Cornis-Pop, M., & Beach, W. A. (2015). Examination of validity in spoken language evaluations: Adult onset stuttering following mild traumatic brain injury. *NeuroRehabilitation, 36*(4), 415–426. https://doi.org/10.3233/NRE-151230

Rothbart, A., & Sohlberg, M. M. (2021). Resilience as a mainstream clinical consideration for speech-language pathologists providing post–acquired brain injury neurorehabilitation. *Perspectives of the ASHA Special Interest Groups, 6*(5), 1026–1032. https://doi.org/10.1044/2021_PERSP-20-00249

Rubin, T. G., Catenaccio, E., Fleysher, R., Hunter, L. E., Lubin, N., Stewart, W. F., . . . Lipton, M. L. (2018). MRI-defined white matter microstructural alteration associated with soccer heading is more extensive in women than men. *Radiology, 289*(2), 478–486. https://doi.org/10.1148/radiol.2018180217

Salvatore, A. P., Cannito, M., Brassil, H. E., Bene, E. R., & Sirmon-Taylor, B. (2017). Auditory comprehension performance of college students with and without sport concussion on Computerized–Revised Token Test subtest VIII. *Concussion, 2*(2), CNC37. https://doi.org/10.2217/cnc-2016-0024

Schneider, A. L. C., Huie, J. R., Boscardin, W. J., Nelson, L., Barber, J. K., Yaffe, K., . . . TRACK-TBI Investigators. (2022). Cognitive outcome 1 year after mild traumatic brain injury: Results from the TRACK-TBI study. *Neurology, 98*(12), e1248–e1261. https://doi.org/10.1212/WNL.0000000000200041

Schneider, E., & Van Auken, S. (2018). Bridging the gap: Pragmatic language group approach for cognitive communication deficits postconcussion. *Perspectives of the ASHA Special Interest Groups, 3*(2), 31–43. https://doi.org/10.1044/persp3.SIG2.31

Schneider, K. J., Leddy, J. J., Guskiewicz, K. M., Seifert, T., McCrea, M., Silverberg, N. D., . . . Makdissi, M. (2017). Rest and treatment/rehabilitation following sport-related concussion: A systematic review. *British Journal of Sports Medicine, 51*(12), 930–934. https://doi.org/10.1136/bjsports-2016-097475

Schönberger, M., Humle, F., & Teasdale, T. W. (2007). The relationship between clients' cognitive functioning and the therapeutic working alliance in post-acute brain injury rehabilitation. *Brain Injury, 21*(8), 825–836. https://doi.org/10.1080/02699050701499433

Schrank, F. A., McGrew, K. S., & Mather, N. (2014). Woodcock-Johnson IV. *Journal of Psychoeducational Assessment, 33*(4), 391–398. https://doi.org/10.1177/0734282915569447

Schwab, K., & Cernich, A. (2011). Comments on "Longitudinal effects of mild traumatic brain injury and posttraumatic stress disorder comorbidity on postdeployment outcomes in National Guard soldiers deployed to Iraq." *Archives of General Psychiatry, 68*, 79–89.

Seiger, A., Goldwater, E., & Deibert, E. (2015). Does mechanism of injury play a role in recovery from concussion? *Journal of Head Trauma Rehabilitation, 30*(3), E52–E56. https://doi.org/10.1097/HTR.0000000000000051

Shafi, R., Crawley, A. P., Tartaglia, M. C., Tator, C. H., Green, R. E., Mikulis, D. J., & Colantonio, A. (2020). Sex-specific differences in resting-state functional connectivity of large-scale networks in postconcussion syndrome. *Scientific Reports, 10*(1), 21982. https://doi.org/10.1038/s41598-020-77137-4

Shenton, M. E., Hamoda, H. M., Schneiderman, J. S., Bouix, S., Pasternak, O., Rathi,

Y., . . . Zafonte, R. (2012). A review of magnetic resonance imaging and diffusion tensor imaging findings in mild traumatic brain injury. *Brain Imaging and Behavior, 6*(2), 137–192. https://doi.org/10.1007/s11682-012-9156-5

Sherer, M., Evans, C. C., Leverenz, J., Irby, J. W., Lee, J. E., & Yablon, S. A. (2009). Therapeutic alliance in post-acute brain injury rehabilitation: Predictors of strength of alliance and impact of alliance on outcome. *Brain Injury, 21*(7), 663–672.

Silverberg, N. D., & Iverson, G. L. (2013). Is rest after concussion "the best medicine?": Recommendations for activity resumption following concussion in athletes, civilians, and military service members. *Journal of Head Trauma Rehabilitation, 28*(4), 250–259. https://doi.org/10.1097/HTR.0b013e31825ad658

Silverberg, N. D., Iverson, G. L., & ACRM Mild TBI Definition Expert Consensus Group and the ACRM Brain Injury Special Interest Group Mild TBI Task Force. (2021). Expert panel survey to update the American congress of rehabilitation medicine definition of mild traumatic brain injury. *Archives of Physical Medicine and Rehabilitation, 102*(1), 76–86. https://doi.org/10.1016/j.apmr.2020.08.022

Silverberg, N. D., Iverson, G. L., ACRM Brain Injury Special Interest Group Mild TBI Task Force, & ACRM Mild TBI Diagnostic Criteria Expert Consensus Group. (2023). The American Congress of Rehabilitation Medicine diagnostic criteria for mild traumatic brain injury. *Archives of Physical Medicine and Rehabilitation,* S0003-9993(23)00297-6. Advance online publication. https://doi.org/10.1016/j.apmr.2023.03.036

Silverberg, N. D., Panenka, W. J., & Iverson, G. L. (2018). Work productivity loss after mild traumatic brain injury. *Archives of Physical Medicine and Rehabilitation, 99*(2), 250–256. https://doi.org/10.1016/j.apmr.2017.07.006

Snell, D. L., Macleod, A. D. S., & Anderson, T. (2016). Post-concussion syndrome after a mild traumatic brain injury: A minefield for clinical practice. *Journal of Behavioral and Brain Science, 6*(6), 227–232. https://doi.org/10.4236/jbbs.2016.66023

Snell, D. L., Martin, R., Surgenor, L. J., Siegert, R. J., & Hay-Smith, E. J. C. (2017). What's wrong with me? Seeking a coherent understanding of recovery after mild traumatic brain injury. *Disability and Rehabilitation, 39*(19), 1968–1975. https://doi.org/10.1080/09638288.2016.1213895

Soble, J. R., Cooper, D. B., Lu, L. H., Eapen, B. C., & Kennedy, J. E. (2018). Symptom reporting and management of chronic post-concussive symptoms in military service members and veterans. *Current Physical Medicine and Rehabilitation Reports, 6*(1), 62–73. https://doi.org/10.1007/s40141-018-0173-1

Sohlberg, M. K. M., Hamilton, J., & Turkstra, L. (2023). *Transforming cognitive rehabilitation: Effective instructional methods.* Guilford.

Sohlberg, M. M. (2000). Psychotherapy approaches. In S. A. Raskin & C. A. Mateer (Eds.), *Neuropsychological management of mild traumatic brain injury* (pp. 137–156). Oxford University Press.

Sohlberg, M. M., Ehlhardt, L., & Kennedy, M. (2005). Instructional techniques in cognitive rehabilitation: A preliminary report. *Seminars in Speech and Language, 26*(4), 268–279. https://doi.org/10.1055/s-2005-922105

Sohlberg, M. M., Griffiths, G. G., & Fickas, S. (2014). An evaluation of reading comprehension of expository text in adults with traumatic brain injury. *American Journal of Speech-Language Pathology, 23*(2), 160–175. https://doi.org/10.1044/2013_AJSLP-12-0005

Sohlberg, M. M., & Ledbetter, A. K. (2016). Management of persistent cognitive symptoms after sport-related concussion. *American Journal of Speech-Language Pathology, 25*(2), 138–149. https://doi.org/10.1044/2015_AJSLP-14-0128

Sohlberg, M. M., & Mateer, C. A. (2005). *Attention Process Training: A program for cognitive rehabilitation to address persons with attentional deficits ranging from mild to severe* (3rd ed.). Lash and Associates.

Sohlberg, M. M., & Turkstra, L. S. (2011). *Optimizing cognitive rehabilitation: Effective instructional methods*. Guilford.

Sollmann, N., Echlin, P. S., Schultz, V., Viher, P. V., Lyall, A. E., Tripodis, Y., . . . Koerte, I. K. (2018). Sex differences in white matter alterations following repetitive subconcussive head impacts in collegiate ice hockey players. *NeuroImage. Clinical*, *17*, 642–649. https://doi.org/10.1016/j.nicl.2017.11.020

Stein, M. B., Kessler, R. C., Heeringa, S. G., Jain, S., Campbell-Sills, L., Colpe, L. J., . . . Army STARRS Collaborators. (2015). Prospective longitudinal evaluation of the effect of deployment-acquired traumatic brain injury on posttraumatic stress and related disorders: Results from the Army Study to Assess Risk and Resilience in Service Members (Army STARRS). *American Journal of Psychiatry*, *172*(11), 1101–1111. https://doi.org/10.1176/appi.ajp.2015.14121572

Stein, T. D., Alvarez, V. E., & McKee, A. C. (2014). Chronic traumatic encephalopathy: A spectrum of neuropathological changes following repetitive brain trauma in athletes and military personnel. *Alzheimer's Research and Therapy*, *6*(1), 4. https://doi.org/10.1186/alzrt234

Stergiou-Kita, M., Mansfield, E., Sokoloff, S., & Colantonio, A. (2016). Gender influences on return to work after mild traumatic brain injury. *Archives of Physical Medicine and Rehabilitation*, *97*(2, Suppl.), S40–S45. https://doi.org/10.1016/j.apmr.2015.04.008

Stillman, A., Madigan, N., & Alexander, M. (2016). Factors associated with prolonged, subjective post-concussive symptoms (P3.325). *Neurology*, *86*(16), 1.

Stockbridge, M. D., Doran, A., King, K., & Newman, R. S. (2018). The effects of concussion on rapid picture naming in children. *Brain Injury*, *32*(4), 506–514. https://doi.org/10.1080/02699052.2018.1429660

Storzbach, D., Twamley, E. W., Roost, M. S., Golshan, S., Williams, R. M., O'Neil, M., . . . Huckans, M. (2017). Compensatory cognitive training for Operation Enduring Freedom/Operation Iraqi Freedom/Operation New Dawn veterans with mild traumatic brain injury. *Journal of Head Trauma Rehabilitation*, *32*(1), 16–24. https://doi.org/10.1097/HTR.0000000000000228

Sufrinko, A., Pearce, K., Elbin, R. J., Covassin, T., Johnson, E., Collins, M., & Kontos, A. P. (2015). The effect of preinjury sleep difficulties on neurocognitive impairment and symptoms after sport-related concussion. *American Journal of Sports Medicine*, *43*(4), 830–838. https://doi.org/10.1177/0363546514566193

Swanson, M. W., Weise, K. K., Dreer, L. E., Johnston, J., Davis, R. D., Ferguson, D., . . . Swanson, E. (2017). Academic difficulty and vision symptoms in children with concussion. *Optometry and Vision Science*, *94*(1), 60–67. https://doi.org/10.1097/OPX.0000000000000977

Talavage, T. M., Nauman, E. A., Breedlove, E. L., Yoruk, U., Dye, A. E., Morigaki, K. E., . . . Leverenz, L. J. (2014). Functionally-detected cognitive impairment in high school football players without clinically diagnosed concussion. *Journal of Neurotrauma*, *31*(4), 327–338. https://doi.org/10.1089/neu.2010.1512

Tator, C. H., Davis, H. S., Dufort, P. A., Tartaglia, M. C., Davis, K. D., Ebraheem, A., & Hiploylee, C. (2016). Postconcussion syndrome: Demographics and predictors in 221 patients. *Journal of Neurosurgery*, *125*(5), 1206–1216. https://doi.org/10.3171/2015.6.JNS15664

Taylor, C. A., Bell, J. M., Breiding, M. J., & Xu, L. (2017). Traumatic brain injury–related emergency department visits, hospitalizations, and deaths—United States, 2007 and 2013. *Morbidity and Mortality Weekly Report. Surveillance Summaries*,

66(9), 1–16. https://doi.org/10.15585/mmwr.ss6609a1

Terrio, H., Brenner, L. A., Ivins, B. J., Cho, J. M., Helmick, K., Schwab, K., . . . Warden, D. (2009). Traumatic brain injury screening: Preliminary findings in a U.S. Army brigade combat team. *Journal of Head Trauma Rehabilitation, 24*(1), 14–23. https://doi.org/10.1097/HTR.0b013e31819581d8

Thiagarajan, P., & Ciuffreda, K. J. (2015). Short-term persistence of oculomotor rehabilitative changes in mild traumatic brain injury (mTBI): A pilot study of clinical effects. *Brain Injury, 29*(12), 1475–1479. https://doi.org/10.3109/02699052.2015.1070905

Thiagarajan, P., Ciuffreda, K. J., & Ludlam, D. P. (2011). Vergence dysfunction in mild traumatic brain injury (mTBI): A review. *Ophthalmic and Physiological Optics, 31*(5), 456–468. https://doi.org/10.1111/j.1475-1313.2011.00831.x

Tiersky, L. A., Anselmi, V., Johnston, M. V., Kurtyka, J., Roosen, E., Schwartz, T., & DeLuca, J. (2005). A trial of neuropsychologic rehabilitation in mild-spectrum traumatic brain injury. *Archives of Physical Medicine and Rehabilitation, 86*(8), 1565–1574. https://doi.org/10.1016/j.apmr.2005.03.013

Toccalino, D., Wiseman-Hakes, C., & Zalai, D. M. (2021). Preliminary validation of the sleep and concussion questionnaire as an outcome measure for sleep following brain injury. *Brain Injury, 35*(7), 743–750. https://doi.org/10.1080/02699052.2021.1906949

Toldi, J., & Jones, J. (2021). A case of acute stuttering resulting after a sports-related concussion. *Current Sports Medicine Reports, 20*(1), 10–12. https://doi.org/10.1249/JSR.0000000000000795

Tulsky, D. S., Kisala, P. A., Victorson, D., Carlozzi, N., Bushnik, T., Sherer, M., . . . Cella, D. (2016). TBI-QOL: Development and calibration of item banks to measure patient reported outcomes following traumatic brain injury. *Journal of Head Trauma Rehabilitation, 31*(1), 40–51.

https://doi.org/10.1097/HTR.0000000000000131

Twamley, E. W., Jak, A. J., Delis, D. C., Bondi, M. W., & Lohr, J. B. (2014). Cognitive symptom management and rehabilitation therapy (CogSMART) for veterans with traumatic brain injury: Pilot randomized controlled trial. *Journal of Rehabilitation Research and Development, 51*(1), 59–70. https://doi.org/10.1682/JRRD.2013.01.0020

Twamley, E. W., Thomas, K. R., Gregory, A. M., Jak, A. J., Bondi, M. W., Delis, D. C., & Lohr, J. B. (2015). CogSMART compensatory cognitive training for traumatic brain injury: Effects over 1 year. *Journal of Head Trauma Rehabilitation, 30*(6), 391–401. https://doi.org/10.1097/HTR.0000000000000076

VA/DoD Clinical Practice Guideline for the Management of Concussion-Mild Traumatic Brain Injury version 2.0. (2016). https://www.va.gov/covidtraining/docs/mTBICPGFullCPG50821816.pdf

Vanderploeg, R. D., Belanger, H. G., & Curtiss, G. (2009). Mild traumatic brain injury and posttraumatic stress disorder and their associations with health symptoms. *Archives of Physical Medicine and Rehabilitation, 90*(7), 1084–1093. https://doi.org/10.1016/j.apmr.2009.01.023

Vanderploeg, R. D., Cooper, D. B., Curtiss, G., Kennedy, J. E., Tate, D. F., & Bowles, A. O. (2018). Predicting treatment response to cognitive rehabilitation in military service members with mild traumatic brain injury. *Rehabilitation Psychology, 63*(2), 194–204. https://doi.org/10.1037/rep0000215

Vanderploeg, R. D., Groer, S., & Belanger, H. G. (2012). Initial development process of a VA semistructured clinical interview for TBI identification. *Journal of Rehabilitation Research and Development, 49*(4), 545–556. https://doi.org/10.1682/jrrd.2011.04.0069

Vander Werff Kathy, R. (2016). The application of the International Classification of Functioning, Disability and Health to functional auditory consequences of mild traumatic brain injury. *Seminars in Hearing, 37*(3), 216–232. https://doi.org/10.1055/s-0036-1584409

Velikonja, D., Ponsford, J., Janzen, S., Harnett, A., Patsakos, E., Kennedy, M., . . . Bayley, M. T. (2023). INCOG 2.0 guidelines for cognitive rehabilitation following traumatic brain injury, Part V: Memory. *Journal of Head Trauma Rehabilitation, 38*(1), 83–102. https://doi.org/10.1097/HTR.0000000000000837

Viola-Saltzman, M., & Watson, N. F. (2012). Traumatic brain injury and sleep disorders. *Neurologic Clinics, 30*(4), 1299–1312. https://doi.org/10.1016/j.ncl.2012.08.008

Voss, J. D., Connolly, J., Schwab, K. A., & Scher, A. I. (2015). Update on the epidemiology of concussion/mild traumatic brain injury. *Current Pain and Headache Reports, 19*(7), 32. https://doi.org/10.1007/s11916-015-0506-z

Wade, S. L., Sidol, C., Babcock, L., Schmidt, M., Kurowski, B., Cassedy, A., & Zhang, N. (2022). Findings from a randomized controlled trial of SMART: An ehealth intervention for mild traumatic brain injury. *Journal of Pediatric Psychology, 48*(3), 241–253. https://doi.org/10.1093/jpepsy/jsac086

Wäljas, M., Iverson, G. L., Lange, R. T., Hakulinen, U., Dastidar, P., Huhtala, H., . . . Öhman, J. (2015). A prospective biopsychosocial study of the persistent post-concussion symptoms following mild traumatic brain injury. *Journal of Neurotrauma, 32*(8), 534–547. https://doi.org/10.1089/neu.2014.3339

Warden, D. (2006). Military TBI during the Iraq and Afghanistan wars. *Journal of Head Trauma Rehabilitation, 21*(5), 398–402. https://doi.org/10.1097/00001199-200609000-00004

Wechsler, D. (2009). *Wechsler Memory Scale* (4th ed.). Pearson.

Weinstein, C. E., Palmer, D., & Schulte, A. C. (1987). *Learning and Study Strategies Inventory (LASSI).* H & H Publishing.

Whyte, J., & Turkstra, L. S. (2021). Building a theoretical foundation for cognitive rehabilitation. *Brain, 144*(7), 1933–1935. https://doi.org/10.1093/brain/awab210

Wickwire, E. M., Williams, S. G., Roth, T., Capaldi, V. F., Jaffe, M., Moline, M., . . . Lettieri, C. J. (2016). Sleep, sleep disorders, and mild traumatic brain injury. What we know and what we need to know: Findings from a national working group. *Neurotherapeutics, 13*, 403–417.

Willer, B. S., Zivadinov, R., Haider, M. N., Miecznikowski, J. C., & Leddy, J. J. (2018). A preliminary study of early-onset dementia of former professional football and hockey players. *Journal of Head Trauma Rehabilitation, 33*(5), E1–E8. https://doi.org/10.1097/HTR.0000000000000421

Wiseman-Hakes, C., Colantonio, A., & Gargaro, J. (2009). Sleep and wake disorders following traumatic brain injury: A systematic review of the literature. *Critical Reviews in Physical and Rehabilitation Medicine, 21*(3–4), 317–374. https://doi.org/10.1615/CritRevPhysRehabilMed.v21.i3-4.70

Wiseman-Hakes, C., Albin, M., & Hardin, K. Y., (2022, April 28-30). *Traumatic brain injury and vulnerable populations: An important role for speech-language pathologists* [Conference presentation]. Speech-Language and Audiology Canada (SAC) Speech-Language Pathology Conference virtual, Canada. https://congresoac.ca

Wiseman-Hakes, C., Foster, E., Langer, L., Chandra, T., Bayley, M., & Comper, P. (2022). Characterizing sleep and wakefulness in the acute phase of concussion in the general population: A naturalistic cohort from the Toronto concussion study. *Journal of Neurotrauma, 39*(1–2), 172–180. https://doi.org/10.1089/neu.2021.0295

Wiseman-Hakes, C., Magor, T., Bauman, N., Colantonio, A., & Matheson, F. I. (2023). Exploring the cognitive communication challenges of adults with histories of traumatic brain injury and criminal justice system involvement: A pilot study. *American Journal of Speech-Language Pathology, 32*, 941–955. https://doi.org/10.1044/2022_AJSLP-22-00086

Wiseman-Hakes, C., Victor, J. C., Brandys, C., & Murray, B. J. (2011). Impact of post-traumatic hypersomnia on functional recovery of cognition and communication. *Brain Injury, 25*(12), 1256–1265. https://doi.org/10.3109/02699052.2011.608215

Wood, R. L., O'Hagan, G., Williams, C., McCabe, M., & Chadwick, N. (2014). Anxiety sensitivity and alexithymia as mediators of postconcussion syndrome following mild traumatic brain injury. *Journal of Head Trauma Rehabilitation, 29*(1), E9–E17. https://doi.org/10.1097/HTR.0b013e31827eabba

Working Group to Develop a Clinician's Guide to Cognitive Rehabilitation in mTBI. (2016). *Clinician's guide to cognitive rehabilitation in mild traumatic brain injury: Application for military service members and veterans.* https://www.asha.org/siteassets/practice-portal/traumatic-brain-injury-adult/clinicians-guide-to-cognitive-rehabilitation-in-mild-traumatic-brain-injury.pdf

World Health Organization. (2001). *ICIDH2: International classification of functioning, disability and health: ICF 2001.*

Wright, A. J., Mihura, J. L., Hadas, P., & McCord, D. M. (2020). *Guidance on psychological tele-assessment during the COVID-19 crisis.* https://www.apaservices.org/practice/reimbursement/health-codes/testing/tele-assessment-covid-19

Ylvisaker, M. (2006). Self-coaching: A context-sensitive, person-centred approach to social communication after traumatic brain injury. *Brain Impairment, 7*(3), 246–258. https://doi.org/10.1375/brim.7.3.246

Ylvisaker, M., & Feeney, T. (2001). Supported behavior and supported cognition: An integrated, positive approach to serving students with disabilities. *Educational Psychology in Scotland, 6*(1), 17–30.

Ylvisaker, M., Turkstra, L. S., & Coelho, C. (2005). Behavioral and social interventions for individuals with traumatic brain injury: A summary of the research with clinical implications. *Seminars in Speech and Language, 26*(4), 256–267. https://doi.org/10.1055/s-2005-922104

Yue, J. K., Upadhyayula, P. S., Avalos, L. N., Phelps, R. R. L., Suen, C. G., & Cage, T. A. (2020). Concussion and mild-traumatic brain injury in rural settings: Epidemiology and specific health care considerations. *Journal of Neurosciences in Rural Practice, 11*(1), 23–33. https://doi.org/10.1055/s-0039-3402581

Zalai, D. M., Girard, T. A., Cusimano, M. D., & Shapiro, C. M. (2020, March 10). Circadian rhythm in the assessment of post-concussion insomnia: A cross-sectional observational study. *CMAJ Open, 8*(1), E142–E147. https://doi.org/10.9778/cmajo.20190137

Zeitzer, M. B., & Brooks, J. M. (2008). In the line of fire: Traumatic brain injury among Iraq War veterans. *AAOHN Journal, 56*(8), 347–353; quiz 354. https://doi.org/10.3928/08910162-20080801-03

Appendix 7–A
Special Population: Service Members/Veterans and mTBI

SLPs are commonly used on rehabilitation teams for military-related mTBI, and consequently, military medicine professionals have created extensive recommendations for SLPs and other providers working in mTBI. These recommendations are often overlooked by civilian-treating SLPs, and we highlight their value to treating veterans/service members as well as civilians, strongly recommending that clinicians consider these resources with civilian patients as well. Information from the Defense and Veterans Brain Injury Center (DVBIC) is free and readily available. These excellent resources are outside the scope of this chapter, but for students and clinicians working with service members and veterans across clinical care settings, these resources are important evidence-based practice resources.

Incidence of mTBI in the U.S. Military

According to the DoD, 383,947 of the more than 2 million troops, who served worldwide between 2000 and 2018, sustained a TBI, with 82.3% classified as mild (DVBIC, 2018). Many service members sustained multiple mTBIs during their two or more deployments in both Iraq and Afghanistan. Military service members are at greater risk for mTBI than civilians, due to their demographics. Most are young healthy males, representing a high-risk group, and they are engaged in risk-related training, operational engagements, and deployments to combat zones (Soble et al., 2018). Deployments to combat theaters of operation put individuals at risk for concussive blast exposures from improvised explosive devices (IEDs), suicide bombers, land mines, mortar rounds, and rocket-propelled grenades. TBI is recognized as the "signature injury" of modern warfare.

Military-related mTBI seems more likely to be accompanied by persistent symptoms than sports injures, with 47% of individuals remaining symptomatic 3 months postinjury or longer (Schwab & Cernich, 2011). Although deployment/combat-related mTBI receives much attention in the media, the majority of recorded TBIs among service members occur in nondeployed contexts (DVBIC, 2018). Military-related activities, including boxing and combat training, put service members at risk for concussion and repeated subconcussive blows. This estimate may be higher among service members with a history of one or more combat deployments, given the frequency of multiple TBI events, concomitant mental health conditions such as depression and PTSD, and other factors unique to combat deployments.

The incidence of military members sustaining TBI ranges from 11% to 23% of post-9/11 service members and veterans who met criteria for TBI, with 87% sustaining mTBI. Half of the respondents with TBI reported multiple TBIs and 46% reported a loss of consciousness, which is far higher than is commonly reported (Lindquist et al., 2017). In the absence of a biomarker for diagnosing TBI, this number is based largely on self-reports. However, even when there is opportunity to self-report, military values of self-sacrifice and "warrior ethos" can lead to under-reporting potential occurrences.

Mechanism of Blast Injuries

Blast injuries result from the impact of a blast overpressurization wave, or a complex pressure wave generated by an explosion, that causes an instantaneous rise in atmospheric pressure, much higher than normal for humans to withstand (Centers for Disease Control and Prevention, 2003). There are four basic mechanisms of blast injuries, classified as primary, secondary, tertiary, and quaternary. Primary blast injuries result directly from the explosion. Blast explosives generate a sudden rise in atmospheric pressure that strikes the individual and pushes on all of the organs of the body. Air-filled organs such as the ears, lungs, gastrointestinal tract, and organs surrounded by fluid-filled cavities, including the brain and spinal cord, are especially susceptible to primary blast injury (Elsayed, 1997; Mayorga, 1997). Secondary blast injuries result from the blast fragments flying through the air or any objects that are set in motion by the blast. IED explosions create debris of glass, wood, or metal that can lodge

in limbs or any exposed surface of the body or cause penetrating brain injury or contusion damage from the impact (Phillips, 1986). Tertiary blast injuries occur when an individual is thrown against other moving or stationary objects by the force of the blast (Finkel, 2006). Quaternary blast-related injuries include all other injuries or medical complications caused by explosions, including burns, toxic inhalation of gases, exposure to radiation, asphyxiation, and inhalation of dust containing coal or asbestos (DePalma et al., 2005; Pennardt & Franke, 2021). Blasts from explosive devices, causing repeated blast-induced neurotrauma over the course of multiple and prolonged deployments (Terrio et al., 2009; Warden, 2006), are responsible for most mTBIs among military service members and veterans. Advances in medical care and technology, including protective equipment, medical evacuation systems, and life-saving procedures, contribute to greater survival rates following combat-related as well as non-combat, training-related injuries sustained by service members previously (Bagalman, 2014; Martin et al., 2008; Owens et al., 2008). The surviving individuals, who in earlier conflicts might have died, are facing a complex combination of impairments in physical, cognitive, and psychosocial functioning (Zeitzer & Brooks, 2008) that requires a comprehensive, coordinated, evidence-based standard of care.

Combat-related primary blast injury is almost always accompanied by psychological and/or blunt trauma. MacDonald, Johnson, Nelson, and colleagues (2014) utilized the term "blast-plus-impact" (or "blast-plus") to describe the frequently reported history of being exposed to multiple blasts as well as impact-related blows during military service; for example, when the power of a blast explosion throws the individual off their feet and against a hard surface, this is known as a blast-plus-impact injury. Blast injuries often are accompanied by the psychological trauma of war in the context fear, anxiety, and emotional shock. Much remains to be learned about the effects of blast injuries and the short- and long-term effects of multiple blast exposures and blast-plus concussions on the brain. The military continues to fund extensive research to further the understanding of the effects of blasts on the brain and how best to diagnose the neurotrauma of mTBI.

Unique Clinical Considerations

When considering clinical care, there are additional unique considerations for veterans and service members for clinicians to consider. Former service members with a history of mTBI often receive subsequent health care in the Veterans Health Administration (Soble et al., 2018).

Because active-duty and reserve service members are at greater risk of TBI than their civilian counterparts (DVBIC, 2018), and many military service members have sustained mTBI prior to military service (Ivins et al., 2009), it is important for clinicians to screen for a history of TBI prior to military service, as well as non-combat-related TBI. The traumatic nature of combat and the co-occurrence of posttraumatic stress increase the complexity of these injuries, and injury characteristics (e.g.,

distance from blast) are often based on self-report that may have questionable accuracy because of the intense psychological stress during the time of injury (Soble et al., 2018).

Hearing loss and tinnitus occur in up to 60% of individuals with blast-related TBI, a rate higher than in non-blast-related TBI (Fausti et al., 2009). When exposed to the primary blast wave of an explosion, the human auditory system is at risk for both peripheral and central damage from the pressure wave. Permanent pure sensorineural hearing loss is the most prevalent type of auditory impairment in blast exposure with a 35% to 100% incidence rate in blast-injured patients (Lew et al., 2007). Rupture of the tympanic membrane, causing a conductive hearing loss, is also common, with incidence ranging from 4% to 79% (de Ceballos et al., 2004; Gondusky & Reiter, 2005; Lucic, 1995).

PTSD, Depression, and Other Psychological Health Considerations in mTBI

U.S. military veterans who deployed post-9/11 were found to have an increased risk of developing posttraumatic stress disorder compared to the general population, with a 23% overall prevalence rate (Fulton et al., 2015). Psychiatric comorbidity, including major depressive disorder and/or generalized anxiety disorder postdeployment, was reported in 18% of post-9/11 veterans following combat-related mTBI relative to other veterans without mTBI (Stein et al., 2015). PTSD is described as the most commonly diagnosed comorbid psychiatric diagnosis in veterans with deployment-related mTBIs (Carlson et al., 2010). Research findings suggest that PTSD and major depressive disorder contribute to cognitive dysfunction. Cooper et al. (2011) reported that post-9/11 service members with PTSD symptoms and major depressive disorder had a high risk for self-reported cognitive dysfunction, even in the absence of a history of mTBI.

A comparison study of measures of psychiatric functioning, postconcussive symptoms, deployment-related PTSD, pain coping, and a brief neuropsychological evaluation demonstrated veterans with comorbid mTBI and PTSD reported significantly higher postinjury symptoms, as well as greater pain intensity and challenges coping, and performed more poorly on measures of recall but not on measures of attention, encoding, or executive functioning (Aase et al., 2018). In summary, research findings across numerous studies suggest neuropsychological deficits and persistent symptoms are driven by PTSD in the context of mTBI, and in the absence of mTBI, neuropsychological deficits can be caused by PTSD and depression.

SLPs and Interdisciplinary Care for Veterans and Service Members

There are several examples of high-profile multiprovider care models for persistent symptoms of mTBI. One such model is the Marcus Institute of Brain Health (MIBH) at the University of Colorado Anschutz medical campus, where care for veterans moves from multiprovider to true interdisciplinary care (Hardin & Kelly, 2019). Interdisciplinary care requires that providers interact regularly and that care planning incorporates all discipline perspectives in client-centered care. At the MIBH, clinicians practice in a co-located group of spaces, allowing for easy communication throughout the day on specific patient performance and concerns. The MIBH intensive outpatient care team is led by neurology with accompanying providers from speech-language pathology, physical therapy, sleep, behavioral health, clinical pharmacy, mind-body medicine, art therapy, and case management. During 3-day evaluations, SLPs participate in a patient-centered group clinical interview, screen auditory processing skills, and assess cognitive and communication factors. Interventionally, speech-language pathology has three roles on the team, providing both individual and group-based care. Individual sessions occur approximately 3 days per week and often target communication strategies, metacognitive strategy instruction, and memory strategies. Patient group sessions are transdisciplinary in nature, where SLPs go with patients outside of the traditional clinic environments to practice strategies from physical therapy, speech, and behavior in a more real-world setting (Hardin & Kelly, 2019). Working with family members, the speech team also co-treats with behavioral health on how mTBI symptoms can impact communication at home and offering strategies to increase success. While the MIBH offers civilian-centered care, similar models for care exist within military medicine, including the National Intrepid Center for Excellence (NICoE) in Bethesda, Maryland, and Intrepid Spirit Centers across the country. SLPs can look to these interdisciplinary programs as examples of rehabilitation for mTBI in practice.

Additional Resources Available for Working With Military-Related Individuals Following mTBI

- Defense Centers of Excellence for Psychological Health and Traumatic Brain Injury (DCoE): https://health .mil/News/Authors/Defense-Centers-of-Excellence-for-Psychological-Health-and-Traumatic-Brain-Injury
- Defense and Veterans Brain Injury Center (DVBIC): http://dvbic.dcoe .mil
- Clinician's Guide to Cognitive Rehabilitation in Mild Traumatic Brain Injury: Application for Military Service Members and Veterans: https://www.asha .org/uploaded Files/ASHA/ Practice_Portal/Clinical_Topics/ Traumatic_Brain_Injury_in_Adults/ CliniciansGuide-to-Cognitive-Reha bilitationin-Mild-Traumatic-Brain-Injury.pdf
- Mild Traumatic Brain Injury Rehabilitation Toolkit: http:// www.cs.amedd.army.mil/File Downloadpublic.aspx?docid= e454f2ce-00ae-4a2d-887d-26d547 4c8d1a

Acknowledgments. The authors would like to acknowledge Ms. Maya Albin for her contributions on trauma-informed practices. The authors would also like to acknowledge Ms. May Johnson for her assistance with manuscript preparation.

8

Traumatic Brain Injury

Kelly Knollman-Porter, Jessica A. Brown,
and Sarah E. Wallace

Chapter Learning Objectives

After reading this chapter you will be able to:

1. Describe traumatic brain injury risk factors, pathophysiology, recovery trajectories, and characteristics.
2. Describe general considerations for assessment and treatment for people with traumatic brain injury.
3. Identify various informal and standardized assessment tools for use with people with traumatic brain injury across multiple domains.
4. Identify various restorative and compensatory treatment strategies for use with people with traumatic brain injury across multiple domains.

Introduction[1]

Traumatic brain injury (TBI) is an acquired injury to the brain due to an applied force that results in widespread damage to cortical and subcortical structures. TBIs often cause a range of symptoms, including cognitive, language, speech, motor, pragmatic, and sensory impairments. No matter the cause, whether from falls, blunt-force injury, motor vehicle crashes, blast injuries, or other mechanisms, the devastating social, emotional, physical, and cognitive effects of the injury often lead to substantial and permanent changes to a person's life. The deficits associated with TBI are devastating to the people who survive the TBI as well as their loved ones and community. In this chapter, we will focus on the cognitive and communication deficits commonly experienced by individuals with TBI

[1]Although the focus of this chapter is primarily adults with TBI, unfortunately, children are also affected by TBI. Much of the strategies and information presented within this chapter may still apply to children with TBI, but readers should seek additional information about TBI rehabilitation within an educational system and developmental issues that affect children with TBI.

and will provide guidelines for assessment and treatment practices.

Incidence and Risk Factors

Estimates suggest that in 2019, there were 223,135 TBI-related hospitalizations in the United States (Centers for Disease Control and Prevention [CDC], 2022a), with even greater numbers of injuries likely occurring without documentation. Furthermore in 2019, TBIs resulted in 60,611 deaths in the United States. This epidemic results in approximately 611 TBI-related hospitalizations and 176 TBI-related deaths per day in the United States. Adults 75 years and older had the highest numbers and rates of TBI-related hospitalizations and deaths, accounting for about 32% of hospitalizations and 28% of deaths related to TBI. During 2018 and 2019, American Indian or Alaska Native, non-Hispanic people had the highest average annual age-adjusted rate of TBI-related deaths when compared to other racial and ethnic groups. People residing in the South are at greatest risk for TBI-related deaths over those living in the Midwest, West, and Northeast (CDC, 2022b).

Information about the prevalence of the effects of TBI is limited; however, estimates suggest that in the United States, between 3.2 million and 5.3 million survivors of TBI are living with varying degrees of permanent disability resulting from their injury (Selassie et al., 2008; Thurman et al., 1999; Zaloshnja et al., 2008). Long-term deficits impair an individual's ability to live independently such that 76% of adults with moderate-to-severe brain injury reside in assisted living facili-

ties or require total support from a care partner for completion of daily living activities (Colantonio et al., 2004). Due to these deficits, the estimated total health care spending, including Medicaid, Medicare, and private health insurance, secondary to nonfatal TBI was more than $46 billion annually (Miller et al., 2021). These data are perhaps an underestimate because TBIs are often underreported due to poor recognition of the symptoms or reluctance to report the injury, although this may be particularly true with mild TBIs rather than moderate or severe (Lovell et al., 2002; McCrea et al., 2004; Sosin et al., 1996; Summers et al., 2009).

A disproportionate number of people with TBIs have preexisting conditions, including substance abuse, a previous TBI, and medical conditions. Alcohol or other controlled substances are often a factor in motor vehicle crashes, pedestrian accidents, assaults, and falls that can result in TBI. Additionally, their continued use and abuse often affect rehabilitation success. Previous TBIs are a risk factor for a second or subsequent TBI due to changes in problem solving, judgment, motor control, and impulsivity. Preexisting medical conditions such as heart disease and high blood pressure, as well as psychiatric illnesses, appear to put people at greater risk for TBI. In addition to these preexisting conditions, as many as 25% to 87% of prisoners report having experienced a head injury or TBI compared to about 8.5% of the general population (CDC, n.d.), with frequency of TBI associated with more convictions, greater violent offenses, decreased mental health, and increased drug use in this population (Williams et al., 2010). Additionally, a South Carolina study provided data suggesting that 60% of men and 72% of women who are incarcerated experienced a TBI (Ferguson et al., 2012). Individuals who are unhoused or have a low socioeconomic status also are at greater risk for TBI and for underreporting TBIs (Stubbs et al., 2020; Topolovec-Vranic et al., 2012). The increased incidence and risk in certain segments of the population highlight the need for screenings and targeted education efforts.

Pathophysiology

To fully appreciate cognitive communication deficits associated with TBI, it is useful to understand the nature of the neurologic damage sustained during and after traumatic events. TBIs are often categorized based on two types of brain damage: penetrating TBI (i.e., open head injury) and nonpenetrating blunt force TBI (i.e., closed head injury).

Penetrating TBI

A penetrating TBI occurs when a foreign object, such as a high-velocity bullet, shrapnel from an explosive device, or a sharp weapon, passes through the skull and meningeal layers. This type of open head injury results in brain tissue destruction from the foreign objects as well as from the generation of a pressure wave within the skull. Additionally, people with TBI may experience secondary complications (e.g., infections) from the presence of foreign material, such as bone fragments embedded in the brain. Penetrating TBIs are more likely than nonpenetrating injuries to result in focal damage to the brain and, therefore, often result in cognitive and

communicative deficits specific to the area of brain damage.

Nonpenetrating TBI

Nonpenetrating injuries, the most frequent cause of TBIs, may occur when a head accelerates and strikes an external object, when an external object hits a stationary head, or when the head experiences significant movement without impact. For example, an injury may occur during a motor vehicle crash when the driver's head accelerates forward and hits the steering wheel. Similarly, a motor vehicle crash can result in extreme forward and backward movement of the head with no significant impact on an external object (i.e., whiplash injuries). Finally, nonpenetrating injuries can result from an external object such as a baseball hitting a stationary head.

People who survive blunt-force injuries are often left with widespread neurological damage resulting in part due to linear acceleration/deceleration and rotational forces. The mechanical forces associated with violent movement of the brain may lead to coup (damage at the point of impact) and contrecoup (damage opposite the original point of impact or acceleration) damage, lacerations of brain tissue, and widespread shearing and tearing of neurons known as diffuse axonal injury resulting from rotational forces (Baron & Jallo, 2007; Figure 8–1). In addition to the brain's response to trauma, additional consequences of the injury can also occur, including but not limited to elevated intercranial pressure secondary to cerebral edema and/or traumatic hydrocephalus and seizure activity. These secondary consequences of TBI

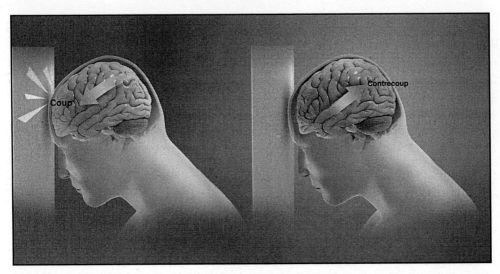

Figure 8–1. Coup and contrecoup damage occurring during brain injury. By manu5 (http://www.scientificanimations.com/wiki-images/), CC By-SA 4.0 (https://commons.wikimedia.org/w/index.php?curid=71496323).

are monitored closely during hospitalization and can negatively influence recovery.

Injury Severity

In addition to the variety of characteristics clinicians might encounter when working with people with TBI, the severity of the injury contributes to the heterogeneous nature of this population. Injury severity has significant implications for prognosis, participation in rehabilitation, and selection of formal assessment tools. Injuries are generally labeled as mild, moderate, and severe (CDC, 2017). Blast-related TBIs, such as those associated with military combat, have a unique signature. The injuries can be described as primary (i.e., resulting from a pressure wave impacting air-filled cavities), secondary (i.e., similar to the injuries found in penetrating TBIs and blunt trauma), tertiary (i.e., resulting from the body being thrown with force at another object), and quaternary (i.e., burns and chemical exposure; DePalma et al., 2005). Some TBIs may be compounded by polytrauma, or multiple traumatic injuries to the body, loss of vision and hearing, and posttraumatic stress disorder. The damaged peripheral sensory and motor systems may have a significant effect on the person's ability to participate in rehabilitation. For this reason, adaptive or modified treatment approaches may be warranted involving a multidisciplinary team of rehabilitation specialists.

The Glasgow Coma Scale (GCS) is often used to determine the severity classification of initial TBI and is the most widely used tool for quantifying comas (Teasdale & Jennett, 1974). This 15-point scale measures behaviors associated with eye opening, as well as the best motor and the best verbal responses within 24 hours of injury

(Table 8–1). A total score of 3 to 8 represents a severe TBI, a score of 9 to 12 represents a moderate TBI, and a score of 13 to 15 represents a mild TBI (CDC, 2017; Teasdale & Jennett, 1974). These results should be interpreted carefully because factors, such as time postinjury, pharmaceutical treatments to control brain swelling or to relax muscles, high blood alcohol levels, paralysis or hemiparesis, and communication disorders such as aphasia and dysarthria may affect performance within each area assessed.

The use of coma length as a measure of TBI severity is complicated primarily by the use of pharmaceutical treatments to induce a coma for medical stabilization and the potential presence of alcohol or drugs at the time of the injury. An additional complication is the use of motor and speech/language-dependent responses to measure coma severity in a population who is likely to have associated damage in one or both areas separate from their cognitive impairments as described previously. For these reasons, coma length alone should not be used as an index of TBI severity. Because of the limitations

inherent to the GCS, additional items are typically considered when classifying TBI severity. Those include results of structural imaging testing, length of time for which the individual has lost consciousness, the length of time the person has experienced posttraumatic amnesia, and the Abbreviated Injury Scale score for the head and neck region (Association for the Advancement of Automotive Medicine, 2016; Baker et al., 1974; Brasure et al., 2012; CDC, 2015).

The Abbreviated Injury Scale is a globally used scoring system that classifies injury to an anatomical structure (in this case, head and neck) according to a 6-point severity scale such that scores of 1 relate to minor injury severity and scores of 6 relate to maximal injury severity. Standardized terminology is used to describe characteristics of each severity rating level in order to maximize fidelity and interrater reliability. Use of the Abbreviated Injury Scale in conjunction with other measures such as the GCS correlates to long-term outcomes better than when these scales are used in isolation (Foreman et al., 2007). The Abbreviated Injury Scale measure

Table 8–1. Glasgow Coma Scale Responses

	Eye-Opening Response	Best Motor Response	Best Verbal Response
1	No response	No response	No response
2	Eye opening to pain	Extension of limbs	Incomprehensible
3	Eye opening to speech	Flexion of limbs	Inappropriate
4	Spontaneous eye opening	Withdraws from stimulus	Confused
5		Localizes sensory stimulus	Oriented ×3
6		Obeys commands	

has been extensively revised over time (1998, 2008, 2015) to reflect international and cross-professional use of quantifying anatomical trauma severity (Loftis et al., 2018).

Another measurement of severity is posttraumatic amnesia (PTA), which is defined as the time between injury and recovery of continuous memory. The individual must demonstrate the ability to remember events for a 24-hour period before being considered out of PTA. There is a relationship between the length of PTA and the severity of the TBI as displayed in Table 8–2 (Levin et al., 1983; Ponsford et al., 2016). Although using a comprehensive approach and considering all these factors is critically important to classification, limitations still exist in using any severity criteria as a predictor of outcome without considering other personal and environmental factors. PTA is commonly measured by the Galveston Orientation and Amnesia Test (Levin et al., 1979) as described below.

Mild TBI

About 75% to 90% of TBIs are categorized as mild TBIs (or concussions) each year based on initial symptoms (Janak, 2015). They are generally described as having normal results on structural imaging and involve the person experiencing less than 30 minutes of loss of consciousness or 0 to 1 day of posttraumatic amnesia. Additionally, mild TBI is classified when the person receives a score between 13 and 15 as their best score on the GCS within 24 hours or a score between 1 and 2 out of 6 on the Abbreviated Injury Scale.

The symptoms associated with mild TBI can be physical (e.g., dizziness), emotional (e.g., depression, irritability), sleep related (e.g., hypersomnia or insomnia), and/or cognitively based (e.g., mental fogginess, difficulty concentrating), impacting the person's ability to return to academic or occupational activities previously performed with ease (CDC, 2022c). While symptom resolution occurs in 80% to 90% of mild TBI, approximately 10% to 20% of individuals experience persistent symptoms (Jotwani & Harmon, 2010). Despite the term "mild," the long-term consequences of these injuries can be substantial. Because of the mildness of the injury, many people neglect seeking medical attention, and if they do seek medical attention, they may not receive complete information about the potential long-term deficits. The purpose of this chapter is to provide an overview

Table 8–2. Length of PTA and Initial Injury Severity

Length of PTA	Initial Injury Severity
Less than 5 minutes	Very mild deficits
5–59 minutes	Mild deficits
1–24 hours	Moderate long-term deficits
1–7 days	Severe long-term deficits
Greater than 7 days	Very severe long-term consequences

of TBI-related information and mostly focus on moderate and severe injuries as Chapter 7 covers mild TBI.

Moderate and Severe TBI

According to the CDC (2017), moderate TBIs result in normal or abnormal structural imaging results and involve the person experiencing between 30 minutes and 24 hours of loss of consciousness and greater than 1 and fewer than 7 days of posttraumatic amnesia. Additionally, moderate TBIs are those that result in characteristics consistent with a GCS scale between 9 and 12 and an Abbreviated Injury Scale score: Head of 3 out of 6. Severe injuries are those during which the structural imaging may be normal or abnormal and the person experiences a loss of consciousness greater than 24 hours and a period of posttraumatic amnesia greater than 7 days. People with severe TBI typically score between 3 and 8 on the GCS and between 4 and 6 out of 6 on the Abbreviated Injury Scale score: Head (Brasure et al., 2012; CDC, 2017).

Impaired Consciousness

When an injury to the brain is severe enough, a person may become unconscious. Varying terms and definitions are used to describe an individual's state of consciousness; such definitions may be based on an individual's level of arousal, time in which specific characteristics have been demonstrated, or awareness of an individual's surroundings. Controversy exists about the exact terminology to use when describing people with prolonged disorders of consciousness. The term "coma" denotes a complete state of unconsciousness (i.e., no environmental interaction) with no eye opening and an absence of sleep/wake cycles. The person does not communicate and does not respond to sound, touch, or pain. There is no purposeful motor activity and no indication of receptive or expressive language skills (American Congress of Rehabilitation Medicine, 1995; Jennett & Teasdale, 1977). A vegetative state is defined as the complete lack of environmental interaction with some eye opening and periods of wakefulness and sleep; however, the person will exhibit a lack of visual tracking, objective recognition, and other environmental interaction. Responses such as smiling or crying as a reaction to visual or auditory stimuli are brainstem reflexes that can be beyond the person's control in the event of extensive cortical damage (Multi-Society Task Force on PVS, 1994a). A person may be determined to be in a minimally conscious state when they demonstrate eye opening and sleep/wake cycles and some visual tracking while exhibiting some behaviors associated with conscious awareness such as contingent smiling (Giacino et al., 2002)—this individual may have preserved arousal and fluctuating levels of awareness. During this state of limited awareness, the person may inconsistently follow some simple instructions or may communicate with yes/no spoken responses or gestures (regardless of accuracy). These types of responses are referred to as purposeful behaviors. Some people may never improve beyond a minimally conscious state, but others may improve to a state of confusion and demonstrate disorientation and severe cognitive impairments. Emergence from a minimally conscious state is characterized as a consistent ability to communicate and purposeful use of at least two objects. The person may follow simple commands.

Recovery Trajectories of TBI

The initial severity of the brain injury can influence the speed and degree of recovery following TBI. Yet not all people who survive TBI follow the same recovery trajectory, with some returning to previous levels of function in a relatively quick state while others experience persistent functional disability impacting occupational, social, and daily living activities despite extensive rehabilitative efforts. Comorbidities, resilience, cognitive reserve, cognitive stressors, and treatment received can influence the degree of recovery from TBI (Iverson et al., 2017; Sullivan et al., 2016). In addition, older age has been associated with greater disability following TBI in terms of physical and cognitive function (Graham et al., 2010). As greater life expectancy and mobility of older adults is increasing, so is the increased risk of falls and the incidence of TBI (Faul & Coronado, 2015).

Two additional factors that may also influence recovery are race and insurance status. A study exploring the discharge destination of patients with moderate or severe TBI found that Hispanic and Black patients were less likely to be discharged to higher-level rehabilitation than non-Hispanic White patients, even when considering older adults for whom uniform insurance coverage existed (i.e., Medicare) (Meagher et al., 2015). These factors may contribute to why Black, Hispanic, and

uninsured people with TBI have worse outcomes when compared to other members of the public (Haider et al., 2008). Finally, inadequate access to and/or the unavailability of specialized TBI-related care that is age appropriate, secondary to rural health disparities, may further contribute to long-term outcomes in people who survive TBI (Eliacin et al., 2018).

Comas are indicative of widespread cortical and subcortical damage; consequently, the length of a coma has previously been used as a useful predictor of long-term disability (Wilson et al., 1991; Zafonte et al., 1996). A coma lasting less than a day is generally associated with a good recovery, whereas coma durations of 1 to 2 weeks may lead to moderate disability. Prolonged comas, those lasting 2 to 5 weeks in duration, are rare; however, people experiencing prolonged comas may progress to statuses indicative of brain death, vegetative state, or locked-in syndrome (Gosseries et al., 2011).

TBI Characteristics

Cognitive Impairments

Cognitive deficits following TBI vary significantly depending on the location and extent of the brain areas damaged. Additionally, although most people with TBI may have deficits in one or many areas of cognition, the extent of impairment in each area may vary. Generally, many people with TBI experience deficits in orientation, attention, memory, pragmatics, executive functions, and awareness. Although many of these aspects of cognition were discussed in Chapters 1, 2, and 3, a review of these deficits as they manifest in people with TBI is provided here.

Orientation

Orientation to the environment is a significant problem for many people with TBI. Orientation is typically measured in terms of person, place, time, and purpose or situation. Orientation may be evaluated daily or multiple times a day while hospitalized or during residential rehabilitation programs. Typically, orientation to person (i.e., self) returns before orientation to place (e.g., town, city, state, facility). Orientation to place is usually followed by an improved orientation to time (e.g., season, year, month, week, day, date). Orientation to purpose or situation (e.g., injury, rehabilitation goals) may return last and continue to be significantly impaired as the result of impaired self-awareness. Measures of orientation can take on varied degrees of specificity and can therefore be somewhat subjective.

Attention

Attention deficits are common in people with TBI regardless of the severity of their injury (Ponsford, Velikonja, et al., 2023). People with TBI may have deficits in all areas of attention, although depending on the model or theoretical framework, these types of attention may have different labels. Specific information about impairments in different types of attention and various models of attention are provided in Chapter 1. Additionally, sometimes people with TBI can be hypervigilant, become overstimulated, and are unable to be redirected (Stierwalt & Murray,

2002). Most people with TBI have difficulty selecting and prioritizing the most important information to which they should attend. These attention deficits are critical to cognitive rehabilitation because attention is believed to be foundational for all other cognitive abilities. Thus, attention deficits in people with TBI are likely to interfere with successful rehabilitation outcomes (Brooks et al., 1987). After consciousness is regained and during states of minimal awareness, attention impairments may be severe and occur across multiple attention types, creating difficulty even orienting to simple stimuli (Stierwalt & Murray, 2002). After some confusion has resolved, higher-level attention skills such as alternating attention are impaired, particularly during complex, demanding tasks.

Memory

As many as 75% of people with TBI report persistent memory problems that may be very mild or may be characterized as permanent amnesia (Thomsen, 1984). Additionally, different types of memory may be impaired in people with TBI (e.g., short-term memory, long-term memory) for various types of information (e.g., declarative memory, nondeclarative memory, visual, verbal). These types of memory are described in more detail in Chapter 2. Despite the multiple potential profiles of memory impairments, most people with TBI have more difficulty storing and retrieving declarative information than procedural information (Sohlberg et al., 2007). Even people with mild or moderate TBI demonstrate deficits in episodic memory (i.e., immediate and delayed verbal memory recall, verbal recognition, immediate and delayed visual memory recall; Miotto et al., 2010).

Executive Functions

As described in Chapter 3, executive functions are a group of cognitive processes that facilitate goal-directed behavior. Much like impairments in attention and memory following TBI, executive functions resulting from TBI deficits vary significantly in severity and type. Two general categories of executive function impairments include initiation related and inhibition related. Some examples of characteristics of executive function impairments exhibited by people with TBI include difficulty setting reasonable goals, planning and organizing their behavior to reach goals, and initiating behaviors that help achieve goals. People with TBI may also experience challenges related to inhibiting behaviors that are incompatible with reaching goals, as well as to monitoring their performance and revising plans as needed. They may also exhibit poor judgment and struggle to anticipate the difficulty of daily tasks.

Awareness and Theory of Mind

Researchers have reported up to 97% of individuals with TBI demonstrate self-awareness impairments (Sherer et al., 1998). Failure to recognize one's deficits can take a significant emotional toll on the person with TBI and their care partners, and act as a barrier to successful rehabilitation outcomes (Robertson & Schmitter-Edgecombe, 2015). Crosson and colleagues (1989) described an awareness pyramid built on a foundation of intellectual awareness, defined as the cognitive capacity to understand that a particular cognitive function is diminished from preinjury levels. They defined the middle level of the pyramid as emergent awareness. Emergent awareness is evident when the person with TBI recognizes a problem or deficits in real time. People with TBI must reach this level to activate situational specific strategies to compensate for their deficits. Crosson and colleagues (1989) suggested that, when a person with TBI reaches the top of the pyramid, they demonstrate anticipatory awareness. Anticipatory awareness is the ability to recognize that because a deficit is present, the person can predict when a problem may happen and take appropriate steps to mitigate the effect or avoid a situation completely through anticipatory compensations.

Awareness deficits may be a precursor to deficits in theory of mind. Impaired theory of mind suggests that a person has difficulty in taking another person's perspective. People who experience theory of mind deficits have difficulty determining the intentions of others, lack understanding about how their behaviors affect others, and struggle with social reciprocity (Happé et al., 1999). These impairments may significantly affect a person's ability to make friends, succeed in school, and return to work.

Communication Impairments

People with TBI experience a variety of types and severities of speech and language impairments (MacDonald, 2017; Sarno et al., 1986). Mutism is common during early stages of recovery, usually due to severe cognitive (e.g., impaired consciousness) or physical impairments (e.g., locked-in syndrome; Levin et al., 1983). Sometimes they may be diagnosed with aphasia, which may present as transient word-finding problems during the early stages of recovery. Incidence of aphasia in people with TBI ranges from 2% to 32% (Braun & Baribeau, 1987; Sarno, 1980; Sarno et al., 1986). Usually, aphasia following TBI is the result of focal damage to the areas responsible for language functions. About one third of people with severe TBI have characteristics of dysarthria. Finally, in addition to dysarthria and aphasia, almost all people with severe TBI experience cognitive communication impairments.

Cognitive communication impairments result in ineffective or inefficient communication due to deficits in areas of cognition that support communication (e.g., attention, memory, executive functions). Cognitive communication deficits may be subtle and therefore may only be detected through analysis of discourse tasks. Discourse produced by people with TBI may be similar to people with right hemisphere disorder as discussed in Chapter 4 and include poor topic maintenance, cohesion, and coherence (Coelho et al., 2005). They may also have difficulty understanding the gist and abstract language. Although deficits in discourse production and comprehension are subtle, these may also significantly affect a person's participation in daily activities as well as return to school or work.

Little is known about the exact trajectory of people with TBI with communication impairments in part because of the variety of impairments and levels of severities that may occur after TBI. For people with severe communication impairments after TBI, recovery of nat-

ural speech may occur over an extended period of time. As a result, clinicians should continue to reassess people with TBI over time, particularly as cognitive abilities change (Light et al., 1988). Of the people with severe TBI who initially cannot use natural speech to meet communication needs, 55% to 59% recover functional natural speech during the middle stages of recovery, which was defined by the authors as Ranchos Los Amigos Scale Levels of Cognitive Functioning–Revised (Hagen, 1982, 2000) Level V on the original scale with the highest level of functioning being Level VIII (Dongilli et al., 1992). By these middle stages, if the person is unable to rely on natural speech, it is often due to severe motor speech or language disorders (Dongilli et al., 1992).

Psychosocial Experiences

A period of PTA can occur following a comatose state for some individuals with TBI. During this time, people with TBI may experience behavioral disturbances such as agitation, disinhibition, impulsivity, aggression, emotional lability, and restlessness (Phyland et al., 2021). Agitation specifically has been associated with poorer outcomes, including longer hospital stays, reduced engagement in therapy, and less frequent return to home independently (Bogner et al., 2001; Singh et al., 2014). In addition, these behavioral disturbances can create stress and a safety risk for care partners (Silver et al., 2004). McKay and colleagues (2020) reported an association between agitation and cooccurring cognitive impairment. Therefore, treatments targeting improvements in cognition during the middle and late stages of posttraumatic amnesia may facilitate reduced agitation in some people with TBI (McKay et al., 2020). Staff, care partners, and clinicians should avoid repeated drill-based questioning at this time and instead use short, simple communication methods with added picture support or visual aids to facilitate understanding and feelings of safety (Ponsford, Trevena-Peters, et al., 2023).

People with TBI may also exhibit deficits in social communication at various stages during recovery. Social communication involves the skills needed to meet social goals in a variety of personally relevant settings (Togher et al., 2023). During social interactions, some people with TBI may not recognize social cues (e.g., person looking at watch suggesting it is time to leave), violate social norms (e.g., standing too close to a stranger), and not understand implied meanings. Failure to recognize social communication norms can negatively impact social and occupational relationships leading to isolation and loneliness, making some people with TBI vulnerable to exploitation and crime (Williams et al., 2018).

Other Relevant Areas of Impairment

In addition to cognitive and communication impairments, many people with TBI experience auditory or vestibular symptoms such as dizziness and vertigo, tinnitus and hyperacusis, hearing loss, and loudness sensitivity (Dennis, 2009). Injuries specifically resulting from a blast may include tympanic membrane rupture, dislocations of the ossicles, or cochlea damage. This damage may be a sign of blast exposure despite the lack of other signs or symptoms. Immediately following blast injury, people may experience temporary hearing loss and tinnitus that should be closely monitored.

In addition to communication impairments, people with TBI often also have dysphagia. The severity of swallowing impairment and prognosis can vary greatly in this population. The primary concern for individuals with swallowing impairments is aspiration, which occurs when food or liquids are present below the vocal folds. Some people may cough or have a wet "gurgly" voice due to aspiration, while others may not exhibit signs or symptoms of aspiration. Assessment and treatment for dysphagia can be complicated by other physical, sensory, and cognitive impairments experienced by many people with TBI.

As the purpose of this chapter is to provide information about cognitive and communication impairments following TBI, readers are referred to resources in Table 8–3 for additional information about hearing loss, visual disturbances, and swallowing after TBI.

Assessment

General Assessment Considerations

As part of a comprehensive TBI evaluation, speech-language pathologists should consider a number of factors. Injury severity is an important factor that is described in detail in the next section. In addition to determining severity, it is important that clinicians consider that poor performance on formal and informal assessment measures

Table 8–3. Resources About Dysphagia, Audiology, and Vision in People With TBI

Audiology
Dennis, K. C. (2009). Current perspectives on traumatic brain injury. *ASHA Access Audiology*. www.asha.org/aud/articles/currentTBI.htm
Dodd-Murphy, J. (2014). Auditory effects of blast exposure: Community outreach following an industrial explosion. http://www.asha.org/aud/Articles/Auditory-Effects-of-Blast-Exposure/?utm_source=asha&utm_medium=enewsletter&utm_campaign=accessaud051214#sthash.zOdcZBFb.dpuf
Myers, P., Henry, J., Zaugg, T., & Kendall, C. (2009). Tinnitus evaluation and management considerations for persons with mild traumatic brain injury. First published in *ASHA Access Audiology*, *8.* http://www.asha.org/aud/articles/TinnitusTBI/
Dysphagia
American Speech-Language-Hearing Association Evidence maps. http://ncepmaps.org/ptbi/tx/
Mackay, L. E., Morgan, A. S., & Bernstein, B. A. (1999). Swallowing disorders in severe brain injury: Risk factors affecting return to oral intake. *Archives of Physical Medicine and Rehabilitation*, *80*, 365–371.
Mandaville, A., Ray, A., Robertson, H., Foster, C., & Jesser, C. (2014). A retrospective review of swallow dysfunction in patients with severe traumatic brain injury. *Dysphagia*, *29*, 1–9.
Morgan, A. S., & Mackay, L. E. (1999). Causes and complications associated with swallowing disorders in traumatic brain injury. *The Journal of Head Trauma Rehabilitation*, *14*, 454–461.
Vision
Hac, N. E. F., & Gold, D. R. (2022). Neuro-visual and vestibular manifestations of concussion and mild TBI. *Current Neurology and Neuroscience Reports*, *22*, 219–229. https://doi.org/10.1007/s11910-022-01184-9
Kelts, E. A. (2010). Traumatic brain injury and visual dysfunction: A limited overview. *NeuroRehabilitation*, *27*, 223–229.
Ripley, D. L., Politzer, T., Berryman, A. Rasavage, K., & Weintraub, A. (2010). The Vision Clinic: An interdisciplinary method for assessment and treatment of visual problems after traumatic brain injury. *NeuroRehabilitation*, *27*, 231–235. https://doi.org/10.3233/NRE-2010-0602

may reflect motor or sensory-perceptual problems, sleep-wake disturbances, pain, medication, preexisting academic difficulties, or emotional-behavioral deficits (e.g., depression and anxiety) (Ponsford, Velikonja, et al., 2023). To ensure assessment results accurately represent accurate cognitive communication levels of performance, accommodations should be made for sensory loss (e.g., glasses and hearing aids). Additionally, during the acute stages of TBI, people often make dramatic performance changes, so it is helpful to use established scales (e.g., Rancho Los Amigos Level of Cognitive Functioning Scale) to describe their overall function and to continue to assess their abilities throughout treatment. Finally, people with TBI tend to perform better within structured tasks in a clinical setting than they do in the real world, thus emphasizing the need for assessment measures that reflect functional performance in the real world.

Interprofessional collaborations may be particularly vital for successfully evaluating and documenting deficits following TBI. The unique challenges faced by people with TBI across a variety of domains (e.g., physical, sensory, cognitive, and emotional) require a team approach to ensure best practice and implementation of evidence-based techniques to serve the individual as a whole rather than as someone experiencing distinct deficits and challenges. Recently, rehabilitation professionals have begun using the term "transdisciplinary efforts" to describe the collaborative and interactive roles of professionals rather than as distinct or siloed domains of care (Karol, 2014). In rehabilitative settings, transdisciplinary assessment practices, including the perspective and expertise of multiple professionals, may include, but are not limited to, audiologists, occupational therapists, physical therapists, respiratory therapists, recreation therapists, nurses, physicians, dieticians, and neuropsychologists. Navigating the team dynamic and determining the various roles and responsibilities of each professional involved is necessary for thorough evaluation and treatment post-injury (Sander et al., 2009).

In addition to these factors for consideration, rehabilitation professionals must consider potential constraints that may serve as barriers to the assessment process. Some such barriers may include time constraints, availability of testing measures, and reimbursement practices. Specifically, depending on the setting in which an evaluation is conducted, time and procedural constraints may inhibit the type and length of assessments chosen by an SLP. Little evidence is available to inform the average length of evaluation in acute, post-acute, outpatient, and skilled nursing settings; however, it is likely that many therapists are encouraged or required to complete a full evaluation of cognitive, communicative, and swallowing competencies in a single, often short 30- to 60-minute session. Co-occurring deficits post-TBI such as decreased processing speed and alertness, motor challenges, sensory challenges (e.g., vision impairments), and neurobehavioral deficits (e.g., agitation) may further contribute to these difficulties. In the early stages of rehabilitation, clinicians may consider the use of informal assessments, which evaluate discrete aspects of cognition in isolation in a controlled environment to refrain from distractions that hinder performance. In contrast, as the person becomes more stable, clinicians should consider selecting assessment subtests or tasks that are reflective of a variety of domains simultaneously, which may require access from more than one assessment tool. Of course, the severity of cognitive deficits may continue to affect the appropriate approach to assessment beyond the early stages of rehabilitation in some situations. A model suggested by the World Health Organization may assist clinicians in developing holistic testing protocols when time and procedural constraints confound testing practices.

Models of Assessment

The World Health Organization's Classification of Functioning, Disability and Health (WHO-ICF) provides a logical, globally recognized model for assessing deficits at the impairment, activity, and functioning levels within the recovery continuum of TBI (McDougall et al., 2010; Wade, 2005); however, a great deal of focus has recently emerged regarding

the evaluation of deficits in real-world, functional settings. According to the WHO-ICF model, a person's functioning ability, including participation in everyday activities, comprises the interaction among the experienced health condition, contextual real-world factors, and personal characteristics. Thus, a variety of factors must be considered when evaluating the outcomes of a disorder or disease given this biopsychosocial health perspective—encompassing both the individual (i.e., personal factors) and societal perspective (i.e., environmental factors). The WHO-ICF model offers a unifying conceptual and terminological framework for rehabilitation professionals (Figure 8–2, used with permission).

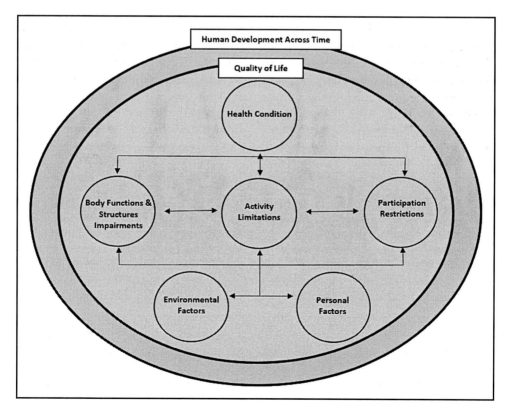

Figure 8–2. World Health Organization's Classification of Functioning, Disability and Health. Used with permission from the World Health Organization (WHO).

Adequately assessing functioning at the individual levels requires an assessment protocol that meets the following five primary objectives (Constantinidou et al., 2012):

- Evaluate strengths and weaknesses and their effect on premorbid abilities.
- Guide the development and implementation of short- and long-term treatment goals.
- Guide the development of remedial and compensatory strategies.
- Steer discussion with people with TBI and family members challenges within the recovery process.
- Serve as an anchor for future changes resulting from recovery and treatment.

In the sections that follow, we will discuss various methods available to rehabilitation professionals attempting to reach these aims during the assessment process. Globally, this will include consideration of injury severity and personal demographics; self-report and quality of life measures; standardized, objective testing methods; and functional, ecologically valid tasks.

Early Assessment Techniques

The following principles are important considerations during assessment and treatment of individuals with altered consciousness (e.g., Ranchos Level I, II, or III) or posttraumatic amnesia. First, the person must always be treated with dignity and respect. Second, it is important to remember that the person may understand what is said near them, so be careful to only say things that you would want them to hear. Finally, the person may be able to perceive pain without a way to respond or communicate about it, so it is important that they are monitored for possible discomfort or pain. For example, watch that the person's limbs are free from any moving parts of a wheelchair or the bed rail before moving them. During these stages of recovery, assessment and monitoring of communication and swallowing should occur. Because individuals with posttraumatic amnesia may experience behavioral disturbances such as disinhibition, lability, aggression, impulsivity, and restlessness, the use of short, simple language is recommended to facilitate clarity of an intended message (Ponsford, Trevena-Peters, et al., 2023). Repeated, drill-based questioning should be avoided, which may lead to frustration and agitation. To facilitate communication between care partners, staff, and the person with TBI, the use of simple supportive communication strategies via picture support may be appropriate for those who are alert and can attend to simple stimuli (Nielsen et al., 2020).

Posttraumatic Amnesia

As stated previously, PTA is another indicator of TBI severity, which also has prognostic utility. PTA can be formally assessed using one of the two following tools.

The Galveston Orientation and Amnesia Test (Levin et al., 1979) was the first test of PTA. The test has 10 questions that are heavily weighted toward orientation but also tap into the person's recall of information. For example, the first few questions require the person to provide their name, place of birth, and place of residence. The examiner also asks the person to describe details about the first event they recall after the injury and the last event they can recall before the injury. This helps the clinician determine what the person remembers about their experience. A person can obtain a maximum score of 100 on the test. Scores between 80 and 100 points indicate performance within normal limits. Scores between 66 and 79 points suggest borderline disability, and scores ranging from 0 to 65 points are representative of clear difficulty with PTA (Levin et al., 1979). An individual who receives a consistent score of 75 or greater three tries in a row is considered to have recovered from PTA. The Children's Orientation and Amnesia Test (Ewing-Cobbs et al., 1990) was normed on 146 children with ages between 3 and 15 years. The 16-item scale assesses general orientation, temporal orientation, and memory (i.e., immediate, short term, and remote) and takes about 5 to 10 minutes to administer. The test can be administered daily. A score of 78 or greater on three consecutive occasions indicates that the child is no longer in a state of PTA.

Scales and Observational Checklists

Severity of injury is also measured through medical chart reviews, case history interviews, and completion of general observational scales. Particularly relevant case history questions for this population include questions about demographics such as age and date of injury (i.e., measures orientation and memory), goals (i.e., measure self-

awareness), occupational demands, level of care partner support, and level of education (i.e., education may correlate with performance on standardized tests). The provided case form (Appendices 8–A and 8–B) serves as a starting point for clinicians when performing medical chart reviews and establishing basic case histories. As a supplement, both person and care partner interviews should be initiated.

With information from the case history, as well as from observational scales or checklists, clinicians may plan an appropriate, comprehensive evaluation for the person with TBI. In particular, the use of formal or structured assessment of some areas of cognition (e.g., attention) may be inappropriate during early stages of cognitive recovery because test results obtained during this phase are typically unreliable and invalid due to the person's state of generalized confusion and agitation. Moreover, formal testing procedures and stimuli may cause overstimulation and increased agitation. Alternatively, reliance on scales and checklists will help speech-language pathologists determine a general sense of severity, thereby conveying the attention and behavioral abilities of the person with TBI. The use of additional, structured measures (formal or informal) in conjunction with scales and checklists may provide a holistic evaluation of the individual's skills and serve as baseline data regarding performance in a variety of areas.

Ranchos Los Amigos Levels of Cognitive Functioning–Revised (RLA-R) (Hagen, 2000; Hagen et al., 1972) is perhaps the most widely used measure of cognitive status of people with TBI. The original scale described eight categories that effectively evaluated a person's level of cognitive ability at a given point in time. Individuals are assigned to a level according to several behavioral variables. The written descriptors capture in detail the behavior and characteristics of a person with TBI as they move from coma to minimally responsive behavioral states to purposeful and independent behavior. This scale was revised from its original 8 points to a 10-point scale to address changes in independence during later rehabilitative stages (Hagen, 2000; "Ranchos Los Amigos Cognitive Scale Revised," 2014). Levels IX and X were added to provide a greater definition of purposeful and appropriate behaviors, which are more sensitive to individuals at the higher end of the recovery spectrum. The revision also provided clearer descriptions of the behaviors at each level, so that it is easier to differentiate people who are high functioning.

This scale is a valid and sensitive measure of the behaviors that are associated with long-term functional improvement and can guide the development of a comprehensive assessment and treatment plan. It is important for clinicians to remember that people progress through the levels at different rates and that at times one person might demonstrate characteristics that are associated with more than one level. In these cases, frequent documentation of an individual's abilities and characteristics across levels and contexts may be appropriate to reflect accurate progress and continued needs.

Another commonly used scale that helps clinicians describe a person's general level of function is the Functional Independence Measure (FIM™; Guide for Uniform Data Set for Medical Rehabilitation, 1996; Wright, 2000; Table 8–4). The purpose of this assessment tool is to capture, based on observation and for-

Table 8–4. Functional Independence Measure Rating Scale and Interpretations

Score	Description
7	100% Functional—independent (I)
6	Functional with assistance of a device or extra time
5	Occasional difficulty, 90% functional—requires assistance less than 10% of the time (supervision)
4	Minimally impaired; 75%–90% functional—requires assistance 10%–25% of the time
3	Moderately impaired; 50%–74% functional—requires assistance 25%–50% of the time
2	Maximally impaired; 25%–49% functional—requires assistance 50%–75% of the time
1	Profoundly impaired; 0%–24% functional—requires assistance 75%–100% of the time

mal assessments, the person's level of disability and the amount of assistance required for them to complete everyday tasks. Five of the 18 items assessed relate to cognitive abilities. The clinician uses a 7-point scale to rate the person as being dependent or independent in that particular activity such that a score of 1 refers to complete dependence and a score of 7 refers to complete independence. The five cognitive items include cognitive comprehension, expression, social interaction, problem solving, and memory. Several benefits exist regarding the implementation of FIM scores in practice. First, this scale provides a common language across rehabilitative disciplines such that professionals in a variety of domains (e.g., occupational therapy and physical therapy) can subjectively rate client independence and supportive needs on a well-established, standardized scale. Furthermore, this assessment measure provides quantifiable data for initial evaluation and progress monitoring for primarily subjective clinical observations.

Finally, the Disability Rating Scale (Rappaport et al., 1982) was designed to measure functional changes in people with moderate and severe TBI as they progress through various stages of recovery. The clinician rates the person's behavior in four categories: consciousness (i.e., eye opening, verbal response, motor response), cognitive abilities (i.e., feeding, toileting, grooming), level of dependence on others, and employability. The Disability Rating Scale yields a score out of 29 points, with higher scores indicating a greater extent of impairment. Because it covers a wide range of recovery, it may not be as sensitive to subtle changes, particularly at the mild end of the scale. Malec

and colleagues' (2012) modified telephone interview protocol, the Disability Rating Scale Post-acute Interview, was found to be an efficient approach to standardized follow-up assessment for people with TBI. Additionally, this modified version was found to be more sensitive and provides more detail for people with mild impairments than the original Disability Rating Scale.

Self-Report and Quality of Life Measures

Many professionals rely on client self-report to diagnose and determine symptomatology for individuals with TBI. This is because performance on standardized, objective measures can be skewed based on a variety of environmental and personal factors and provide inconsistent identification of deficits (Wood & Liossi, 2006). Current suggested models from the WHO encourage rehabilitation professionals and researchers to collect information from the perspective of individuals themselves, as well as from other sources. Additionally, self-report elicited through structured screening tools or client interviews is increasingly recognized as the best, or perhaps only, way to estimate TBI incidence and chronic TBI prevalence (Dams-O'Connor et al., 2014). In fact, a 2010 panel of rehabilitation specialists documented the importance of self-report measures, indicating that a multidimensional approach to patient-reported outcomes was a promising evaluative tool across the brain injury severity spectrum (Wilde et al., 2010).

Initiation of person-centered care relies on the involvement of the client during both the assessment and treatment process. Thus, the inclusion of measures that solicit perspectives of patients, family members, and care partners is vital to selecting functional, real-world treatment goals. Many self-report measures are available to professionals working with individuals with TBI. The following sections briefly highlight some of the available tools.

Behavior Rating Inventory of Executive Function– Adult (BRIEF-A)

This self-rating scale captures the participants' executive functions and self-regulation in everyday environments (Roth et al., 2005). This 75-item measure includes nine nonoverlapping scales that measure various aspects of executive functioning (i.e., inhibition, self-monitoring, planning/organization, shifting, initiation, task monitoring, emotional control, working memory, and organization). Three scores are comprised from this measure: Behavioral Regulation, Metacognition, and the Global Executive Composite. This self-report scale is normed on U.S. adults from a variety of ethnic, geographical, and educational backgrounds. Higher raw scores, T scores, and percentile ranks indicate a greater degree of executive dysfunction (Roth et al., 2005).

Quality of Life After Brain Injury (QOLIBRI)

The Quality of Life After Brain Injury (QOLIBRI) is the first instrument specifically developed to assess health-related quality of life of individuals after TBI (https://qolibrinet.com/).

This questionnaire is designed to measure physical, psychological, daily life, and psychosocial changes typical of brain injury. Questions are coded as "satisfaction" or "feeling bothered" items and are queried using a 5-point Likert-type scale. The comprehensive measure includes 37 items covering six health-related dimensions of quality of life following TBI—cognition, self, daily life and autonomy, social relations, emotions, and physical problems. The questionnaire provides a profile of quality of life through a total score value and domain scores ranging from zero to 100; scores of zero indicate very poor quality of life, and scores of 100 equal very high quality of life.

National Institutes of Health Toolbox

The National Institutes of Health (NIH) created a validated, standardized toolbox for the evaluation of deficits across a variety of cognitive domains (i.e., the NIH Toolbox). Within this collection of instruments are several self-report measures that may be useful in documenting symptomatology postinjury and the effect on daily functioning. Two such examples are the Neuro-QOL Cognitive Function measure (National Institute of Neurological Disorders and Stroke, 2015) and the PROMIS Cognitive Function measure (Health Measures, 2018). The Neuro-QOL queries individuals regarding current difficulties with cognitive functions as well as difficulties experienced over the previous 7-day period. Questions are formed in a manner to provide example activities relative to distinct cognitive functions. Participants are tasked with responding on a 5-point Likert-type scale indicating the frequency with which a symptom occurs from very often (1) to never (5). Similarly, the PROMIS item bank queries individuals regarding cognitive function across the previous 7-day period using a 5-point Likert-type scale; however, the PROMIS differs from the Neuro-QOL in that it does not provide contextual examples of cognitive deficits but rather explicitly queries respondents regarding particular cognitive domains.

Brain Injury Screening Questionnaire (BISQ)

The three-part tool is an evidence-based, self-report instrument designed to screen for and document history related to TBI (Dams-O'Connor et al., 2014). The Brain Injury Screening Questionnaire (BISQ) was developed based on the mild TBI diagnosis criteria set by the American Congress of Rehabilitation Medicine with the goal of creating a screening tool that could document lifetime histories of self-reported TBI and symptoms. The BISQ, which is divided into three distinct parts (TBI History, Symptoms, and Other Health Conditions), rules out alternative explanations for symptoms (e.g., neurological or developmental conditions). The inventory includes 100 possible cognitive, physical, emotional, and behavioral symptoms for endorsement. When the BISQ is used in evaluations, inferences can be made regarding the extent to which symptoms are specifically attributable to TBI. Furthermore, the BISQ reportedly has increased sensitivity compared to other commonly used self-assessment measures for the mild TBI population.

Mayo-Portland Adaptability Inventory

The Mayo-Portland Adaptability Inventory–Fourth Edition (MPAI-4; Malec et al., 2003; Malec & Lezak, 2008) is a subjective rating form that can be completed by a single professional, professional consensus, the person with brain injury, or a care partner. Each part of the scale queries the respondent on various domains associated with daily living and specifically targets an individual with brain injury's abilities, adjustment, and participation using a 5-point Likert-type scale. Additionally, the scale takes into consideration preexisting and associated conditions that may be substantially contributing to results. The obtained raw scores are converted to standard scores and can be used clinically to judge the level of impairment such that a higher score indicates a more advanced level of impairment and increased reliance on others for daily task completion.

Motivational Interview Techniques

Motivational interview techniques combine a supportive and empathic counseling style with a conscious, directive method for client self-analysis (Hettema et al., 2005; Medley & Powell, 2010). Motivational interviewing emphasizes and honors client autonomy through clinician and client co-construction of challenges and needs. Motivational interview techniques involve the clinician beginning with an open-ended question (e.g., "What can I help you with?"). The clinician then follows client responses with open-ended, directive prompts (e.g., "Tell me more about why that bothers you."), reflects on client responses (e.g., "It's hard to stay focused for long periods of time."), and summarizes/synthesizes client remarks (e.g., "So what I hear you saying is . . . "). Such techniques assist in developing client-centered care plans and enhancing client buy-in for therapy goals and targets.

Standardized Assessment Measures

In addition to self-report tools and observational scales, clinicians use standardized, objective assessment tools to measure the cognitive and communicative abilities of people with TBI. These may take the form of screening tools, subtests, or holistic testing batteries. Due to the extensive number of tests available and the challenges faced by clinicians in determining the most appropriate formal assessment tools for people with TBI, the Academy of Neurological Communication Disorders and Sciences created a committee to review the evidence for commonly used assessment tools (Turkstra et al., 2005). As described in Chapter 3, only seven tests met the committee's criteria. Additionally, the committee emphasized that standardized assessments, although valuable for identifying cognitive and communication deficits, should only be one component of a comprehensive evaluation.

Benefits include procurement of a standardized score, potential comparison of patient performance to age and gender norms, commonalities among test-taking procedures and questions, and provision of a quantitative diag-

nosis of a problem. However, the adequacy of these measures when utilized in isolation is substantially lacking. A recent survey of speech-language pathologists (Brown, 2018) revealed that on average, approximately 80% of respondents reported less than complete satisfaction and/or dissatisfaction with available assessment tools across cognitive domains from people with all severities of TBI. Furthermore, when asked to provide cons to assessments, respondents commonly reported issues such as (a) lack of norm-referenced data, poor psychometrics, and poor standardization; (b) problems with test length or administration ease; and (c) challenges related to the functional, realistic, or patient-specific nature of assessments. In fact, of the 467 reported cons, a staggering 32% related to challenges with the functional, realistic nature of assessments. Thus, at this time, an ideal approach to assessing cognition and communication in individuals with neurogenic disorders likely includes administering a variety of tools and developing personally relevant, functional tasks.

Screening Tools

As an initial step in the assessment process, clinicians may wish to administer screening tools. Such tests are meant to detect the presence of a disorder and serve to alert clinicians as to whether in-depth exploration and assessment in each area is a necessary next step. Screening tools do not provide information regarding deficit severity, nor do they elucidate the specific characteristics of challenges faced by individuals with TBI. For example, completion of a screening tool for left neglect may reveal a potential deficit in visual attention and processing and provide guidance for the clinician to initiate in-depth assessment in these areas. A variety of screening tools are available to rehabilitation professionals working with individuals with TBI that highlight a variety of cognitive, linguistic, and visuospatial domains. Such tools include, but are not limited to, the Mini Mental State Exam (MMSE; Folstein et al., 1975), Montreal Cognitive Assessment (MOCA; Nasreddine et al., 2005), and St. Louis University Mental Status Examination (SLUMS; Morley & Tumosa, 2002). Such tools are intended to be administered in a short time frame (e.g., 30 minutes or less) and provide an initial evaluation of deficits in areas such as orientation, visuospatial skills, attention, memory (immediate and delayed), language comprehension and expression, and executive functioning skills. Additional brief assessments for consideration include the Repeatable Battery for the Assessment of Neuropsychological Status (RBANS; Randolph, 2012) and the Cognitive Linguistic Quick Test–Plus (CLQT+; Helm-Estabrooks, 2017). Although useful in settings where initial deficit detection is vital (e.g., acute care), brief assessments and screening tools should only be used as a component of a comprehensive evaluation and should not replace in-depth, holistic deficit testing postinjury.

Cognitive Subtests and Batteries

Often speech-language pathologists may evaluate people with TBI using subtests from various batteries or by selecting measures related to specific areas of deficits. For example, the clinicians might combine subtests from the Functional Assessment of Verbal Reasoning and Executive Strategies (MacDonald, 2005) for assessment of executive functioning, the Test of Everyday Attention (Robertson et al., 1994) for attention, and the Rivermead Behavioural Memory Test Third Edition (Wilson et al., 2008) for memory. Please refer to previous chapters for descriptions of assessment tools that are appropriate for these areas. Two batteries specifically designed for people with TBI are the Brief Test of Head Injury (Helm-Estabrooks & Hotz, 1991) and the Scales of Cognitive Ability for Traumatic Brain Injury (Adamovich & Henderson, 1992). The Brief Test of Head Injury may be most appropriate for people at RLA-R Levels IV to VI, particularly because its administration lasts about 20 to 30 minutes, so attention deficits will be less impactful, and because it scores gestural and verbal responses. In contrast, the Scales of Cognitive Ability for Traumatic Brain Injury (Adamovich & Henderson, 1992) may be most appropriate for people at RLA-R Levels VI and above. This battery takes 30 to 120 minutes and progresses to levels of difficulty that will likely be challenging for some adults without brain injury.

Communication Subtests and Batteries

Speech-language pathologists may also wish to administer standardized tests aimed at evaluating various components of communication. Although we will not discuss physical deficits associated with TBI in detail in this book, it is important to note that clinicians should complete thorough motor speech and swallowing evaluations on all people with a history of TBI. As a focus of this chapter, we provide suggestions for assessment practices relative to various aspects of communication (e.g., aphasia, reading, writing, social communication). Evaluating communication at an appropriate stage in recovery is crucial for an accurate representation of linguistic ability such that a person's current cognitive status may interfere with assessment results. For example, evaluating communicative functioning may be inappropriate for people at RLA-R Level V or below given their continued agitation, confusion, and

severe attention and memory deficits. Thus, consideration of language and communication evaluation for individuals at RLA-R Level VI or above may be most appropriate. Table 8–5 provides potential standardized measures for clinicians to evaluate communication in individuals following TBI. Because the evidence related to some areas of assessment following TBI is limited (American Speech-Language-Hearing Association, 2019), clinicians may consider tools that are validated with other populations; however, further research examining their use is needed. These areas may also be evaluated using informal measures until validated tools are available.

Table 8–5. Standardized Assessments for Evaluation of Communication Deficits Following TBI

Communicative Domain	Measure
Aphasia Diagnosis	Western Aphasia Battery–Revised (WAB-R)
	Boston Naming Test (BNT)
	Comprehensive Aphasia Test (CAT)
	Test of Adolescent/Adult Word Finding (TAWF)
Holistic Language Evaluation	American Speech Language Hearing Association Functional Assessment of Communication Skills for Adults (ASHA FACS)
	Communication Activities of Daily Living–Third Edition (CADL-3)
	Scales of Cognitive and Communicative Ability for Neurorehabilitation (SCCAN)
Reading	Wechsler Test of Adult Reading (WTAR)
Writing	Western Aphasia Battery–Revised Part II
Social Skills	Mini Inventory of Right Brain Injury–Second Edition (MIRBI-2)
	Scales of Cognitive Ability for Traumatic Brain Injury (SCATBI)
Apraxia & Motor Speech Disorders	Frenchay Dysarthria Assessment–Second Edition
	Assessment of Intelligibility of Dysarthric Speech (AIDS)

Functional Assessment Measures

Given some of the challenges described in the above sections, ecologically valid assessments are critically important to a thorough TBI assessment. These evaluations may include, among other things, observational reports, discourse analysis, and completion of functional, personally relevant tasks that may or may not reflect a set of standardized, objective procedures. Understanding the contribution of real-world constraints to the performance of individuals with TBI is vital. In fact, a wealth of research exists documenting that individuals with TBI perform relatively well given structured and routine tasks (e.g., standardized tests) but may perform poorly during novel functional tasks. Specifically, ample evidence exists to suggest that cognitive and executive difficulties are often more pronounced when a reminder cue must be self-generated, when the cognitive load of the ongoing task is high, or when distractors are present (Carlesimo et al., 2004; Knight et al., 2006; Maujean et al., 2003). These factors are indicative of naturalistic, real-world settings and, thus, important to note. Inclusion of tasks during the assessment process that attempt to mimic personally relevant, real-world situations are necessary in order to select and implement effective treatment plans for a return to functional status postinjury.

The literature investigating the ecological validity of common neuropsychological tests of cognition in particular is inconsistent (Chaytor et al., 2006). However, many researchers and clinicians have acknowledged the usefulness of ecologically valid assessments to (a) determine competency when standardized assessments do not exist for a particular skill, (b) identify unique demands of a client's personal contexts, (c) describe performance within natural contexts, and (d) evaluate the effectiveness of potential supports to enhance competency (Coelho et al., 2005). Past researchers have assessed ecological validity using a variety of measurement tools, including self-questionnaires, clinician rating scales, and observation of simulated everyday tasks (Chaytor et al., 2006). The following sections highlight functional assessment tools available to rehabilitation professionals across a variety of cognitive and communicative domains.

Observational Reports

Observational reports may assess general behaviors (e.g., alertness, restlessness) during standardized assessments, simulated situations (e.g., role-play, phone calls, ordering food), or real-world situations (e.g., grocery store, bank). Behaviors to evaluate include those related to social appropriateness (e.g., proxemics, turn taking, eye contact), as well as fatigue (i.e., how long it takes performance to decline) and emotional lability (e.g., uncontrollable emotional displays). Role-play tasks can be simple (e.g., look up a phone number and call for a pet store's hours) or complex (e.g., budget and plan a trip to Italy for two couples). The opportunity to select personally relevant tasks may enable the speech-language pathologist to get a complete picture of how the person's constellation of strengths and deficits affects their daily functioning. This type of assessment may also help the clinician detect subtle deficits that may not be identified using standardized assessments.

Discourse Analysis

People with TBI may have communicative deficits not readily captured by standardized testing methods. Discourse analysis is another approach that may identify these subtle deficits. Implementation and assessment of discourse analysis should be culturally responsive and consider preinjury variables, including gender identity; native, first, and preferred languages; literacy and language proficiency; and communication style based on culture and background (Togher et al., 2023).

Discourse analysis can be particularly powerful because it can measure various areas of deficits ranging from those less likely to be affected in TBI (e.g., topic maintenance) to those likely to be affected (e.g., organization). Coelho and colleagues (2005) reviewed several types of discourse analysis used with people with TBI including both noninteractive (e.g., description, procedural) and conversational. Noninteractive discourse is elicited through story retelling, story generation, personal event retelling, and procedural descriptions. Coelho and colleagues (2005) recommended the analysis of the following elements because they produced the most consistent findings: verbal output, content accuracy and organization, story grammar, and coherence. Measures of syntax, grammatical complexity, and cohesion resulted in inconsistent findings across studies. Conversational analyses often made use of rating scales such as Damico's Clinical Discourse Analysis (1992), but training is required and the four basic psychometric properties should be considered (Coelho et al.,

2005). Two categories of measurements (i.e., measures of initiation and manipulation of content) are appropriate for the analysis of conversational discourse, with content and topic management probably being the most useful. Conversational discourse analyses appear to better distinguish people with TBI from people without brain injury than noninteractive analyses.

Additional analyses may focus on the coherence and cohesion of expressive language output produced by individuals with TBI. Cohesion refers to the linking of meaning across sentences that occur through the use of cohesive markers. Such markers are words that lead the listener to information elsewhere in the conversation. Coherence, on the other hand, refers to the relation of an expressed utterance to the overall content or topic and is defined in two ways—that is, local and global. Local coherence is established by relating the content of one utterance to the content of the previous utterance; global coherence occurs by relating the content of one utterance to the general theme or topic of conversation (Glosser & Deser, 1990). In both instances of cohesion and coherence deficits, underlying cognitive issues associated with skills such as attention, memory, organization, and theory of mind may play a role. Objectively analyzing expressive language for these characteristics may shed light on communication difficulties attributable, in part, to common cognitive deficits following brain injury (Van Leer & Turkstra, 1999).

Functional, Personally Relevant Tasks

The development of ecologically valid tools in addition to standardized measurements is necessary to successfully evaluate clients at the participation level and within their natural contexts (Constantinidou et al., 2012; Eslinger et al., 2011; Wood & Liossi, 2006). Several methods exist to aid clinicians in administering functionally, personally relevant assessments that do not require development for each individual. For example, the Multiple Errands Test, available in many forms, both paper based and electronically (e.g., Dawson et al., 2009; Knight et al., 2002; Raspelli et al., 2012), requires the individual with TBI to perform tasks similar to those experienced in daily life while outside of the therapy room setting (e.g., in a mall, within a rehabilitation facility campus). Similarly, the Party Planning Task (Shanahan et al., 2011) facilitates the planning of a party while following various restrictions and guidelines—again, a task that may be relevant to functional, real-world needs. Furthermore, other researchers have developed and evaluated functional tasks that include both planning and execution and encompass constraints for both immediate and prospective memory (Brown & Hux, 2016, 2017) and have been specifically created for use with individuals with TBI. However, many researchers and clinicians have acknowledged the usefulness of functional assessments to (a) determine competency when standardized assessments do not exist for a particular skill, (b) identify unique demands of an individual's personal contexts, (c) describe performance within natural contexts, and (d) evaluate the effectiveness of potential supports to enhance competency (Coelho et al., 2005). Thus, in times when functionally relevant tools are not readily available to clinicians, the creation of client-specific tasks may be of value to the assessment process.

Treatment

Treatment of TBI ideally involves a team of rehabilitation professionals; thus, it is critical that services are carefully coordinated. Researchers and clinicians have addressed the concept of interprofessional practices for decades, citing models such as the creation of multidisciplinary and interdisciplinary teams. The use of a transdisciplinary model of care is considered the current gold standard, where team members engage in shared decision-making (and treatment practices) to enhance communication and create a maximally person-centered approach (Karol, 2014). Within this approach, all team members are responsible for an individual's well-being and overall rehabilitative goals. To build a therapeutic plan, professionals first look at the person's needs or concerns to be addressed in therapy and create a hierarchy of needs. The team works together to identify how much or what aspects of each need will be addressed by a given professional domain or team member. This rehabilitative concept posits that no team member may opt out of addressing a goal area or need, but some professionals may have more influence on a goal than others. Such a care model is particularly important in neurorehabilitation given the complexity of neurobiology and trauma recovery.

Additionally, although interventions emphasized through this section focus on cognitive and communication impairments, consideration of potential impairments in swallowing, hearing, and visual processing are important to the development of a successful, comprehensive intervention program. Finally, for people with TBI, evidence suggests comprehensive neuropsychological programs are beneficial. These programs are often interdisciplinary in nature and may offer group and individual interventions during postacute rehabilitation (Cicerone et al., 2011).

Multiple systematic reviews examining the evidence for cognitive rehabilitation have been conducted (e.g., Cicerone et al., 2011; Jeffay et al., 2023; Kennedy et al., 2008; Ponsford, Trevena-Peters, et al., 2023; Ponsford, Velikonja, et al., 2023; Togher et al., 2023; Velikonja et al., 2023). Many of these reviews have examined interventions within the areas of attention, memory, executive functions, and communication. Although it is difficult to isolate cognitive impairments during interventions due to multiple areas of overlap, each is discussed in separate sections below. Typically, in clinical practice, a group of intervention strategies may be implemented with consideration of the specific needs of the client. In 2022, members of an interdisciplinary panel established by the American Speech-Language-Hearing Association reviewed literature published between 1980 and 2020 relative to the treatment of cognitive disorders following acquired brain injury (Guideline Development Panel et al., 2022). Despite differences in literature findings, the panel recommended an overarching consensus that individuals should receive holistic, integrated cognitive rehabilitation postinjury that is person centered and evidence based. Eleven additional recommendations related to cognitive rehabilitation were provided. Results of this literature review indicated that both compensatory and restorative intervention methods are warranted for functional and domain-specific goals

postinjury dependent on the unique individual needs of the client.

A variety of methods are available to treat cognitive and communicative deficits in individuals with TBI such that no one, standard approach should be utilized. Selection of a specific approach may depend on several factors (e.g., timeline for treatment, client preference, research evidence) and, thus, understanding the underlying principles of treatment is a vital clinical skill. Following the completion of in-depth assessments, clinicians and their clients should initiate co-construction of goals, when possible, to enhance the treatment process and maintain personal relevance during therapy. Other chapters in this textbook describe various methods available to clinicians when selecting cognitive communication goals and personalizing treatment activities post-TBI (e.g., Goal Attainment Scaling). Subsequently, clinicians may wish to decide whether a selected goal and subsequent treatment is aimed at restoring functioning and remediating deficits (e.g., drill and practice), compensating for present deficits (e.g., strategy training), or environmental management. The sections below highlight some potential treatment approaches for various cognitive and communicative deficits typically experienced by individuals with TBI.

Attention

Treatment approaches implemented for attentional deficits should be considered based on the severity of the cognitive deficits exhibited by the person with TBI. Implementation of environmental modification by staff and trained care partners can reduce the impact of attentional deficits for individuals with severe deficits who lack awareness and use of compensatory strategies (Ponsford, Velikonja, et al., 2023). Environmental modifications can include removing distractions (e.g., turn off cellphone), reducing the amount and complexity of information presented during treatment, and providing redirection prompts. For individuals with mild to moderate deficits, with some self-awareness, the use of metacognitive skill training is appropriate when directly tied to everyday personally relevant tasks (Ponsford, Velikonja, et al., 2023). For example, Time Pressure Management is a method used to compensate for slow information processing by breaking down functional tasks into hierarchical levels for analysis prior to completion (Fasotti et al., 2000). Through the review of the task in advance of implementation, the time pressure demands experienced can be reduced, allowing the person with TBI greater success. However, generalization to tasks not trained should not be expected. In addition, computer- or drill-based decontextualized attention training tasks lack evidence supporting carryover to everyday attentional activities (Ponsford, Velikonja, et al., 2023). Direct attention training (as described in Chapter 1) includes improvement of the neurocognitive system through repetition of exercises that stimulate attention. Attention Process Training is one well-known example of direct attention training that targets multiple areas of attention (Sohlberg & Mateer, 2001a). During postacute care and for individuals with mild impairments, Sohlberg and colleagues (2007) recommend combining direct attention training with metacognitive strategy instruction (e.g., goal setting, feedback, self-monitoring) (as described in Chapters 1 and 3). In this way, direct attention training can be combined with compensatory strategy instruction, perhaps increasing the overall effect. There is limited evidence that these strategies automatically generalize to improvements in functional attention; thus, the guidelines provided within Chapter 1 for direct attention training and self-management strategies warrant careful consideration (Sohlberg & Mateer, 2001b). Additionally, little evidence is available to explain the effect of these interventions during acute rehabilitation (Cicerone et al., 2011). Computer-based interventions may be added as a supplement to other clinician-guided treatments but should not be implemented as the sole intervention (Cicerone et al., 2011).

Memory

Memory interventions for TBI can be categorized as external memory aids and internalized strategies. In 2003, written communication notebooks or daily planners were reported to be the most commonly used external memory aid, while electronic memory aids were reported to be infrequently used, perhaps due to their complexity (Evans et al., 2003). Given the many advances in computerized memory aids and the increased presence of technology in society, electronic aids are increasing in use. It may be most helpful to match the memory intervention to the type and severity of memory impairment. Evidence suggests that external memory aids (described in Chapter 2) are appropriate intervention strategies for people with mild to severe memory impairments (Cicerone et al., 2011). Additional factors considered before selecting an external aid may include previous use of technology, physical limitation, affordability, portability, cognitive strengths and challenges, and functional needs (Velikonja et al., 2023). People with severe memory impairments may most easily use external aids to complete a specific task. Instruction in the use of external aids is critical to successful use (Velikonja et al., 2023). Sohlberg and colleagues (2023) described the importance of teaching the mechanics of using the aids along with the supports and reinforcement required to use the aid in functionally relevant environments. A three-stage approach is used to facilitate this process that includes acquisition (i.e., procedures and motivations for using the aid), mastery (i.e., increase the fluency and automaticity of aid in functional context), and retention (i.e., treatment methods to facilitate long-term use of the aid). Many studies have modified this approach for use with external memory aids with incorporation of massed practice and an errorless learning approach, as described in other chapters in this text (e.g., Donaghy & Williams, 1998; Schmitter-Edgecomb et al., 1995).

For people with mild memory impairments, long-standing evidence supports the use of internalized strategies such as visual imagery (Cicerone et al., 2011), verbal rehearsal (Harris, 1996), storytelling, or mnemonics (Gianutsos & Gianutsos, 1979; Richardson, 1995). However, current evidence regarding the use of internal memory strategies does not delineate for whom and under what conditions such strategies are most beneficial (O'Neil-Pirozzi et al., 2015). Regardless, a systematic review of such techniques with the TBI population supports interventions that encompass internal memory strategies as one component to the therapeutic plan. For people with severe memory impairments, the use of errorless learning for specific skills or information (e.g., taking medication at a meal) may also be effective; however, it is important to note that carryover to other memory tasks may be limited. One such method is to initiate spaced retrieval techniques in therapy (Schacter et al., 1985). Spaced retrieval involves the selection of distinct pieces of information for later recall. In this method, the clinician systematically increases the amount of time between which a client successfully recalls the target information. This is completed using an errorless learning approach such that if a person incorrectly recalls the target information, the correct answer is provided and the time interval is reduced. A recent systematic review by Lambez and Valkil (2021) found that interventions using both internal strategies and external memory aids resulted in the greatest degree of effectiveness.

Group memory interventions might also be appropriate for individuals with TBI at all severity levels and should focus primarily on teaching compensatory strategies (Cicerone et al., 2011). Group participants can discuss memory problems and generate multiple solutions with real-time feedback from other group members (Thickpenny-Davis & Barker-Collo, 2007). Often this discussion focuses on prospective memory tasks, but discussion of memory for information at shorter intervals may also be useful. Time spent in group therapy can also be used to practice implementing memory strategies learned through errorless learning strategies (Thickpenny-Davis & Barker-Collo, 2007). Clinicians may use multiple methods for presenting information in groups to support the retention of learned strategies.

Executive Functions

In a review of the literature examining executive function interventions for TBI, Kennedy and colleagues (2008) found that although the interventions focused on different aspects of executive functions, three general intervention approaches were used: metacognitive strategy instruction, training strategic thinking, and multitasking instruction. Metacognitive strategies can increase participation and improve problem solving, planning, and organization skills for personally relevant activities (Jeffay et al., 2023). Although specific instructional programs for metacognition may differ, they typically involve solving a problem or achieving a goal through the deliberate use of multistep instructions such as "go-plan-do" (Kennedy et al., 2008). Generally, the steps of a metacognitive program include creating goals, self-monitoring and documenting performance, and adjusting plans based on feedback. Goal management training (Levine et al., 2000) and goal attainment scaling (Webb & Glueckauf, 1994) are examples of metacognitive interventions that use variations of these steps and are described in detail in Chapter 2. These strategies emphasize the inclusion of the client in developing treatment goals. Additionally, evidence for goal

management training suggests that it should be integrated into a comprehensive treatment plan to maximize effectiveness (Krasny-Pacini et al., 2014).

Few studies have examined the use of strategic thinking and multitasking instruction. Strategic thinking interventions typically have the clinician prompt the person with TBI to engage in verbal reasoning and then provide feedback. This strategy is described in the Interactive Strategy Modeling Training section in Chapter 3 (Marshall et al., 2004). Another such example is to initiate the IDEAL approach. This method prompts the client to evaluate different components of the problem in order to generate a variety of solutions while recalling the acronym IDEAL. This acronym refers to identifying a problem, defining the problem, exploring alternative approaches, acting on a plan, and looking at the effects. Despite the potential usefulness of these tools, it is important to note that people with TBI, particularly those with significant communication impairments, may struggle to use these language-mediated problem-solving strategies.

Multitasking interventions are designed to improve the person's ability to do two things at once or dual-task. These studies provide instruction in multitasking during simulated real-life activities or through the use of a computerized program that requires a response to different and changing features of stimuli.

Finally, increasing self-awareness requires self-reflection and self-monitoring of behaviors across tasks requiring different cognitive skills. Schmidt and colleagues (2015) examined methods of facilitating awareness through three types of feedback: video + verbal,

verbal only, and experiential feedback only. Their findings revealed video + verbal feedback were superior to other methods, with maintenance exhibited 10 weeks postimplementation.

Communication

Communication interventions for people with TBI may aim to address aphasia, dysarthria, or apragmatism. There is limited evidence concerning specific treatments for people with TBI who have aphasia (e.g., Massaro & Tompkins, 1994). Many people with TBI are included in studies that have examined interventions for stroke-induced aphasia (e.g., Ballard & Thompson, 1999; Hinckley & Craig, 1992); however, rarely do the results indicate what worked best for the people with TBI separate from the people with aphasia from a stroke. However, interventions grounded in the current best available evidence should be considered for people with cognitive and communication challenges related to TBI. This can include the development of communication strategies and supports (e.g., use of multimodal communication supports to facilitate expression and comprehension) for training and use in situations relevant to the person with TBI including school, work, and social activities (e.g., textbook reading, notetaking strategies, ordering groceries online). Furthermore, communication partner training (e.g., care partner, teachers, employers) should be employed to provide guidance and structure to facilitate expressive and receptive communication activities (e.g., positive question asking, scaffolding, providing background) (Togher et al., 2023).

Motor Speech and Voice

Similarly, studies examining motor speech interventions for people with TBI are limited. Typically, treatments for dysarthria following TBI would be selected based on the specific speech characteristics (e.g., vocal weakness or fatigue, slurred speech, impaired intonation and rate). Thus, these treatments have been included in systematic reviews for dysarthria that included other etiologies such as Parkinson's disease (e.g., Yorkston et al., 2007). For example, Solomon and colleagues (2001) found that Lee Silverman Voice Treatment, when combined with respiratory exercises, was effective for a person with moderate to severe hypokinetic-spastic dysarthria resulting from TBI. Additionally, one systematic review found that external pacing strategies, such as a metronome or pacing board, increase intelligibility by reducing the rate of speech (Teasell et al., 2012).

Discourse and Pragmatics

Individuals with brain injury typically display two variations of discourse deficits: (a) problems in narrative and conversational discourse and (b) social disconnection and reduced awareness. For individuals with deficits in narrative and conversational discourse, challenges with inferences, quantity and quality of expressed language, and recognition of alternative meanings may be apparent. Targeting these domains directly or through compensatory approaches (e.g., strategy implementation) may result in improved outcomes (Gabbatore et al., 2015). Individuals with TBI may also experience difficulties connecting in social situations and may benefit from treatment aimed at various pragmatic goals (e.g., increasing awareness of listener needs, improving use of social conventions, reducing theory of mind deficits). Available evidence related to communication skills for people with TBI suggests the benefits of specific interventions aimed at improving pragmatic conversational skills (e.g., turn taking, initiating a conversation, prosodic comprehension and expression). Additionally, group-based interventions, sometimes called social communication skills training, have been found to increase effective communication skills after TBI (e.g., Dahlberg et al., 2007; McDonald et al., 2008). Such treatments appear to achieve gains that are maintained over time and enhance overall life satisfaction for clients (Dahlberg et al., 2007). Included in this type of therapy should be counseling with the person and family members to assist with increasing deficit awareness and focusing on potential strategy implementation during social interactions. Potential effective methods for increasing awareness of social deficits could include, but are not limited to, video recording client conversations (Bornhofen & McDonald, 2008) and asking family members to record or document socially inappropriate situations (McDonald et al., 2008). An example compensatory strategy may include encouraging the individual to explicitly state or label their emotions to reduce confusion (e.g., "I feel angry.").

Augmentative and Alternative Communication

People who cannot meet their communication needs through natural speech often rely on augmentative and alternative communication (AAC) strategies (Beukelman & Mirenda, 2013). People with TBI may use AAC to supplement or replace insufficient or ineffective expressive or receptive communication (Togher et al., 2023). When considering AAC methods to support or replace oral communication, clinicians should include occupational and physical therapists to assist with access and positioning of such systems.

Strategies used by people with TBI range significantly based on the characteristics of the individuals as well as the severity of their deficits (Wallace, 2010). Speech-language pathologists should consider the evolution of AAC strategy use during recovery in the development of an AAC treatment plan for people with TBI (Doyle & Fager, 2011; Fager & Karantounis, 2011; Light et al., 1988). The framework of AAC strategies for people with TBI based on cognitive stage appears in Table 8–6. This framework highlights AAC strategies for each of three stages: Early Stage (RLA-R I–III), Middle Stage (RLA-R IV–VI), and Late Stage (RLA-R VII–X) and can provide a starting point for clinicians to determine appropriate strategies.

Cognitive considerations are important aspects of an AAC assessment for people with TBI. Cognitive abilities affect how people with TBI learn to use an AAC device or strategy, as well as the selection of appropriate organizational approaches. For many people with TBI, clinicians should develop strategies that avoid new learning and tap residual knowledge. For example, people with TBI who do not have aphasia may prefer to use text-to-speech devices that make use of overlearned

Table 8–6. Staging of AAC Strategies Using the Ranchos Los Amigos Scale Levels of Cognitive Functioning–Revised as Described by Fager and Karantounis (2011)

Early Stage	Middle Stage	Late Stage
RLA-R I-III	*RLA-R IV-VI*	*RLA-R VII-X*
• Simple choice-based systems • Yes/no systems • Eye gaze or direct selection	• Complex choice making with picture, letter, or word board • Written Choice Communication Strategy • Simple voice output for basic information	*Familiar listeners:* • Alphabet board for supplemented speech • Gestures combined with natural speech *Unfamiliar listener and specific contexts:* • Text-to-speech • Stored message complex voice output systems

spelling and typing skills (Fager et al., 2006). Investigation of organizational approaches for high-technology AAC devices used by people with TBI suggests that accuracy and efficiency increase with the use of an alphabetically organized device but that people with TBI tend to prefer a topical (i.e., semantic) organization strategy (Burke et al., 2004). Similarly, other studies have identified idiosyncratic organizational strategies and significant heterogeneity in the use and preference of organizational strategies (Brown et al., 2015; Snyder & Hux, 2000). Additionally, cognitive flexibility affects the accuracy and efficiency with which people with TBI navigate dynamic display AAC devices with semantic organizations (Wallace et al., 2010). Training on the use of AAC devices should also be ongoing and evolve based on advances in technology. These results highlight the need for individualized

assessments of AAC organization with multiple trials with various organizations, as well as instruction in the use of strategies and devices.

The instruction clinicians provide to teach people with TBI and their facilitators to use AAC is critical to eventual successful communication participation. Recommendations include providing a structured environment for practice (e.g., therapy room) before expecting functional use in a natural setting, using errorless learning (described in previous chapters) to support strategy initiation as well as navigation of high-technology devices (Baddeley & Wilson, 1994), and encouraging repetitive practice to facilitate overlearning (e.g., at least four times the amount of practice required by individuals without brain injury; Wilson et al., 1994). Finally, facilitator instruction and buy-in are critically important to the eventual success of AAC strategies with people with TBI. Lack of facilitator support is the primary reason for device abandonment (Fager et al., 2006).

Models of Service Delivery

Group Treatment

As described in previous sections, group therapy for people with TBI and/or their care partners can support various areas of cognition and communication (Cicerone et al., 2011) and may focus on intervention of skills, counseling and education, or psychosocial support. Clinicians can implement group therapy with people with TBI across different severity levels and lengths of time postonset; however, clinicians should carefully assess cognitive and communication abilities prior to placing people with TBI in a particular group (Velikonja et al., 2023). Additional considerations include fatigue, behavioral challenges, age, and interest in group theme, which may impact an individual's engagement with and performance in a particular group.

Clinicians may wish to structure group treatment for individuals with TBI based on the overall group goal. For example, a group that focuses on direct treatment of skills would likely be highly structured, be clinician directed, and target specific language processes (e.g., a group aimed at improving naming and word retrieval abilities). Conversely, a group whose goal is indirect treatment of skills might be low in structure, provide a rich cognitive communicative environment, and focus on facilitating general involvement of

group members (e.g., conversation, role-playing activities). Additional foci of group treatment include sociolinguistic groups (i.e., emphasize interaction among group participants), transition groups (i.e., intended to ease the transition from treatment to discharge and emphasize a person's independence), or maintenance groups (i.e., opportunities to practice skills to prevent deterioration). Additionally, groups may be structured based on a common theme or therapeutic goal, with some group themes being more appropriate for outpatient or community-based settings and some being better implemented during inpatient rehabilitation (Gillis, 1999a, 1999b). For instance, group interventions that emphasize executive function skills and problem solving may be appropriate after TBI (Cicerone et al., 2011). Other ideas for group themes appear in Table 8–7.

Telepractice and TBI

Telepractice involves using Internet technology via tablet, computer, or phone to implement assessment, treatment,

Table 8–7. Group Therapy Themes

- Problem-Solving Group
- Psychosocial Adjustment Group
- Job Skills Group
- Parenting Group
- Money Management Group
- Orientation Group
- Meal Planning Group
- Communication Skills Group
- External Memory Aid Group

and educational practices between a clinician, person with TBI, and care partner (American Speech-Language-Hearing Association, n.d.). Teleprac-tice, employed by a trained clinician, can provide accessibility to individual or group services, especially for those living in rural or remote areas or for others who lack reliable and accessible transportation options. Currently, the validity and reliability of results from online administration of traditional in-person assessment for cognitive and communication assessments have not been determined. As a result, clinicians should be cautious when administer-ing these assessments online. How-ever, evidence is beginning to emerge regarding the effectiveness of teleprac-tice service delivery for individuals with TBI. Riegler and colleagues (2013) implemented a web-based cognitive intervention for veterans with a his-tory of nonadherence, which resulted in increased compliance in completing the treatment program. Participants also exhibited improvements in standard-ized memory and learning test results comparable to those participating in in-person treatments. A systematic review found that structured telephone cogni-tive interventions were feasible and effective in improving outcomes for individuals with mild and moderate-to-severe TBI (Ownsworth et al., 2018). In addition, social skills training, admin-istered to persons with TBI and their care partner, resulted in similar posi-tive gains in conversational proficiency as those receiving the same service in person (Rietdijk et al., 2020a; 2020b; Rietdijk et al., 2022). Decisions regard-ing the feasibility and effectiveness of telepractice at this time for individuals with TBI should be made on a case-by-case basis with careful consideration of the person's unique cognitive and com-munication strengths and challenges.

Summary

Cognitive communication deficits re-sult in permanent and profound social-emotional, educational, and vocational challenges for people with TBI and their family members. The unique nature of generalized brain damage and the resul-tant deficits in attention, memory, and executive function paired with deficits in awareness and theory of mind lead to reduced participation in daily activities. Speech-language pathologists are faced with the challenge of identifying defi-cits primarily through informal non-standardized tests and treating deficits with an array of creative approaches. More research is needed to identify the relationships between communication skills and various cognitive functions (e.g., attention, memory, and executive functions). Increased understanding of these relationships will facilitate the development of interventions that can best address the complex constellation of symptoms in people with TBI.

References

Adamovich, B. B., & Henderson, J. (1992). *Scales of Cognitive Ability for Traumatic Brain Injury*. Pro-Ed.

American Congress of Rehabilitation Med-icine. (1995). Recommendations for use of uniform nomenclature pertinent to patients with severe alterations in con-sciousness. *Archives of Physical Medicine and Rehabilitation, 76*(2), 205–209.

American Speech-Language-Hearing Association. (n.d.). Telepractice advocacy in states. https://www.asha.org/advocacy/telepractice/

American Speech-Language-Hearing Association. (2019). The practice portal. https://www.asha.org/practice-portal/

Association for the Advancement of Automotive Medicine. (2016). *Abbreviated Injury Scale (AIS)*.

Baddeley, A., & Wilson, B. A. (1994). When implicit learning fails: Amnesia and the problem of error elimination. *Neuropsychologia, 32*, 53–68.

Baker, S. P., O'Neill, B., Haddon, W., Jr., & Long, W. B. (1974). The injury severity score: A method for describing patients with multiple injuries and evaluating emergency care. *Journal of Trauma and Acute Care Surgery, 14*(3), 187–196.

Ballard, K. J., & Thompson, C. K. (1999). Treatment and generalization of complex sentence production in agrammatism. *Journal of Speech, Language, and Hearing Research, 42*, 690–707.

Baron, E., & Jallo, J.I. (2007). TBI: Pathology, pathophysiology, acute care and surgical management, critical care principles, and outcomes. In N. D. Zasler, D. Katz, & R. D. Zafonte (Eds.), *Brain injury medicine: Principles and practice* (pp. 265–282). Demos.

Beukelman, D., & Mirenda, P. (2013). *Augmentative and alternative communication: Supporting children and adults with complex communication needs*. Brookes.

Bogner, J. A., Corrigan, J. D., Fugate, L., Mysiw, W. J., & Clinchot, D. (2001). Role of agitation in prediction of outcomes after traumatic brain injury. *American Journal of Physical Medicine and Rehabilitation, 80*(9), 636–644.

Bornhofen, C., & McDonald, S. (2008). Treating deficits in emotion perception following traumatic brain injury. *Neuropsychological Rehabilitation, 18*, 22–44.

Brasure, M., Lamberty, G. J., Sayer, N. A., Nelson, N. H., MacDonald, R., Ouellette, J., . . . Wilt, T. J. (2012). *Multidisciplinary postacute rehabilitation for moderate to severe traumatic brain injury in adults*. https://www.ncbi.nlm.nih.gov/books/NBK98993/pdf/Bookshelf_NBK 98993 .pdf

Braun, C. M., & Baribeau, J. (1987). Subclinical aphasia following closed head injury: A response to Sarno, Buonaguro, and Levita. *Clinical Aphasiology, 17*, 326–333.

Brooks, N., McKinlay, W., Symington, C., Beattie, A., & Campsie, L. (1987). Return to work within the first seven years of severe head injury. *Brain Injury, 1*, 5–19.

Brown, J. A. (2018, Nov.). *Cognitive assessment for adults with acquired neurological disorders: Speech-language pathologist practices*. Poster presentation at the American Speech-Language-Hearing Association Annual Convention. Boston, MA.

Brown, J. A., & Hux, K. (2016). Functional assessment of immediate task planning and execution by adults with acquired brain injury. *NeuroRehabilitation, 39*, 191–203.

Brown, J. A., & Hux, K. (2017). Ecologically valid assessment of prospective memory task planning and execution by adults with acquired brain injury. *American Journal of Speech-Language Pathology, 26*, 819–831.

Brown, J. A., Hux, K., Kenny, C., & Funk, T. (2015). Consistency and idiosyncrasy of semantic categorization by individuals with traumatic brain injuries. *Disability and Rehabilitation: Assistive Technology, 10*(5), 378–384.

Burke, R., Beukelman, D. R., & Hux, K. (2004). Accuracy, efficiency, and preferences of survivors of traumatic brain injury when using three organization strategies to retrieve words. *Brain Injury, 18*, 497–507.

Carlesimo, G. A., Casadio, P., & Caltagirone, C. (2004). Prospective and retrospective components in the memory for actions to be performed in patients with severe closed-head injury. *Journal of the International Neuropsychological Society, 10*, 679–688.

Centers for Disease Control and Prevention (CDC). (n.d.). *Traumatic brain injury in prisons and jails: An unrecognized problem.* http://www.cdc.gov/traumaticbraininjury/pdf/Prisoner_TBI_Prof-a.pdf

Centers for Disease Control and Prevention (CDC). (2015). *Heads up: Concussion signs and symptoms.* https://www.cdc.gov/headsup/basics/concussion_symptoms.html

Centers for Disease Control and Prevention (CDC). (2017). *Severe traumatic brain injury.* https://www.cdc.gov/traumaticbrain injury/severe.html

Centers for Disease Control and Prevention (CDC). (2022a). *National Center for Health Statistics: Mortality Data on CDCWONDER.* https://wonder.cdc.gov/mcd.html

Centers for Disease Control and Prevention (CDC). (2022b). *Surveillance report of traumatic brain injury-related deaths by age group, sex, and mechanism of injury—United States, 2018 and 2019.* Centers for Disease Control and Prevention, U.S. Department of Health and Human Services.

Centers for Disease Control and Prevention (CDC). (2022c). *National Center for Injury Prevention and Control.* https://www.cdc.gov/traumaticbraininjury/concussion/symptoms.html

Chaytor, N., Schmitter-Edgecombe, M., & Burr, R. (2006). Improving the ecological validity of executive functioning assessment. *Archives of Clinical Neuropsychology, 21,* 217–227.

Cicerone, K. D., Langenbahn, D. M., Braden, C., Malec, J. F., Kalmar, K., Fraas, M., . . . Ashman, T. (2011). Evidence-based cognitive rehabilitation: Updated review of the literature from 2003 through 2008. *Archives of Physical Medicine and Rehabilitation, 92,* 519–530.

Coelho, C., Ylvisaker, M., & Turkstra, L. (2005). Nonstandardized assessment approaches for individuals with traumatic brain injuries. *Seminars in Speech and Language, 26,* 223–241.

Colantonio, A., Ratcliff, G., Chase, S., Kelsey, S., Escobar, M., & Vernich, L. (2004). Long-term outcomes after moderate to severe traumatic brain injury. *Disability and Rehabilitation, 26*(5), 253–261.

Constantinidou, F., Wertheimer, J. C., Tsanadis, J., Evans, C., & Paul, D. R. (2012). Assessment of executive functioning in brain injury: Collaboration between speech-language pathology and neuropsychology for an integrative neuropsychological perspective. *Brain Injury, 26,* 1549–1563.

Crosson, B., Barco, P. P., Velozo, C. A., Bolesta. M. M., Cooper, P. V., Werts, D., & Brobeck, T. (1989). Awareness of compensation in postacute head injury rehabilitation. *Journal of Head Trauma Rehabilitation, 4*(3), 46–54.

Dahlberg, C. A., Cusick, C. P., Hawley, L. A., Newman, J. K., Morey, C. E., Harrison-Felix, C. L., & Whiteneck, G. G. (2007). Treatment efficacy of social communication skills training after traumatic brain injury: A randomized treatment and deferred treatment controlled trial. *Archives of Physical Medicine and Rehabilitation, 88,* 1561–1573.

Damico, J. S. (1992). Systematic observation of communicative interaction: A valid and practical descriptive assessment technique. *Best Practice in School Speech-Language Pathology, 2,* 133–144.

Dams-O'Connor, K., Cantor, J. B., Brown, M., Dijkers, M. P., Spielman, L. A., & Gordon, W. A. (2014). Screening for traumatic brain injury: Findings and public health implications. *Journal of Head Trauma Rehabilitation, 29,* 479–489.

Dawson, D. R., Anderson, N. D., Burgess, P., Cooper, E., Krpan, K. M., & Stuss, D. T. (2009). Further development of the Multiple Errands Test: Standardized scoring, reliability, and ecological validity for the Baycrest version. *Archives of Physical Medicine and Rehabilitation, 90,* S41–S51.

Dennis, K. C. (2009). Current perspectives on traumatic brain injury. *ASHA Access*

Audiology. http://www.asha.org/aud/articles/currentTBI.html

DePalma, R. G., Burris, D. G., Champion, H. R., & Hodgson, M. J. (2005). Blast injuries. *New England Journal of Medicine, 352,* 1335–1342.

Dodd-Murphy, J. (2014). *Auditory effects of blast exposure: Community outreach following an industrial explosion.* http://www.asha.org/aud/Articles/Auditory-Effects-of-Blast-Exposure/?utm_source=asha&utm_medium=enewsletter&utm_campaign=accessaud051214#sthash.zOdcZBFb.dpuf

Donaghy, S., & Williams, W. (1998). A new protocol for training severely impaired patients in the usage of memory journals. *Brain Injury, 12*(12), 1061–1076.

Dongilli, P. A., Hakel, M. E., & Beukelman, D. R. (1992). Recovery of functional speech following traumatic brain injury. *Journal of Head Trauma Rehabilitation, 7*(2), 91–101.

Doyle, M., & Fager, S. (2011). Traumatic brain injury and AAC: Supporting communication through recovery. *The ASHA Leader 16*(2). https://doi.org/10.1044/leader.FTR8.16022011.np

Eliacin, J., Fortney, S., Rattray, N.A., & Kean, J. (2018). Access to health services for moderate to severe TBI in Indiana: Patient and caregiver perspectives. *Brain Injury, 32*(12), 1510–1517.

Eslinger, P., Zappala, G., Chakara, F., & Barrett, A. (2011). Cognitive impairments after TBI. In N. D. Zasler, D. I. Katz, & R. D. Zafonte (Eds.), *Brain injury medicine* (2nd ed., pp. 779–790). Demos.

Evans, J. J., Wilson, B. A., Needham, P., & Brentnall, S. (2003). Who makes good use of memory aids? Results of a survey of people with acquired brain injury. *Journal of the International Neuropsychological Society, 9*(6), 925–935.

Ewing-Cobbs, L., Levin, H. S., Fletcher, J. M., Miner, M. E., & Eisenberg, H. M. (1990). The Children's Orientation and Amnesia Test: Relationship to severity of acute head injury and to recovery of memory. *Neurosurgery, 27,* 683–691.

Fager, S., Hux, K., Beukelman, D. R., & Karantounis, R. (2006). Augmentative and alternative communication use and acceptance by adults with traumatic brain injury. *Augmentative and Alternative Communication, 22*(1), 37–47.

Fager, S., & Karantounis, R. (2011). AAC assessment and interventions in TBI. In K. Hux (Ed.), *Assisting survivors of traumatic brain injury* (2nd ed., pp. 227–254). Pro-Ed.

Fasotti, L., Kovacs, F., Eling, P. A., & Brouwer, W. H. (2000). Time pressure management as a compensatory strategy training after closed head injury. *Neuropsychological Rehabilitation, 10*(1), 47–65. https://doi.org/10.1080/096020100389291

Faul, M., & Coronado, V. (2015). Chapter 1: Epidemiology of traumatic brain injury. In J. Grafman & A. M. Salazar (Eds.), *Handbook of clinical neurology* (Vol. 127, pp. 3–13). Elsevier.

Ferguson, P. L., Pickelsimer, E. E., Corrigan, J. D., Bogner, J. A., & Wald, M. (2012). Prevalence of traumatic brain injury among prisoners in South Carolina. *Journal of Head Trauma Rehabilitation, 27*(3), E11–E20.

Folstein, M. F., Folstein, S. E., & McHugh, P. R. (1975). "Mini-Mental State": A practical method for grading the cognitive state of patients for the clinician. *Journal of Psychiatric Research, 12*(3), 189–198.

Foreman, B. P., Caesar, R. R., Parks, J., Madden, C., Gentilello, L. M., Shafi, S., . . . Diaz-Arrastia, R. R. (2007). Usefulness of the abbreviated injury score and the injury severity score in comparison to the Glasgow Coma Scale in predicting outcome after traumatic brain injury. *Journal of Trauma and Acute Care Surgery, 62*(4), 946–950.

Gabbatore, I., Sacco, K., Angeleri, R., Zettin, M., Bara, B. G., & Bosco, F. M. (2015). Cognitive pragmatic treatment: A rehabilitative program for traumatic brain injury individuals. *Journal of Head Trauma Rehabilitation, 30*(5), E14–E28.

Giacino, J. T., & Cicerone, K. D. (1998). Varieties of deficit unawareness after brain injury. *Journal of Head Trauma Rehabilitation, 13,* 1–15.

Gianutsos, R., & Gianutsos, J. (1979). Rehabilitating the verbal recall of brain injured patients by mnemonic training: An experimental demonstration using single-case methodology. *Journal of Clinical and Experimental Neuropsychology, 1,* 117–135.

Gillis, R. J. (1999a). Traumatic brain injury: Cognitive-communicative needs and early intervention. In R. J. Elman (Ed.), *Group treatment of neurogenic communication disorders: The expert clinician's approach* (pp. 141–151). Butterworth-Heinemann.

Gillis, R. J. (1999b). Cotreatment and community-oriented group treatment for traumatic brain injury. In R. J. Elman (Ed.), *Group treatment of neurogenic communication disorders: The expert clinician's approach* (pp. 153–163). Butterworth-Heinemann.

Glosser, G., & Deser, T. (1990). Patterns of discourse production among neurological patients with fluent language disorders. *Brain and Language, 40,* 67–88.

Gosseries, O., Vanhaudenhuyse, A., Bruno, M., Demetrzi, A., Schnakers, C., Boly, M. M., . . . Laureys, S. (2011). Disorders of consciousness: Coma, vegetative and minimally conscious states. In D. Cvetkovic & I. Cosic (Eds.), *States of consciousness.* Springer-Verlag. https://doi .org/10.1007/978-3-642-18047-7_2

Graham, J. E., Radice-Neumann, D. M., Reistetter, T. A., Hammond, F. M., Dijkers, M., & Granger, C. V. (2010). Influence of sex and age on inpatient rehabilitation outcomes among older adults with traumatic brain injury. *Archives of Physical Medicine and Rehabilitation, 91*(1), 43–50. https://doi.org/10.1016/j .apmr.2009.09.017

Guide for Uniform Data Set for Medical Rehabilitation. (1996). *Guide for the use of the uniform data set for medical rehabilitation, Version 5.0.* State University of New York at Buffalo Research Foundation.

Guideline Development Panel, Brown, J., Kaelin, D., Mattingly, E., Mello, C., Miller, E. S., . . . Bowen, R. (2022). American Speech-Language-Hearing Association Clinical Practice Guideline: Cognitive rehabilitation for the management of cognitive dysfunction associated with acquired brain injury. *American Journal of Speech-Language Pathology, 31*(6), 2455–2526. https://doi.org/10.1044/2022_AJSLP-21-00361

Hagen, C. (1982). Language-cognitive disorganization following closed head injury: A conceptualization. In L. E. Trexler (Ed.), *Cognitive rehabilitation* (pp. 131–151). Plenum.

Hagen, C. (2000, February). *Rancho Levels of Cognitive Functioning–Revised.* Presentation at TBI Rehabilitation in a Managed Care Environment: An Interdisciplinary Approach to Rehabilitation, Continuing Education Programs of America.

Hagen, C., Malkmus, D., & Durham, P. (1972). *Rancho Los Amigos Levels of Cognitive Functioning Scale.* Professional Staff Association.

Haider, A. H., Chang, D. C., Efron, D. T., Haut, E. R., Crandall, M., & Cornwell, E. E., III. (2008). Race and insurance status as risk factors for trauma mortality. *Archives of Surgery, 143*(10), 945–949. https://doi .org/10.1001/archsurg.143.10.945

Happé, F., Brownell, H., & Winner, E. (1999). Acquired theory of mind impairments following stroke. *Cognition, 70,* 211–240.

Harris, J. R. (1996). Verbal rehearsal and memory in children with closed head injury: A quantitative and qualitative analysis. *Journal of Communication Disorders, 29,* 79–93.

Health Measures. (2018). *Patient-Reported Outcomes Measurement Information System–Cognitive Function.* http://www .healthmeasures.net/images/PROMIS/ manuals/PROMIS_Cognitive_Function _Scoring_Manual.pdf

Helm-Estabrooks, N. (2017). *Cognitive Linguistic Quick Test–Plus (CLQT+)*. Pearson.

Helm-Estabrooks, N., & Hotz, G. (1991). *Brief Test of Head Injury*. Pro-Ed.

Hettema, J., Steele, J., & Miller, W. R. (2005). Motivational interviewing. *Annual Review of Clinical Psychology, 1*, 91–111.

Hinckley, J. J., & Craig, H. K. (1992). A comparison of picture-stimulus and conversational elicitation contexts: Responses to comments by adults with aphasia. *Aphasiology, 6*, 257–272.

Iverson, G. L., Gardner, A. J., Terry, D. P., Ponsford, J. L., Sills, A. K., Broshek, D. K., & Solomon G. S. (2017). Predictors of clinical recovery from concussion: A systematic review. *British Journal of Sports Medicine, 51*(12), 941–948.

Janak, J. C., Pugh, M. J., & Langlois Orman, J. A. (2015). Epidemiology of TBI. In D. X. Cifu & B. C. Eapen (Eds.), *Traumatic brain injury rehabilitation medicine* (pp. 6–35). Elsevier.

Jeffay, E., Ponsford, J., Harnett, A., Janzen, S., Patsakos, E., Douglas, J., . . . Green, R. (2023). INCOG 2.0 guidelines for cognitive rehabilitation following traumatic brain injury, Part III: Executive function. *Journal of Head Trauma Rehabilitation, 38*(1), 52–64. https://doi.org/10.1097/HTR.0000000000000834

Jennett, B., & Teasdale, G. (1977). Aspects of coma after severe head injury. *Lancet, 309*(8017), 878–881.

Jotwani, V., & Harmon, K. G. (2010). Post-concussion syndrome in athletes. *Current Sports Medicine Reports, 9*(1), 21–26.

Karol, R. L. (2014). Team models in neurorehabilitation: structure, function, and culture change. *NeuroRehabilitation, 34*(4), 655–669.

Kennedy, M. R., Coelho, C., Turkstra, L., Ylvisaker, M., Moore Sohlberg, M., Yorkston, K., . . . Kan, P. F. (2008). Intervention for executive functions after traumatic brain injury: A systematic review, meta-analysis, and clinical recommendations. *Neuropsychological Rehabilitation, 18*, 257–299.

Knight, C., Alderman, N., & Burgess, P. W. (2002). Development of a simplified version of the Multiple Errands Test for use in hospital settings. *Neuropsychological Rehabilitation, 12*, 231–255.

Knight, R. G., Titov, N., & Crawford, M. (2006). The effects of distraction on prospective remembering following traumatic brain injury assessed in a simulated naturalistic environment. *Journal of the International Neuropsychological Society, 12*, 8–16.

Krasny-Pacini, A., Chevignard, M., & Evans, J. (2014). Goal Management Training for rehabilitation of executive functions: A systematic review of effectiveness in patients with acquired brain injury. *Disability and Rehabilitation, 36*(2), 105–116.

Lambez, B., & Valkil, E. (2021). The effectiveness of memory remediation strategies after traumatic brain injury: Systematic review and meta-analysis. *Annals of Physical and Rehabilitation Medicine, 64*(5), 101530. https://doi.com/10.1016/j.rehab.2021.101530

Levin, H. S., Madison, C. F., Bailey, C. B., Meyers, C. A., Eisenberg, H. M., & Guinto, F. C. (1983). Mutism after closed head injury. *Archives of Neurology, 40*(10), 601–606.

Levin, H. S., O'Donnell, V. M., & Grossman, R. G. (1979). The Galveston Orientation and Amnesia Test: A practical scale to assess cognition after head injury. *Journal of Nervous and Mental Disease, 167*, 675–684.

Levine, B., Robertson, I. H., Clare, L., Carter, G., Hong, J., Wilson, B. A., . . . Stuss, D. T. (2000). Rehabilitation of executive functioning: An experimental-clinical validation of goal management training. *Journal of the International Neuropsychological Society, 6*(3), 299–312.

Light, J., Beesley, M., & Collier, B. (1988). Transition through multiple augmentative and alternative communication systems: A three-year case study of a head injured adolescent. *Augmentative and Alternative Communication, 4*, 2–14.

Loftis, K. L., Price, J., & Gillich, P. J. (2018). Evolution of the abbreviated injury scale: 1990–2015. *Traffic Injury Prevention, 19*(Suppl. 2), S109–S113.

Lovell, M. R., Collins, M. W., Maroon, J. C., Cantu, R., Hawn, M. A., Burke, C. J., & Fu, F. (2002). Inaccuracy of symptom reporting following concussion in athletes. *Medicine & Science in Sports & Exercise, 34*(5), S298.

MacDonald, S. (2005). *Functional Assessment of Verbal Reasoning and Executive Strategies.* CCD.

MacDonald, S. (2017). Introducing the model of cognitive-communication competence: A model to guide evidence-based communication interventions after brain injury. *Brain Injury, 31*(13/14), 1760–1780. https://doi.org/10.1080/02699052.2017.1379613

Mackay, L. E., Morgan, A. S., & Bernstein, B. A. (1999). Swallowing disorders in severe brain injury: Risk factors affecting return to oral intake. *Archives of Physical Medicine and Rehabilitation, 80,* 365–371.

Malec, J. F., Hammond, F. M., Giacino, J. T., Whyte, J., & Wright, J. (2012). Structured interview to improve the reliability and psychometric integrity of the Disability Rating Scale. *Archives of Physical Medicine and Rehabilitation, 93*(9), 1603–1608.

Malec, J. F., Kragness, M., Evans, R. W., Finlay, K. L., Kent, A., & Lezak, M. D. (2003). Further psychometric evaluation and revision of the Mayo-Portland Adaptability Inventory in a national sample. *The Journal of Head Trauma Rehabilitation, 18*(6), 479–492.

Malec, J. F., & Lezak, M. D. (2008). *Manual for the Mayo-Portland Adaptability Inventory (MPAI-4) for adults, children and adolescents.* http://www.tbims.org/mpai/manual.pdf

Mandaville, A., Ray, A., Robertson, H., Foster, C., & Jesser, C. (2014). A retrospective review of swallow dysfunction in patients with severe traumatic brain injury. *Dysphagia, 29,* 1–9.

Marshall, R., Karow, C., Morelli, C., Iden, K., Dixon, J., & Cranfill, T. (2004). Effects of interactive strategy modelling training on problem-solving by persons with traumatic brain injury. *Aphasiology, 18,* 659–673.

Massaro, M., & Tompkins, C. A. (1994). Feature analysis for treatment of communication disorders in traumatically brain-injured patients: An efficacy study. *Clinical Aphasiology, 22,* 245–256.

Maujean, A., Shum, D., & McQueen, R. (2003). Effect of cognitive demand on prospective memory in individuals with traumatic brain injury. *Brain Impairment, 4,* 135–145.

McCrea, M., Hammeke, T., Olsen, G., Leo, P., & Guskiewicz, K. (2004). Unreported concussion in high school football players: Implications for prevention. *Clinical Journal of Sport Medicine, 14*(1), 13–17.

McDonald, S., Tate, R., Togher, L., Bornhofen, C., Long, E., Gertler, P., & Bowen, R. (2008). Social skills treatment for people with severe, chronic acquired brain injuries: A multicenter trial. *Archives of Physical Medicine and Rehabilitation, 89,* 1648–1659.

McDougall, J., Wright, V., & Rosenbaum, P. (2010). The ICF model of functioning and disability: Incorporating quality of life and human development. *Developmental Neurorehabilitation, 13*(3), 204–211.

McKay, A., Love, J., Trevena-Peters, J., Gracey, J., & Ponsford, J. (2020). The relationship between agitation and impairments of orientation and memory during the PTA period after traumatic brain injury. *Neuropsychological Rehabilitation, 30*(4), 579–590. https://doi.org/10.1080/09602011.2018.1479276

Meagher, A. D., Beadles, C. A., Doorey, J., & Charles, A. G. (2015). Racial and ethnic disparities in discharge to rehabilitation following traumatic brain injury. *Journal of Neurosurgery, 122*(3), 595–601. https://doi.org/10.3171/2014.10.JNS14187

Medley, A. R., & Powell T. (2010). Motivational interviewing to promote self-awareness and engagement in rehabilitation following acquired brain injury: A conceptual review. *Neuropsychological Rehabilitation, 20*(4), 481–508.

Miller, G. F., DePadilla, L., & Xu, L. (2021). Costs of non-fatal traumatic brain injury in the United States, 2016. *Medical Care, 59*(5), 451–455. https://doi.org/10.1097/MLR.0000000000001511

Miotto, E. C., Cinalli, F. Z., Serrao, V. T., Benute, G. G., Lucia, M. C. S., & Scaff, M. (2010). Cognitive deficits in patients with mild to moderate traumatic brain injury. *Arquivos de Neuro-psiquiatria, 68*, 862–868.

Morgan, A. S., & Mackay, L. E. (1999). Causes and complications associated with swallowing disorders in traumatic brain injury. *Journal of Head Trauma Rehabilitation, 14*, 454–461.

Morley, J. E., & Tumosa, N. (2002). Saint Louis University Mental Status Examination (SLUMS). *Aging Successfully, 12*(1), 4.

Multi-Society Task Force on PVS. (1994a). Medical aspects of the persistent vegetative state. *New England Journal of Medicine, 330*, 1499–1508.

Multi-Society Task Force on PVS. (1994b). Medical aspects of the persistent vegetative state (second of two parts). *New England Journal of Medicine, 330*, 1572–1579.

Myers, P., Henry, J., Zaugg, T., & Kendall, C. (2009). Tinnitus evaluation and management considerations for persons with mild traumatic brain injury. *Access Audiology, 8*. http://www.asha.org/aud/articles/TinnitusTBI/

Nasreddine, Z. S., Phillips, N. A., Bédirian, V., Charbonneau, S., Whitehead, V., Collin, I., . . . Chertkow, H. (2005). The Montreal Cognitive Assessment, MoCA: A brief screening tool for mild cognitive impairment. *Journal of the American Geriatrics Society, 53*, 695–699.

National Institute of Neurological Disorders and Stroke (NINDS). (2015). *User manual for the Quality of Life in Neurological Disorders (Neuro-QOL) Measures, Version 2.0.* https://www.sralab.org/sites/default/files/2017-06/Neuro-QOL_User_Manual_v2_24Mar2015.pdf

Nielsen, A. I., Power, E., & Jensen, L. R. (2020). Communication with patients in posttraumatic confusional state: Perceptions of rehabilitation staff. *Brain Injury, 34*(4), 447–455. https://doi.org/10.1080/02699052.2020.1725839

O'Neil-Pirozzi, T. M., Kennedy, M. R. T., & Sohlberg, M. M. (2015). Evidence-based practice for the use of internal strategies as a memory compensation technique after brain injury: A systematic review. *Journal of Head Trauma Rehabilitation, 15*, 32–42.

Ownsworth, T., Arnautovska, U., Beadle, E., Shum, D. H. K., & Moyle, W. (2018). Efficacy of telerehabilitation for adults with traumatic brain injury: A systematic review. *Journal of Head Trauma Rehabilitation, 33*(4), E33–E46. https://doi.org/10.1097/HTR.0000000000000350

Phyland, R. K., Ponsford, J. L., Carrier, S. L., Hicks, A. J., & McKay, A. (2021). Agitated behaviours following traumatic brain injury: A systematic review and meta-analysis of prevalence by posttraumatic amnesia status, hospital setting and agitated behavior type. *Journal of Neurotrauma, 38*(22), 3047–3067. https://doi.org/10.1089/neu.2021.0257

Ponsford, J., Spitz, G., & McKenzie, D. (2016). Using post-traumatic amnesia to predict outcome after traumatic brain injury. *Journal of Neurotrauma, 33*(11), 997–1004.

Ponsford, J., Trevena-Peters, J., Janzen, S., Harnett, A., Marshall, S., Patasakos, E., . . . McKay, A. (2023). INCOG2.0 Guidelines for cognitive rehabilitation following traumatic brain injury, Part I: Posttraumatic amnesia. *Journal of Head Trauma Rehabilitation, 38*(1), 24–37. https://doi.org/10.1097/HTR.0000000000000840

Ponsford, J., Velikonja, D., Janzen, S., Harnett, A., McIntyre, A., Wiseman-Hakes, C., . . . Bayley, M. T. (2023). INCGOG 2.0 Guidelines for cognitive rehabilitation following traumatic brain injury,

Part II: Attention and information processing speed. *Journal of Head Trauma Rehabilitation, 38*(1), 38–51. https://doi.org/10.1097/HTR.0000000000000839

Rancho Los Amigos Cognitive Scale Revised. (2014). https://www.neuroskills.com/education-and-resources/rancho-los-amigos-revised/

Randolph, C. (2012). *Repeatable Battery for the Assessment of Neuropsychological Status: Manual.* Pearson.

Rappaport, M., Hall, K. M., Hopkins, K., Belleza, T., & Cope, D. N. (1982). Disability Rating Scale for severe head trauma: Coma to community. *Archives of Physical Medicine and Rehabilitation, 63,* 118–123.

Raspelli, S., Pallavicini, F., Carelli, L., Morganti, F., Pedroli, E., Cipresso, P., . . . Riva, G. (2012). Validating the Neuro VR-based virtual version of the Multiple Errands Test: Preliminary results. *Presence: Teleoperators and Virtual Environments, 21,* 31–42.

Richardson, J. T. (1995). The efficacy of imagery mnemonics in memory remediation. *Neuropsychologia, 33,* 1345–1357.

Riegler, L. J., Neils-Strunjas, J., Boyce, S., Wade, S. L., & Scheifele, P. M. (2013). Cognitive Intervention results in web-based videophone treatment adherence and improved cognitive scores. *Medical Science Monitor, 19,* 269–275.

Rietdijk, R., Power, E., Attard, M., Heard, R., & Togher, L. (2020a). Improved conversation outcomes after social communication skills training for people with traumatic brain injury and their communication partner: A clinical trial investigating in-person and telehealth delivery. *Journal of Speech Language and Hearing Research, 63*(2), 615–634. https://doi.org/10.1044/2019_JSLHR-19-00076

Rietdijk, R., Power, E., Attard, M., Heard, R., & Togher, L. (2020b). A clinical trial investigating telehealth and in-person social communication skills training for people with traumatic brain injury: Participant reported communication outcomes. *Journal of Head Trauma Rehabilitation, 35*(4), 241–253. https://doi.org/10.1097/HTR.0000000000000554

Robertson, I. H., Ward, T., Ridgeway, V., & Nimmo-Smith, I. (1994). *Test of Everyday Attention.* Thames Valley Test Company.

Robertson, K., & Schmitter-Edgecombe, M. (2015). Self-awareness and traumatic brain injury outcome. *Brain Injury, 29,* 848–858. https://doi.org/10.3109/02699052.2015.1005135

Roth, R. M., Isquith, P. K., & Gioia, G. A. (2005). *Behavior Rating Inventory of Executive Function–Adult version (BRIEF-A).* PAR.

Sander, A. M., Raymer, A., Wertheimer, J., & Paul, D. (2009). Perceived roles and collaboration between neuropsychologists and speech-language pathologists in rehabilitation. *The Clinical Neuropsychologist, 23,* 1196–1212.

Sarno, M. T. (1980). The nature of verbal impairment after closed head injury. *Journal of Nervous and Mental Disease, 168*(11), 685–692.

Sarno, M. T., Buonaguro, A., & Levita, E. (1986). Characteristics of verbal impairment in closed-head injured patients. *Archives of Physical Medicine and Rehabilitation, 67*(6), 400–405.

Schacter, D. L., Rich, S. A., & Stampp, M. S. (1985). Remediation of memory disorders: Experimental evaluation of the spaced-retrieval technique. *Journal of Clinical and Experimental Neuropsychology, 7,* 79–96.

Schmidt, J., Fleming, J., Ownsworth, T., & Lannin, N. A. (2015). Maintenance of treatment effects of an occupation-based intervention with video feedback for adults with TBI. *NeuroRehabilitation, 36*(2), 175–186. https://doi.org/10.3233/NRE-151205

Schmitter-Edgecombe, M., Fahy, J. F., Whelan, J. P., & Long, C. J. (1995). Memory remediation after severe closed-head injury: Notebook training versus supportive therapy. *Journal of Consulting and Clinical Psychology, 63*(3), 484.

Selassie, A. W., Zaloshnja, E., Langlois, J. A., Miller, T., Jones, P., & Steiner, C. (2008). Incidence of long-term disability following traumatic brain injury hospitalization, United States, 2003. *Journal of Head Trauma and Rehabilitation*, 23(2), 123–131.

Shanahan, L., McAllister, L., & Curtin, M. (2011). The Party Planning Task: A useful tool in the functional assessment of planning skills in adolescents with TBI. *Brain Injury*, 25, 1080–1090.

Sherer, M., Boake, C., Levin, E., Silver, B. V., Ringholz, G., & High, W. M. (1998). Characteristics of impaired awareness after traumatic brain injury. *Journal of the International Neuropsychological Society*, 4(4), 380–387.

Silver, J. M., & Yudofsky, S. C. (2004). Aggressive disorders. In J. M. Silver & S. C. Yudofsky (Eds.), *Neuropsychiatry of traumatic brain injury* (pp. 313–353). American Psychiatric Press.

Singh, R., Venkateshwara, G., Nair, K. P., Khan, M., & Saad, R. (2014). Agitation after traumatic brain injury and predictors of outcome. *Brain Injury*, 28(3), 336–340. https://doi.org/10.3109/02699 052.2013.873142

Snyder, C., & Hux, K. (2000). Traumatic brain injury survivors' ability to reduce idiosyncrasy in semantic organization. *Journal of Medical Speech-Language Pathology*, 8, 187–197.

Sohlberg, M., Avery, J., Kennedy, M. R. T., Coelho, C., Ylvisaker, M., Turkstra, L., & Yorkston, K. (2003). Practice guidelines for direct attention training. *Journal of Medical Speech-Language Pathology*, 11, xix–xxxix.

Sohlberg, M. M., Hamilton, J., & Turkstra, L. S. (2023). *Transforming cognitive rehabilitation: Effective instructional methods*. Guilford.

Sohlberg, M. M., Kennedy, M., Avery, J., Coelho, C., Turkstra, L., Ylvisaker, M., & Yorkston, K. (2007). Evidence-based practice for the use of external aids as a memory compensation technique. *Journal of Medical Speech Language Pathology*, 15, xv–li.

Sohlberg, M. M., & Mateer, C. A. (2001a). Improving attention and managing attentional problems. *Annals of the New York Academy of Sciences*, 931, 359–375.

Sohlberg, M. M., & Mateer, C. A. (Eds.). (2001b). *Cognitive rehabilitation: An integrative neuropsychological approach*. Guilford.

Solomon, N. P., McKee, A. S., & Garcia-Barry, S. (2001). Intensive voice treatment and respiration treatment for hypokineticspastic dysarthria after traumatic brain injury. *American Journal of Speech-Language Pathology*, 10, 51–64.

Sosin, D. M., Sniezek, J. E., & Thurman, D. J. (1996). Incidence of mild and moderate brain injury in the United States, 1991. *Brain Injury*, 10, 47–54.

Stierwalt, J. A., & Murray, L. L. (2002). Attention impairment following traumatic brain injury. *Seminars in Speech and Language*, 23, 129–138.

Stubbs, J. L., Thornton, A. E., Sevick, J. M., Silverberg, N. D., Barr, A. M., Honer, W. G., & Panenka, W. J. (2020). Traumatic brain injury in homeless and marginally housed individuals: A systematic review and meta-analysis. *The Lancet Public Health*, 5(1), e19–e32. https://doi.org/ 10.1016/S2468-2667(19)30188-4

Sullivan, K. A., Kempe, C. B., Edmed, S. L., & Bonanno, G. A. (2016). Resilience and other possible outcomes after mild traumatic brain injury: A systematic review. *Neuropsychology Review*, 26(2), 173–185.

Summers, C. R., Ivins, B., & Schwab, K. A. (2009). Traumatic brain injury in the United States: An epidemiologic overview. *Mount Sinai Journal of Medicine*, 76, 105–110.

Teasdale, G., & Jennett, B. (1974). Assessment of Coma and Impaired Consciousness: A practical scale. *The Lancet*, 304(7872), 81–84.

Teasell, R., Marshall, S., Cullen, N., Bayley, R., Rees, L., Weiser, M., . . . Aubut, J. (2012). *Evidence-based review of moderate to*

severe acquired brain injury. http://www
.abiebr.com/pdf/executiveSummary.pdf

Thickpenny-Davis, K. L., & Barker-Collo,
S. L. (2007). Evaluation of a structured
group format memory rehabilitation
program for adults following brain
injury. *Journal of Head Trauma Rehabilitation*, 22, 303–313.

Thomsen, I. V. (1984). Late outcome of very
severe blunt head trauma: A 10–15 year
second follow-up. *Journal of Neurology,
Neurosurgery & Psychiatry*, 47, 260–268.

Thurman, D. (2001). The epidemiology and
economics of head trauma. In L. Miller
& R. Hayes (Eds.), *Head trauma: Basic,
preclinical, and clinical directions* (pp. 327–
347). Wiley and Sons.

Thurman, D. J., Alverson, C., Dunn, K. A.,
Guerrero, J., & Sniezek, J. E. (1999). Traumatic brain injury in the United States:
A public health perspective. *Journal of
Head Trauma and Rehabilitation*, 14(6),
602–615.

Togher, L., Douglas, J., Turkstra, L. S.,
Welch-West, P, Janzen, S., Harnett, A.,
. . . Wiseman-Hakes, C. (2023). INCOG
2.0 guidelines for cognitive rehabilitation following traumatic brain injury,
Part IV: Cognitive-communication and
social cognition disorders. *Journal of
Head Trauma Rehabilitation*, 38(1), 65–82.
https://doi.org/10.1097/HTR.00000000
00000835

Topolovec-Vranic, J., Ennis, N., Colantonio,
A., Cusimano, M. D., Hwang, S. W., Kontos, P., . . . Stergiopoulos, V. (2012). Traumatic brain injury among people who
are homeless: A systematic review. *BMC
Public Health*, 12(1), 1059.

Turkstra, L., Ylvisaker, M., Coelho, C., Kennedy, M., Sohlberg, M. M., & Avery, J.
(2005). Practice guidelines for standardized assessment for persons with traumatic brain injury. *Journal of Medical
Speech-Language Pathology*, 13, ix–xxvii.

Van Leer, E., & Turkstra, L. (1999). The effect
of elicitation task on discourse coherence
and cohesion in adolescents with brain

injury. *Journal of Communication Disorders*, 32, 327–349.

Velikonja, D., Ponsford, J., Janzen, S., Harnett, A., Patsakos, E., Kennedy, M., . . .
Bayley, M. T. (2023). INCOG 2.0 Guidelines for cognitive rehabilitation following traumatic brain injury, Part V: Memory. *Journal of Head Trauma Rehabilitation*,
38(1), 83–102. https://doi.org/10.1097/
HTR.0000000000000837

Wade, D. T. (2005). Applying the WHO
ICF framework to the rehabilitation of
patients with cognitive deficits. In P. W.
Halligan & D. T. Wade (Eds.), *Effectiveness of rehabilitation for cognitive deficits*
(pp. 31–42). Oxford University Press.

Wallace, S. E. (2010). AAC use by people
with TBI: Effects of cognitive impairments. *Perspectives on Augmentative and
Alternative Communication*, 19, 79–86.

Wallace, S. E., Hux, K., & Beukelman, D. R.
(2010). Navigation of a dynamic screen
AAC interface by survivors of severe
traumatic brain injury. *Augmentative and
Alternative Communication*, 26, 242–254.

Webb, P. M., & Glueckauf, R. L. (1994). The
effects of direct involvement in goal setting on rehabilitation outcome for persons with traumatic brain injuries. *Rehabilitation Psychology*, 39, 179.

Wilde, E. A., Whiteneck, G. G., Bogner, J.,
Bushnik, T., Cifu, D. X., Dikmen, S., . . .
von Steinbuechel, N. (2010). Recommendations for the use of common outcome measures in traumatic brain injury
research. *Archives of Physical Medicine and
Rehabilitation*, 91, 1650–1660. https://doi
.org/10.1016/j.apmr.2010.06.033

Williams, W. H., Chitsabesan, P., Fazel., S.,
McMillan, T., Hughes, N., Parsonage, M.,
& Tonks, J. (2018). Traumatic brain injury:
A potential cause of violent crime? *Lancet Psychiatry*, 5(10), 836–844. https://doi
.org/10.1016/s2215-0366(18)30062-2

Williams, W. H., Cordan, G., Mewse, A. J.,
Tonks, J., & Burgess, C. N. (2010). Self-reported traumatic brain injury in male
young offenders: A risk factor for reoff-

ending, poor mental health and violence. *Neuropsychological Rehabilitation*, *20*(6), 801–812.

Wilson, B., Vizor, A., & Bryant, T. (1991). Predicting severity of cognitive impairment after severe head injury. *Brain Injury*, *5*(2), 189–197.

Wilson, B. A., Baddeley, A., Evans, J., & Shiel, A. (1994). Errorless learning in the rehabilitation of memory impaired people. *Neuropsychological Rehabilitation*, *4*, 307–326.

Wilson, B. A., Greenfield, E., Clare, L., Baddeley, A., Cockburn, J., Watson, P., . . . Nannery, R. (2008). *The Rivermead Behavioural Memory Test–Third edition*. Thames Valley Test Company.

Wood, R. L., & Liossi, C. (2006). The ecological validity of executive tests in a severely brain injured sample. *Archives of Clinical Neuropsychology*, *21*, 429–437.

Wright, J. (2000). *The FIM™*. The Center for Outcome Measurement in Brain Injury. http://www.tbims.org/combi/FIM

Yorkston, K. M., Hakel, M., Beukelman, D. R., & Fager, S. (2007). Evidence for effectiveness of treatment of loudness, rate or prosody in dysarthria: A systematic review. *Journal of Medical Speech-Language Pathology*, *15*, xi–xxxvi.

Zafonte, R. D., Hammond, F. M., Mann, N. R., Wood, D. L., Black, K. L., & Millis, S. R. (1996). Relationship between Glasgow Coma Scale and functional outcome. *American Journal of Physical Medicine & Rehabilitation*, *75*(5), 364–369.

Zaloshnja, E., Miller, T., Langlois, J. A., & Selassie, A. W. (2008). Prevalence of long-term disability from traumatic brain injury in the civilian population of the United States. *Journal of Head Trauma Rehabilitation 23*, 394–400.

Appendix 8–A

Case History Example

SPEECH-LANGUAGE THERAPY CASE HISTORY

NAME: Thomas Casler (he/him)	ONSET DATE: 11/30/22 (6 months ago)
ADDRESS: 593 E. Spencer Boulevard, Columbus, OH	PHONE: (555) 555-8735

EMERGENCY CONTACT: Jordan (parent) 248-555-1212 Power of Attorney: Jordan (parent) 248-555-1212	AGE: 21 years	DATE OF BIRTH: 5/11/2001

SOCIAL HISTORY	MEDICAL HISTORY
PARTNER: N/A (single)	DIAGNOSES: History of ADHD managed with medication. Diffuse axonal injury; subdural hematoma on 11/30/22. No other remarkable medical history.
FAMILY: Younger sister who also lives at home	
LIVING SITUATION: Lived with parent (Jordan—age 51 years) prior to accident.	PAST MEDICAL HISTORY: Survived a motor vehicle accident 6 months ago. Upon intake to the intensive care unit, he had a GCS of 5: eyes = 1; motor = 2; verbal = 2. He was in a medically induced coma for 13 days. Upon waking up from his coma he was oriented ×1 (person only) and was in a state of PTA as determined by the GOAT for 25 days postinjury. Ranchos Level upon waking was 4. Remained in acute care for 15 days before being transferred to inpatient rehabilitation to participate in physical therapy, occupational therapy, and speech-language therapy.
EMPLOYMENT: Worked part-time at a grocery store approximately 20 hours per week.	
EDUCATION: Was recently enrolled as a full-time student in community college studying art history.	

HOBBIES/INTERESTS: Pottery, running, video games, volunteers for YMCA			GLASSES?	YES	(NO)	
HANDEDNESS?	Left	(Right)				
PREVIOUSLY DRIVING?	(YES)	NO	HEARING AIDS?	YES	(NO)	
LITERATE – READING?	(YES)	NO		Left	Right	
LITERATE – WRITING?	(YES)	NO	DENTURES?	YES	(NO)	
RESPONSIBLE FOR FINANCES?	(YES)	NO				

ACUTE CARE INFORMATION

DIET LEVEL: No modifications	HOSPITAL: Southwestern Medical
PREVIOUS MODIFIED BARIUM SWALLOW STUDY: 1/10/23 showed silent aspiration on thin liquids, impulsivity was noted; recommended diet modification and initiation of dysphagia management. 2/10/23 no signs or symptoms of aspiration; recommend return to regular diet.	RANCHOS LEVEL: 6
	PREVIOUS IMAGING RESULTS: A noncontrast computed tomography (CT) scan was conducted at the time of injury. A skull fracture and subdural hematoma were identified in the scan.

INPATIENT REHABILITATION ASSESSMENT RESULTS

Scales of Cognitive Ability for Traumatic Brain Injury: Overall Cognitive Severity Rating 8/17 suggesting moderate cognitive impairment. Concerns noted across cognitive domains:

Summary	Attention: Perception/ Discrimination	Orientation	Organization	Recall	Reasoning
Raw Score	50/58	16/20	24/30	31/52	26/55
Percentile Rank	32	27	32	37	30
Standard Score	93	91	93	95	92

Test of Everyday Attention: Greatest deficits were noted in selective attention and sustained attention.

Summary	Map Search Subtest (1 minute)	Map Search Subtest (2 minutes)	Elevator Counting with Distraction	Lottery
Raw Score	25	46	6/10	8/10
Percentile	1	1	5	7
Scaled Score	4	1	25	5

Assessment of Intelligibility of Dysarthric Speech: Determined to be 55% intelligible to unfamiliar listeners when topic is known.

Informal Discourse Sample: Three samples were collected: personal narrative, picture description, and procedural task. Using criteria, characteristics, and procedures from Van Leer and Turkstra (1999) and Hux et al. (2008) no areas of concerns were noted (e.g., intact local and global coherence, adequate number of content units, appropriate use of cohesive markers, and no abnormal presence of redundancies). However, he does exhibit superficial awareness of his cognitive limitations and the limits they place on his safety. He occasionally overestimates his abilities and is unable to think about the consequences of a decision or action.

AUGMENTATIVE AND ALTERNATIVE COMMUNICATION/SUPPLEMENTAL SUPPORTS: None at this time but plan includes introducing letterboard to supplement speech intelligibility challenges.

continues

CURRENT PLAN OF CARE	
SAMPLE SHORT-TERM THERAPY GOALS: 1. Thomas will use a letter board and/or over articulation strategies to resolve 65% of communication breakdowns with unfamiliar communication partners with verbal prompts. 2. Thomas will be oriented to time with the use of an external aid with min visual cues and 95% accuracy. 3. Thomas will use an external strategy to manage internal distractions at least two times during a 15-minute conversation in a minimally distracting environment with minimal verbal or visual cues. 4. Thomas will use an electronic calendar to schedule daily tasks (e.g., work, school) with 80% accuracy with moderate verbal cues. 5. Thomas will use external aid to document daily events completed with min verbal cues and 85% accuracy.	CURRENT FUNCTIONAL STATUS: Rancho Level = 7; Transitional rehab with a patient goal of discharging to home environment to live with his parent (father). Completes activities of daily living with minimal cues (verbal cues). Thomas and his family state goal related to him returning to audit one community college course.

Appendix 8–B

Treatment Protocol Description

Short-Term Goal: Thomas will use an external strategy to manage internal distractions at least two times during a 15-minute conversation in a minimally distracting environment with minimal verbal or visual cues.

Long-Term Goal: Thomas will independently use an external strategy to manage internal distractions at least two times during a 45-minute conversation in a minimally distracting environment with minimal verbal or visual cues.

Protocol: This activity will involve teaching Thomas to use compensatory strategies to manage his attention deficits. The clinician will provide instruction on three strategies and include spoken and written description of the strategies. One strategy will be a Key Ideas Log.

Key Ideas Log

At the beginning of each session, the clinician will ask Thomas to write down any ideas or persistent thoughts that were present in his head or things he wanted to comment on. Items that could be dealt with quickly (i.e., a person with blue hair that he saw) were addressed at that time. Other items that might lead to broader discussion were kept until later. The clinician indicates that they will save 5 minutes at the end of each session to discuss what was written in the log. The key ideas log is kept on the table or another visible location during the therapy session, and if other thoughts or ideas (unrelated to therapy) come to his mind, he can write them in the log. The client will then be able to focus on the therapy tasks because he knows that (a) he will not forget to mention the ideas that are important to him, and (b) he will be given time to talk about them. The introduction of a key ideas log can substantially reduce negative effects of distractibility in therapy. This strategy can generalize to other tasks and can assist with participation in school and work activities.

Appendix 6-9
Treatment Protocol Description

9

Implementing Culturally Responsive and Trauma-Informed Care in Acquired Cognitive Communication Disorders:
SLP Considerations for Marginalized and Underserved Populations

Catherine Wiseman-Hakes, Kathryn Y. Hardin, and Maya Albin

Chapter Learning Objectives

After reading this chapter you will be able to:

1. Identify the cognitive and social communication impairments that may contribute to marginalization and vulnerability for individuals with traumatic brain injury (TBI) and other neurodisabilities.
2. Summarize the prevalence of TBI as the primary etiology of acquired cognitive communication disorders among marginalized and underserved populations.
3. Explain how the sequalae of acquired cognitive communication disorders, including the associated cognitive and social communication impairments, can be both a risk factor for TBIs, and a barrier to successful community reintegration.
4. Describe the intersection of psychological trauma, in concert with physical and brain trauma, with considerations for speech-language pathology (SLP) clinical practice.

5. Explain the role of SLPs in assessing and treating cognitive communication disorders for marginalized and underserved populations with acquired brain injury.

Overview

Speech-language pathologists (SLPs) assess and treat individuals with acquired cognitive communication disorders (CCDs) subsequent to acquired brain injury (ABI), damage to the brain that occurs after birth. ABI etiologies include stroke, brain hemorrhage, tumor, neurological illness or disorder, progressive degenerative brain disorder, and traumatic brain injury (TBI) (Brain Injury Canada, n.d.). ABI from traumatic and nontraumatic causes is a leading cause of disability worldwide and data estimates that approximately 34% to greater than 75% of people with ABI have residual cognitive and communication impairments (Lannoo et al., 2004; MacDonald, 2017).

Acquired CCDs frequently result from TBI, and while the prevalence of TBI among the general population globally is 8.4% (Nguyen et al., 2016), it has a higher prevalence among several groups who are often considered marginalized and underserved. While SLPs have historically not been involved with these groups, there is growing acknowledgment that the communication impairments commonly associated with TBI (as well as other neurodisabilities) may contribute to emotional and behavioral challenges, lack of agency, impaired self-advocacy, and lack of health equity and social justice. Communication challenges create unique barriers, needs, and challenges for these individuals, and SLPs can, and should, play an important role.

Recognizing the importance of the phrase, "individuals are not populations" (Sackett et al., 1996), meaning that individuals within each of these groups have their own stories, strengths, and challenges, we suggest specific considerations for SLPs working with the following groups:

- Women survivors of Intimate Partner Violence (IPV)
- Persons intersecting with the criminal justice system, including those who are incarcerated
- Refugees and asylum seekers
- Indigenous persons
- Persons who are precariously housed

These groups are not mutually exclusive as they can and often do intersect.

It has been well recognized that people with TBI can live positive and meaningful lives, however, factors that facilitate positive outcomes such as health equity, timely access to diagnosis and care, more years of education, positive social integration, family support, and the ability to return to employment in some capacity (Grace et al., 2015), are often not readily available to marginalized and underserved communities. These disparities have been further exacerbated in the context of the COVID-19 pandemic, which has also created new inequities (Kantamneni, 2020). Therefore, these underserved communities and their unique needs and challenges are the focus of this chapter.

Why "Marginalized" and "Underserved"?

The terminology used within this chapter evolved throughout its writings, and, when the title was first proposed, the term "vulnerable" populations was considered. We were aware that in a public health and social context, "vulnerable" often refers to those who lack, or have restricted access to, the social determinants of health and face inherent societal and structural barriers (Katz et al., 2019). Furthermore, this term is commonly used in both health care and public health literature to attract public concern, policy change, and resources (Katz et al., 2019). However, there is little to no consensus as to what this term specifies (Katz et al., 2019; Levine et al., 2004). The term "vulnerable" is inherently vague, particularly about the causes of the inequities. According to Katz et al. (2019), this term can lead to incorrect and damaging narratives whereby inadvertent blame is placed upon groups with "preventable" health conditions or life situations that are attributed to their choices and behaviors. Thus, upon reflection, "vulnerable" was deemed to be stigmatizing, and would negatively impact our aim to provide information and guidance.

Marginalized was also a term we considered that is commonly used in the literature. According to the definition of the National Collaborating Centre for Determinants of Health (NCCDH) these are "groups and communities that often experience discrimination and exclusion (social, political, and economic) because of unequal power relationships across economic, politi-cal, social, and cultural dimensions" (NCCDH, 2022). Underserved was also considered as this term is utilized by the U.S. federal governmental health care agencies to describe groups of individuals that "receive fewer health care services, face economic, cultural, and/ or linguistic barriers to accessing health care services . . . [and] lack familiarity with the health care systems" (Centers for Medicare & Medicaid Services, n.d., p.12). Therefore, ultimately, we agreed that the terms "marginalized" and "underserved" best reflected the groups we were addressing.

A Model of Intersectionality and TBI Among Marginalized and Underserved Communities

While there are other etiologies that can result in CCDs, TBI is the primary cause of neurodisability and CCDs among marginalized and underserved groups and communities. Furthermore, these groups mandate special consideration relating to social justice and health inequities as they are often overlooked and underserved. Moreover, many intersectionalities exist among these groups that may stem directly from their TBI(s) and subsequent lack of support, placing them at a high risk of additional challenges. The concept of "intersectionality" is defined as "intersectional oppression that arises out of the combination of various oppressions (i.e., the opposite of privilege, such as racism, sexism, TBI, or neurodiversity, precarious housing) which together, produce something distinct from any one form of oppression or discrimination standing alone" (OHRC, n.d., p. Intersectional Approach). To illustrate this, we propose a model of intersectionality through which TBI and the associated sequelae can cause risks of further marginalization, and where experiences both prior to and post-TBI create barriers and inequities to diagnosis and care. The model is centered by certain groups who are at high risk for TBI. Factors located on the right side of the model represent the increased risks and social justice inequities that can occur to individuals after sustaining TBI (e.g., increased risks of crimi-

nalization, re-injury) while factors on the left represent systemic barriers to accessing care for their TBI (e.g., lack of culturally appropriate care, history of colonization, racism), that lead to greater health inequities. Lack of access to the social determinants of health falls under both categories and is therefore a risk factor and a barrier to accessing care. These factors are nested within a ring reflecting the lack of access to social determinants of health and the constructs of sex and gender (Figure 9–1).

Clinicians working with these communities may, and likely will, see indi-

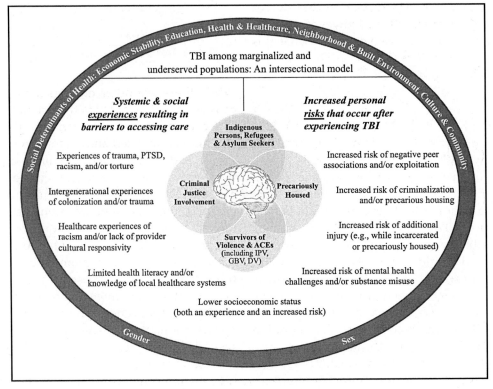

Figure 9–1. TBI among marginalized and underserved populations: A model of intersectionality. The inner circles represent groups who are most at risk of TBI. The arrows and text on the left illustrate the increased risks that often occur with greater incidence after TBI for individuals from these groups. The arrows and text on the right illustrate pre- and post-TBI experiences and systemic injustices that act as barriers to quality care. The bottom circle, lower socioeconomic status, is both a barrier and a risk factor. IPV= intimate partner violence; GBV = gender-based violence; DV = domestic violence; ACEs = adverse childhood events.

viduals who have experienced many of these interacting conditions and face the cumulative impacts of these conditions. For example, a refugee and/or asylum seeker may have sustained a TBI by means of trauma/torture in addition to lacking appropriate care, while also struggling to access care given the cultural and linguistic differences from their home country. There may be different legal rights available to asylum seekers and refugees in the host country, as well as limited access to the social determinants of health. These issues, in combination with possible mental health challenges and precarious housing, intersect to create additional complexities, all of which must be considered when working with underserved and marginalized people.

Introduction to Marginalized and Underserved Communities and TBI Prevalence

Intimate Partner Violence

There is a growing body of research highlighting the prevalence of TBI among women who experience intimate partner violence (between romantic partners; IPV), in heterosexual, queer, and non-binary relationships. Studies indicate that between 75% to 87% of IPV survivors sustain a TBI from repeat hits to the head, face, and neck, as well as anoxic injuries from attempted strangulation (Toccalino et al., 2022; Valera & Kucyi, 2017; Zieman et al., 2017). Many reported a lifetime history of abuse with physical and sexual violence and emotional mistreatment (Manoranjan et al., 2022), and there may be experience of domestic violence (i.e., between household members; e.g., parent and child, siblings, roommates) in the home. There is also an emerging awareness of the prevalence of gender-based violence (GBV) resulting in TBI among cisgender and transgender women who are sex workers (Baumann et al., 2019). GBV is a global public health issue and has been referred to as the "shadow pandemic" within the COVID-19 pandemic by the United Nations Women (UN Women, 2022). Since the outbreak of COVID-19, emerging data and reports have identified an increase in domestic violence, GBV, and IPV against women and girls (UN Women, 2022). While most research has focused upon women survivors of IPV, there is emerging evidence of IPV among men, although the prevalence of TBI among this group is unknown (Canadian Association for Equality, n.d.).

IPV is a form of GBV, and is highly correlated with poverty, precarious housing, mental health challenges, and substance use (Canadian Association for Equality, n.d.). Many survivors of IPV report using substances to cope with their IPV victimization (Canadian Association for Equality, n.d.). Furthermore, factors such as race, disability, age, and sexual orientation directly impact the experiences of individuals who identify as women experiencing IPV. Moreover, these factors intersect to shape experiences of violence, precarious housing, support seeking, as well as responses from service providers (Learning Network, 2022).

Survivors of IPV also may experience isolation, stigma, and shame due to psychological abuse, self-blame, and lack of perceived understanding and awareness of IPV (i.e., cultural stigma) and that this shame can negatively affect help-seeking behavior (Overstreet & Quinn, 2013). There is also a lack of understanding among first responders on how to support survivors, as well fears of being judged by family members and health care providers (Overstreet & Quinn, 2013). Furthermore, many survivors of IPV are unaware that they have sustained a TBI or multiple TBIs (Haag et al., 2019). All individuals who have experienced IPV and TBI, regardless of gender, require appropriate supports and intervention that may include support from SLPs.

Criminal Justice System

Additionally, there is a high prevalence of TBI among jail and prison inmates who have encountered the criminal justice system. Individuals with TBI are 2.5 times more likely to be incarcerated compared to the general population (Matheson et al., 2020) and as many as 80% of incarcerated adults report a history of TBI (Durand et al., 2017; Moynan & McMillan, 2018). Findings from two systematic reviews indicate that the prevalence of TBI ranged from 35.7% to 88% among studies that employed a validated TBI screening tool (Allely, 2016; O'Rourke et al., 2016). For youth within the justice system, findings from a systematic review identified the prevalence rate of TBI as ranging from 16.5% to 72% (Hughes et al., 2015). For many individuals, their injury (or first injury) was sustained during the teenage years, and prior to their first contact with the criminal justice system (Ferguson et al., 2012; Matheson et al., 2020). Furthermore, data show that many individuals sustain multiple injuries and may be unaware of the relationship between earlier injuries

and the circumstances that led to their incarceration (Ferguson, 2012). Consistent with our model of intersectionality, evidence indicates a high prevalence of adverse early life experiences among persons with TBI who are incarcerated. For example, incarcerated women with TBI experienced greater physical and sexual abuse compared to incarcerated women without TBI (Colantonio et al., 2014). There is also a higher prevalence of mental health challenges, housing instability, and substance use in the 5 years prior to incarceration for women with TBI (Matheson et al., 2020). The cognitive-communication challenges associated with TBI are often superimposed upon preexisting language and literacy impairments, which are also highly prevalent among persons who are incarcerated. Research from the United Kingdom indicates that approximately 60% to 90% of youth involved with the criminal justice system have significant deficits in both understanding and expressing language (Bryan et al., 2015; Gregory & Bryan, 2011; Hughes et al., 2012; Snow, 2019), as well as low literacy rates (Bryan et al., 2007; Snow & Powell 2011; Snowling et al., 2000). Cognitive-communication and language impairments increase the potential for misunderstanding the complex language used in legal interactions, spanning from the first contact with police officers to dealings with corrections staff (Wszalek & Turkstra, 2019). Communication impairments may also play a role in recidivism and poor community integration. SLPs play a critical role in mitigating these challenges through screening, assessment, provision of services, and education and training of justice personnel (Wiseman-Hakes et al., 2020). Additionally, SLPs can provide support for the understanding of the specific and often abstract terminology used in the justice system, including development of a glossary of terms in simple language.

Precariously Housed

Over six million people annually are precariously housed in the United States and European Union (Fazel et al., 2014), with numbers reaching over 100 million individuals globally. Additionally, over one billion people, predominantly in developing nations, experience inadequate housing (UN Commission on Human Rights, 2005). Being precariously housed, also described as homelessness, is predicated on many misconceptions within the general public. It is a commonly believed that individuals who are precariously housed sleep primarily outside in locations such as doorways, under bridges, or overnight in shelters; however, in the United States and Canada, many people who are inadequately housed may have intermittent stays on couches in others' homes, or temporary accommodations such as inexpensive motels. Many with stable housing perpetuate a damaging narrative, that "being homeless" is a choice that reflects past drug use/abuse, lacking interest in employment, and/ or choosing to live unmedicated for possible concurrent behavioral health needs. Not only are these ideas incorrect, they marginalize those who are precariously housed. It is important to note, however, that some of these misperceptions are changing with increasing levels of public compassion (Tsai & Wilson, 2020).

It is well documented that the experience of being precariously housed is multifactorial, including confounding factors of adverse childhood events such as abuse/neglect, TBI, sexual assault, substance use disorder, psychiatric comorbidities, food insecurity and hunger, and limited access to adequate resources such as healthcare (Bransford & Cole, 2019). A systematic review and meta-analysis by Stubbs and colleagues (2020) examined "homelessness" in developed nations and concluded that the lifetime prevalence of TBI was 53.1%, with a 22.5% prevalence of moderate-severe injury. Importantly, the average age of initial TBI was 15 years of age, and the majority of respondents sustained their initial TBI prior to experiencing precarious housing, similar to individuals in the criminal justice system. These early brain injuries can directly impact academic and vocational functioning, and is a clear factor related to precarious housing (Stubbs et al., 2020; Zeiler et al., 2021). Consistent with our model, TBI has doubly impactful consequences in regard to housing; the functional socioeconomic results of a TBI may result in unstable housing, and the long-term impacts of the TBI, including CCDs, may prevent individuals from acquiring stable housing once lost. In essence, TBI can be "both a cause and consequence of homelessness" (Young & Hughes, 2020).

In addition to housing concerns, the presence of TBI is associated with poorer self-reported physical and mental health, exacerbated sleep disturbance, higher rates of suicidality and suicide risk, memory concerns, increased health service use, and criminal justice involvement (Stubbs et al., 2020), as is consistent with an intersectionality model. Persons experiencing precarious housing with TBI and/or

CCDs require additional considerations and trauma-informed supports.

Indigenous Persons

In North America, Australia, and New Zealand, there is a long history of colonization that has done great injustice to generations of Indigenous communities through trauma that is historical (Cox et al., 2021; Lakhani et al., 2017; Nutton & Fast, 2015), but extends to contemporary experiences. This contributes to a significant burden of structural inequalities and health disparities, including a high prevalence of TBI among Indigenous persons in the United States, Canada, Australia, and New Zealand (Lakhani et al., 2017).

Indigenous people have a higher prevalence of TBI as compared to non-Indigenous people, yet they are less likely to present to the emergency department for diagnosis and care (Bohanna et al., 2019). This is directly related to a number of factors including a general lack of trust in a medical system that is based on the dominant culture and a product of the settler society. Furthermore, there are several health determinants such as rural location (physical environment), female gender (interpersonal and intimate partner violence), lack of availability of rehabilitation (health services), and lack of family and/or friend support (social) (Lasry et al., 2016; Zeiler & Zeiler, 2017), as well as prior encounters of discrimination and stigma with health care practitioners (Rehman et al., 2023. Indigenous Australians who sustain a TBI are more likely to be injured through an assault, to be female, to live remotely, and to have co-morbidities (Lakhani et al.,

2017). Indigenous peoples are the most over-represented ethnicity in Canadian prisons. Indigenous women account for over 40% of the female prison population, yet only 4.9% of the Canadian population identifies as Indigenous (Department of Indigenous Services Act, 2020). The lived experiences of Indigenous people with TBI intersect with many of the barriers and risk factors identified in the model, and warrant additional culturally safe, responsive, and trauma-informed support to navigate and address TBI-related communication disorders.

Refugees and Asylum Seekers

The UN has estimated that 68.5 million people globally have been displaced from their homes (Burton, 2019), with over one-third having crossed international borders, and are officially considered refugees (UN Refugee Agency, 2016). Asylum seekers, alternatively, are individuals seeking refugee status but awaiting formal verification; a process that can be significantly impacted by cultural and linguistic differences (Blommaert, 2009). Experiences of refugees and asylum seekers are marked by a lack of comfort with local languages and challenges with understanding local health care systems (Deora et al., 2019). As refugees adjust to a new environment, they may lack awareness that disabilities such as TBI could qualify for specific services. They also may maintain expectations of care from their past medical communities and apply those standards to their new environment (Mirza & Heinemann, 2012; Worabo et al., 2016). For example, their home countries may not have provided rehabilitation services in any form. Therefore, knowledge of the concept of rehabilitation may be a barrier to accessing care. Conversely, Western views of "disability" may conflict with an individual's personal and cultural views of illness or injury (McPherson, 2019; Mirza & Heinemann, 2012). It is also important to note that humanitarian care providers and interpreters for refugees and asylum seekers may have limited understanding of communication disorders, resulting in additional barriers to care (Marshall & Barrett, 2018).

Rates of TBI for adult refugees have been found to range from 51% to 69%, primarily resulting from direct traumas including: assault, IPV, torture, and human trafficking (Doherty et al., 2016; McPherson, 2019). Torture has been reported in over 50% of refugees across multiple continents (McPherson, 2019). TBI and accompanying CCDs co-occur with PTSD in adults and children, up to 86% and 46% respectively, as well as high rates of care for epilepsy and stroke (McPherson, 2019). As with IPV, refugees and asylum seekers may not report TBI-related injuries due to the significant stigma and shame associated with TBI in some cultures, which can be compounded by a desire to avoid discussing past traumatic events (McPherson, 2019, p. 1240). Their lived experiences frequently intersect with each of the aforementioned underserved groups: IPV, interactions with local legal systems, and unstable housing, partnered with the marked access barrier of non-native language demands within an unfamiliar health care system. Each of these issues and their compounding intersections require additional considerations and support when addressing communication disorders.

In conclusion, as authors, we acknowledge that the prevalence data among these groups is likely to be underestimated given, in many instances, lack of access to timely diagnosis or any diagnosis, possible cultural and linguistic barriers, issues regarding stigma, as well as barriers to accessing the basic social determinants of health. In addition to the cognitive-communication and social communication challenges associated with TBI, the prevalence of co-occurring mental health challenges, precarious housing, as well as substance use in some cases, create additional challenges in accessing care.

The Intersection of Cognitive-Communication Disorders and Marginalized Communities

Cognitive-Communication Disorders

As this chapter has described in detail, neurogenic CCDs occur in individuals from diverse backgrounds, and factors associated with these backgrounds directly impact how clinical care is delivered. Importantly, care considerations for CCDs associated with neurodisability becomes even more complex when persons from marginalized and under-served populations experience these challenges. It is well documented that neurogenic communication disorders, including aphasia, dysarthria, and right hemisphere disorder, as well as ADHD and autism spectrum disorder do occur in under-served populations; however, the exceptionally high incidence of TBI in these groups, as described earlier, mandates that SLPs be particularly cognizant of potential CCDs when serving these clients. According to Katz and Kennedy (2002), CCDs occur when there are disruptions in:

> Underlying cognitive processes (e.g., attention, memory, self-monitoring, executive function) as they interact and are manifested in communication behavior, broadly understood (listening, reading, writing, speaking, gesturing), and at all levels of language (phonological, morphologic, syntactic, semantic, pragmatic). (p. ix)

Pathophysiological disruptions to cognitive channels in both the gray and white matter can affect any communication modalities, including receptive, expressive, nonverbal, and social communication. As such, CCDs are formally defined as challenges with communication (i.e., listening, understanding spoken language, speaking, reading, writing, conversational interaction, and social communication) that occur as a result of underlying deficits in cognition, in the areas of attention, memory, information processing, reasoning, problem solving, executive functions, or self-regulation (CASLPO, n.d.). CCDs may directly impact success in all communicative environments, such as at home, work, and school. (MacDonald, 2017).

Changes in cognitive-communication competence after acquired neurogenic injury may be overt or quite subtle, transient or chronic, and these heterogeneous signs may be difficult to identify (Covington & Duff, 2021). ASHA describes how individuals with CCDs often have decreased conversational initiation, limited awareness of communicative struggles, and challenges with incorporating feedback or repair strategies in interactions (Wiseman-Hakes et al., 2019, 2023). Cornis-Pop and colleagues (2012) created an outstanding reference table describing the effects of TBI on varying areas of cognition and possible changes in communication functionality (p. xiii). For example, an individual struggling with attention may be distracted in conversation by background noise or have difficulties maintaining focus while reading; while slowed processing can manifest itself in delayed responses to questions. Those struggling with memory may seem repetitive in conversation or struggle recalling details. Changes in executive functioning and social communication can result in individuals having disorganized language, being tangential and hyperverbose, making inappropriate comments, or struggling to interpret higher level language (Cornis-Pop et al., 2012; ASHA, n.d.).

Identification and diagnosis of acquired CCDs can be challenging given the breadth of possible presentations, and, importantly, access to services is often even a greater barrier for individuals from underserved and marginalized backgrounds. Furthermore, acquired CCDs are often misinterpreted as either behavioral or as mental health conditions (Stanford, 2020). Individuals who are precariously housed are frequently misjudged and their communication disorders may be misattributed to changes solely in psychological health. For those facing the language-heavy, high-stakes justice system, memory problems, seemingly inappropriate "nervous" laughter, or minimal responsiveness to questions, may negatively influence judicial outcomes. Individuals experiencing IPV or seeking asylum may not endorse cognitive and communication deficits for fear of retribution and may lack awareness that intervention for such functional changes even exists. Each of these situations becomes exponentially more complex co-occurring with health care racialization and limited health literacy.

There are commonalities in communication dysfunction resulting from TBI in marginalized and underserved groups; however, when providing clinical care, SLPs must also consider there are unique elements for each community and person without making assumptions or overgeneralizing.

Functional Implications of CCDs for Marginalized and Underserved Communities

It is well-established that the language, speech, cognitive communication, and social communication challenges faced by individuals with TBI impact their life participation (Meulenbroek & Keegan, 2021). We encourage clinicians to consider the impacts of communication disorders through the lens of the International Classification of Functioning, Disability and Health (ICF) (World Health Organization, 2001), as an individual's personal factors, environment, activities of daily living, and participation goals directly influence how their communication challenges impact daily life. When working with marginalized and underserved individuals, we must consider the additional participation barriers related to their environment and personal factors. For example, individuals who are precari-

ously housed may need to look for shelters or rental units, read complex legal documents such as leases, or coordinate moving their belongings. Individuals who are at risk of or have been in conflict with the law will need to navigate the legal system or interactions with police. Survivors of IPV/GBV may also need to interact with first responders, health care providers, and the legal system (Wiseman-Hakes et al., 2020). For those who intersect with the justice system, the communication demands are critical as:

Verbal communication is the primary interface with the justice system in almost every jurisdiction, from the moments leading up to and following apprehension and questioning by police, to discussions with lawyers, court hearings, and throughout any restorative justice and/or rehabilitation processes . . . Therefore, any barriers to being able to participate fully—be it through impaired cognitive abilities, language or cultural barriers, and/or difficulties with hearing, auditory processing, or language skills—have implications for the offender's basic rights and access to justice. (Lambie, 2020)

Barriers Faced by Underserved and Marginalized Populations:

Although underserved and marginalized groups face unique barriers to life participation, SLPs should be aware that many clients from these groups will also experience stigma, trauma, oppression, as well as poor access to the social determinants of health.

Assumptions, Stigma, and Biases

Individuals with TBI generally face stigma as it is most often an "invisible injury," and thus misunderstood. However, those who are underserved and marginalized face additional stigma (Johnstone et al., 2015). Unfortunately, those from different cultural and ethnic backgrounds are often subjected to stigma and bias, which has been perpetuated during the COVID-19 pandemic (American Psychological Association, 2020; Kantamneni, 2020). These groups often describe experiences of being judged, or "put into a box," which may lead to the dismissal of other aspects of their identity. For example, it may be assumed that a well-dressed individual could or would not be precariously housed, that an individual who speaks English fluently would not be a refugee or asylum seeker, or that a woman without visible physical injuries would not be a victim of IPV/GBV.

Clinicians must also challenge the biases they may hold to best serve their clients. As well as being generally harmful, stereotypes or biases imposed upon clients, purposefully or implicitly, may impact the care they receive from us or other health care professionals. If clinicians assume that their client has stable housing, they may suggest an in-home service delivery model without considering whether that is possible. If they assume that clients have safe and trusting relationships with their intimate partners or family members,

they may cause harm by assuming that partners or family members should be involved in care.

Clinicians working with marginalized and underserved individuals with TBI should consider stigma as an environmental factor that can influence success. SLPs must ponder the stereotypes or implicit biases they may have about their clients, and ensure that they are creating a clinical environment that is free of judgment and stigmatization. Failing to do this work before meeting clients can cause significant harm.

Privilege and Oppression

All clinicians must consider how their own experiences of privilege and oppression influence their clients. Underserved individuals with TBI face many intersecting barriers and forms of oppression. The Coin Model of Privilege and Critical Allyship (Nixon, 2019) is a useful framework to conceptualize privilege and oppression generally, and specifically as it relates to health inequities faced by underserved individuals. This model conceptualizes each system of inequality in society as a coin. The top of the coin represents unearned advantage (privilege), and the bottom represents unearned disadvantage (oppression). Everyone's intersecting identities fall on either side of the coin, "tipping" it further towards oppression or privilege. Many individuals from the aforementioned underserved and marginalized groups have identities falling on the bottom of the coin, including neurodisability, lower socioeconomic status, precarious housing situations, not identifying as male, or mental health diagnoses. Experiences of racism and discrimination are also aspects of trauma that must be addressed and considered.

Specific Considerations for SLPs Serving Marginalized and Underserved Communities

SLPs are trained to screen for and diagnose communication and swallowing disorders, and to develop and implement treatment to address these disorders. Through the lens of the ICF, these refer to the health condition or disease (TBI) and the associated body structures (the brain). However, it is imperative that we move beyond the diagnosis or impairments and consider the definition of health according to Huber et al. (2011), as "the ability to adapt and self-manage" (p. 2) in the face of social, physical, and emotional challenges. For many individuals with TBI, and particularly those from marginalized and/or underserved populations, their challenges have left them without the tools, skills, and support to adapt and self-manage. Therefore, SLPs must look at the impact of TBI and intersecting personal and environmental factors on a person's functioning and life participation. We need to understand the storied truths and circumstances that act as facilitators and barriers to the person's ability to adapt and self-manage. To this end, the development of a trusting relationship whereby we can work together with clients to answer the questions "what do you need?" and "how can we help?"

is paramount. We also have an ethical responsibility to communicate the risks and benefits related to pursuing or refusing treatment. Therefore, in addition to assessing and treating CCDs in a structured, clinic setting, we strongly suggest that where possible, this takes place in natural contexts. Further, SLPs play an important role as advocates for adequate funding, representation in court (i.e., communication intermediaries), or navigating life transitions, as well as training of frontline staff regarding communication disorders and TBI.

It has also been our experience in these contexts that the clinical relationship with clients from underserved and/or marginalized groups may be more personal, and require constant evaluation of our scope of practice and ethical responsibilities. SLPs working in this area often walk a fine line between establishing a trusting relationship with clients and ensuring that their scope of practice and limitations are made clear. SLPs may wish to receive additional training on counseling, keeping in mind that clients who feel safe may share their traumatic experiences or relive past traumas when discussing their injury or working on highly personal goals. All of these steps are critical to serving our clients ethically and in a culturally safe and responsive manner. We also acknowledge that hearing the stories of our clients may be hard or even shocking, however, according to nurse practitioner and Indigenous health researcher Dr. Amy Wright, we need to "sit with that discomfort in order to rid ourselves of old perceptions and learn about what is culturally safe care" (University of Toronto, n.d., p. 2).

In light of this, clinicians must also ensure that they have support systems in place to protect their own mental health in order to best serve their clients. Experiences of burnout and secondary traumatization, defined as "indirect exposure to trauma through a firsthand account or narrative of a traumatic event," can commonly occur (Zimering & Gulliver, 2003). There is a fine line between sitting with discomfort and experiencing vicarious trauma. While clinicians providing behavioral health intervention often receive formal education to prevent burnout and secondary trauma, this is less common in SLPs. Therefore, we encourage practicing clinicians to be aware of their own emotional and psychological health and to discuss concerns of burnout or traumatization with their clinical leadership and/or seek support from workplace mental health services as these feelings arise or, whenever the complexities associated with work follow a clinician away from work. These supports should be available to all individuals involved in SLP care, including support personnel, clinical placement students, volunteers, and researchers.

Considerations for Trauma Informed and Culturally Responsive Practice

Culturally Informed Practice

In addition to thinking about systems of inequity for our clients, SLPs must practice cultural humility and consider how these systems relate to their lives and may influence their clinical relationships. Cultural humility involves recognizing that culturally-responsive care requires lifelong learning and consideration of factors such as health care power dynamics and implicit biases (Gregory, 2020). To be culturally responsive with clients we must develop culturally safe models of rehabilitation (Bohanna et al., 2019). In order to do this, we suggest the following: First, ask the questions—during the intake and history with the client, politely and warmly ask clients to tell you about linguistic and cultural traditions that are important to them in their day-to-day lives. We also suggest the following cultural and linguistic factors be considered:

- Do they come from an individualistic culture, such as North America, that values and prioritizes independence and freedom, or a collectivist culture that values and prioritizes relationships and solidarity?
- Do they come from a cultural and linguistic background that espouses humility and listening first, or speaking up?
- Is eye contact appropriate, and in which contexts?
- Do they focus on nonverbal communication as much as verbal?
- What is the role of family and friends in their culture?
- Are there sex and gender-based differences in communication style and manner?

Second, is there an opportunity to connect the client (or involve them) with culturally similar communities, and or extended family, who could be involved in facilitating communication goals? Ask what is important to them in terms of their cultural identity and practices.

For example, many Indigenous cultures have deep connections to land and nature that are important in the healing process. They may be guided by the teachings of traditional healers, elders and medicine people, and so you may wish to ask Indigenous clients how that may be incorporated in therapy.

Further, it is recommended that SLPs confer with Indigenous organizations to determine best practices. Clients may utilize services in both traditional Indigenous health structures and non-Indigenous ones that would require collaboration with Indigenous health organizations.

Use culturally responsive therapy materials where appropriate. For example, stories, music, and lyrics and materials that celebrate Black excellence or Indigenous resilience, leadership, and cultural practices. Culturally-responsive practice requires the clinician to be open, respectful, to listen, and to consider the earlier text when choosing therapy goals and therapy materials.

Trauma-Informed Practice

It has been our experience that most of the clients we have worked with from underserved and marginalized communities have experienced trauma and often-repeated trauma, and many from a young age. As a result, many of these individuals may have low self-esteem and may have had negative and disrespectful experiences with health care providers. Given that TBI typically results in slowed processing, many clients find interacting with busy clinicians to be extremely challenging. The intake process, including history taking, can be particularly difficult and

triggering as clients are often asked to retell their stories of violence and abuse. Furthermore, there is an inherent power imbalance in any clinical relationship; for example, the reports we write for our clients may influence their access to funding, or how future health care professionals reading these reports will view them.

There are many things SLPs can do to provide trauma responsive care that acknowledges what has happened to an individual, rather than what is wrong with them. First, we suggest that whenever possible, SLPs complete additional training in trauma-informed practice. We also suggest that sessions be conducted in an environment that is as safe, non-threatening, and comfortable as possible for the client to create a space where they can be brave in sharing their stories. This may involve meeting the client at their shelter or in the community. For those providing telehealth services, where some body language cues are absent, a warm and smiling face, moderate speech rate, soft tone of voice, and use of simple language is encouraged.

Clinicians may wish to listen more than speak during the first sessions where relationship-building is critical. When mindfulness and breathwork are part of the client's background, beginning each session with some grounding practices should be a consideration. Even clients who have not experienced these practices are likely to find them beneficial with time and practice. For clinicians working in person, a soothing, sensory kit may be helpful that may include calming tactile items (e.g., squishy ball, soft blanket, blowing bubbles to help calm a rapid breathing rate), or anything that the client finds useful.

Clinicians should intentionally select the language they use with clients. Using invitational language can also be helpful; clinicians may use the phrase "I invite you to tell me" or "I invite you to try." However, if this concept is too abstract for clients with CCDs, consider "would you be able to tell me?" or "would you be willing to try?" This shift in language can help reduce any dynamics where clients perceive that they must accommodate or respond to the clinician's demands. Clinicians may wish to use principles from "motivational interviewing," which is a communication style that promotes collaboration and change with clients (Miller & Rollnick, 2013). Motivational interviewing principles are consistent with many themes discussed in this chapter, including equal partnership between clinicians and clients, providing care compassionately, helping clients discover the skills they already have to achieve their goals, and nonjudgmental acceptance (Miller & Rollnick, 2013). Motivational interviewing strategies, such as using open-ended questions, sharing positive affirmations, reflective listening, and providing summaries, are often useful for empowering clients to achieve their goals. Finally, conducting sessions using a strengths-based approach with compassion and kindness will go a long way to create a safe, therapeutic environment.

Assessment and Intervention Through the Lens of the ICF

Assessment With a Purpose

Given that most individuals from underserved and marginalized groups are likely to have complex histories and limited access to funds for services, it is critical that there be a clearly defined purpose for assessment and intervention. In addition to formal testing, when appropriate, to determine language and cognitive-communication strengths and challenges, we suggest a functional evaluation of discourse, along with a survey of the person's life roles and demands. This involves a cognitive-communication skills task analysis. For example, if an individual is struggling with precarious housing, the clinician can assess the communication demands involved in completing forms, negotiating with landlords, and reading and understanding the terms of a lease. This also involves an assessment of environmental and personal factors, guided by the ICF. In accordance with culturally-responsive and trauma-informed practice, choose assessment measures that lack cultural bias whenever possible and reassure clients that the assessment process is not something that one passes or fails. We often introduce assessment tasks by explaining to clients that some tasks are supposed to be challenging to determine specific areas of strength, and areas of challenge, so that we can work together to address them. Keep in mind that the experience of completing an assessment may be triggering for clients, as it often reveals challenges about which they feel negatively.

Finally, we suggest that assessment, without offering any solutions or access to therapy, may be harmful to the client. We recognize that some service-delivery models have SLPs providing assessments without subsequent treatment, however, at minimum, assessment findings should be paired with education and strategies that the client may implement effectively. In these scenarios, clinicians must be mindful about not flooding the client with too many strategies or strategies with only limited introductions.

Social Determinants of Health

The social determinants of health (SDH) are nonmedical factors influencing health and impacting conditions of daily life (Datto, n.d.). Many SDH are important to consider for the groups discussed in this chapter, including housing, social inclusion and nondiscrimination, access to affordable health services, income and social protection, job security, and language and literacy skills. These factors are identified to account for between 30% to 55% of health outcomes and can be more important than health care or lifestyle choices (Datto, n.d.).

When assessing and treating clients from marginialized and underserved groups, SLPs should be aware of the impact that intersecting SDHs have on a client's readiness for services. Clinicians should aim to "meet the individual where they are." To do so, Maslow's hierarchy of needs is a useful framework that outlines physiologic needs as being foundational to progression to the higher-level needs of safety, belongingness/love, esteem, and, finally, self-actualization (Maslow, 1970). Many underserved and marginalized individuals do not have basic physiological or safety needs met, such as access to nutritious food, rest, safety, and security. This hierarchy was applied in 2015 to community-based interventions, identifying basic services such as food banks, legal aids, or domestic violence shelters, as necessary before embarking on any job training or rehabilitative work (Henize et al., 2015). For example, when clients lack basic physiologic needs, it is likely not appropriate to focus on cognitive-communication skills such as discourse, or social communication as they relate to self-actualization tasks such as obtaining employment. Rather, it may be more relevant to focus on functional goals such as developing scripts and communication supports to navigate food insecurity, support to complete forms, and to liaise with the local brain injury association. Before SLP sessions, clinicians should consider whether their clients are nourished, have had enough sleep, and if they feel safe in the clinical encounter.

Targeted Intervention With a Purpose

To this end, intervention should be about enhancing participation through functional goals, self-management, provision of strategies, self-education, education of close others, and education of frontline staff. Clinicians should take time to develop goals with the client based on their environmental and personal factors (e.g., culture) according to the ICF. Clinicians should also ensure that goals consider the specific demands of the client's communicative life roles, identified through a cognitive-communication skills task analysis. We also suggest that SLPs introduce their clients to local brain injury associations and any available support groups or peer-mentors, as these are a positive way to expand social circles, help with coping, and share lived experiences with others (Hughes et al., 2020).

Culturally Responsive Care in Action

Specialized Interprofessional Care Teams

At this time, there are limited models of care that directly address people with TBI from underserved and marginalized communities. To our knowledge, The Barrow Institute in Phoenix, Arizona, is the first facility to develop and implement a domestic violence (DV) program within the Barrow Concussion, Brain Injury, and Sports Medicine Center. It was founded in 2012 by social worker Ashley Bridwell and Dr. Javier Cardenas, former Barrow Director, to provide medical care, community outreach support, and research for survivors of DV with brain injuries. Individuals at participating shelters are screened using the HELPS TBI Screening Tool and are then offered a referral to the Barrow Concussion, Brain Injury, and Sports Medicine Center for comprehensive medical care, regardless of insurance status. An additional outreach program is offered at participating shelters by the Barrow neurorehabilitation SLP and occupational therapist. The program is currently led by neurologist Dr. Glynnis Zieman with continued support from Ms. Bridwell and the Center's team.

Emerging Resources and Care Models

In addition to articulated models of care, there are emerging resources that can benefit marginalized and underserved individuals with TBI. The Brain Injury Society of Toronto (Ontario, Canada) has created an online toolkit for those involved with the criminal justice system. This toolkit (see Resources) has two sections, one for survivors navigating the justice system, and one for legal and justice professionals working with survivors. Groups within the United Nations are working to improve identification of communication disorders for refugees and asylum seekers (United Nations High Commissioner for Refugees, 2021), and interprofessional communication recommendations derived from this work can be found online (Physiopedia, n.d.).

Wiseman-Hakes and Turkstra (2021) created a publicly available online educational advocacy video regarding youth with TBI in the criminal justice system, and the associated communication challenges and suggestions for communication partners (see Resources).

Also in Toronto, Canada, The ABI Research Lab under the direction of Dr. Angela Colantonio and doctoral candidate Halina (Lin Haag) created an online toolkit "Abused and Brain Injured: Understanding the Intersection of Intimate Partner Violence and Traumatic Brain Injury" (see Resources).

Clinicians should also feel empowered to explore additional non-TBI-centric information on underserved and marginalized communities, such as the work of Dr. Shameka Stanford, and apply these principles in their practices. Dr. Stanford has created an excellent workbook for SLPs working in juvenile justice and communication disorders. (See Resources.) Similarly, the Centers for Medicare & Medicaid Services have developed free training materials for working with marginalized and underserved groups to help them better understand U.S. governmentally-sponsored health care. These materials cover communication strategies and considerations to assist with low health care literacy, specifically related to Medicare and Medicaid coverage, but can be applied across settings (see Resources).

Talking Trouble-Aotearota New Zealand is a website developed by SLPs for SLPs working to support the speech, language and communication needs experienced by many children, youth, and adults involved with care and protection, justice, mental health, and behavior services (see Resources). Finally, The TBI-Youth-Justice website is an additional resource with information regarding the communication challenges of children and youth in the criminal justice system (see Resources).

Conclusions

There is an increasing awareness and understanding of the intersection between CCDs and issues of social justice and health inequities for marginalized and underserved communities. Acquired CCDs can increase risks of further intersectionalities and can also be an additional barrier to accessing the social determinants of health and accessing justice within the legal system. SLPs can play an important role in addressing inequities by providing meaningful, culturally-responsive, and trauma-informed assessment, intervention, education, and advocacy.

Acknowledgments. We gratefully acknowledge the review and thoughtful comments provided by Ms. Katie Almond, a retired Probation and Parole Officer who worked for many years with marginalized communities, and

Ms. Lori-Davis Hill Reg. CASLPO, speech language pathologist and (Acting) Executive Director of the Indigenous Health Learning Lodge at McMaster University in Hamilton, ON, Canada.

Resources

ABI Justice: http://abijustice.org

ABI Youth Justice Video: Addressing the needs of young people with TBI in the criminal justice system: http://youtube.com/watch?v=CA2oOL1ipyk&ab_channel=OntarioNeurotraumaFoundation

Abused and Brain Injured: ABI Toolkit: http://www.abitoolkit.ca

Centers for Medicare & Medicaid Services. (n.d.). Serving Vulnerable and Underserved

Dr. Shameka Stanford; The SLP Solution: https://www.slpsolution.com/dr-shameka-stanford-juvenile-forensic-speech-language-pathologist/ https://www.juvforensicslp.com/

Populations: https://marketplace.cms.gov/technical-assistance-resources/training-materials/vulnerable-and-underserved-populations.pdf

Talking Trouble NZ: http://talking-troublenz.org

TBI-Youth Justice: A web-based toolkit on the topic of children and youth in the criminal justice system with information and resources regarding communication and CCDs. http://TBI-youth-justice.org

United Nations Communication Accessibility: http://www.unhcr.org60e5ad650.pdf

Wiseman-Hakes, C. & Turkstra, L. (2021): https://www.youtube.com/watch?v=CA2oOL1ipyk

References

Allely, C. S. (2016). Prevalence and assessment of traumatic brain injury in prison inmates: A systematic PRISMA review. *Brain Injury, 30*(10), 1161–1180. https://doi.org/10.1080/02699052.2016.1191674

American Psychological Association. (2020). Combating bias and stigma related to COVID-19. https://www.apa.org/topics/covid-19/bias

ASHA. (n.d.). *Cognitive-communication referral guidelines for adults.* https://www.asha.org/slp/cognitive-referral/

Baumann, R., Hamilton-Wright, S., Riley, D., Brown, K., Hunt, C., Michalak, A., & Matheson, F. (2019). Experiences of violence and head injury among women and transgender women sex workers. *Sexuality Research and Social Policy,* (3). https://www.springerprofessional.de/en/experiences-of-violence-and-head-injury-among-women-and-transgen/15758516

Blommaert, J. (2009). Language, asylum, and the national order. *Current Anthropology, 50*(4), 415–441. https://doi.org/10.1086/600131

Bohanna, I., Cullen, J., & Fleming, J. (2019). Brain impairment in Indigenous populations. *Brain Impairment, 20*(2), 105–106. https://doi.org/10.1017/BrImp.2019.22

Brain Injury Canada. (n.d.). What is an acquired brain injury—Traumatic brain injury. https://braininjurycanada.ca/en/survivor/traumatic-brain-injury/about-brain-injury

Bransford, C., & Cole, M. (2019). Trauma-informed care in homelessness service settings: Challenges and opportunities. In *Homelessness prevention and intervention in social work: Policies, programs, and practices* (pp. 255–277). Springer Nature Switzerland AG. https://doi.org/10.1007/978-3-030-03727-7_13

Bryan, K., Freer, J., & Furlong, C. (2007). Language and communication difficulties in juvenile offenders. *International Journal of Language & Communication Disorders, 42*(5), 505–520. https://doi.org/10.1080/13682820601053977

Bryan, K., Garvani, G., Gregory, J., & Kilner, K. (2015). Language difficulties and criminal justice: The need for earlier identification. *International Journal of Language & Communication Disorders, 50*(6), 763–775. https://doi.org/10.1111/1460-6984.12183

Burton, A. (2019). Meeting the neurological needs of refugees and other forcibly displaced people. *The Lancet Neurology, 18*(6), 524–525. https://doi.org/10.1016/S1474-4422(19)30164-4

Canadian Association for Equality. (n.d.). *An analysis of the correlations between intimate partner violence and homelessness in a Canadian urban centre.* https://equalitycanada.com/report/

CASLPO. (n.d.). *CASLPO resource section Lsearch—Caslpo—College of Audiologists and Speech-Language Pathologists of Ontario.* https://caslpo.com/members/resources

Centers for Medicare & Medicaid Services. (n.d.). https://marketplace.cms.gov/technical-assistance-resources/training-materials/vulnerable-and-underserved-populations.pdf

Colantonio, A., Kim, H., Allen, S., Asbridge, M., Petgrave, J., & Brochu, S. (2014). Traumatic brain injury and early life experiences among men and women in a prison population. *Journal of Correctional Health Care, 20*(4), 271–279. https://doi.org/10.1177/1078345814541529

Cornis-Pop, M., Mashima, P. A., Roth, C. R., MacLennan, D. L., Picon, L. M., Hammond, C. S., . . . Frank, E. M. (2012). Guest editorial: Cognitive-communication rehabilitation for combat-related mild traumatic brain injury. *Journal of Rehabilitation Research and Development, 49*(7), xi–xxxii.

https://doi.org/10.1682/jrrd.2012.03.0048

Covington, N. V., & Duff, M. C. (2021). Heterogeneity is a hallmark of Traumatic Brain Injury, not a limitation: A new perspective on study design in rehabilitation research. *American Journal of Speech-Language Pathology*, *30*(2S), 974–985. https://doi.org/10.1044/2020_AJSLP-20-00081

Cox, G. R., FireMoon, P., Anastario, M. P., Ricker, A., Escarcega-Growing Thunder, R., Baldwin, J. A., & Rink, E. (2021). Indigenous standpoint theory as a theoretical framework for decolonizing social science health research with American Indian communities. *AlterNative: An International Journal of Indigenous Peoples*, *17*(4), 460–468. https://doi.org/10.1177/11771801211042019

Datto, A. (n.d.). *Social determinants of health.* World Health Organization website: https://www.who.int/westernpacific/health-topics/social-determinants-of-health

Deora, H., Agrawal, A., Pal, R., Moscote-Salazar, L. R., Alothman, M. H., & Satyarthee, G. D. (2019). Burden of traumatic brain injury in refugee population: Unmet need of care and gaps in knowledge. *Romanian Neurosurgery*, 449–454. https://doi.org/10.33962/roneuro-2019-071

Department of Indigenous Services Act. (2020). *Annual Report to Parliament 2020* [Report]. Government of Canada. https://www.sac-isc.gc.ca/eng/1602010609492/1602010631711

Doherty, S. M., Craig, R., Gardani, M., & McMillan, T. M. (2016). Head injury in asylum seekers and refugees referred with psychological trauma. *Global Mental Health*, *3*, e28. https://doi.org/10.1017/gmh.2016.23

Durand, E., Chevignard, M., Ruet, A., Dereix, A., Jourdan, C., & Pradat-Diehl, P. (2017). History of traumatic brain injury in prison populations: A systematic review. *Annals of Physical and Rehabilitation Medicine*, *60*(2), 95–101. https://doi.org/10.1016/j.rehab.2017.02.003

Fazel, S., Geddes, J. R., & Kushel, M. (2014). The health of homeless people in high-income countries: Descriptive epidemiology, health consequences, and clinical and policy recommendations. *Lancet (London, England)*, *384*(9953), 1529–1540. https://doi.org/10.1016/S0140-6736(14)61132-6

Ferguson, P. L., Pickelsimer, E. E., Corrigan, J. D., Bogner, J. A., & Wald, M. (2012). Prevalence of traumatic brain injury among prisoners in South Carolina. *The Journal of Head Trauma Rehabilitation*, *27*(3), E11-20. https://doi.org/10.1097/HTR.0b013e31824e5f47

Grace, J. J., Kinsella, E. L., Muldoon, O. T., & Fortune, D. G. (2015). Post-traumatic growth following acquired brain injury: A systematic review and meta-analysis. *Frontiers in Psychology*, *6*, 1162. https://doi.org/10.3389/fpsyg.2015.01162

Gregory, J., & Bryan, K. (2011). Speech and language therapy intervention with a group of persistent and prolific young offenders in a non-custodial setting with previously undiagnosed speech, language and communication difficulties. *International Journal of Language & Communication Disorders*, *46*(2), 202–215. https://doi.org/10.3109/13682822.2010.490573

Gregory, K. (2020). From my perspective/opinion: moving forward as a profession in a time of uncertainty. *Leader Live.* https://leader.pubs.asha.org/do/10.1044/leader.FMP.25082020.8/full/

Haag, H. (Lin), Sokoloff, S., MacGregor, N., Broekstra, S., Cullen, N., & Colantonio, A. (2019). Battered and brain injured: Assessing knowledge of Traumatic Brain Injury among intimate partner violence service providers. *Journal of Women's Health*, *28*(7), 990–996. https://doi.org/10.1089/jwh.2018.7299

Henize, A. W., Beck, A. F., Klein, M. D., Adams, M., & Kahn, R. S. (2015). A road map to address the Social Determinants of Health through community collaboration. *Pediatrics, 136*(4), e993-1001. https://doi.org/10.1542/peds.2015-0549

Huber, M., Knottnerus, J. A., Green, L., van der Horst, H., Jadad, A. R., Kromhout, D., . . . Smid, H. (2011). How should we define health? *BMJ (Clinical Research Ed.), 343*, d4163. https://doi.org/10.1136/bmj.d4163

Hughes, N., Williams, W., Chitsabesan, P., Walesby, R., & Mounce, L. (2012). *Nobody made the connection: Neurodisability in the youth justice system.* Office of the Children's Commissioner for England.

Hughes, N., Williams, W. H., Chitsabesan, P., Walesby, R. C., Mounce, L. T. A., & Clasby, B. (2015). The prevalence of traumatic brain injury among young offenders in custody: A systematic review. *The Journal of Head Trauma Rehabilitation, 30*(2), 94–105. https://doi.org/10.1097/HTR.0000000000000124

Hughes, R., Fleming, P., & Henshall, L. (2020). Peer support groups after acquired brain injury: A systematic review. *Brain Injury, 34*(7), 847–856. https://doi.org/10.1080/02699052.2020.1762002

Johnstone, M., Jetten, J., Dingle, G. A., Parsell, C., & Walter, Z. C. (2015). Discrimination and well-being amongst the homeless: The role of multiple group membership. *Frontiers in Psychology, 6*, 739. https://doi.org/10.3389/fpsyg.2015.00739

Kantamneni, N. (2020). The impact of the COVID-19 pandemic on marginalized populations in the United States: A research agenda. *Journal of Vocational Behavior, 119*, 103439. https://doi.org/10.1016/j.jvb.2020.103439

Katz, A. S., Hardy, B.-J., Firestone, M., Lofters, A., & Morton-Ninomiya, M. E. (2019). Vagueness, power and public health: Use of 'vulnerable' in public health literature. *Critical Public Health, 30*(5), 601–611. https://doi.org/10.1080/09581596.2019.1656800

Katz, R., & Kennedy, M. R. T. (2002). Evidence-based practice guidelines for cognitive-communication disorders after traumatic brain injury: Initial committee report. (ANCDS Bulletin Board). *Journal of Medical Speech-Language Pathology, 10*(2), x.

Lakhani, A., Cullen, J., & Townsend, C. (2017). The cost of disability for indigenous people: A systematic review. *Journal of Social Inclusion, 8*(1), 34–45. https://doi.org/10.36251/josi.116

Lambie, I. (2020). *What were they thinking? A discussion paper on brain and behaviour in relation to the justice system in New Zealand.* https://doi.org/10.17608/k6.OPMCSA.12279278.v1

Lannoo, E., Brusselmans, W., Van Eynde, L., Van Laere, M., & Stevens, J. (2004). Epidemiology of acquired brain injury (ABI) in adults: Prevalence of long-term disabilities and the resulting needs for ongoing care in the region of Flanders, Belgium. *Brain Injury, 18*(2), 203–211. https://doi.org/10.1080/02699050310001596905

Lasry, O., Dudley, R. W., Fuhrer, R., Torrie, J., Carlin, R., & Marcoux, J. (2016). Traumatic brain injury in a rural indigenous population in Canada: A community-based approach to surveillance. *Canadian Medical Association Open Access Journal, 4*(2), E249–E259. https://doi.org/10.9778/cmajo.20150105

Learning Network. (2022). *Learning network.* http://www.vawlearningnetwork.ca//our-work/index.html

Levine, C., Faden, R., Grady, C., Hammerschmidt, D., Eckenwiler, L., & Sugarman, J. (2004). The limitations of "vulnerability" as a protection for human research participants. *The American Journal of Bioethics, 4*(3), 44–49. https://doi.org/10.1080/15265160490497083

MacDonald, S. (2017). Introducing the model of cognitive-communication competence: A model to guide evidence-based communication interventions after brain injury. *Brain Injury, 31*(13–14), 1760–1780. https://doi.org/10.1080/02699052.2017.1379613

Manoranjan, B., Scott, T., Szasz, O. P., Bzovsky, S., O'Malley, L., Sprague, S., . . . Turkstra, L. S. (2022). Prevalence and perception of intimate partner violence-related Traumatic Brain Injury. *The Journal of Head Trauma Rehabilitation, 37*(1), 53–61. https://doi.org/10.1097/HTR.00 00000000000749

Marshall, J., & Barrett, H. (2018). Human rights of refugee-survivors of sexual and gender-based violence with communication disability. *International Journal of Speech-Language Pathology, 20*(1), 44–49. https://doi.org/10.1080/17549507.2017 .1392608

Maslow, A. H. (1970). *New introductions: Religions, values, and peak experiences* (New ed., p. 8).

Matheson, F. I., McIsaac, K. E., Fung, K., Stewart, L. A., Wilton, G., Keown, L. A., . . . Moineddin, R. (2020). Association between traumatic brain injury and prison charges: A population-based cohort study. *Brain Injury, 34*(6), 757–763. https://doi.org/10.1080/02699052.2020 .1753114

McPherson, J. I. (2019). Traumatic brain injury among refugees and asylum seekers. *Disability and Rehabilitation, 41*(10), 1238–1242. https://doi.org/10.1080/096 38288.2017.1422038

Meulenbroek, P., & Keegan, L. C. (2021). The life participation approach and social reintegration after traumatic brain injury. In *Neurogenic communication disorders and the life participation approach: The Social Imperative in supporting individuals and families* (pp. 181–207). Plural Publishing.

Miller, W. R., & Rollnick, S. (2013). *Motivational interviewing: Helping people change* (3rd ed.). Guilford Press.

Mirza, M., & Heinemann, A. W. (2012). Service needs and service gaps among refugees with disabilities resettled in the United States. *Disability and Rehabilitation, 34*(7), 542–552. https://doi.org/10 .3109/09638288.2011.611211

Moynan, C. R., & McMillan, T. M. (2018). Prevalence of head injury and associated disability in prison populations: A systematic review. *The Journal of Head Trauma Rehabilitation, 33*(4), 275–282. https://doi .org/10.1097/HTR.0000000000000354

NCCDH. (2022). National Collaborating Centre for Determinants of Health. *Marginalized populations.* https://nccdh.ca/glos sary/entry/marginalized-populations

Nguyen, R., Fiest, K. M., McChesney, J., Kwon, C.-S., Jette, N., Frolkis, A. D., . . . Gallagher, C. (2016). The international incidence of Traumatic Brain Injury: A systematic review and meta-analysis. *The Canadian Journal of Neurological Sciences. Le Journal Canadien Des Sciences Neurologiques, 43*(6), 774–785. https://doi .org/10.1017/cjn.2016.290

Nixon, S. A. (2019). The coin model of privilege and critical allyship: Implications for health. *BMC Public Health, 19*(1), 1637. https://doi.org/10.1186/s12889-019-7884-9

Nutton, J., & Fast, E. (2015). Historical trauma, substance use, and Indigenous peoples: Seven generations of harm from a "Big Event." *Substance Use & Misuse, 50*(7), 839–847. https://doi.org/10.3109/ 10826084.2015.1018755

OHRC. (n.d.). Ontario Human Rights Commission. *An introduction to the intersectional approach.* https://www.ohrc.on.ca/ en/intersectional-approach

O'Rourke, C., Linden, M. A., Lohan, M., & Bates-Gaston, J. (2016). Traumatic brain injury and co-occurring problems in prison populations: A systematic review. *Brain Injury, 30*(7), 839–854. https://doi .org/10.3109/02699052.2016.1146967

Overstreet, N. M., & Quinn, D. M. (2013). The Intimate Partner Violence stigmatization model and barriers to help-seeking. *Basic and Applied Social Psychology, 35*(1), 109–122. https://doi.org/10.1080/01973 533.2012.746599

Physiopedia. (n.d.). *Effective communication for people with refugee experience.* https:// www.physio-pedia.com/Effective_Com munication_for_People_with_Refugee_ Experience

Rehman, L., Kim, E., Shirt, C. & Jo-Hardy, B. (2023). An overview of Traumatic Brain & Spinal Cord Injuries (TBI/TSCI) among Indigenous populations in Canada, United States, Australia, and New Zealand. *University of Toronto, Journal of Public Health, 4*(1). DOI: 10.33137/utjph .v4i1.40708 https://utjph.com/index .php/utjph/article/view/40708

Sackett, D. L., Rosenberg, W. M., Gray, J. A., Haynes, R. B., & Richardson, W. S. (1996). Evidence based medicine: What it is and what it isn't. *BMJ (Clinical Research ed.), 312*(7023), 71–72. https:// doi.org/10.1136/bmj.312.7023.71

Snow, P. C. (2019). Speech-Language Pathology and the youth offender: Epidemiological overview and roadmap for future Speech-Language Pathology research and scope of practice. *Language, Speech, and Hearing Services in Schools, 50*(2), 324– 339. https://doi.org/10.1044/2018_LSH SS-CCJS-18-0027

Snow, P. C., & Powell, M. B. (2011). Oral language competence in incarcerated young offenders: Links with offending severity. *International Journal of Speech-Language Pathology, 13*(6), 480–489. https://doi.org/ 10.3109/17549507.2011.578661

Snowling, M. J., Adams, J. W., Bowyer-Crane, C., & Tobin, V. (2000). Levels of literacy among juvenile offenders: The incidence of specific reading difficulties. *Criminal Behaviour and Mental Health, 10*(4), 229–241. https://doi.org/10.1002/ cbm.362

Stanford, S. (2020). The school-based speech-language pathologist's role in diverting the school-to-confinement pipeline for youth with communication disorders. *Perspectives of the ASHA Special Interest Groups, 5*(4), 1057–1066. https://doi .org/10.1044/2020_PERSP-20-0002

Stubbs, J. L., Thornton, A. E., Sevick, J. M., Silverberg, N. D., Barr, A. M., Honer, W. G., & Panenka, W. J. (2020). Traumatic brain injury in homeless and marginally housed individuals: A systematic review and meta-analysis. *The Lancet. Public Health, 5*(1), e19–e32. https://doi .org/10.1016/S2468-2667(19)30188-4

Toccalino, D., Haag, H. (Lin), Estrella, M. J., Cowle, S., Fuselli, P., Ellis, M. J., . . . Colantonio, A. (2022). The intersection of Intimate Partner Violence and Traumatic Brain Injury: Findings from an emergency summit addressing system-level changes to better support women survivors. *The Journal of Head Trauma Rehabilitation, 37*(1), E20. https://doi.org/10 .1097/HTR.0000000000000743

Tsai, J., & Wilson, M. (2020). COVID-19: A potential public health problem for homeless populations. *The Lancet Public Health, 5*(4), e186–e187. https://doi .org/10.1016/S2468-2667(20)30053-0

UN Commission on Human Rights. (2005). OHCHR | 61st session of the commission. https://www.ohchr.org/EN/HR Bodies/CHR/61/Pages/Session61.aspx

UN Refugee Agency. (2016). *UNHCR global trends—Forced displacement in 2016.* https:// www.unhcr.org/globaltrends2016/

UN Women. (2022). *The shadow pandemic: Violence against women during COVID-19.* https://www.unwomen.org/en/news/ in-focus/in-focus-gender-equality-in-covid-19-response/violence-against-women-during-covid-19

United Nations High Commissioner for Refugees. (2021). *Improving communication accessibility for refugees with communication disabilities through capacity building—A case study from Rwanda.* https:// www.unhcr.org/protection/operations/ 60e5ad650/improving-communication-accessibility-refugees-communication-disabilities.html

Valera, E., & Kucyi, A. (2017). Brain injury in women experiencing intimate partner-violence: Neural mechanistic evidence of an "invisible" trauma. *Brain Imaging and Behavior, 11*(6), 1664–1677. https://doi .org/10.1007/s11682-016-9643-1

Wiseman-Hakes, C., Colantonio, A., Ryu, H., Toccalino, D., Balogh, R., Grigorovich, A.,

... Chan, V. (2020). Research to integrate services for individuals with traumatic brain injury, mental health, and addictions: Proceedings of a multidisciplinary workshop. *Canadian Journal of Community Mental Health, 39*(1), 133–150. https://doi .org/10.7870/cjcmh-2020-001

Wiseman-Hakes, C., Magor, T., Bauman, N., Colantonio, A., & Matheson, F. I. (2023). Exploring the cognitive-communication challenges of adults with histories of traumatic brain injury and criminal justice system involvement: A pilot study. *American Journal of Speech-Language Pathology, 32*(2S), 941–955. https://doi.org/ 10.1044/2022_AJSLP-22-00086

Wiseman-Hakes, C., Ryu, H., Lightfoot, D., Kukreja, G., Colantonio, A., & Matheson, F. I. (2019). Examining the efficacy of communication partner training for improving communication interactions and outcomes for individuals with traumatic brain injury: A systematic review. *Archives of Rehabilitation Research and Clinical Translation, 2*(1), 100036. https:// doi.org/10.1016/j.arrct.2019.100036

Wiseman-Hakes, C. & Turkstra, L. (2021). https://www.youtube.com/watch?v= CA2oOL1ipyk

Worabo, H., Hsueh, K.-H., Yakimo, R., Worabo, E., Burgess, P., & Farberman, S. (2016). Understanding refugees' perceptions of health care in the United States. *The Journal for Nurse Practitioners, 12*, 487–494. https://doi.org/10.1016/j .nurpra.2016.04.014

World Health Organization. (2001). *International Classification of Functioning, Disability and Health (ICF)*. https://www.who .int/standards/classifications/interna tional-classification-of-functioning-dis ability-and-health

University of Toronto. (n.d.). *Healing the Hurt—campaign led by Indigenous women and U of T Nursing researcher aims to educate health care providers on culturally safe care.* https://bloomberg.nursing.utoronto .ca/news/healing-the-hurt-campaign-led-by-indigenous-women-and-u-of-t-researcher-aims-to-educate-health-care-providers-on-culturally-safe-care/

Wszalek, J. A., & Turkstra, L. S. (2019). Comprehension of legal language by adults with and without traumatic brain injury. *The Journal of Head Trauma Rehabilitation, 34*(3), E55–E63. https://doi.org/10.1097/ HTR.0000000000000434

Young, J. T., & Hughes, N. (2020). Traumatic brain injury and homelessness: From prevalence to prevention. *The Lancet Public Health, 5*(1), e4–e5. https://doi .org/10.1016/S2468-2667(19)30225-7

Zeiler, K. J., Gomez, A., Mathieu, F., & Zeiler, F. A. (2021). Health determinants among North Americans experiencing homelessness and traumatic brain injury: A scoping review. *Neurotrauma Reports, 2*(1), 303–321. https://doi.org/10.1089/ neur.2021.0010

Zeiler, K. J., & Zeiler, F. A. (2017). Social determinants of traumatic brain injury in the North American Indigenous population: A review. *The Canadian Journal of Neurological Sciences. Le Journal Canadien Des Sciences Neurologiques, 44*(5), 525–531. https://doi.org/10.1017/cjn.2017.49

Zieman, G., Bridwell, A., & Cárdenas, J. F. (2017). Traumatic brain injury in domestic violence victims: A retrospective study at the Barrow Neurological Institute. *Journal of Neurotrauma, 34*(4), 876–880. https://doi.org/10.1089/neu.2016 .4579

Zimering, R., & Gulliver, S. (2003). *Secondary traumatization in mental health care providers*. https://www.psychiatrictimes.com/ view/secondary-traumatization-mental-health-care-providers

Glossary

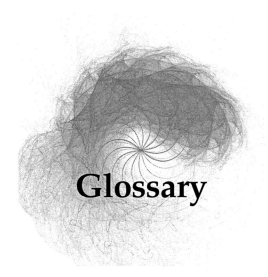

alerting: The ability to prepare for, and sustain alertness to, relevant stimuli.

allocate: The ability to assign cognitive resources to various tasks.

alternating attention: The ability to flexibly switch back and forth between different tasks and task instructions.

amnestic: Mild Cognitive Impairment (MCI) that initially only affects memory.

apply the framework: Training a person to execute a specific, discrete routine using a framework to structure the routines.

appropriate interpretation: The ability to integrate multiple cues to generate the most accurate inference.

apragmatism: A previously suggested diagnostic label that encompasses the communication-specific impairments that occur following RHD. The term was not adopted for general clinical use after being proposed over 20 years ago, although a group of international researchers working

collaboratively recently renewed the proposal to use it as a label.

attention for outcomes: The process by which we connect stimuli (input) with a response to that stimuli (output).

Auditory Elevator With Reversal: A subtest of the Test of Everyday Attention in which the test-taker is asked to keep track of what floor they are on by counting medium auditory tones. In this task, high and low tones indicate a change in direction.

auditory neglect: An impairment in processing sounds that originates from the left side of the brain.

awareness of impairment, or self-awareness: Metacognitive knowledge or self-knowledge, which includes stored knowledge and beliefs about task characteristics and understanding personal strengths and limitations (intellectual awareness), as well as an online awareness of performance, which includes self-appraisal and self-monitoring during a task or situation (emergent awareness) and anticipating future difficulties (anticipatory awareness).

capacity limitation: The ability of the human attention system to only process a limited number or amount of stimuli at once.

client's preferences: The client's choices for how they would like to approach their rehabilitation and life.

cognitive flexibility, or set-shifting: A core executive function process; it is the ability to intentionally move between tasks, mental sets, or goals as well as reacting to changing circumstances.

contextual features: The economic and social circumstances that might influence a client's decisions for treatment.

design test: A subtest of the Cognitive-Linguistic Quick Test–Plus (CLQT+) that requires the patient to create unique designs by using exactly four straight lines to make connections among 10 dots without a set-shifting condition.

divided attention: The ability to engage in multiple tasks simultaneously.

dual-tasking, or multi-tasking: Involves performing two or more tasks at the same time, which results in decreased working memory capacity.

early filter theory: Suggests that all stimuli receive a preliminary analysis of general features such as location or intensity, but that irrelevant or unattended stimuli are filtered out at a relatively early stage of processing, while the attended stimulus is selected

and goes on to receive additional processing.

Elevator Counting: A subtest of the Test of Everyday Attention in which the test-taker is instructed to pretend they are in an elevator in which the visual floor number indicator is not working. In this auditory task, they are presented with a series of tones and asked to count these tones and asked to count these tones to determine what floor they are "on."

Elevator Counting With Distraction: A subtest of the Test of Everyday Attention in which the test-taker is instructed to pretend they are in an elevator in which the visual floor number indicator is not working. In this auditory task, two types of tones (medium-pitched and high-pitched) are presented. The test-taker is asked to count the medium tones and ignore the high ones to determine what floor they are "on."

environmental factors: Many factors including society's services, systems, and policies as well as the attitudes and beliefs of others.

evaluating: The stage of systematic instruction when the effectiveness of the instructional technique and the specific outcome needs to be identified.

executive control of attention: The skill of attending to two tasks simultaneously represented by alternating attention.

executive control system, or target detection: The effortful control of attention, which includes processes such as conflict resolution and error detection.

extinction: A sensory neglect phenomenon where an individual with RHD may accurately localize visual or tactile input when each side of the body is touched independently or objects are shown in each visual field separately but may not report sensation or the presence of visual stimuli on the left when the stimuli are presented bilaterally at the same time.

filter attenuation model: Posits that relevant stimuli are selected early on for further processing; however, unselected stimuli are not completely filtered out but rather are attenuated, making them potentially available for further analysis later on.

focus: The ability to select target stimuli from an array.

focused attention: A fundamental, low-level ability to orient and respond to specific stimuli in any modality.

general attention deficits: Forms of impaired attention, including focused, sustained, alternating, divided attention, and neglect.

generative naming test: A subtest of the Cognitive-Linguistic Quick Test–Plus (CLQT+) in which individuals must generate as many words as they can in a specified category within 1 minute without a set-shifting condition.

implementation stage: The stage of systematic instruction when the ingredients are applied depending on the specific target.

inference failure: Inefficient or incomplete inferencing processes observed through difficulties with inferring meanings in both verbal and visual modalities.

inhibitory control, or response inhibition: A core executive function process, it is the ability to deliberately control or inhibit an automatic response, behavior, or thought and instead do what is more appropriate or needed in a given situation.

intra-individual: Abilities within a person.

intra-individual variability: The concept that if an individual is given the same task to complete on several different days, performance may fluctuate to some degree from day to day.

late filter model, or late selection model: Theorized that all stimuli are analyzed in the early stages of processing, and that selection of the target stimulus occurs later and is based on "importance weighting."

linguistic prosody: The ability to interpret and produce grammatical and pragmatic prosodic features that convey meaning in speech acts.

Lottery: A subtest of the Test of Everyday Attention in which the test-taker is presented with a series of spoken letters and numbers. They are instructed to listen for a target number and, each time they hear it, to write down the preceding two letters.

major/minor neurocognitive disorders: A diagnostic category that includes a number of more specific etiologies, including neurocognitive disorder due to Alzheimer's disease, dementia with Lewy bodies, vascular neurocognitive disorder, and frontotemporal neurocognitive disorder. Previously known as delirium, dementia, amnestic, and other cognitive disorders.

Major Neurocognitive Disorders:
A diagnostic category of dementia in which there must be evidence of significant cognitive decline and this observed, quantifiable cognitive decline must be severe enough to disrupt independent completion of activities of daily living.

Map Search: A subtest of the Test of Everyday Attention in which the test-taker is given a map of Philadelphia and asked to find and circle as many restaurant symbols (a knife and fork) as they can in 2 minutes. Two scores are taken from this task: the number of symbols circled in 1 minute and the number of symbols circled in 2 minutes.

Mazes: A subtest of the Cognitive-Linguistic Quick Test–Plus (CLQT+) in which participants must create a path through two mazes (easy and difficult) without going into any dead ends or crossing lines.

medical indications: The clinician's interpretation of a client's condition, including the diagnosis and prognosis (e.g., stable vs. progressive condition) and how this might influence progress and expectations.

mental representations: A cognitive rehabilitation treatment target focused on training awareness (e.g., increasing knowledge or changing an attitude).

Mild Neurocognitive Disorders:
A diagnostic category of dementia in which persons demonstrate subtle yet measurable cognitive impairment with minimal impairment of instrumental activities of daily living.

multi-tasking, or dual-tasking:
Involves performing two or more tasks at the same time, which results in decreased working memory capacity.

neglect: A decreased ability to process information.

nonamnestic: Mild Cognitive Impairment (MCI) in which cognitive functions such as language, visuospatial function, or executive function are initially affected.

orienting: The direction of attention toward a specific location.

personal beliefs: A patient's self-advocacy, empowerment, work/academic activities, and performance which should be evaluated in a patient interview.

personal expectations: A patient's goals and motivation for rehabilitation which should be evaluated in a patient interview.

personal factors: A patient's knowledge and opinion about their diagnosis which should be evaluated in a patient interview.

planning: Involves thinking about an end goal and determining a course of action, or a "road map" to achieve that goal.

planning stage: The stage of systematic instruction when the target is identified by considering who the learner is, what type of information is to be trained, where the skill will be used, why is the skill being trained, and how the outcome will be evaluated.

pragmatic aphasia: A previously suggested diagnostic label for communication deficits associated with RHD that highlighted the centrality of pragmatic deficits to communication problems. The term was not adopted for general clinical use after being proposed over 20 years ago.

problem solving: Involves determining whether there is a problem, identifying the specific problem, generating potential solutions, choosing a solution, evaluating the outcome, and trying another solution if the expected outcome is not achieved.

quality of life: The impact of a diagnosis on a client's activities and social interactions.

reasoning: The process of using existing knowledge to draw conclusions, make predictions, or construct explanations.

resource allocation theory: Posits that humans are able to flexibly allocate resources from a single cognitive pool to various cognitive tasks. This cognitive pool of resources is considered to be limited in capacity, such that when more resources are taken up by one task, fewer resources remain to be allocated.

selection: The ability to focus on stimuli that are most relevant to its behavior, goals, or interests, while ignoring or filtering out stimuli that are less relevant while continuing to monitor these less-relevant stimuli to some extent in case they should become relevant again.

selective attention: The ability to sustain attention to a target stimulus in the presence of irrelevant or distractor stimuli.

self-awareness, or awareness of impairment: Metacognitive knowledge or self-knowledge, which includes stored knowledge and beliefs about task characteristics and understanding personal strengths and limitations (intellectual awareness), as well as an online awareness of performance,

which includes self-appraisal and self-monitoring during a task or situation (emergent awareness) and anticipating future difficulties (anticipatory awareness).

shift: The ability to flexibly adapt attentive focus, and attention for action is the process by which we connect stimuli (input) with a response to that stimuli (output).

skills and habits: A cognitive rehabilitation treatment target focused on training an automatic routine with practice, in which "practice makes perfect."

slowed: Cognitive impairment relative to healthy controls of processing and attention.

social cognition skills: The ability to form social judgments, such as theory of mind, emotion recognition, and emotional empathy.

suppressing: The inhibition of meanings to allow rapid selection of the most appropriate meaning for a given context.

sustain: The ability to maintain focus on selected stimuli, as well as alertness.

sustained attention: The ability to maintain attention to an ongoing, repetitive task for a period of time.

Symbol Trails: A subtest of the Cognitive-Linguistic Quick Test–Plus (CLQT+) in which participants connect shapes in order from smallest to largest.

target detection, or executive control system: The effortful control of attention, which includes processes such as conflict resolution and error detection.

Telephone Search: A subtest of the Test of Everyday Attention in which the test-taker is given a telephone directory and asked to cross out specific symbols.

Telephone Search Dual Task: A subtest of the Test of Everyday Attention in which the test-taker is asked to cross out specific symbols in a telephone directory; however, they are also asked to simultaneously count auditory tones. Scores on Telephone Search and Telephone Search Dual Task can be compared to determine the decrement in performance when a second task is added.

Unilateral Visual Neglect (UVN), or visuospatial neglect: A decreased ability to process spatial information.

verbal fluency: Cognitive control related to communication tested by asking the test-taker to list words starting with a particular letter or category within a one-minute period.

Visual Elevator: A subtest of the Test of Everyday Attention in which the test-taker is presented with a series of pictured stimuli including elevator doors and arrows pointing up or down and is asked to keep track of what floor they are on (with the arrows indicating a switch in the up/down direction).

visuospatial neglect, or Unilateral Visual Neglect (UVN): A decreased ability to process spatial information.

working memory: A core executive function process, it is the ability to maintain a task or idea in mind and mentally manipulate it.

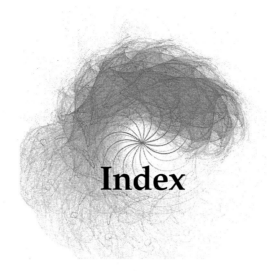

Index

Note: Page numbers in **bold** reference non-text material

Black, Indigenous, and People of Color
(BIPOC), concussion and, 365
Black ethnic group
dementia in, 319
TBI (Traumatic brain injury), recovery
and, 437
Blast injuries, 362, 426–427
clinical considerations, 427–428
described, 737
mechanism of, 426–427
Blow flow, cerebral, concussion and, 363
Blunt-force trauma, concussion and, 362
Bottom-up stimulus, 9
Brain
aphasia and, 16
death, coma and, 438
edema, concussion and, 363
females, concussion and, 365
frontal lobes, memory and, 59
games, computer, **398–399**
infections, memory and, 64
injury
acquired, 112–113, 458
cognitive impairments following,
communication, 116
communication impairments
following, models, 115
memory and, 56
neglect and, 16
resource allocation/organizing and,
62
tumors, RHD (Right hemisphere
damage) and, 206
resource allocation/organizing and,
62
Brain Injury Screening Questionnaire
(BISQ), 451
Brain Injury Society of Toronto, 500
BrainHQ, **398**
BRAVE trial, **398–399**
Bridwell, Ashley, 500
BRIEF (Behavior Rating Inventory of
Executive Function), 76, 384
A (Behavior Rating Inventory of
Executive Function–Adult), 136,
450
Brief Cognitive Assessment Tool
(BCAT), 30

Brief Test of Attention (BTA), **23**, 26–27
Broadbent, D.E., 6
BTA (Brief Test of Attention), 26–27
Burns Brief Inventory of
Communication and Cognition,
229

C

CADL (Communication Activities for
Daily Living), 336–337
California Verbal Learning Test (CVLT),
79–80
Cambridge Semantic Memory Test
Battery, 298
CAN (Concussion Awareness Now),
American Speech-Language-
Hearing Association (ASHA), 360
Canada, indigenous people, concussion
and, 366
Capacity limitation, 8–9
described, 4
theories/models of, 8–9
Cardenas, Javier, 500
Care
culturally responsive, 500–501
models, 500–501
specialized teams, 500
Case study
attention, 37–39
Brian, **124–125**, 149
assessment results, 141–144
history, **124–125**
treatment plan, 172–176
Carmi, **126–128**
assessment results, 144–148
change statements, **152**
motivational interviewing
questions, **129–130**
treatment plan, 176–179
cognitive impairment, 84–88
dementia, 344–348
executive function, 122–130
Mrs. V, 344–348
Ms. Smith, 306–307
right hemisphere damage, Patrick,
257–261
CAT (Comprehensive Aphasia Test), 296